MEDICAL SERVICE IN THE EUROPEAN THEATER OF OPERATIONS

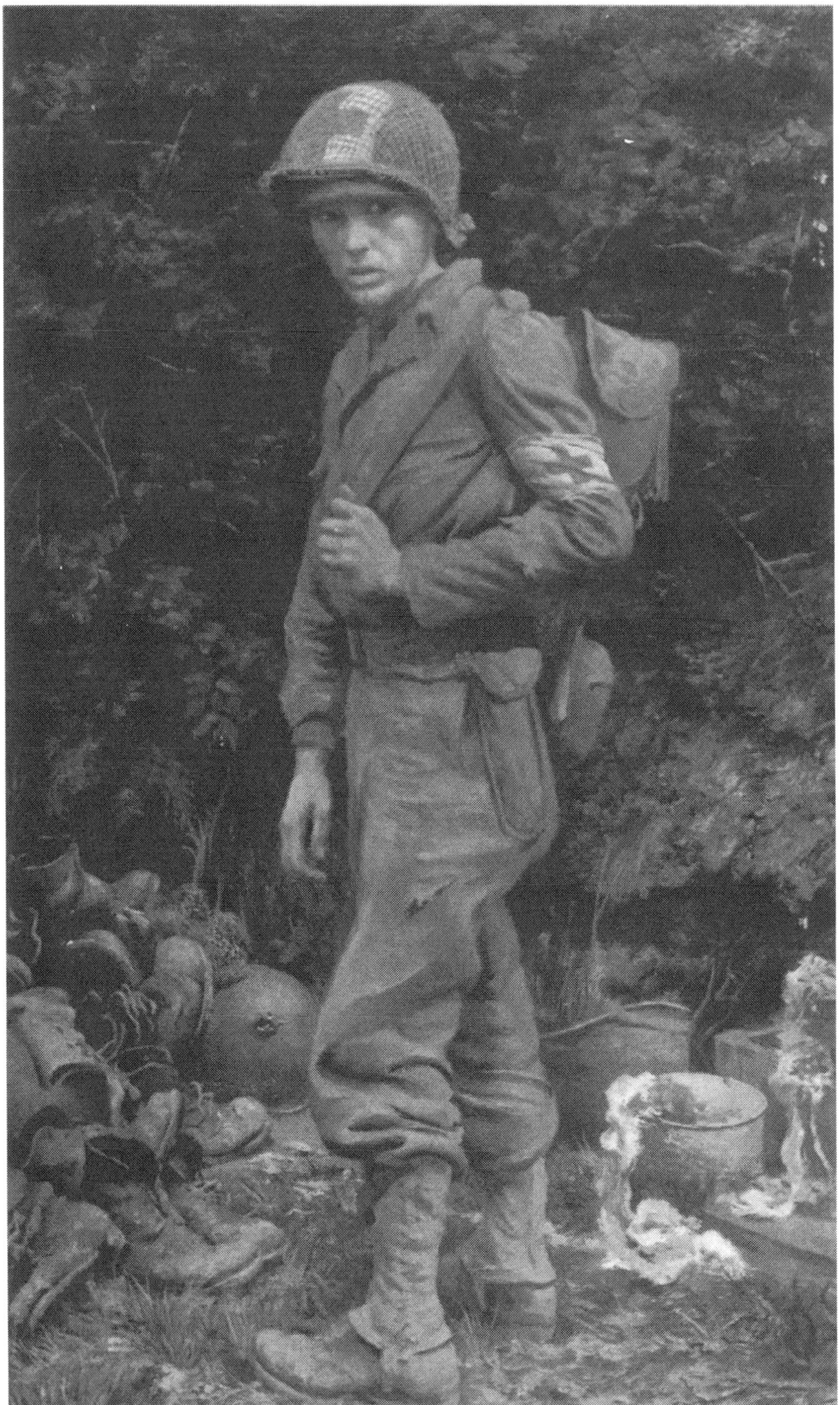

THE MAN WITHOUT A GUN

UNITED STATES ARMY IN WORLD WAR II

The Technical Services

THE MEDICAL DEPARTMENT:

MEDICAL SERVICE IN THE EUROPEAN THEATER OF OPERATIONS

by
Graham A. Cosmas
and
Albert E. Cowdrey

CENTER OF MILITARY HISTORY
UNITED STATES ARMY
WASHINGTON, D.C., 1992

Library of Congress Cataloging-in-Publication Data

Cosmas, Graham A.
The medical department: medical service in the European theater of operations / by Graham A. Cosmas and Albert E. Cowdrey.
p. cm. — (United States Army in World War II. The technical services)
Includes bibliographical references.
Includes index.
1. World War, 1939–1945—Medical care—United States. 2. World War, 1939–1945—Campaigns—Western. I. Cowdrey, Albert E. II. Title. III. Series: United States Army in World War II. Technical services.
[DNLM: 1. Military Medicine—history—Europe. 2. War—history—Europe.]
D806.U6C67 1991
940.54"7573—dc20
DLC
for Library of Congress 90-2452
CIP

First Printing—CMH Pub 10–23

For sale by the Superintendent of Documents, U.S. Government Printing Office
Washington, D.C. 20402

UNITED STATES ARMY IN WORLD WAR II

. . . to Those Who Served

Foreword

Although readily admitting the importance of combat service support forces, military students and historians alike tend to concentrate on combat and combat support units when studying operations, giving only passing attention to the vital work of the logisticians, signalmen, transport troops, and the rest. This is regrettable, for the operations of combat service support units—especially in a global conflict like World War II with its vast distances and varied terrains—have much to teach us about modern warfare, lessons that remain of surpassing importance to our profession. *The Medical Department: Medical Service in the European Theater of Operations* supports the proposition that the experience of medical personnel in war directly stimulates advances in medical science. More importantly, it demonstrates that the organization of health care in the combat zones, including evacuation of the wounded, control of disease among troops and civilian populations, and care of prisoners of war, contributed directly to the Allied victory. The exploits of the doctors, corpsmen, and medical support units provide a model for the planning and organization of medical support in today's Army.

This volume continues a subseries begun in 1966 with the study of medical support of the Army in the Mediterranean Theater. The Center of Military History will soon complete this project with the publication of a similar study of the very different challenges faced by the Medical Department in the Pacific. I urge our officers and noncommissioned officers to consult these histories and to use them, not only because they provide a clear example of the best in combat service support in wartime but because the principles of medical organization that they examine remain of vital importance to today's military planners and students.

Washington, D.C.
1 September 1990

HAROLD W. NELSON
Brigadier General, USA
Chief of Military History

The Authors

Graham A. Cosmas was born in Weehawken, New Jersey, and received his education from the schools of Leonia, New Jersey, and from Columbia University, Oberlin College, and the University of Wisconsin. After teaching at the Universities of Texas (Austin) and of Guam he joined the staff of the U.S. Marine Corps' History and Museums Division and, since 1979, that of the U.S. Army Center of Military History, serving in 1984–85 as the Harold Keith Johnson Visiting Professor of Military History at the U.S. Army Military History Institute, Carlisle Barracks, Pennsylvania. Dr. Cosmas is the author of *An Army for Empire: The U.S. Army in the Spanish-American War, 1898–1899,* and coauthor of *U.S. Marines in Vietnam: Vietnamization and Redeployment, 1970–71.* He also has published numerous journal articles and book reviews.

Albert E. Cowdrey was born in New Orleans, Louisiana, and received his education from the schools of that city and from Tulane and Johns Hopkins Universities. He served in the Army as an enlisted man during the years 1957–59. After teaching at Tulane University and at Louisiana State University he entered the government historical programs, working for the Corps of Engineers historical office and, since 1978, for the U.S. Army Center of Military History. His continuing interest in southern history brought him the 1984 Herbert Feis Award of the American Historical Association for his book *This Land, This South.* His prizewinning history of Army medicine in the Korean war, *The Medics' War,* has been widely adopted as a text in military medical schools. He also has contributed articles on a variety of historical topics to American, British, Canadian, and international journals.

Preface

The Medical Department: Medical Service in the European Theater of Operations is the second of three volumes recounting the overseas activities of the U.S. Army Medical Department in World War II. Charles M. Wiltse's volume on the Mediterranean and minor theaters was published in 1963, and a completed manuscript dealing with the war against Japan now exists in the Center of Military History. These volumes deal primarily with the operational and organizational history of Army medicine in the theaters, as distinguished from the clinical volumes published by the Office of the Surgeon General. In each case the combat narrative has been drawn from relevant volumes in the United States Army in World War II series, as well as from the large body of subsequent scholarship. Our aim has been to show how the military medical system organized itself in a combat theater; how medical planning was integrated with logistical and tactical planning; how medical troops were organized, trained and deployed; how hospitals were built and supplies assembled and moved forward; and how casualties were treated and evacuated from the field of battle. The volume deals only peripherally with medical support for the Army Air Forces, in view of the fact that a lengthy published official history already exists.

Army medicine has long possessed a consciousness of its own history. ETO medics were especially concerned with recording their achievements in the largest and most complex American land campaign of World War II. Well before D-Day the theater chief surgeon established a historical section in his office under Col. Sanford V. Larkey. The manuscript history that Colonel Larkey's office produced during and immediately after the war formed the starting point for an extended effort by the Office of the Surgeon General to publish a history of the campaign. Among the various manuscripts written during the subsequent three decades, a study by George Garand, Hubert E. Potter, and Pauline Vivette stands out for its length and detail. Nevertheless, the present volume in many ways represents a new start; a fresh conception of the theme and organization led us into much additional research in manuscripts, recent secondary works, and interviews with participants.

Yet we gladly acknowledge our debts to the many people who contributed their efforts and expertise to this volume. Members of the review panel included Col. Richard O. Perry, David F. Trask, Tom F. Whayne, MD, Charles B. MacDonald, Col. Roger H. Wichelt, MC, and Arnold G. Fisch, Jr. Their comments and suggestions contributed much to the final form of this volume. We are especially grateful to the following veterans of the campaign interviewed by us and other members of the Medical History Branch: Honorable Elliot Richardson, Maj. Gen. Thomas J. Hartford, Maj. Gen. Collin F. Vorder Bruegge, Brig. Gen. Sam F. Seeley, Brig. Gen. Crawford F. Sams, Col. Virginia Brown, Col. Tom F. Whayne, Joseph A. Gosman, M.D., Lester Wallman, M.D., Herbert G. Wing, and Jane A. Lee. Their reminiscences added color and human detail to the documentary record. We are grateful to Dr. Gosman for allowing us to consult his manuscript "War Without Blood" and to Mrs. Lee for providing us with personal snapshots of nurses and hospitals in Great Britain. Robert J. T. Joy, M.D., and Col. Charles J. Simpson contributed expert knowledge, encouragement, and counsel.

Archivists in the Washington, D.C., area and at Carlisle Barracks, Pennsylvania, provided unstinting help during our research. Among the many to whom we owe our gratitude, Fred W. Pernell, Richard L. Boylan and Victoria Washington of the National Archives, and Richard Sommers of the Military History Institute, were particularly generous with their time and expertise. Among our present and former colleagues at the Center of Military History, Hannah M. Zeidlik, Charles Ellsworth, Geraldine K. Harcarik, Carol I. Anderson, James B. Knight, and Mary J. Sawyer helped us obtain needed materials. Arthur S. Hardyman and Linda M. Cajka oversaw the preparation of maps and charts, and Howell C. Brewer searched out photographs. Mr. Hardyman was in overall charge of the visual aspects of the volume. Terrence L. Offer was our rapid and helpful manuscript typist.

Our greatest debt, of course, is owed to our meticulous and hardworking editor, Joanne M. Brignolo, whose technical proficiency and attention to detail contributed immeasurably to the smooth flow of the manuscript and the accuracy of its citations. Any errors of fact or interpretation remaining in the book, however, are ours alone.

Washington, D.C.
1 September 1990

GRAHAM A. COSMAS
ALBERT E. COWDREY

Contents

Tables

Charts

Diagrams

Maps

Illustrations

Illustrations courtesy of the following sources: p. 7, National Library of Medicine; pp. 11, 32, 34, 47, 66, 67, 138, 145 (top/bottom), 187 (right), 244, and 254, Armed Forces Institute of Pathology; pp. 115 (bottom) and 121, Mrs. Jane Lee; p. 185, National Archives and Records Administration; and p. 333, Smithsonian Institution. All other illustrations are from the files of the Department of the Air Force, the Department of the Army, and the U.S. Army Center of Military History.

The works of Lawrence Beall Smith (1909–) depicted on p. ii—*The Man Without a Gun,* 1944, oil on masonite, 36½" x 22"—and on the paperback cover—*Normandy Sabbath,* 1944, oil on masonite, 23¾" x 37"—are from the Army Art Collection.

1

MEDICAL SERVICE IN THE EUROPEAN THEATER OF OPERATIONS

PROLOGUE

The Onset of War

In the late summer of 1939, as World War II opened in Europe, the Medical Department of the United States Army comprised medical field units, fixed hospitals, laboratories, and schools, a complex whose center was the Office of the Surgeon General in Washington, D.C. The surgeon general commanded his own office and the general hospitals. He advised the chief of staff and the secretary of war on all matters relating to the health and medical care of the Army, and he provided technical guidance to all the men and women of the department in the continental United States and its overseas possessions.

By later standards the Medical Department was few in numbers, comprising about 10,000 officers and men. Its officers were organized into Medical, Dental, Veterinary, and Medical Administrative Corps; members of the Army Nurse Corps, exclusively female, held quasi-officer status known as relative rank. Another 23,000 doctors, dentists, administrators (a title which included specialists in some ancillary fields, such as pharmacists), and sanitarians made up the Medical Department Reserve Corps. In the laboratories and general hospitals a small elite group of physicians preserved the department's traditional devotion to medical science, which derived from the days of Walter Reed and William C. Gorgas.[1] But most Army doctors were in the broadest sense general practitioners. They guarded the public health of the Army, gave aid to injured soldiers, and provided treatment at unit sick calls, at dispensaries, and at unit and post hospitals. In addition, Army doctors were soldiers who commanded medical units, advised their commanders, sat on courts-martial, stood formations, conducted inspections, and—if considered worthy—attended Army schools like the Infantry School at Fort Benning or the Command and General Staff School at Fort Leavenworth. They participated in the active if somewhat stiff and formal social life of the officer corps, with its teas, its balls, and its near-obsessive devotion to sports and horsemanship. Many practiced a kind of medicine that was elementary and repetitive, but developed a broad grasp of Army ways and

[1] Walter Reed (1851–1902) was the Army doctor who headed and supervised the work of the U.S. Army Yellow Fever Commission that proved mosquitoes carried yellow fever. William C. Gorgas (1854–1920) was the Army doctor who systematically applied this discovery in public health campaigns that rid Havana and later the Panama Canal Zone of the disease.

wide acquaintance with their fellow officers. Even for junior officers, military medicine offered definite rewards, especially during the Depression years of the 1930s—a secure paycheck, travel, a round of usually undemanding duties, and slow advance up the ladder of rank.

The limited mobilization proclaimed by President Franklin D. Roosevelt in September 1939 brought quick and drastic changes to this insular life. During the twenty-one years since the end of World War I, the Medical Department had supported a garrison army of less than 200,000 men, and the field medical establishment had dwindled to only five units—four medical regiments and a medical squadron. Tables of organization and equipment (T/O&Es) for both fixed and mobile medical units had remained unchanged for a decade. The military buildup, escalating into full mobilization and conscription as France fell and England stood alone, transformed the Medical Department along with the rest of the Army. In the seventeen months before Pearl Harbor medical strength grew to 131,586 officers and men, a rate of increase slightly more rapid than that of the Army as a whole. Concurrently, the surgeon general, Maj. Gen. James C. Magee, and his staff reworked the medical annexes to national mobilization plans, expanded training programs, and revised unit T/O&Es. Among other changes they replaced horse-drawn with motor vehicles. Reviving a successful World War I expedient, the Medical Department formed affiliated reserve hospital units of both fixed and mobile types, each staffed and sponsored by a civilian hospital or medical school. By 7 December 1941 the Medical Department had created the cadre of an organization able to care for a vastly expanded national Army.[2]

Although the Japanese attack on Pearl Harbor unexpectedly confronted the United States with an immediate crisis in the Pacific, President Roosevelt continued to view Nazi Germany as the principal enemy. Attempts to inform the American military about the British war effort and to assist Prime Minister Winston S. Churchill's government in resisting the common foe predated U.S. entry into the war. It was through these early moves to aid Britain that the foundations of the European Theater of Operations and its medical support system were first laid.

[2] For details on mobilization, see Clarence McKittrick Smith, *The Medical Department: Hospitalization and Evacuation, Zone of Interior* (hereafter cited as *Hospitalization and Evacuation*), United States Army in World War II (Washington, D.C.: Office of the Chief of Military History, Department of the Army, 1956), pp. 3–43.

CHAPTER I

Beginnings

The European Theater of Operations, which was to conduct the United States Army's largest and most complex land campaign of the Second World War and complete the destruction of Nazi Germany, had modest beginnings. Its initial objectives were to establish Army forces in the British Isles in order to protect them from invasion; to relieve British troops for operations in the Mediterranean; and to reinforce the Royal Air Force (RAF) Bomber Command in its strategic air offensive against the Third Reich.

Preparation for establishment of the theater began early in 1941. At that time, almost a year before Pearl Harbor, the United States, which had undertaken limited mobilization soon after the outbreak of war in September 1939, advanced its support of Great Britain to the stage of direct materiel aid and combined contingency planning. While Congress debated and passed the Lend-Lease Act, authorizing direct government transfers of American military equipment to anti-Axis nations, American and British staff officers met secretly in Washington. They drew up an agreement, known as ABC–1, outlining Anglo-American worldwide strategy in the event the United States entered the war. Under ABC–1 and the subsequent War Department RAINBOW–5 plan of April 1941, the U.S. Army initially would play a limited role in the North Atlantic and Western Europe. Army troops were to replace the British garrison in Iceland. An Army air force would deploy to Great Britain to join the Royal Air Force in bombing Germany, while ground elements protected U.S. Navy bases in Scotland and Northern Ireland and a reinforced regiment took station to help defend southern England. Altogether, the contingents in the United Kingdom were to include about 87,000 officers and men, almost half of them in the bomber command.[1]

[1] Maurice Matloff and Edwin M. Snell, *Strategic Planning for Coalition Warfare, 1941–1942*, United States Army in World War II (Washington, D.C.: Office of the Chief of Military History, Department of the Army, 1953), pp. 43–46; Roland G. Ruppenthal, *Logistical Support of the Armies*, United States Army in World War II, 2 vols. (Washington, D.C.: Office of the Chief of Military History, Department of the Army, 1953–59), vol. 1, *May 1941–September 1944* (1953), pp. 2 and 19–20; An. 2, ABC–1 (American-British Conversations), 27 Mar 41, quoted in Historical Section, ETO, "The Special Observer Group Prior to the Activation of the European Theater of Operations" (hereafter cited as "SPOBS Hist"), October 1944, p. 13. Depository codes used in citations in this volume are as follows: CMH (U.S. Army Center of Military History, Washington, D.C.); MHI (U.S. Army Military History Institute, Carlisle

Continued

Early Activities in Britain

While President Roosevelt justified early mobilization measures in terms of Western Hemisphere defense, the United States from the beginning based its preparations on the probability that, if drawn into the war, it would fight as the ally of Great Britain. For this reason, as well as to keep abreast of wartime technical developments, the armed services and other government agencies sent official observers to study the British war effort. British medical problems and achievements drew their share of attention. Military and naval attaches at the London embassy transmitted medical information along with other intelligence. The National Research Council, part of the U.S. National Academy of Sciences, which advised the surgeon general on medical research and therapy, pooled information with counterpart British and Canadian organizations. The Army Medical Department dispatched its own observer, Col. Raymond W. Bliss, MC, who went to London during late 1940. Although injured in a November air raid, Bliss sent back reports on subjects ranging from hospitalization and evacuation of bombing casualties to the incidence of combat fatigue among RAF flight officers.[2]

These American observers found in Great Britain a medical profession as fully developed and highly institutionalized as that in the United States, and one ahead of its American counterpart in many war-related areas of research and clinical practice. British medicine—part of a nation which German bombers had made into a single combat zone—was fully mobilized for war. Under the Ministry of Health the Emergency Medical Services (EMS) controlled about 300,000 beds in existing private and governmental hospitals and in newly constructed semipermanent plants. Working closely with the civil defense organization, it evacuated and treated civilian air raid casualties and provided most station and general hospitalization for the armed services.[3]

The medical services of the British Army, Royal Navy, and Royal Air Force paralleled in structure and functions, though not in nomenclature, those of the United States armed forces. The Royal Army Medical Service, with which the U.S. Army medical establishment was to work most closely, was headed by Lt. Gen.

Barracks, Penn.); NARA (National Archives and Records Administration, Suitland, Md.); and NLM (National Library of Medicine, Bethesda, Md.) Manuscript sources cited without any depository code are in the custody of CMH and, upon publication of this volume, will be returned to the collection of Army records in the custody of NARA. See Bibliographical Note.

[2] For a summary of early contacts, see Sanford V. Larkey, "Administrative and Logistical History of the Medical Service, Communications Zone, European Theater of Operations" (hereafter cited as Larkey "Hist") (Historical Division, United States Forces, European Theater, 1945), ch. 1, pp. 1-3; Col R. W. Bliss, MC, Compiled Reports of Medical Observer in London, October-December 1940 (hereafter cited as Bliss Rpts), file ETO 7/1.

[3] The EMS secured beds by discharging or moving patients, crowding more beds into wards and buildings, and adding hut annexes to permanent hospitals. The British radically overestimated air raid losses, expecting 35,000 dead and injured a day for the first two weeks of heavy bombing. In fact, they suffered about 43,000 civilians killed and 50,400 severely injured in the entire period June 1940-May 1941. See C. L. Dunn, *The Emergency Medical Services* (hereafter cited as *EMS*), History of the Second World War, United Kingdom Medical Series, 2 vols. (London: Her Majesty's Stationery Office, 1952-53), vol. 1, *England and Wales* (1952), pp. 114-15 and passim; Bliss Rpts, file ETO 7/1.

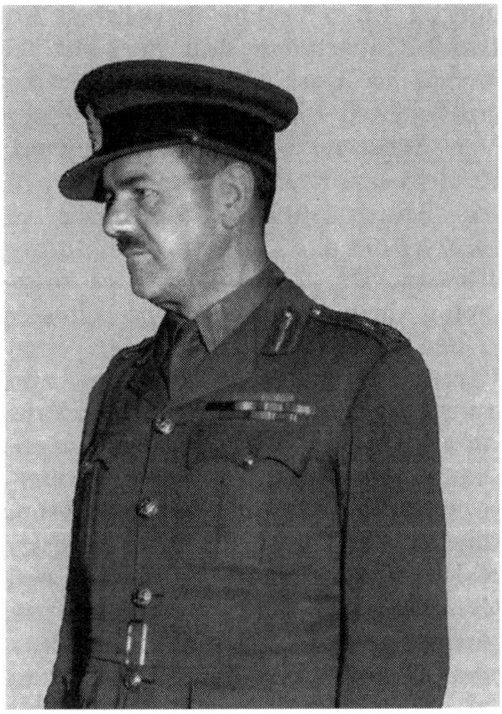

LT. GEN. SIR ALEXANDER HOOD

Sir Alexander Hood, director general of Army Medical Services. General Hood served on the staff of the adjutant general, who in turn sat on the Army Council, the British Army's central administrative body. General Hood's office consisted of a number of functional directorates, with responsibilities much like those of the divisions of the U.S. Army's Office of the Surgeon General. In geographical area commands and field armies a deputy or assistant director of Medical Services, depending on the size of the organization, advised the commander on medical matters and exercised technical and administrative control over hospitals and medical units. Tactical medical units, from field ambulances to general hospitals, made up a chain of evacuation similar in operations and principles to that of the U.S. Army. The British in 1940–41 were in the process of reorganizing these elements to achieve greater mobility and to bring emergency surgery closer to the firing line. For home base fixed hospitals, the British Army, like the other services, had to rely primarily on the Emergency Medical Services, since the Cabinet in 1939 had all but forbidden construction of new military hospitals in the United Kingdom. EMS hospitals cared for the sick and injured of units stationed in Britain, and they were the final link in the chain of evacuation from overseas battlefields.[4]

By late 1940 the Royal Army Medical Service was suffering from a shortage of medical officers, and throughout the British war effort the demand for qualified practitioners had begun to exceed the supply. The British, accordingly, welcomed American and other foreign civilian doctors and employed these volunteers in the Emergency Medical Services to release British doctors for military service. American medical people came to Britain as individuals, and they also came in organized hospitals, two of which were destined for close association with the U.S. Army. The first of these, the American Hospital in Great Britain, which was organized by New

[4] In May 1940 the British Army had 9,000 beds available in Great Britain in its own hospitals, all enlarged prewar plants. See Dunn, *EMS*, 1:96. For army medical organization and its wartime development, see F. A. E. Crew, *The Army Medical Services* (hereafter cited as *AMS*), History of the Second World War, United Kingdom Medical Series, 2 vols. (London: Her Majesty's Stationery Office, 1953–55), vol. 1, *Administration* (1953), chs. 3, 8 and pp. 458–79.

York City doctors and laymen and financed by the British War Relief Society in America, went into operation late in 1940. Its British-American-Canadian staff occupied a 300-bed wing of an EMS hospital at Basingstoke and specialized in orthopedics and plastic surgery. In January 1942 the unit, renamed the Churchill Hospital, moved to a larger facility, taking over an entire new 600-bed EMS hospital near Oxford.[5]

At the time the American Hospital was taking shape, the Harvard Medical School and the American Red Cross, in cooperation with the Ministry of Health, established a contagious disease treatment and control unit. Named the American Red Cross–Harvard Field Hospital Unit, this facility included a laboratory, mobile investigating teams, and a 125-bed hospital, staffed except for nurses by Harvard and equipped largely by the Red Cross, which also recruited the nurses. The unit's director, Dr. John E. Gordon, professor of Epidemiology at Harvard, and many of the professional staff began work in Britain in mid-1940. They assisted the Ministry of Health in combating disease outbreaks, which were a constant threat in the crowded and bomb-damaged cities; they also completed plans for the hospital. The rest of the unit arrived in Britain during early 1941. Five of the staff's Red Cross nurses and their chaperone died at sea when a U-boat torpedoed their ship in the North Atlantic. Dr. Gordon also became a war casualty, injured when bombs demolished his London apartment, but he soon returned to work. In September the unit opened its 22-building complex near Salisbury in southern England. Its field teams and laboratory helped the British suppress outbreaks of paratyphoid and scabies, among other diseases. Dr. Gordon, besides overseeing the unit, advised the minister of health on epidemiology, served on Ministry of Health committees, and transmitted information between British and American public health agencies. After the unit had been in operation for a year, Sir Wilson Jameson, chief medical officer of the Ministry of Health, declared that Gordon and his colleagues "have come to be regarded not as a group of workers from America but more as a part of the general public health staff of this country" and that the volunteer unit would be "a model for the post-war development of epidemiological studies" in Britain.[6]

Medical Department activity in Britain expanded and became more systematic after the signing of ABC–1. To execute and maintain that agreement, the United States and Great Britain exchanged military missions. The members of these missions collectively represented their country's chiefs of staff. Individually, each mission member exchanged information and developed contacts with counterparts in his own branch of service.

[5] Larkey "Hist," ch. 1, pp. 3–7; Sheila M. Dwyer, "A Base Hospital in England," *The American Journal of Nursing 41* (August 1941): 877–79; Bliss Rpts, file ETO 7/1.

[6] Ltr, Sir Wilson Jameson to Dean Burwell, Harvard Medical School, 16 Sep 42, in *The American Red Cross–Harvard Field Hospital Unit* (Cambridge, Mass.: Harvard University, 1943), pp. 38–40. This publication sketches the history of the unit. On Gordon's injury, see *New York Times*, 7 May 41, p. 6.

The United States Army mission to England established its headquarters in London on 19 May 1941, setting up offices in the United States Embassy on Grosvenor Square. Maj. Gen. James E. Chaney, an Air Corps officer who earlier had observed the Battle of Britain for the War Department, headed the delegation, designated the Special Observers Group (SPOBS) to conceal its actual, unneutral functions. Chaney's seventeen subordinates, called special assistant Army observers, were carefully selected field-grade officers whose branches and specialties included most of those required to staff a theater headquarters. Wearing civilian clothes and carring British identification and ration cards, they collected much military information while carrying out their primary task of making preliminary preparations for the Army forces earmarked for Great Britain in ABC–1 and RAINBOW–5; they selected locations for bomber bases and other installations and surveyed transportation facilities and supply sources. General Chaney, who reported directly to Army Chief of Staff General George C. Marshall, had responsibility for recommending changes in the details of the basic plan. At the proper time he was to advise the chief of staff on actual force deployments.[7]

Initially, Maj. Arthur B. Welsh, MC, represented the Medical Department in the Special Observers Group. A Regular Army medical officer since 1926, Welsh had attended the Command and General Staff College and

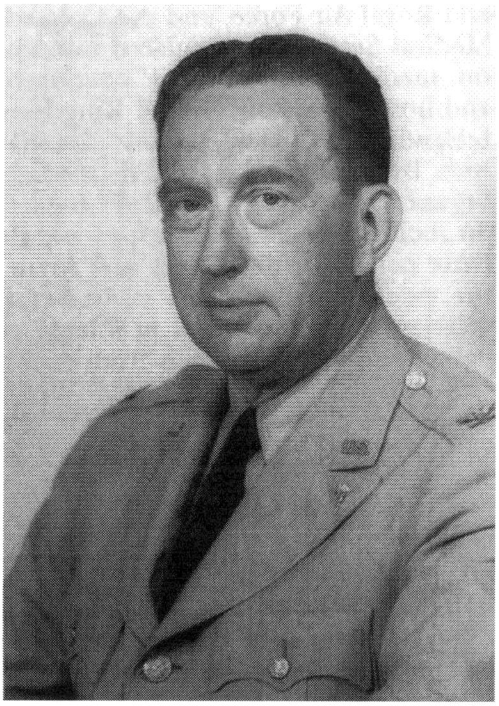

COL. ARTHUR B. WELSH
(1953 photograph)

taught at the Medical Field Service School at Carlisle Barracks. Since October 1939, as assistant chief of the Planning, Plans, and Training Division, Office of the Surgeon General, he had helped make Medical Department emergency and war plans. He was thus a logical choice for the SPOBS assignment.[8]

Welsh spent much of his time at first meeting with British civil and military medical officials and collecting information as preparation for his medical planning tasks. He conferred regularly with counterparts from the Ministry of Health, the British Army

[7] The operations of this group, which also included coordinating the allocation of lend-lease equipment and participation in early military discussions with the Soviet Union, are described in ETO, "SPOBS Hist," passim.

[8] Biographical data from Name-Rank file, CMH; Interv, OSG with Col A. B. Welsh, 28–29 Oct 47, file HD 000.71, CMH.

and Royal Air Force, and the Colonial Medical Service; accumulated material on medical and sanitary conditions and hospitals in the United Kingdom, Iceland, and Africa; became familiar with British Army and RAF medical organization; and compiled reports on such subjects as the proper goggle lense colors for the desert and Arctic, the most common types of bombing injuries, and the special problems of evacuating wounded men from tanks. During July and August 1941 Welsh completed his medical plans for the U.S. Army forces to be stationed in Iceland, Northern Ireland, Scotland, and England. These plans, in accord with ABC-1 and RAINBOW-5, provided for static garrison and antiaircraft defense units and for air commands operating from fixed bases. Because of their limited scale, they soon became obsolete by the rush of events.

Welsh's medical plans, despite their quick demise, contained hospitalization and evacuation principles that were to reappear in subsequent more elaborate programs. For example, Welsh emphasized that the Army in the British Isles should establish "its own complete medical service with 10% fixed beds and sufficient medical units and transport to collect and evacuate sick and wounded. . . ." While he arranged for the initial care of American casualties in British hospitals, his plans called for early construction of U.S. Army hospitals for the entire command. Welsh outlined a hospitalization scheme based on unit dispensaries, station hospitals with 250 to 750 beds, and general hospitals with 1,000 beds. Under his proposed evacuation policy units would treat sick and wounded needing less than 72 hours of care in their own dispensaries, more serious cases would go to station hospitals, and those needing over 120 days of hospitalization would be evacuated to the United States by air or hospital ship. In addition to these hospitalization and evacuation programs Welsh submitted lists of medical units for the ABC-1 and RAINBOW-5 forces, as well as a proposed table of organization for a small theater chief surgeon's office; recommended the use of American rations to feed U.S. troops stationed in Great Britain and the need for various preventive medicine measures, such as venereal disease suppression; and warned that all hospital equipment and medical supplies would have to come from the United States, an assumption which turned out to be wrong.[9]

In mid-September illness forced the relief of Major Welsh.[10] To replace him, the War Department, on Welsh's recommendation, selected Col. Paul R. Hawley, MC, at that time assistant commandant of the Medical Field Service School at Carlisle Barracks, Pennsylvania. Fifty years old in 1941, Hawley had served in France in World War I as a regimental surgeon

---

[9] Larkey "Hist," ch. 1, pp. 11-15, 19-26, 30-31. Ch. 1, app. 1, reproduces Welsh's major plans. See also ETO, "SPOBS Hist," pp. 30-31 and 34-35. Army medical service in the Iceland occupation, which began in late 1941, is covered in an earlier volume of this series. See Charles M. Wiltse, *The Medical Department: Medical Service in the Mediterranean and Minor Theaters* (hereafter cited as *Mediterranean*), United States Army in World War II (Washington, D.C.: Office of the Chief of Military History, Department of the Army, 1965), pp. 10-18.

[10] Welsh spent the rest of the war in the Office of the Surgeon General in high-level planning and supervisory assignments.

and as sanitary inspector of the Intermediate Sector, Services of Supply. Between the wars he held varied assignments in the United States, the Philippines, and Nicaragua; taught biostatistics and epidemiology at the Army Medical School; and earned a doctorate in Public Health from Johns Hopkins University. Hawley also possessed military staff training, having attended both the Command and General Staff School, at Fort Leavenworth, Kansas, and the Army War College in Washington, D.C. Genial but strong-willed, Hawley, more than any other one man, was to dominate medical service in the European Theater of Operations.[11]

Hawley received a hectic introduction to the Special Observers Group. Departing for England on less than two days' notice, he took along little spare clothing and no passport. He crossed the Atlantic in a B–24 bomber being ferried over for the Royal Air Force. "The pilot and I shared the same experience," he recalled. "Neither one of us had flown over the ocean before." Having traveled in uniform, Hawley bought a civilian suit off the rack in a London department store in order to conceal his military identity. By this time, he observed, the group's disguise had worn thin. Even a woman passerby who directed the Americans back to their hotel in the blackout seemed to know who they were.[12]

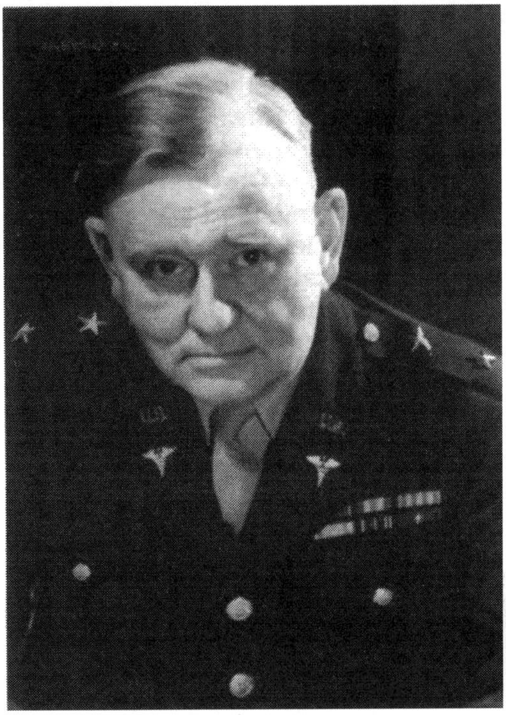

MAJ. GEN. PAUL R. HAWLEY
(Rank as of 27 February 1944)

As Welsh had done, Hawley worked out of a single small room in the American embassy without even a personal secretary to assist him. Quickly, he picked up the threads of Welsh's activities. He revised the Northern Ireland medical plan to relieve the Navy of any responsibility for medical care of Army troops near naval bases, and he recommended establishment of fewer and larger fixed hospitals than Welsh had proposed. Hawley drafted a medical plan of his own for the Army forces to be stationed in Scotland, generally following the principles of Welsh's earlier England and Scotland plans. Late in November, he completed tentative plans for medical support of the

[11] Biographical data from Name-Rank file, CMH; Memo, Maj A. B. Welsh to Gen McNarney, 11 Sep 41; AGO Orders to Col Paul R. Hawley, 16 Sep 41, box 1, Paul R. Hawley Papers, MHI.

[12] Interv, OSG with Maj Gen Paul R. Hawley, 16 and 18 Jun 62 (hereafter cited as Hawley Interv, 1962), pp. 5–7, CMH.

American bomber command, which was to operate from airfields in eastern England already designated for turnover by the Royal Air Force. For this command, then expected to include about 36,000 officers and men, Hawley recommended provision of hospital beds for 1 percent of troop strength in local dispensaries, 4 percent in area station hospitals, and 3 percent in general hospitals, with beds for another 1.3 percent in convalescent facilities.[13] Besides making plans, Hawley arranged for the turnover of British Army medical supplies to American troops in Iceland. He negotiated informally with the War Office and the Ministry of Health for free-of-charge treatment of American personnel in British military and EMS hospitals, promising the British reciprocal privileges in U.S. Army hospitals if and when such were built in the United Kingdom.[14]

Hawley assiduously cultivated his British counterparts. Except when out of London on inspection trips, he paid daily visits to General Hood, Army Medical Services, and to Hood's directorate chiefs; he also attended Hood's weekly staff conferences. The British gave Hawley their equivalent of a Top Secret security clearance, admitting him to the deliberations of their most sensitive medical research committees. In return, the British drew on Hawley's knowledge of the U.S. Army's field medical organization to aid their own army medical service reorganization planning. Outside London Hawley visited British Army regional commands and became the "good friend" of their medical officers. Hawley was junior to the British generals with whom he had to deal. Nevertheless, he said, "the British just adopted me down in the Surgeon's Office. . . . These were major generals and I was just an unknown colonel [but] they took me in."[15]

Early in the morning of 8 December 1941 Hawley, who intended to visit the British Army Southern Command that day, walked from his London apartment to the nearby Baker Street tube station on his way to Waterloo Station. He had not had his radio on the night before. As he entered the subway, large black newspaper headlines told him that the Japanese had bombed Pearl Harbor, ending American neutrality. Hawley abruptly changed plans. "I went right back to my apartment . . . [and] got into uniform. That morning, Monday morning, was always conference in the [Director] General's office—all of his department heads. . . . And I walked into that conference room in uniform and they got up and yelled and cheered. . . ."[16]

Chief Surgeon, USAFBI

As Colonel Hawley had signified by donning his uniform, Pearl Harbor

[13] Medical planners usually established hospital requirements in terms of beds, assuming that each bed carried with it a proportional amount of personnel, supplies, and equipment.

[14] Hawley Interv, 1962, p. 12, CMH; Larkey "Hist," ch. 1, pp. 15, 26–29, and ch. 2, pp. 11–12; Memo, Hawley to AG, SPOBS, 4 Dec 41, file HD ETO 400.22 Exchanges, Shipments, & Transfers; Ltr, OofCSurg, SOS, ETO, to General Purchasing Agent, SOS, 29 Jul 43, file HD 008 ETO O/CS (Policy Book); An. 10 (Medical) to Rpt, U.S. Army in Scotland, 6 Oct 14, file 091–711 ETO.

[15] Quotation in Hawley Interv, 1962, pp. 10–11, CMH. See also Larkey "Hist," ch. 1, pp. 31–32.

[16] Hawley Interv, 1962, pp. 11–12, CMH.

permitted the Army observers to reveal their true military colors. When the War Department, on 8 January 1942, activated Headquarters, United States Army Forces in the British Isles (USAFBI), the observers became the nucleus of a theater staff. General Chaney assumed command of this new headquarters, which was to control all Army elements sent to the United Kingdom under ABC-1 and RAINBOW-5. Chaney's SPOBS subordinates took corresponding general and special staff positions. Colonel Hawley, for example, switched designation from Chief Surgeon, SPOBS, to Chief Surgeon, USAFBI.[17]

The plans that USAFBI was to carry out also changed. During late December 1941 and early January 1942 President Roosevelt, Prime Minister Churchill, and their chiefs of staff met in Washington at the ARCADIA conference. Among other decisions, they agreed to deploy a large American ground combat force to Northern Ireland. In contrast to the 30,000-man garrison and antiaircraft contingent contemplated in RAINBOW-5 this new force, designated MAGNET, was to consist of one armored and three infantry divisions with support elements, in all about 105,000 men. MAGNET was to replace British combat troops in Northern Ireland, allowing their redeployment to North Africa and other active theaters. At the same time American armor and infantry were to be ready to move into the neighboring Republic of Eire if the Germans invaded that weak neutral country.[18]

While the War Department enlarged the Northern Ireland force and revised its mission, it scrapped plans for the Army garrison in Scotland and for the token mobile regiment in southern England. The Army Air Forces buildup, however, remained a firm commitment. Late in January the War Department activated in the United States the Eighth Air Force, which was to be the senior American air headquarters in Great Britain, as well as subordinate bomber, fighter, and base commands. On 20 February the bomber commander, Brig. Gen. Ira C. Eaker, and six staff officers arrived in England to begin plans and preparations for the air offensive. General Chaney two days later established an Advance Detachment, VIII Bomber Command, under General Eaker.[19]

As USAFBI chief surgeon, Colonel Hawley had to revise medical plans to conform to the overall changes in the RAINBOW-5 deployment, as well as prepare for medical support of the troops soon to arrive. He had to do this in the first months, without even the semblance of an adequate staff. Hawley's first assistant, 1st Lt. Dean S. Fleming, MC, a reservist activated from the Red Cross-Harvard unit, reported on 7 January. On 10 March, when Hawley formally organized his office, he had a staff of three: Lieu-

[17] GO Nos. 1 and 2, HQ, USAFBI, 8 Jan 42; Ruppenthal, *Logistical Support,* 1:21-22. Chaney and his staff at the same time assumed the title of Army Members, U.S. Military Mission, London, and were supposed to continue their liaison and observation activities, but these functions quickly declined in importance and the mission went out of existence in mid-1942. See GO No. 13, HQ, ETOUSA, 20 Jul 42.

[18] Matloff and Snell, *Strategic Planning,* pp. 108-09; Ruppenthal, *Logistical Support,* 1:21. ARCADIA was the code name for the Allied summit conference.

[19] GO No. 5, HQ, USAFBI, 22 Feb 42.

tenant Fleming and two other Medical Corps officers, Capt. John T. Martin and 1st Lt. Barron D. Knox, both fresh from the United States. Knox initially assumed the tasks of executive officer, liaison officer, and supply officer. Fleming, an epidemiologist, took charge of preventive medicine, personnel, physical standards, and medical reports and returns; and Martin, a recent Medical Field Service School graduate, became flight surgeon.[20]

With the exception of Fleming, whom Hawley considered a "very good young epidemiologist," Hawley's first assistants were of only limited use. Martin and Knox, Hawley reported, "are both good youngsters and will make someone a good assistant; but they are quite incapable of taking over any section of this office and operating it, and there simply isn't time to devote long hours to training them from the ground up." Repeated pleas to the surgeon general's office for experienced executive and supply officers elicited little but promises, as the Medical Department as a whole was short of qualified men in these fields. As a result, until late April, Colonel Hawley had to do most of his planning and administration himself. He lamented: "I can do the administration, the preventive medicine, the medical planning. But I can't keep on doing all of them. And . . . I am not qualified to do the detailed supply planning." [21]

Additional officers gradually straggled in. By mid-May Hawley's commissioned staff had grown to nine, including an executive officer of field rank, a dentist, a veterinarian, and a supply officer, the latter transferred from duty with the Canadian Army. With these reinforcements Hawley was able to place at least one man in seven of the planned nine divisions of his office (*Chart 1*). Many of his new assistants, nevertheless, lacked experience in their jobs, and the staff shortage would continue to grow worse as the chief surgeon's responsibilities expanded.[22]

Medical Plans and Programs

During early 1942 Hawley revised his Air Force medical support plans to conform to the evolving requirements of General Eaker's projected bomber command. Hawley reiterated his recommendation that each air station have an infirmary with enough beds for 1 percent of the troops located there, while a base command serving all ground and air forces furnished station and general hospitals and supply depots. By 13 March Hawley had selected locations for three station hospitals to support the first bombardment groups scheduled for deployment. Additional site selections had to await completion of Eighth Air Force plans and the arrival

[20] Office Order No. 2, OofCSurg, USAFBI, 10 Mar 42.

[21] Quoted words from Ltr, Hawley to TSG, 4 Apr 42. See also Ltrs, Hawley to TSG, 12 Feb and 29 Apr 42; Ltr, Col F. A. Blesse, MC, to Hawley, 21 Mar 42. All in file HD 024 ETO O/CS (Hawley-SGO Corresp). Hawley shared his staff shortage with the rest of USAFBI, which included a total of twenty-four officers and thirteen enlisted men in January 1942 and received no significant augmentation until April. See Ruppenthal, *Logistical Support,* 1:31–32, and Msg, Chaney to TAG, WD, 17 Jan 42, file ETO Admin 388.

[22] Office Orders Nos. 5, 7, 12, OofCSurg, USAFBI, 29 Apr, 11 May, and 19 May 42, respectively; Larkey "Hist," ch. 3, pp. 3–5.

CHART 1—ORGANIZATION OF THE OFFICE OF THE CHIEF SURGEON, USAFBI, MAY 1942

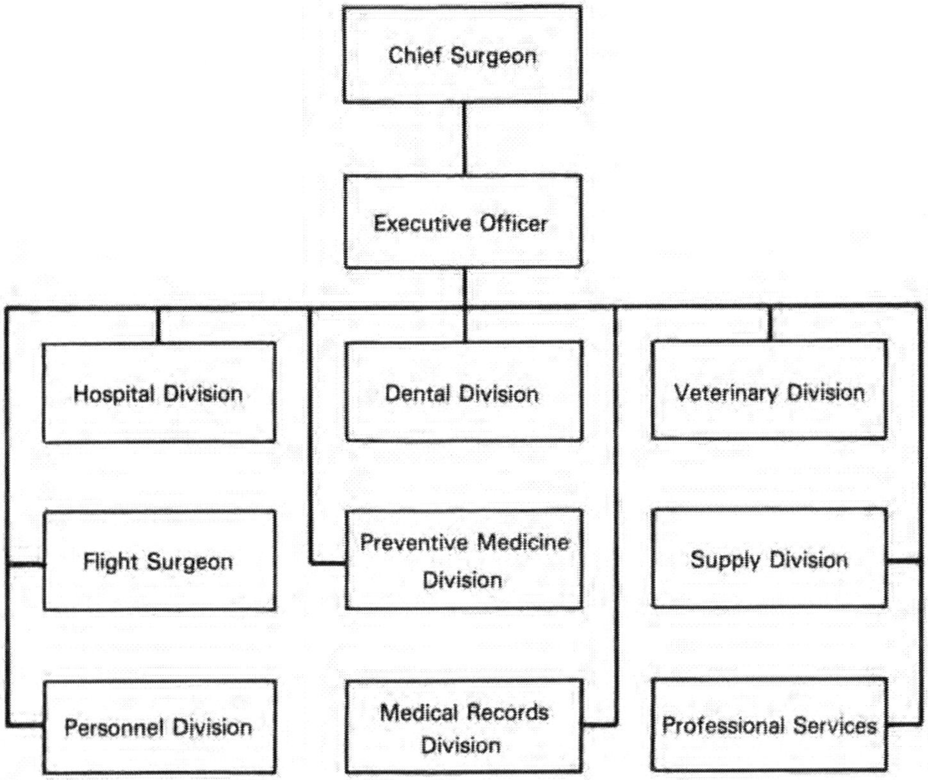

Source: Adapted by authors from George Garand, Hubert E. Potter, and Pauline Vivette, "Medical Service in ETOUSA" (Washington, D.C.: Historical Unit, Office of the Surgeon General, 1976), ch. I, p. I-35.1, on file in CMH.

of troops. The latter were slow in coming, due to shipping shortages and the diversion of men and aircraft to meet urgent needs in the Pacific. The first contingent of 1,800 Air Force soldiers did not reach England until 11 May, and major movements of men, equipment, and aircraft were delayed until June.[23]

Besides reworking his Air Force medical plans, Hawley expanded upon his overall hospital program for the United Kingdom. On 16 January he recommended provision of hospitals for the entire command on the formula earlier established for the Air Force: infirmary beds for 1 percent of strength, station hospital beds for 4 percent, general hospital beds for 3 percent, and convalescent beds for 1.3 percent. He declared that few British hospitals would be available for transfer to the American Army and ruled out conversion of other buildings as expensive and unlikely to produce satisfactory results. Hawley favored instead constructing new semipermanent hospitals from the ground up. He advocated use of the British 20-by-40-foot wood and metal Nissen hut as the basic unit for such hospitals, as the hut could be adapted for wards, operating rooms, mess halls, or any other purpose and afforded some protection against bombing. By late February Hawley had established definite hospital requirements for the forces in England. The Air Force would need thirty-seven battalion-size infirmaries and five station hospitals, each with 125 to 500 beds. The base command, for logistics and support troops, would require twenty-five battalion infirmaries; two station hospitals; two general hospitals, each with 1,000 beds; and one convalescent hospital, with 2,000 beds. The general and convalescent hospitals were to serve both the base and the bomber commands.[24]

Throughout the short organizational life of USAFBI, reception and accommodation of the MAGNET force absorbed much of the effort of all staff sections. Plans called for the initial MAGNET troop contingent—the first significant American force to reach the United Kingdom—to arrive late in January. More troops were to follow as rapidly as the limited amount of shipping and the demands of global war permitted.

Colonel Hawley quickly revised his and Major Welsh's Northern Ireland medical plans. Between 6 and 15 January Hawley surveyed British medical facilities in Northern Ireland. He arranged with the commander of British troops in Northern Ireland for MAGNET to take over the hospitals and medical supplies of redeploying British units and also secured an agreement that this force would treat MAGNET casualties in its hospitals until the Americans established their own. Hawley set the MAGNET hospital requirements on the same 1-4-3-per-

[23] Larkey "Hist," ch. 2, pp. 12–16. For the beginning of the Air Force buildup, see Ruppenthal, *Logistical Support,* 1:26–31, and Wesley F. Craven and James Lea Cate, eds., *The Army Air Forces in World War II (hereafter cited as AAF)*, 7 vols. (Chicago: University of Chicago Press, 1948–58), vol. 1, *Plans and Early Operations, January 1939 to August 1942* (1948), pp. 618–42.

[24] Memo, Hawley to CEngr, HQ, USAFBI, via G–4, 16 Jan 42, in Larkey "Hist," ch. 2. app. 1; Ltr, Hawley to CSurg, GHQ, WD, 12 Feb 42, file HD 024 ETO O/CS (Hawley-SGO Corresp); Msg, USAFBI to AGWAR, 28 Feb 42, file ETO Admin 388.

cent basis as he had recommended for England. He estimated that the British hospitals to be taken over would provide about 2,000 general and perhaps 170 station hospital beds, while U.S. Navy hospitals at Londonderry and Lough Erne, to be acquired by the Army, would account for another 600 station beds. The rest of the approximately 7,000 fixed beds needed would have to come from new construction of 1,000-bed general and 500-bed station hospitals. In addition, the existing British hospitals would require some construction to bring operating theaters, X-ray facilities, mess hall refrigeration, and staff quarters up to American standards.

Because MAGNET was to be a mobile field force, Hawley proposed that three of the projected 500-bed station hospitals be occupied by 750-bed evacuation hospitals. Each evacuation hospital so employed would keep its field equipment in storage and use a separate set of station hospital equipment. During active operations the evacuation hospital would pick up its stored equipment and follow the troops, while a station hospital complement, sent from the United States, took over the fixed facility. Hawley advocated this arrangement as a way of economizing on scarce hospital units, but the War Department delayed approval until further changes in MAGNET plans made the proposal obsolete.[25]

On 19 January a 36-man (18 officers and 18 enlisted men) headquarters advance party from the V Corps, the principal MAGNET command, arrived in Great Britain. The group included Lt. Col. Charles E. Brenn, MC, the corps surgeon. Brenn went to London with the rest of the party and at once conferred with Hawley. The two surgeons discovered an embarrassing misunderstanding. Brenn, before leaving for England, had spent several days at the surgeon general's office developing his own Northern Ireland medical plan in consultation with Major Welsh. Surgeon General Magee had directed Brenn to do so on the mistaken assumption that MAGNET was to be a separate force, independent of USAFBI. A similar misunderstanding of their position prevailed among other MAGNET officers who, according to Hawley, considered USAFBI "a bunch of interlopers trying to usurp the divine authority of MAGNET." In spite of these difficulties Hawley and Brenn at once developed a smooth working relationship. They adopted Hawley's plan for Northern Ireland, because it was based on current firsthand information and included agreements with the British. Once established in Belfast, Brenn exercised much independent authority, but he deferred to Hawley as theater chief surgeon. Hawley later said of Brenn: "He is completely proper and he is doing a fine job." [26]

---

[25] Memo, Hawley to CEngr, HQ, USAFBI, via G-4, 16 Jan 42, in Larkey "Hist," ch. 2, app. 1; An. 6 (Medical Plan) MAGNET, 19 Jan 42, in Larkey "Hist," ch. 2, app. 2 (see also ch. 2, pp. 4-6); Msg, USAFBI to AGWAR, 3 and 28 Feb 42, file ETO Admin 388; Ltr, Hawley to CSurg, GHQ, WD, 12 Feb 42, file HD 024 ETO O/CS (Hawley-SGO Corresp); Memo, Surg, V Corps, to TSG, sub: Medical History, 10 Jan 44; "History of Medical Service, SOS, ETOUSA, from Inception to 31 December 1943" (hereafter cited as "Med Svc Hist, 1942-43"), ex. C, file HD 314.7-2 ETO.

[26] First quotation in Ltr, Hawley to Blesse, 18 Apr 42, and second quotation in Ltr, Hawley to

Continued

On 24 January Hawley and Brenn left London for Belfast to meet the first MAGNET troop contingent. That same day General Chaney issued orders creating the U.S. Army Northern Ireland Force (USANIF) to control all MAGNET troops under USAFBI. Two days later about 4,000 United States soldiers, most of them members of the 34th Infantry Division, became the first American fighting men of World War II to disembark in the United Kingdom. The division commander, Maj. Gen. Russell P. Hartle, who accompanied the troops, assumed command of both USANIF and V Corps.[27]

This initial MAGNET contingent brought with it the first Army medical troops to enter the European Theater of Operations. They included the 10th Station Hospital; an element of the 136th Medical Regiment; and medical detachments of the 133d Infantry, the 151st Field Artillery, the 109th Quartermaster Regiment, the 112th Engineer Battalion, and the 63d Signal Battalion—in all 41 officers, 42 nurses, and 322 enlisted men. As a result of mismanagement at the New York Port of Embarkation and a shortage of shipping, these units landed at Belfast without most of their equipment. Hence, the first MAGNET troops had to depend on the British for all medical services. While the Allies provided generously, the Americans' total dependency, according to Hawley, "made a very bad impression upon the British." A second MAGNET contingent of about 7,000 men, including the 7th General Dispensary and elements of the 109th Medical Battalion, arrived on 2 March no better supplied, although "driblets" of medical equipment addressed to units in the Caribbean and Iceland came in on various transports.[28]

With extensive British assistance the first MAGNET contingents settled in. The troops crowded into Nissen huts in camps turned over by the British. Initially, the Americans ate British Army rations, received their mail from the British postal service, and had their clothes cleaned and shoes repaired in local establishments. Field artillerymen, sent over without their 105-mm. howitzers, learned to fire and maintain the British 25-pounder. Gradually, as supply ships arrived, USANIF established its own mail, laundry, and post exchange services. By late March the mess halls were beginning to serve American rations instead of the unfamiliar and nutritionally less satisfactory British menu.[29]

As rapidly as possible, USANIF set up its own hospitals. On 9 March the 10th Station Hospital took over a British military hospital at Ebrington Barracks, Londonderry, complete with its existing equipment and patients. By rearranging the wards and acquiring additional buildings the American staff increased the capacity of this plant from 150 to 350 beds. To furnish additional fixed hospitals, USANIF pressed mobile medical units

CSurg, GHQ, WD, 12 Feb 42 (see also Ltr, Blesse to Hawley, 21 Mar 42), all in file HD 024 ETO O/CS (Hawley-SGO Corresp); Larkey "Hist," ch. 2, p. 9.

[27] Ruppenthal, *Logistical Support,* 1:22–26.

[28] An. 6 (Medical Plan) MAGNET, 19 Jan 42, in Larkey "Hist," ch. 2, app. 2; Ltrs, Hawley to CSurg, GHQ, WD, 12 Feb 42, Blesse to Hawley, 21 Mar 42, and Hawley to TSG, 4 Apr 42, all in file HD 024 ETO O/CS (Hawley-SGO Corresp).

[29] Ruppenthal, *Logistical Support,* 1:23–26.

into service. The clearing company of the 34th Division's 109th Medical Battalion and later those of the 1st Armored Division's 47th Medical Battalion and the V Corps' 503d Medical Battalion all operated small temporary station hospitals. The 109th's company staffed a former U.S. Navy hospital at Lough Erne until September, when the newly landed 160th Station Hospital relieved it (*see Map 1*).[30]

The 5th General Hospital, the first unit of its kind scheduled for deployment with MAGNET, had been included in the second troop contingent; but it did not open in Belfast until late May, after a long, frustrating odyssey. A 500-bed affiliated unit sponsored by Harvard University, the hospital embarked at New York on 19 February with its equipment and a staff of 37 officers, 60 nurses, and 275 enlisted men.[31] Most of the personnel, including the hospital commander, Lt. Col. Maxwell G. Keeler, MC, embarked on a single vessel; but 7 officers, 28 nurses, and 14 enlisted men sailed on other ships to provide medical care on the voyage. Soon after leaving port, a mechanical breakdown crippled the transport carrying the main body, forcing the ship to turn back to Halifax, Nova Scotia, and eventually to Boston, Massachusetts, where the 5th disembarked; the group spent the next month and a half at Camp Edwards awaiting space on another ship. The rest of the unit landed at Belfast early in March. While the nurses assisted in various American and British hospitals, the officers and enlisted men collected the hospital's equipment at the intended location, the British Army's 31st General Hospital at Musgrave Park on the outskirts of Belfast.

The main body embarked again on 30 April and reached Belfast on 12 May. Nine days later the 5th General Hospital opened it first wards at Musgrave Park. The unit's plant, a three-story brick building formerly used as a boys' reformatory with attached Nissen-hut wards, had room for about 800 beds. At the outset, crated equipment and supplies filled most of the wards. About the time of the hospital's opening a major serum hepatitis epidemic hit the Northern Ireland forces. As a result, according to Colonel Keeler, "it was just a constant run-around to see whether we could get beds set up fast enough each day to accommodate the number of patients that had to be admitted. . . ." Within two weeks, the staff had twelve wards in operation, caring for over 400 patients. In June, as the Musgrave Park facility filled to its 800-bed capacity, the 5th opened a 900-bed convalescent annex in a nearly completed former EMS hospital in Waringfield, about 20 miles away. The hospital's patient load reached a peak of 1,500 in the two facilities during late August. Supporting some 60,000 American and British troops, the 5th General Hospital provided training as

[30] 10th Station Hospital Annual Rpt, 1942; "Med Svc Hist, 1942–43," ex. C, file HD 314.7-2 ETO.

[31] The unit initially was overstaffed for its 500-bed capacity, and the commanding general of the New York Port of Embarkation attempted to transfer its 28 excess officers to tactical units of the 34th Division that lacked medical officers. The unit bitterly resisted this, on grounds that the Office of the Surgeon General had promised affiliated units, when organized, that they would serve together. Eventually, the OSG resolved the problem by transferring the excess officers in a body to Walter Reed Army Medical Center. See 5th General Hospital Annual Rpt, 1942.

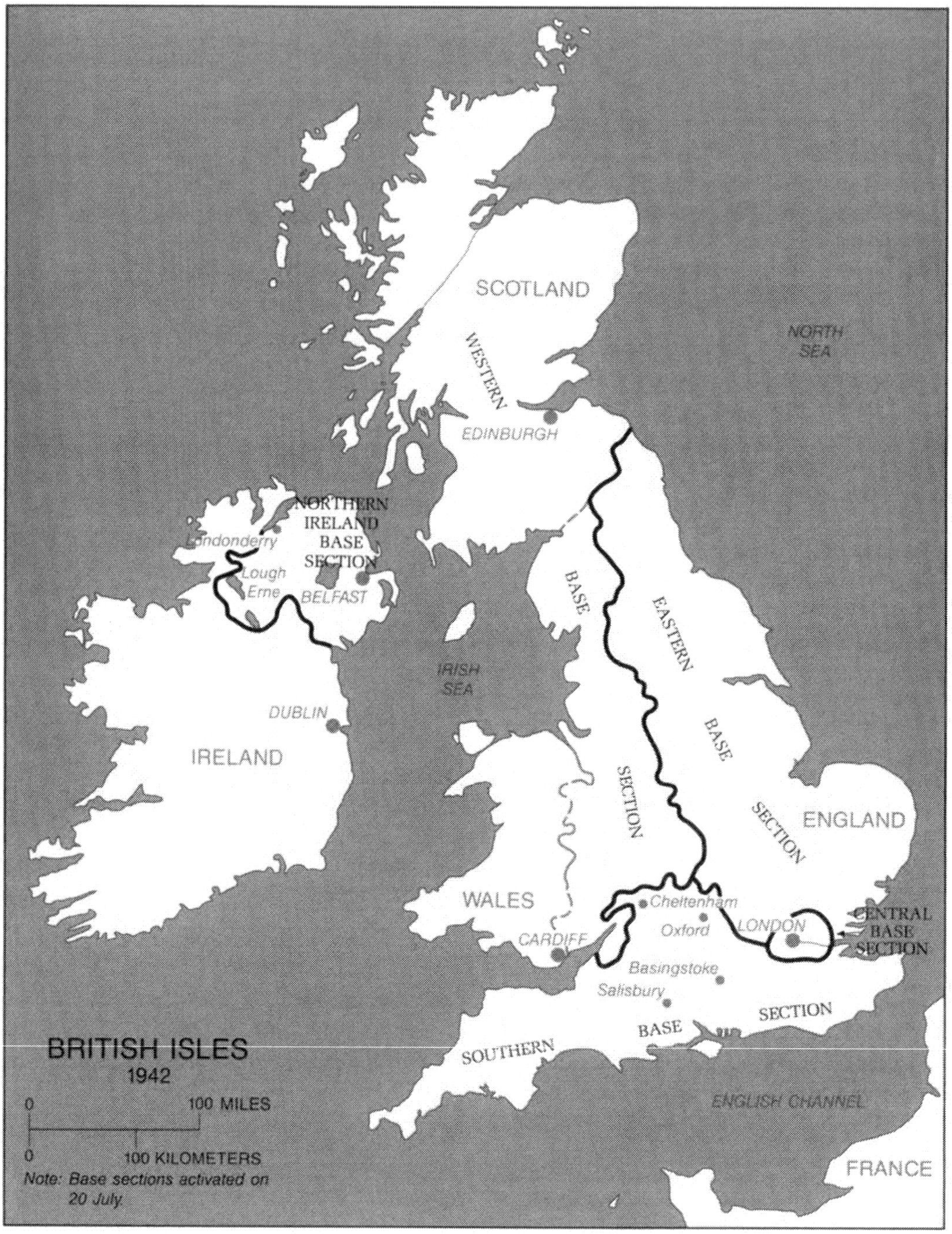
SCOTLAND
NORTH SEA
WESTERN
EDINBURGH
NORTHERN IRELAND BASE SECTION
Londonderry
Lough Erne
BELFAST
BASE
EASTERN
IRISH SEA
DUBLIN
IRELAND
BASE
SECTION
SECTION
SECTION
ENGLAND
WALES
Cheltenham
Oxford
LONDON
CENTRAL BASE SECTION
CARDIFF
Basingstoke
Salisbury
SECTION
BASE
SOUTHERN
BRITISH ISLES
1942
0
100 MILES
0
100 KILOMETERS
Note: Base sections activated on 20 July.
ENGLISH CHANNEL
FRANCE

MAP 1

well as medical care. Under an exchange program, division medical officers worked for brief periods in the wards and hospital staff members were temporarily assigned to units. This arrangement "gave those medical officers of the 5th . . . who had come straight from civilian life a much better understanding of what the soldier goes through within his own organization," while affording unit officers a chance for hospital and professional experience.[32]

For USANIF Colonel Brenn established an evacuation policy on the principles earlier prescribed by Hawley. As soon as they could, unit medical detachments set up dispensaries to treat patients requiring less than 72 hours of care. Using ambulances, organic vehicles, and sometimes buses and trains, units sent men requiring more extended treatment to British hospitals; to the 10th Station and 5th General Hospitals; or to the smaller facilities operated by the clearing companies. A disposition board of medical officers established by order of USAFBI determined which sick and injured men should be evacuated to the United States. Initially located at the 10th Station Hospital and later moved to the 5th General Hospital, the board sent some psychotics, patients needing locally unavailable special therapies or diets, and men unable to return to duty within 180 days. Evacuees who could care for themselves crossed the Atlantic on returning troopships, usually the fast liners *Queen Mary* and *Queen Elizabeth*. Mental and litter patients traveled on British or Canadian hospital ships, as the United States had no such vessels of its own in the Atlantic.[33]

Early in the Northern Ireland occupation Colonel Brenn issued elaborate sanitary regulations, based on the plans Colonel Hawley had developed in January. Brenn emphasized the responsibility of unit commanders and medical officers for protecting troop health. He banned the use of locally produced fresh milk, because Irish cattle often were infected with tuberculosis and few dairies practiced proper pasteurization, and the use of private water supplies, enjoining troops to treat them as polluted until proven otherwise. He also prescribed procedures for keeping mess halls and kitchens clean and for disposing sewage and garbage. ("Garbage removal by pig keepers in adjacent areas will be arranged for.") Troops were to bathe and change clothing "at least twice a week," and units were to make every effort to keep their men in dry clothes to reduce the incidence of respiratory ailments in the damp climate. Venereal disease prevention received Brenn's special attention. Convinced of the need to provide cheap, plentiful prophylactic devices for the troops, he directed units, in cooperation with municipal authorities and the Royal Ulster Constabulary, to establish off-base prophylactic stations and to trace the contacts of men who became infected.

---

[32] Ibid.; Interv, OSG with Col Maxwell G. Keeler, MC (hereafter cited as Keeler Interv), 17 Jul 45, box 223, RG 112, NARA.

[33] "Med Svc Hist, 1942–43," pp. 18–19, file HD 314.7-2 ETO; Ltr, Hawley to TSG, 25 Apr 42, file HD 024 ETO O/CS (Hawley-SGO Corresp), in which the chief surgeon expresses his determination to keep helpless patients off transports subject to U-boat attacks.

Mindful of local sensitivities, Brenn warned that such arrangements must be made "tactfully and unostentatiously" by using, for example, such terms as "Aid Station, U.S. Army," rather than more descriptive ones, on the signs identifying prophylactic stations.[34]

The Army force in Northern Ireland never reached its full projected strength. Two more contingents arrived during May, including the rest of the 34th Division and the entire 1st Armored Division, as well as the bulk of the V Corps headquarters and corps troops. Their arrival brought USANIF to its peak strength of about 32,000 officers and men. On 30 May, however, the War Department dropped the other two divisions from MAGNET. On 1 June USANIF and V Corps headquarters merged into Headquarters, U.S. Army Northern Ireland Forces and V Corps (Reinforced). USANIF at the same time established a provisional Northern Ireland Base Command, staffed as an additional duty by officers from the main headquarters. Colonel Brenn served as chief surgeon of both new commands.[35]

As the medical service in Northern Ireland took shape, Colonel Hawley in London negotiated for the U.S. Army's acquisition of the American Red Cross–Harvard Unit and the Churchill Hospital. During April Hawley reached an understanding with the Emergency Medical Services and the Harvard unit. The unit, with its doctors and nurses given Army commissions, was to become a general medical laboratory as soon as American forces in the United Kingdom expanded enough to need its full-time services. The Army absorbed the unit on 15 July. Until then, Dr. Gordon and his staff informally assisted Hawley in epidemiology and preventive medicine.[36]

Concurrent negotiations for the Churchill Hospital, newly moved into its EMS-constructed facility near Oxford, went less well. The hospital director, Dr. Harlan Wilson, refused to deal with any American authority in Britain below the ambassador. Hawley at the same time became disenchanted with the Churchill staff, which, he reported, had "played more with the 'Lords and Lydies' than with the E.M.S." Yet he wanted their hospital plant. Eventually, Hawley arranged with the surgeon general to have a 500-bed general hospital sent from the United States to take over the Churchill building and incorporate some members of the civilian staff. This plan broke down. In July the War Department sent the 1,000-bed 2d General Hospital to occupy the Oxford facility; however, the unit was too large for the hospital building and had no personnel vacancies for the volunteer doctors and nurses. Most of the eligible members of the Oxford staff, who were unwilling to be dispersed to other units, there-

[34] Quotation in GO No. 6, HQ, USANIF, 2 Feb 42. See also ETO, "SPOBS Hist," p. 149; An. 6 (Medical Plan) MAGNET, 19 Jan 42, in Larkey "Hist," ch. 2, app. 2.

[35] ETO, "SPOBS Hist," pp. 134–39; GO No. 28, HQ, USANIF, 31 May 42, and SO No. 1, HQ, USANIF, and V Army Corps (Reinf), 1 Jun 42, in file Orders (GO, SPO), HQ, V Corps, USANIF, USAFBI, 1942.

[36] ETO, "SPOBS Hist," pp. 169–70; Ltr, Hawley to TSG, 29 Apr 42, file HD 024 ETO O/CS (Hawley-SGO Corresp); Larkey "Hist," ch. 1, pp. 10–11.

upon refused to join the Army. The 2d General Hospital finally established itself in the Oxford plant, which the British enlarged to accommodate the unit.[37]

The 2d General Hospital arrived in time to help USAFBI and USANIF cope with their first major medical crisis, an epidemic of serum hepatitis. This epidemic had begun in February and quickly incapacitated large numbers of troops in the United States and overseas. By late April the Preventive Medicine Service, Office of the Surgeon General, had traced the source of the epidemic to several lots of contaminated yellow fever vaccine made with human serum. The Army at once stopped using vaccine from that particular manufacturer, but by that time men who had received the vaccine earlier in the year were coming down with hepatitis,[38] including many who arrived in Northern Ireland in the May troop shipments.

Before the epidemic passed its peak in late July 1,950 soldiers in the European Theater were stricken, 2 of whom died. About 100 suffered permanent liver damage, which rendered them unfit for further military service, and those who recovered required long periods of recuperation. To help care for the sudden influx of sick, Colonel Hawley in July sent part of the 2d General Hospital staff, who were awaiting expansion of their Oxford plant, to Belfast to reinforce the 5th General Hospital. The 2d General Hospital personnel helped operate the 5th's convalescent facility at Waringfield. With this augmentation and with continued British help, the Northern Ireland hospitals satisfactorily met the emergency. At USAFBI direction, the Red Cross-Harvard Unit and the 5th General Hospital conducted their own search for the source of the epidemic. They independently reached the same conclusion as investigators in the United States, that it was a post-vaccinal infection. This finding reassured British health authorities, who feared the spread of a possible infectious hepatitis epidemic to the civilian population.[39]

While the epidemic ran its course, more ambitious deployment plans superseded RAINBOW-5 and MAGNET, and USAFBI gave way to a new theater command. These changes nullified most of the plans and many of the preparations of Colonel Hawley and his slowly expanding medical establishment. The chief surgeon and his staff would have to do most of their work over again on a grander scale.

[37] Larkey "Hist," ch. 1, pp. 3-8; ETO, "SPOBS Hist," p. 170; Ltrs, Hawley to TSG, 29 Apr and 17 Jul 42, and TSG to Hawley, 25 May 42, file HD 024 ETO O/CS (Hawley-SGO Corresp); Ltr, Maj Gen J. C. H. Lee to CG, SOS, WD, 21 Sep 42, file HD 024 ETO CS (Hawley Chron); file 322.15 (Churchill Hospital, Misc. Papers) on Churchill transfer.

[38] Serum hepatitis has an incubation period of 60-154 days.

[39] The course of the epidemic, which caused over 49,000 cases in the Army throughout the world, is recounted in Ebbe Curtis Hoff, ed., *Communicable Diseases Transmitted Through Contact or by Unknown Means*, Medical Department, United States Army in World War II (Washington, D.C.: Office of the Surgeon General, Department of the Army, 1960), ch. XVII. See also "Med Svc Hist, 1942-43," p. 37, file HD 314.7-2 ETO; Interv, Harlan B. Phillips with Dr. Stanhope Bayne-Jones, 21 Mar-28 Jul 66 (hereafter cited as Bayne-Jones Interv, 1966), vol, 3, p. 692, NLM; Keeler Interv, 17 Jul 45, box 223, RG 112, NARA; Ltrs, Hawley to TSG, 9 Jun, 1 and 17 Jul, and 7 Aug 42, file HD 024 ETO O/CS (Hawley-SGO Corresp).

Yet they had gained valuable experience in these first months of war, especially in supporting the MAGNET force. They had worked out the general principles for organizing an Army medical service in Great Britain. Most important, they had established a close cooperative relationship, based on mutual professional respect and, in many cases, personal friendship, with British military and civilian medical officials.

CHAPTER II

From BOLERO to TORCH

From the start of war preparations the United States intended to make its major military effort in the Atlantic, with the aim of destroying Nazi Germany. RAINBOW-5 and MAGNET were only preliminary steps toward that end. During March 1942, searching for a more decisive course of action and for definite goals to guide Army mobilization, Chief of Staff Marshall and the Operations Division of the General Staff drafted a proposal for a full-scale assault on Nazi-occupied Europe. Their plan called for expansion of the bomber offensive and for deployment of 1 million American combat and support troops in Britain by April 1943. The buildup was to proceed rapidly enough to permit small cross-Channel attacks in late summer 1942. It was to culminate in the spring of the following year in an invasion of France, followed by a drive into Germany.

President Roosevelt approved this plan and in mid-April sent Harry L. Hopkins, his personal troubleshooter, and Marshall to London to present it to the British. Marshall and Hopkins secured tentative British assent. The two governments at once set up Anglo-American combined committees in Washington and London to direct the huge troop buildup, code-named BOLERO. Other committees began planning the late-1942 attack (SLEDGEHAMMER), to be launched if necessary to relieve pressure on the Russians, and the major invasion (ROUNDUP) for early 1943.[1]

Theater Reorganization

To carry out these new plans, the War Department reorganized the Army command structure in the United Kingdom. On 14 May 1942 it directed USAFBI to establish a services of supply, which was to control all the technical services and assume most theater logistics functions. The Services of Supply (SOS) in Britain would be the counterpart of the War Department Serices of Supply (later renamed Army Service Forces), formed earlier under Maj. Gen. Brehon B. Somervell as one of three

[1] BOLERO initially referred to the entire buildup and invasion plan; but, to avoid confusion, President Roosevelt in July restricted use of that code name to measure for the establishment of American forces in the United Kingdom. Development of the BOLERO plan is traced in Matloff and Snell, *Strategic Planning*, pp. 174–91. See also Ruppenthal, *Logistical Support*, 1:52–55, and Gordon A. Harrison, *Cross-Channel Attack*, United States Army in World War II (Washington, D.C.: Office of the Chief of Military History, Department of the Army, 1951), pp. 11–19.

overall Army functional commands.[2] On 8 June USAFBI itself ceased to exist. The War Department redesignated it the European Theater of Operations, United States Army (ETOUSA), and included within the boundaries of this new theater Great Britain, Western Europe, and Iceland. Providing an explicit definition of authority that USAFBI had lacked, the War Department gave ETOUSA operational control of all United States military forces within its boundaries, as well as administrative and logistical authority over the Army elements. ETOUSA, under the strategic direction of the Anglo-American Combined Chiefs of Staff, was to "prepare to carry on military operations in the European Theater against the Axis Powers and their Allies." General Chaney headed the new command until 24 June, when Maj. Gen. Dwight D. Eisenhower replaced him.[3]

While the new theater command structure was taking shape, Allied war plans again changed. The British had agreed to attempt SLEDGEHAMMER and ROUNDUP only with hesitation and many reservations. As planners in Washington and London studied the tactical and logistical problems involved, the feasibility of SLEDGEHAMMER and even of a 1943 ROUNDUP came increasingly into question, confirming earlier British doubts.[4] At the same time the military situation demanded some sort of Anglo-American initiative. The Russians were pressing for the opening of a European "second front," and British forces in North Africa were retreating under heavy German-Italian attack. During June Churchill and his chiefs of staff began urging President Roosevelt to drop plans for SLEDGEHAMMER in favor of an invasion of Northwest Africa (GYMNAST), a project long advocated by the British. The American chiefs of staff fought hard to save SLEDGEHAMMER, but the British eventually convinced Roosevelt—who above all wanted an offensive somewhere in Europe or the Mediterranean in 1942—to undertake the North African attack. By the end of July the Allies had decided to launch a combined assault on Northwest Africa (Morocco, Algeria, and Tunisia) before December 1942, even though this meant the cancellation of SLEDGEHAMMER and the probable postponement of ROUNDUP for up to a year. At the same time the Allies would continue the BOLERO buildup, drawing from it part of the troops and supplies for the African campaign, now renamed Operation TORCH.

To direct the new operation, the Americans and British late in July selected the ETO commander, General Eisenhower, and enlarged ETOUSA to include North Africa. Under Eisen-

[2] The other two were the Army Air Forces and Army Ground Forces.

[3] The basic directive establishing the Services of Supply is Memo, CofS, U.S. Army, to CG, USAFBI, 14 May 42, sub: Organization of Services of Supply, file HQ ETOUSA AGO 320.3 SOS. See also Ruppenthal, *Logistical Support*, 1:33–40, 43, 47–48. Quotation on p. 40. Chaney had disagreed with the War Department on, among other things, Air Force organization in Britain, and General Marshall preferred a commander in closer touch, as Eisenhower was, with Washington thinking and plans.

[4] For the medical difficulties of attempting to support SLEDGEHAMMER, see Larkey "Hist," ch. 4, pp. 2–6 and apps. 2–3.

hower an Anglo-American staff in London, later designated Allied Force Headquarters (AFHQ), planned and organized the invasion. American personel for this headquarters came from ETO and SOS headquarters, which were responsible for supporting TORCH until the invasion force secured its North African lodgement. For the European Theater of Operations and the Services of Supply, this double effort—simultaneously to receive large forces in Britain and mount an invasion of Africa—led to months of confusion and improvisation. The theater medical service would undergo its share of the strain.[5]

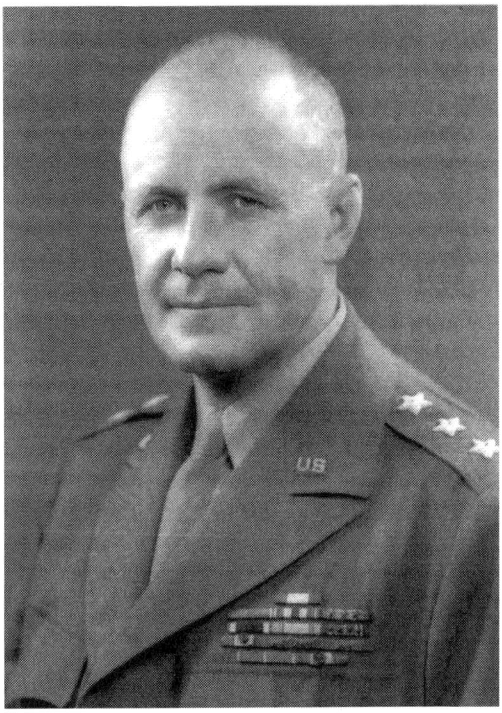

LT. GEN. JOHN C. H. LEE
(1945 photograph)

The Office of the Chief Surgeon

For Colonel Hawley theater reorganization brought both personal and institutional challenges in 1942. Formation of the theater Services of Supply at first threatened him with loss of his position as ETO chief surgeon. The War Department permitted the newly designated SOS commander, Maj. Gen. John C. H. Lee, an experienced Engineer officer, to select key members of his staff from men recommended by the various War Department chiefs of services. Surgeon General Magee proposed Hawley as "best fitted" for the position of SOS chief surgeon, the equivalent of the job Hawley then was filling; but Lee, before he left for London late in May, chose Magee's recommended first alternate, Col. John F. Corby, MC, previously surgeon of the Fourth Army. Corby arrived in England early in June but promptly succumbed to the hepatitis epidemic and spent his first two weeks in the theater in a London hospital. Lee in the meantime became acquainted with Hawley and with the extent of Hawley's knowledge of the theater and preparatory work. He also discovered that Hawley was senior to Corby. Lee, therefore, invited Hawley, who had expected to be relieved and sent home, to stay on as both the ETO and SOS chief surgeon. Hawley, not surprisingly, agreed to do so. Corby, after a brief period as medical liaison officer to the British Southern Command, became deputy force surgeon of

[5] Harrison, *Cross-Channel*, pp. 21–32; Ruppenthal, *Logistical Support*, 1:91–92.

Allied Force Headquarters and eventually went to North Africa.[6]

Chain-of-Command Problems

Less easily resolved were the questions of authority and jurisdiction arising from the interposition of another headquarters—the Services of Supply—between special staff section heads, such as the chief surgeon, and the theater commander. The chiefs of the technical services now were in a different echelon from the commander they were supposed to advise. Further, being incorporated within one of several coordinate commands under the theater, the service chiefs lacked the authority to give technical direction to subordinate elements operating outside the Services of Supply, for example, medical units attached to the Eighth Air Force or the ground armies.

This latter problem especially concerned Colonel Hawley. Even before formation of the Services of Supply, Hawley had maintained that the ETO chief surgeon required theater-wide technical control in at least four areas. First, the theater surgeon must be able to supervise medical unit operations and training in all echelons to ensure adequate, uniform treatment of casualties throughout the chain of evacuation. Second, he should have authority to coordinate evacuation between the several echelons of command. Casualties, Hawley pointed out, "are perishable. . . . They require continuous care and treatment during the entire journey from front to rear; and this can only be accomplished if one agency coordinates the entire operation." Third, the theater surgeon also should supervise preventive medicine, because "communicable diseases recognize no echelon of command" and because it was not practicable to establish the necessary expert staff at every headquarters. Finally, he should collect medical reports and statistics, to avoid burdening nonmedical channels with this information. Commenting early in June on a draft general order defining SOS functions, Hawley warned that subordination of the ETO chief surgeon to the SOS commander effectively would prevent him from performing any of the aforementioned tasks, unless the commander himself were empowered to issue theater-wide directives on some matters. Privately, he expressed himself bluntly: "From where I set [*sic*], everybody seems to have gone completely nuts in the field of staff organization." [7]

[6] Memo, TSG to Maj Gen J. C. H. Lee, 7 May 42, file SPMC 322.051-1; Hawley Interv, 1962, pp. 12-14, CMH; MFR, Col Joseph T. McNinch and Dr. Nora V. Lewison, 24 May 49, sub: Interview With Col James B. Mason, MC (Ret.), file HD 000.71, CMH; Ltrs, Hawley to TSG, 10 and 15 Jun 42, HD 024 ETO O/CS (Hawley-SGO Corresp). Hawley was a close friend of Dr. Frederick W. O'Donnell, with whom Lee had served in the 89th Division in World War I, and the sentimental tie weighed heavily with Lee. See Lt Gen J. C. H. Lee, "Service Reminiscences," pp. 82, 97, P-1, box 1, Hawley Papers, MHI. Corby, who lacked staff experience and suffered from emotional problems, was relieved from the Allied Force Headquarters in early February 1943. See Interv, OSG with Maj Gen Albert W. Kenner, MC (Ret.), 9 Jan 52 (hereafter cited as Kenner Interv, 1952), file HD 000.71, CMH.

[7] Chief surgeon's views on his authority, including quotations in body of paragraph, from: Memo, Hawley to Gen Larkin, 29 May 42, sub: Definition of Medical Responsibility, Hawley Big Picture file, SGO HistDivFiles; and Memos, Hawley to G-1, USAFBI, 17 Apr 42, Hawley to AG, USAFBI, 1 Jun 42, sub: Comments on Draft of General Order Es-

Continued

Relocation of the SOS headquarters complicated the question of the special staff's status. In mid-July, to obtain space for his growing establishment, General Lee moved the Services of Supply from crowded London to an unused British office complex at Cheltenham, a resort and retirement community of about 50,000 people, 90 miles northwest of the capital. This relocation included all sections (except the Procurement Branch) and their chiefs. It physically separated Hawley and his colleagues from the ETO headquarters, which remained in London.[8]

During June and July General Chaney and his successor, General Eisenhower, issued a series of orders and circulars attempting to clarify the dual position of the special staff. On 20 July, as the Services of Supply was completing its move to Cheltenham, Eisenhower established the policy that would prevail until early 1943. His General Order No. 19 reaffirmed General Lee's broad responsibility for logistics planning and operations in the theater and authorized Lee to communicate directly with the War Department and the British on supply matters. Within ETOUSA Eisenhower set up eighteen staff sections. The heads of eight were to be stationed at theater headquarters in London. The other chiefs, including Hawley, also were considered members of the theater staff, but they were to stay at Cheltenham and "for the time being, will operate under the immediate direction of the Commanding General, SOS." Each Cheltenham-based staff section was to maintain a liaison officer at the ETO headquarters, and its chief was to advise the theater commander as required. On the question of supervision of the technical services Eisenhower authorized the service chiefs to correspond directly with their subordinates in other commands "insofar as technical instructions, requests for technical reports, and matters of general routine . . . are concerned"; but they would have to send proposed "orders, policies, or other instructions, pertaining to the services for the theater as a whole," first to SOS headquarters for approval and then to the ETO adjutant general for issue in the name of the theater commander.[9]

While General Order No. 19 in principle established theater-wide technical auhority for the service chiefs, Colonel Hawley remained dissatisfied with both his physical location and his position in the chain or command. The stationing of a liaison

tablishing the Service of Supply, and Hawley to G-1, USAFBI, 8 Jun 42, sub: Comments on Directive for SOS, USAFBI, all in Hawley File of Memos, Letters, etc., 1941-1942. Final quotation from Ltr, Hawley to TSG, 6 Jul 42, HD 024 ETO O/CS (Hawley-SGO Corresp). See also Ruppenthal, *Logistical Support,* 1:37-39. The establishment of a War Department-level SOS had similar effects on the position of the surgeon general. See Blanche B. Armfield, *Organization and Administration in World War II,* Medical Department, United States Army in World War II (Washington, D.C.: Office of the Surgeon General, Department of the Army, 1963), pp. 72-83.

[8] Memo, Acting AG, SOS, to Chiefs of Sections, HQ, SOS, 17 Jul 42, sub: Change of Station of Headquarters, SOS; Ruppenthal, *Logistical Support,* 1:81-83. The new office complex consisted of two groups of one-story temporary buildings with over 500,000 square feet of space. Built by the British to house the War Office if it were bombed out of London, it was never fully occupied.

[9] Quotations from GO No. 19, HQ, ETOUSA, 20 Jul 42, in Larkey "Hist," ch. 3, app. 18. See also Ruppenthal, *Logistical Support,* 1:40-44; Ltr, Hawley to TSG, 11 Sep 42, file HD 024 ETO O/CS (Hawley-SGO Corresp).

officer in London only partially overcame the separation of theater and SOS staffs, for the ETO chief surgeon's representative was out of touch with day-to-day activities and decisions at Cheltenham and lacked independent authority of his own. In addition, Hawley found it difficult to deal from Cheltenham with the British medical services in London. "Many time-consuming trips," he reported, "have not effected proper liaison." More fundamentally, Hawley continued to complain of "the difficulty, if not complete inability, of controlling the technical operations of medical units in echelons of ETOUSA other than SOS." Other commands, and even the theater staff, persistently misunderstood Hawley's position. "Regardless of published directives," he declared in mid-November, "the Chief Surgeon is rather generally regarded as solely a staff officer of the S.O.S commander." At the ETO headquarters it was "common practice . . . to refer direct recommendations of the Chief Surgeon to his representative at ETO 'for remark and recommendation.'"[10]

On 14 November, therefore, Hawley proposed that he, as ETO chief surgeon, be moved to London and given his own staff to oversee medical operations, training, and preventive medicine. A separate SOS chief surgeon, with his own staff, Hawley suggested, should take charge of such theater-wide functions as hospital construction and administration, supply, personnel procurement, and medical records. Several ETO staff section heads, who themselves found the service chiefs' exile to Cheltenham an obstacle to business, endorsed Hawley's proposal. General Lee, however, vetoed it, arguing that the theater surgeon "can best perform his primary mission of coordination, supply and evacuation from HQ, SOS," while maintaining a London deputy of the "highest obtainable quality" for ETO planning and liaison. Lee on 30 November presented a reorganization plan of his own with the opposite objective to Hawley's. The SOS commander wanted to concentrate all but a few theater staff sections and all supply and administrative responsibilities in the Services of Supply. The theater staff, in turn, rejected this plan, insisting that theater headquarters had to retain certain administrative and logistics functions, especially in Great Britain, where clearly defined geographical combat and communications zones did not exist. With this stalemate General Order No. 19 remained in effect, and Hawley stayed at Cheltenham.[11]

Within the Services of Supply General Lee delegated operational responsibility to geographical base sections. On 20 July he designated the Northern Ireland Base Command (Provisional) as the Northern Ireland Base Section and ordered establishment of Eastern, Western, and Southern Base Sections. Each of these

[10] Memo, Hawley to Brig Gen Ray W. Barker, 14 Nov 42, box 1, Hawley Papers, MHI; Memo, Hawley to CEngr, CCWOff, CSigOff, COrdOff, and CQM, 10 Nov 42, file HD 024 ETO CS (Hawley Chron).

[11] Quotations from Memo, Lee to CG, ETOUSA, 10 Dec 42, file HD 320 ETO (Reorganization). See also Ruppenthal, *Logistical Support,* 1:159; Memo, Hawley to Barker, 14 Nov 42, box 1, Hawley Papers, MHI; Memos, Barker to CofS, ETO, 30 Nov 42, sub: Reorganization, Medical Services, and Col Ralph Pulsifer to CG, SOS, 22 Dec 42, file HD 320 ETO (Reorganization).

territorial divisions encompassed that portion of the United Kingdom implied by its name, and the boundaries of each roughly coincided with those of the British regional administrative and defense commands. Each base section commander, directly under General Lee, controlled all SOS troops, installations, and activities within his area; served as SOS point of contact for U.S. ground and air forces; and maintained liaison with British authorities.

Lee gave his base section commanders operational control over all general and station hospitals, medical supply depots, and SOS medical units and personnel within their boundaries. This authority brought the section commanders into conflict with Colonel Hawley, who was supposed to direct technical activities of SOS medical units through the base section staff surgeons. In practice, Hawley declared, "every instruction of a base section commander interferes with technical operations. No person can serve two masters; and with technical instructions requiring time and effort to follow coming from one source and other instruction from another . . . , confusion is inevitable." As American forces increased in size during the second half of 1942, Hawley complained that base section commanders were imposing inappropriate training and detrimental extra duties on his hospitals. He agitated continuously for centralized control by his office of all general hospitals, insisting that "when battle casualties begin to arrive, complete control . . . is imperative" to ensure rapid distribution of patients and efficient employment of staffs. General Lee rejected Hawley's pleas on this point, in accord with Army regulations that vested authority over general hospitals outside the United States in the geographical department or tactical commander. Instead, Lee urged Hawley and the other service chiefs to establish informal cooperation with the base sections. The conflict of authority remained unsettled in principle, with each new problem requiring another ad hoc compromise.[12]

The theater command structure established in mid-1942, especially that part of it affecting the medical and other technical services, thus had conflict of authority built into it. In spite of this fact the commanders involved made it work, more by informal cooperation than by following the organization chart. Colonel Hawley excelled at this kind of personal give-and-take. He collaborated effectively, if not cordially, with General Lee, although they had occasional disagreements. He later said of Lee, whom many in the European Theater regarded as arrogant and difficult to deal with, "He's nobody I'd ever want to go fishing with for a week. . . . But . . . I never went to . . . Lee with a problem that I didn't get complete support." Hawley established cordial relations with the other SOS special staff sections. "Whatever success we

[12] Quotations from Note, Hawley, 10 Oct 42, and Ltr, Hawley to AG, SOS, 15 Oct 42, both in file HD 024 ETO CS (Hawley Chron). See also Ruppenthal, *Logistical Support*, 1:84–87; Armfield, *Organization and Administration*, pp. 317–18. Authority over general hospitals is established in AR No. 40–600, 6 Oct 42, Medical Department: General Hospitals. Hawley had alled early for central control of general hospitals. See Larkey "Hist," ch. 2, p. 6. Base section commanders in their turn complained of interference by service chiefs. See Interv, ETO with Brig Gen Leroy P. Collins, CG, Northern Ireland Base Section (hereafter cited as Collins Interv), 8 Apr 44, CMH.

had as a staff," he recalled, "was due entirely to personalities. We were all friends. We all were mutually helpful." Eventually, he developed a similar rapport with the base section commanders. Wide acquaintanceship among the Engineer officers who held many key SOS positions—the result of a tour as surgeon of the Army Nicaragua canal survey in the 1930s—greatly assisted Hawley in all these relationships, as did his command and general staff training, which enabled him to discuss medical requirements in terms soldiers understood.[13]

Hawley set up his own line of communication to the Office of the Surgeon General, an action made necessary by the latter's submergence in the War Department Services of Supply and consequent removal from the main flow of reports from overseas theaters. In mid-June Hawley began a series of weekly letters to General Magee, describing his activities and calling attention to problems on which he needed help from Washington. "I feel that I can say more in a personal letter than I can in an official letter," he declared in the first of these communications, "and I shall be quite frank and chatty in my personal letters. . . ." Hawley more than kept this promise, for he continued these semiofficial reports until the end of the war in Europe.[14]

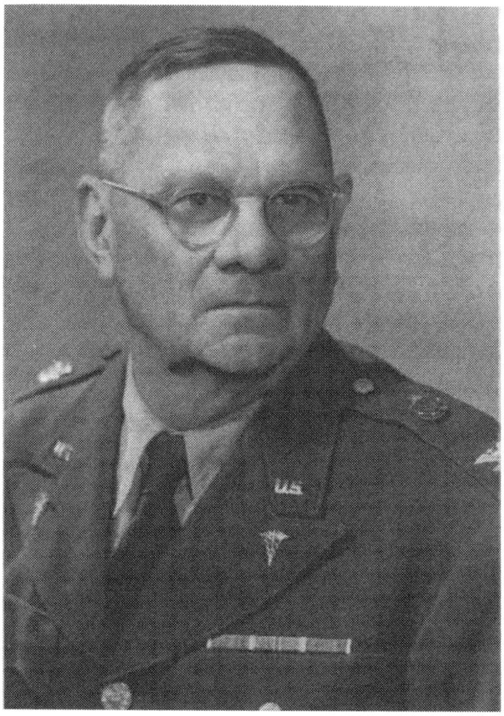

COL. JAMES C. KIMBROUGH
(1959 photograph)

Office Organization

As the European Theater of Operations and the Services of Supply began to function, the Office of the Chief Surgeon expanded and took more elaborate formal shape. A number of medical officers came over with Colonel Corby early in June and stayed on with Hawley, and the surgeon general sent a few others at Hawley's special request. By 20 July, when the office moved to Cheltenham, Hawley's staff had grown to

[13] Quotations from Hawley Interv, 1962, pp. 12-13 and 74-77, CMH. See also Ltr, Lee to Hawley, 16 Jun 44, box 2, Hawley Papers, MHI. Lee's "Reminiscences," passim, reveal his character.

[14] Quotations from Ltr, Hawley to TSG, 9 Jun 42, HD 024 ETO O/CS (Hawley-SGO Corresp). See also, in same file, Ltr, TSG to Hawley, 26 Jun 42, and MFR, Conference with Gen Hawley, 18 Apr 50, file HD 000.71, CMH. Armfield, *Organization and Administration,* p. 83, discusses the surgeon general's difficulty in obtaining up-to-date information on theater medical affairs.

twenty-two officers and fourteen enlisted men.[15]

These June and July reinforcements included some capable administrators. Col. Charles B. Spruit, MC, who headed a newly formed Operations Division and then represented Hawley on the theater staff in London, proved especially valuable. He had worked on war plans in the surgeon general's office and, like Hawley, had been through command and general staff training. The two men "thought alike" so that Hawley "was able to turn over to [Spruit] the planning and training." Although Spruit had an abrasive personality, Hawley considered him "good, . . . loyal [and] unquestionably the ablest officer I have." [16]

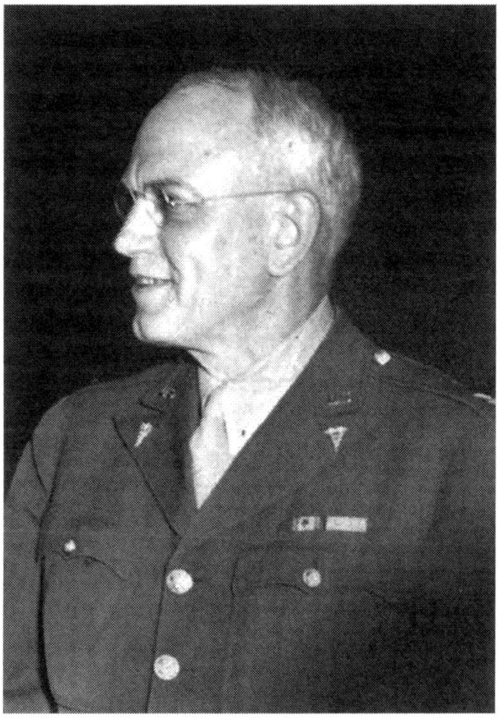

COL. CHARLES B. SPRUIT

In June Dr. Gordon of the Red Cross–Harvard Unit, now commissioned a lieutenant colonel, MC,[17] took charge of the Preventive Medicine Division, bringing to the staff his invaluable contacts with the British medical profession. Lt. Col. James C. Kimbrough, MC, whom Hawley described as a "tower of strength," arrived to organize the Professional Services Division; he headed a growing staff of medical and surgical consultants, all eminent in their fields. Lt. Col. Eli E. Brown, MC, displayed initial promise as head of the Hospitalization Division. In Medical Records Lt. Col. Joseph H. McNinch, MC, "worked into his job very quickly" so that the chief surgeon "stopped worrying about medical records." With these and other competent subordinates on hand, Hawley began to delegate much of the planning and administration he hitherto had had to do himself. One area that remained weak, however, was leadership in key functions, including supply, and some staff members were to prove unequal

[15] Larkey "Hist," ch. 3, pp. 7–8, 11–21, 52–53, apps. 2–7, and ch. 5, pp. 3–4.

[16] Quotations from Ltrs, Hawley to TSG, 17 Jul 42, and Hawley to Brig Gen Charles C. Hillman, 5 Feb 43, file HD 024 ETO O/CS (Hawley-SGO Corresp). See also Interv, OSG with Col C. B. Spruit, MC, 31 Oct 47, and MFR, Conference with Gen Hawley, 18 Apr 50, both in file HD 000.71, CMH; Hawley Interv, 1962, p. 15, CMH.

[17] Gordon's appointment ran into both military and academic seniority problems. Hawley at first wanted to commission him a colonel in recognition of his ability and unique relationship with the British; however, this would have made Gordon senior on the staff to Col. Elliott C. Cutler, who had been appointed ETO chief surgical consultant and was senior to Gordon on the Harvard faculty. Hence, Gordon had to come into the Army at the lower rank, with Hawley's promise of promotion later. See Ltrs, Hawley to TSG, 13 Jun 42, and TSG to Hawley, 27 Jun 42, file HD 024 ETO O/CS (Hawley-SGO Corresp).

to the steadily increasing demands of the BOLERO buildup.[18]

On 26 August, with his staff further enlarged to thirty-two officers, one warrant officer, and eighty-three enlisted men, Hawley issued a directive formally constituting eleven divisions in the chief surgeon's office and defining the responsibility of each (*Chart 2*). The Administration Division had charge of office routine and record-keeping. The Personnel Division dealt with promotions and reductions in rank, reclassified medical officers and enlisted people, requested individual orders, and drafted requisitions for additional manpower. The Operations Division, organized by Colonel Spruit and later headed by Lt. Col. James B. Mason, MC, oversaw medical unit allocations and movements; controlled SOS medical units not assigned to base sections; made medical operational plans; and supervised training. The Finance and Supply Division performed fiscal and accounting functions and coordinated receipt, storage, and issue of medical supplies. Colonel Gordon's Preventive Medicine Division looked after troop health, diet, and sanitation and maintained contact with British public health and preventive medicine agencies. The Hospitalization Division oversaw hospital construction and arranged for care of American troops in U.S. Army and British facilities; it supervised all but the professional aspects of hospital administration and coordinated medical evacuation. The Medical Records Division, besides preparing and collating reports and returns, made statistical analyses of theater medical experience. Kimbrough's Professional Services Division directed the activities of the medical and surgical consultants and kept in touch with British medical research and development. The Dental, Nursing, and Veterinary Divisions supervised the activities and training of the members of their respective corps and were responsible for liaison with their counterpart British organizations.

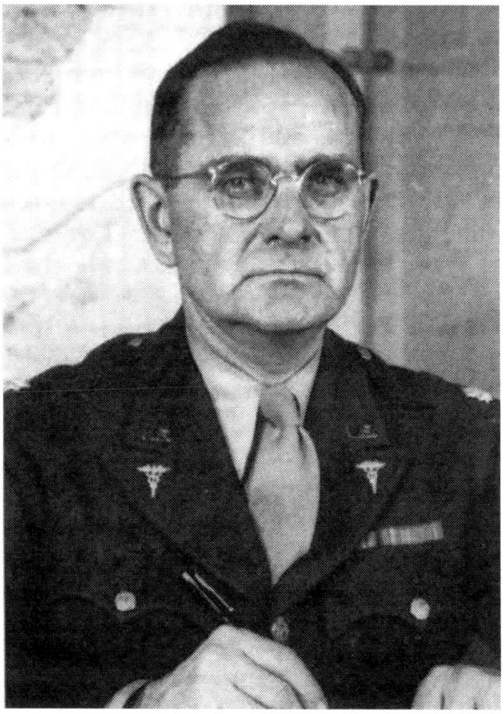

LT. COL. JAMES B. MASON

Colonel Hawley gave his division chiefs broad authority and responsibility and expected them to take initiative in their areas of activity. He encouraged his subordinates to consult directly with each other on the inevitable problems that cut across divi-

[18] For evaluations see Ltrs, Hawley to TSG, 1 Jul, 17 Jul, and 7 Aug 42, file HD 024 ETO O/CS (Hawley-Corresp).

CHART 2—ORGANIZATION OF THE OFFICE OF THE CHIEF SURGEON, ETOUSA–SOS, SEPTEMBER 1942

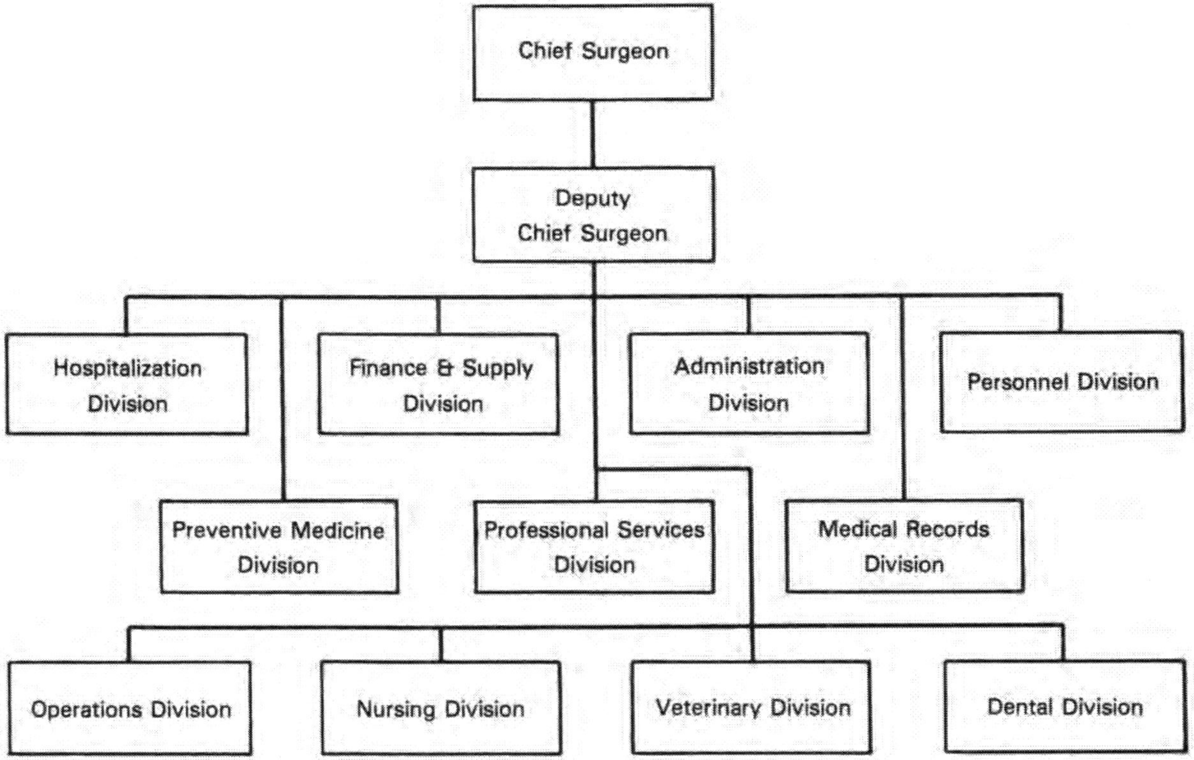

Source: Adapted by authors from Garand, Potter, and Vivette, "Medical Service in ETOUSA," ch. I, p. I–36.1, on file in CMH.

sion lines, "submitting to the Chief Surgeon for decision . . . cases in which the Chiefs concerned are unable to agree." He especially stressed the need for cooperation, declaring:

It is . . . fatal to attempt a military operation without complete cooperation between responsible officers. Although a cooperate and friendly spirit will not compensate for want of ability in an officer, inability to play in a team renders an officer useless, regardless of his other qualification. Each officer must study the individual characteristics of the other officers with whom he deals and adjust his approach accordingly. . . . Each officer must study his own peculiarities and curb such traits that interfere with his relations with his fellows. . . .[19]

The organization established in Hawley's 26 August memorandum remained stable in structure for the rest of the year, although some divisions underwent one or more changes of chief and all received driblets of additional personnel. Hawley himself received a brigadier general's star on 10 September. He needed both the additional staff and the rank, first to negotiate with the British on medical plans for BOLERO and then to cope with the demands of TORCH upon an inexperienced, undermanned, undersupplied medical service.

The Hospital Program

As BOLERO planning began, provision of hospitals for the million-man ETOUSA force claimed much of the chief surgeon's time and attention. This medical challenge had two parts. First, the army required a garrison medical establishment to care for its sick and injured during the buildup and waiting period before the invasion, as well as additional hospitals for Air Force battle casualties. Second, when the cross-Channel assault began, it would need almost as many hospitals again to accommodate the expected flood of wounded from the decisive—and hence undoubtedly the bloodiest—campaign of the war. All of these hospitals would have to be fitted into overcrowded Britain and, if possible, combined with the additional housing required for the American troops.

The exact number, size, and location of hospitals depended on the overall plans developed by the Washington and London BOLERO Combined Committees. The Washington committee, in consultation with ETO headquarters, determined the force structure and set movement schedules and shipping priorities. The London committee, consisting of representatives of ETOUSA and the British armed forces and civilian ministries, decided on ports of entry and troop billeting areas and arranged for housing, transportation, storage facilities, and hospitals. This committee reported to the administrative heads of the British armed forces and relied on the War Office and other ministries to implement its recommendations.

Working with the strength estimates and shipping schedules from the Washington committee, and on what little had been decided thus far about the tactics of ROUNDUP, the London Combined Committee between May and July 1942 developed the First and Second Key Plans for

[19] Memo No. 7, OofCS, HQ, SOS, 26 Aug 42, filed 519 Admin Med Hist (ETO), in Larkey "Hist," ch. 3, app. 19.

BOLERO. These plans were comprehensive programs, embodied in directives to British civilian and military agencies, for the reception of American troops and supplies and for the building of the British invasion base. The First Key Plan, issued on 31 May, and the Second Key Plan, issued on 25 July, differed in the troop numbers used as the basis for planning (1,049,000 versus 1,147,000) but were similar in assumptions and principles. Both plans assumed that in the cross-Channel invasion U.S. troops would constitute the Allied right wing and the British the left. Hence, the Americans, entering England through the west coast ports, would concentrate the bulk of their ground forces in southwestern England and eventually embark for the assault from ports in that region. Under the Key Plans, accordingly, the British Army was to turn over its Southern Command to the Americans, complete with all camps, hospitals, and supply depots. To accommodate the American ground troops in southern England, as well as the Air Force in the northeast, the British would construct additional facilities as required, using their own labor and both their own and American materials. Hospitals were to be a major element of this new construction.[20]

Colonel Hawley began his hospital planning before the formal establishment of the BOLERO committees. During late April Hawley, in consultation with the medical chiefs of the British Army, the Canadian Expeditionary Force, and the Emergency Medical Services, surveyed existing hospital facilities. The survey reaffirmed his earlier conclusion that U.S. forces in Great Britain would have to rely for hospitals primarily on new construction. He also evaluated a flood of offers of English country houses, whose owners wanted to turn them over to the Army for hospitals, either out of patriotism or to escape real estate taxes. Hawley disappointed most of these gentry. He rejected their mansions as too small or requiring too much alteration for efficient use.[21]

During May Hawley and his British colleagues reached a number of significant understandings. The British already had turned over two hospitals—those at Musgrave Park and Ebrington Barracks in Northern Ireland—to the U.S. Army and had agreed to turn over three more—the American Red Cross-Harvard Unit and the EMS plants at Oxford (the Churchill Hospital) and Mansfield. These facilities contained in all about 2,200 beds. On the eleventh the British Army promised to transfer all its Southern Command hospitals to the Americans—another 4,500 beds in units of 50 to 1,000. The Emergency Medical Services at the same time offered three more 600-bed hospitals, then under construction, at Odstock, Taunton, and Bristol. Hawley accepted all these facilities.

In a conference on 21 May Hawley, the USAFBI chief engineer, and representatives of the British Ministry of

[20] Ruppenthal, *Logistical Support*, 1:53–74, describes the general course of BOLERO planning.

[21] Ltr, Hawley to TSG, 29 Apr 42, file HD 024 ETO O/CS (Hawley-SGO Corresp); Hawley Interv, 1962, p. 25, CMH; Ltr, Hawley to Surg, HQ, Eighth Air Force, 28 Sep 42, file HD 024 ETO CS (Hawley Chron).

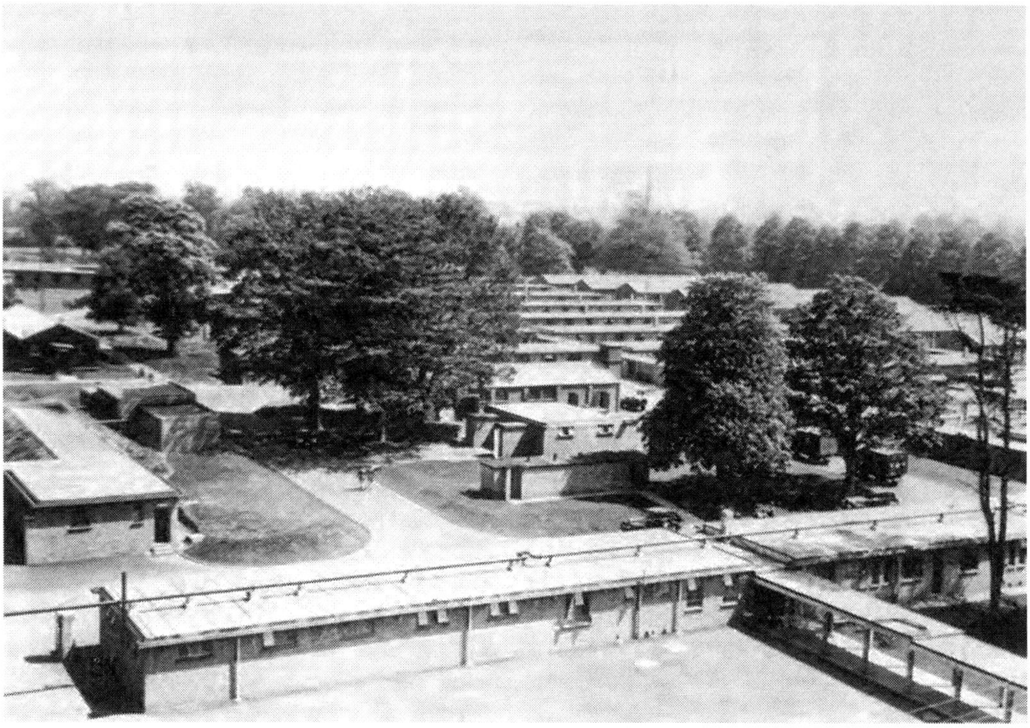

EMS HOSPITAL AT BRISTOL

Works decided to enlarge the five EMS hospitals earmarked for the Americans to 1,000 beds each. At the same time Hawley secured British concurrence on the nine proposed locations for new station hospitals, and he and the British established procedures for selecting additional sites. The Allies also agreed on the agencies and methods of BOLERO hospital construction. Hawley initially had wanted American hospitals built by U.S. Army Engineers following standard plans made by the surgeon general's office. In the face of limited transatlantic shipping for men and materiel, however, he accepted a plan under which British civilian contractors, employed by the Ministry of Works, would erect the plants using British designs and specifications modified to meet American requirements.[22]

On 27 May the London Combined Committee established the Provision of Medical Services Subcommittee to take charge of hospital planning. This action merely gave formal status to the consultations already under way between Hawley, the British military medical chiefs, and the EMS director—all members of the subcommittee. Later, representatives of the Canadian Army medical service and the

[22] Larkey "Hist," ch. 2, pp. 22–30, and ch. 7, pp. 2–3 and app. 1; Hawley Interv, 1962, p. 24, CMH.

Department of Health for Scotland joined the group.[23]

During the drafting of the First and Second Key Plans Hawley worked out the total number of hospital beds that would be needed to support both BOLERO and ROUNDUP. He based his estimate on U.S. Army experience in World War I and on British Army casualty rates in the interwar years and in the French, Norwegian, and North African fighting. Hawley assumed that before the invasion, the Army would have 2.25 sick and nonbattle injured per day for each 1,000 troops. Active operations would result in at least another 2.5 combat casualties per 1,000 men per day. Hawley then calculated the probable patient accumulation in hospitals under a 180-day theater evacuation policy and established his bed requirement as a percentage of total troop strength.

For the static preinvasion period Hawley asked for dispensary beds sufficient for 1 percent of the entire force and station hospital beds for 3 percent. On top of this, the Air Force should have beds for an additional 1.5 percent of its strength for its battle casualties. Black troops, whom Hawley expected to have a higher sick rate than whites, would need beds for an extra 2.5 percent of their total numbers. For ROUNDUP and the ensuing continental operations Hawley wanted beds for 10 percent of the number of men actually committed to combat. In all, he requested about 90,000 station and general hospital beds, about half of which—mostly in station hospitals—would be needed before the invasion.[24]

The Medical Services Subcommittee, after what Hawley described as "a lot of diplomacy," accepted his statement of requirements as the basis for planning. Disagreements developed, however, about ways and means. Hawley insisted, correctly, that the British were overestimating the bed capacity of the hospitals they were turning over and hence underestimating the amount of new building needed. The extent of new construction worried the British quartermaster general, who not only expressed concern at the cost in scarce funds, materials and labor but also urged more use of converted camps, requisitioned buildings, and tent hospitals. Hawley firmly rejected the latter two alternatives, but he decided that some troop housing, existing and to be built, could be adapted for hospitals after the units left for France.[25]

The medical annex of the Second Key Plan incorporated the agreement reached by Hawley and the British on

[23] Larkey "Hist," ch. 2, p. 25. Initial members of the subcommittee were: Maj. Gen. H. M. Gale, MGA Home Forces, Chairman (replaced in September by Maj. Gen. R. H. Lorie, MGA Home Forces); Surgeon Vice Admiral S. F. Dudley, MDG, Admiralty; Lt. Gen. A. Hood, DGAMS, War Office; Air Marshal Sir H. W. Whittingham, DGMS, Air Ministry; Brigadier W. Hartgill, DDG Operations, War Office; Prof. F. R. Fraser, DGEMS, Ministry of Health; and Col. P. R. Hawley, Chief Surgeon, HQ, USAFBI. At this time separate planning committees began work on medical aspects of SLEDGEHAMMER and ROUNDUP. This planning, in which Colonel Spruit was heavily involved, is covered in Chapter VI of this volume.

[24] Memos, Hawley, 1 Jun 42, sub: Hospitalization Required by USAFBI, and Hawley to Provision of Medical Services Subcommittee, 14 Jun 42, sub: Restatement of U.S. Requirements, in Larkey "Hist," ch. 2, apps. 3–4; Ltr, Hawley to TSG, 9 Jun 42, file HD 024 ETO O/CS (Hawley-SGO Corresp).

[25] Quotation from Ltr, Hawley to TSG, 9 Jun 42, file HD 024 ETO O/CS (Hawley-SGO Corresp). See also Larkey "Hist," ch. 2, pp. 26–36 and app. 4, and Memo, Hawley to CG, SOS, 20 Jan 43, in ibid., ch. 7, app. 1.

the number of hospital beds needed and the means of providing them (*Table 1*). Following Hawley's percentage-of-strength requirements, the Second Key Plan called for provision of 40,240 beds during the buildup to accommodate sick, nonbattle injured, and Air Force combat casualties. Roughly 12,000 of these beds were to be in enlarged former British Army and EMS hospitals; newly constructed beds in thirty-five 750-bed station hospitals and two 1,000-bed general hospitals would account for the rest. To support ROUNDUP, the Allies agreed to furnish 50,750 additional beds—18,000 of them in new general hospitals to be built before D-Day and the remainder after D-Day in vacated British militia camps and American hut cantonments. These installations would have structures for operating rooms, clinics, and laboratories added to them before the invasion so that they could be converted quickly into 750-bed station or 1,000-bed general hospitals.[26]

Separately from the BOLERO discussions, Hawley and Surgeon General Magee decided to use, as far as possible, only 750-bed station and 1,000-bed general hospitals in the United Kingdom. Hawley asked for inclusion of a few 250- and 500-bed station hospitals in the early troop shipments, to occupy small facilities taken over from the British or designed before BOLERO to serve the Air Force, but for the new plants he desired only the larger units.[27]

Selection of sites for station and general hospitals had begun before publication of the Second Key Plan in July and accelerated during the following month. For station hospitals Hawley, after obtaining troop locations from the ETO G–3, asked the British War Office for a site within 5 miles of each center of concentration. The War Office and the Ministry of Agriculture then chose the ground, usually in a park or estate to avoid building over farmland. By mid-August Hawley and the British had agreed on sites for thirty-three of the projected thirty-five station hospitals, most of them in southern England and East Anglia. Hawley wanted to group his general hospitals in centers of four or five units for greater efficiency. He allowed the British to determine locations for these centers so as to ensure adequate rail connections for hospital trains without disrupting overall traffic patterns. After consulting the railway authorities, the War Office placed the first three centers in the west of England—at Cirencester, Great Malvern, and Whitchurch.

Construction also got under way. By the end of July the War Office had given orders for all the required expansions of military and EMS plants and for one 750-bed and two 1,000-bed Nissen-hut installations. In addition, the British began building ten 1,250-man troop camps in Southern Command, designed for conversion into hospitals, and they made plans and preparations for altering a number of existing camps. During August the British promised to have the five EMS hospitals, each enlarged to 1,000 beds, ready for American occupancy between 1 October and 31

[26] Larkey "Hist," ch. 2, pp. 36–40, and ch. 7, app. 1.

[27] Ltr, Hawley to TSG, 6 Jul 42, file HD 024 ETO O/CS (Hawley-SGO Corresp).

TABLE 1—HOSPITAL BED REQUIREMENTS AND PROVISIONS, SECOND KEY PLAN, JULY 1942

Phase I (pre-ROUNDUP)		Phase II (ROUNDUP and post-ROUNDUP)	
Requirements		Requirements	
3% of 1,147,000 troops	34,410	10% of 770,000 troops [a]	77,000
1.5% of 195,000 AAF troops	2,925	3% of 377,000 troops [b]	11,310
2.5% of 100,000 blacks	2,500	2.5% of 100,000 blacks	2,500
	39,835		90,810
		Furnished pre-ROUNDUP	–40,240
		Additional needed	50,570
Provisions		Provisions	
Transferred British military hospitals	3,870	Conversion of existing barracks	25,000
Expansion of British military hospitals	1,170	Conversion of 1,250-man camps	7,500
Expansion of British hospitals	1,170	New general hospitals (1,000-bed)	18,070
Transferred EMS hospitals	2,900		50,570
Expansion of EMS hospitals	2,100		
Hospitals in Northern Ireland	1,950		
New 1,000-bed Nissen-hut hospitals (2)	2,000		
New 750-bed Nissen-hut hospitals (35)	26,250		
	40,240		

[a] For battle casualties of forces on the Continent.
[b] For nonbattle casualties of forces in the United Kingdom.
Source: Adapted by authors from Larkey "Hist," ch. 2, pp. 36–40.

December. The War Office ordered construction of fifteen general hospitals in groups of five at the three previously chosen locations. By the end of the month the British Army had evacuated twelve of its hospitals for turnover to the Americans.[28]

After the decision to attack Northwest Africa, the United States gradually scaled down its short-range BOLERO deployment objectives. In October, with TORCH preparations under way on both sides of the Atlantic, the War Department decided to base troop and supply shipments to Britain on a post-TORCH maximum strength there of only 427,000 men, which might be increased later. The authorities in Great Britain, nevertheless, at first tried to keep the full BOLERO construction program going. Around midmonth, in the face of the cutback in American deployment goals, General Lee and the British deputy quartermaster general (liaison), who represented the War Office, agreed to continue construction at the levels established in the First and Second Key Plans. This construction was primarily a British task in any event, and both sides assumed that the million-man buildup eventually would resume.

General Hawley, in accord with this approach, continued to press for his full requirement of over 40,000 pre-ROUNDUP and of nearly 51,000 post-ROUNDUP hospital beds. He increased

[28] Hospitalization Division, OofCSurg, HQ, ETOUSA, Annual Rpt, 1942; Larkey "Hist," ch. 2, pp. 38–44, and ch. 7, pp. 7–13; Hawley Interv, 1962, pp. 45–46, CMH; Ltr, Hawley to TSG, 15 Jun 42, file HD 024 ETO O/CS (Hawley-SGO Corresp).

his station hospital capacity request from 3 percent of strength to 4 percent, citing as justification the absence of convalescent facilities, troop overcrowding in camps and the concomitant higher sick rate, and the lack of hospital ships to carry out a 180-day theater evacuation policy. The London Combined Committee, in its initial revision of the Key Plans to take into account the slower U.S. buildup, reaffirmed Hawley's 90,000-bed hospital request.[29]

The demands of the North African expedition for shipping and supplies forced retreat from these ambitious intentions. On 19 November General Eisenhower, implementing a decision reached jointly with Marshall and Somervell, announced that the European Theater would use its men and materiel only for construction actually needed for the 427,000-man force. Construction by the British in excess of American requirements, he declared, must be accomplished with their own labor and materials, with no use of lend-lease materiel.

The London Combined Committee's Third Key Plan of that same day, while it incorporated Hawley's 4 percent-of-strength request for station hospitals, accordingly reduced the total construction program to 37,900 beds, including 5,000 for expected TORCH casualties. Final provision plans, issued on 3 January 1943, called for about 7,000 beds in British military and EMS hospitals, 19,000 in twenty-three new 750-bed station hospitals, 13,000 in twelve 1,000-bed general hospitals, and 2,000 in two converted militia camps. In these plans Hawley, at British insistence, included in his calculations the fact that, as built to British specifications, a 750-bed station hospital actually had a capacity of 834 beds while a 1,000-bed general hospital had room for 1,084. Hawley previously had rated the capacity of these plants strictly by the table-of-organization bed strength of the units slated to occupy them. Now he gave way to the British in order to obtain more beds for the same amount of construction and planned to reinforce units to operate the odd-size hospitals.[30]

In spite of these reductions in American goals, the British informally promised to keep on with the entire BOLERO hospital program. Their promises exceeded their performance. During the last months of 1942 hospital construction by the Ministry of Works fell steadily farther behind even the reduced schedule of the Third Key Plan. Not a single hospital promised for October or November came anywhere near completion during those months. The construction delays resulted in large part from unavoidable shortages of labor and material and from inclement weather, but British administrative sluggishness and lack of a sense of urgency also retarded progress. With troop transports in limited supply Hawley had to cut back shipment of hospital units because he had no buildings in which to put them, assuring the theater a unit shortage later on when the delayed plants were finished. Making

[29] Ruppenthal, *Logistical Support*, 1:89 and 104–06; Larkey "Hist," ch. 2, pp. 41–45.

[30] Ruppenthal, *Logistical Support*, 1:106–10; Larkey "Hist," ch. 2, pp. 45–48, and ch. 7, pp. 14–15; Ltr, Hawley to CG, SOS, ETO, 7 Dec 42, file HU 312 (Corresp File, Hospitalization Div, O/CS, ETO) 1942.

the situation still worse, changes in military plans forced the British Army to slow down the turnover of its hospitals.

Concerned about the delays, Hawley forced a confrontation with the Ministry of Works. On 22 October he asked for a special meeting of the Medical Services Subcommittee, which had discontinued regular sessions at the onset of TORCH preparations, to discuss hospitals. The subcommittee chairman, Maj. Gen. R. H. Lorie of the British Home Forces, evaded Hawley's request with a promise to refer the problem to the War Office. The chief surgeon persevered with a second—and, ultimately, a move convincing—request to General Lorie on 13 November. Emphasizing the disruptive effect of the delay on the entire American medical buildup, Hawley added a few words of polite blackmail when he reminded the chairman that

> above all else . . . the American people demand in war . . . that their soldiers be given superior medical service. No one thing can cause such a furor in the United States as the knowledge that adequate and proper hospital facilities are not being provided for their troops. Thus far, the status of provision of hospitals has been kept a confidential matter; but I am afraid that I shall not be able to conceal the situation much longer. Already certain news correspondents are inquiring when hospitals will be ready for U.S. troops.[31]

The subcommittee finally met on 25 November, with representatives of the Ministries of Works and Labor in attendance. Hawley expressed concern at the construction lag and asked for firm completion dates on which he could plan. The Ministry of Works representatives offered what Hawley called the "most amazing statement," that all projects were on schedule and those due for December were nearing completion. Hawley, who had visited the sites in question and obtained accurate assessments of progress—or the absence of it—from the local construction superintendents, quickly refuted this argument. The subcommittee in the end agreed in principle that "the demands at present submitted by Brigadier General Hawley must be met." It invited Hawley to prepare a new set of completion deadlines for the BOLERO Accommodations Subcommittee, which set construction priorities. Through this submission Hawley and the Ministry of Works negotiated a revised schedule, which Hawley accepted as "the best I could possibly get," although it was still far less than what he considered necessary. The Ministry of Works, however, failed to meet even these deadlines.[32]

By the end of 1942 four U.S. Army general hospitals, four station hospitals, and one evacuation hospital tem-

[31] Ltr, Hawley to Chairman, Provision of Medical Services Subcommittee, BOLERO Combined Committee, 13 Nov 42, file HD 024 ETO CS (Hawley Chron). The same file contains Hawley's request for 22 Oct 42. See also Memo, Hawley to CG, SOS, 20 Jan 43, in Larkey "Hist," ch. 7, app. 1.

[32] First and second quotations from BOLERO Combined Committee (London) Provision of Medical Services Subcommittee M.P.S. (42) 12th Meeting—25 Nov 42—Minutes of Meeting, and Memo, Hawley to CG, SOS, 20 Jan 43, both in Larkey "Hist," ch. 7, pp. 15–16 and app. 1. Third quotation from Memo, Hawley to CEngr, SOS, 7 Dec 42, file HD 024 ETO CS (Hawley Chron). See also, in same file, Ltr, Hawley to Chairman, Provision of Medical Services Subcommittee, BOLERO Combined Committee, 30 Nov 42.

porarily serving as a station hospital were in operation in the British Isles (*Map 2*). They occupied former British Army plants and fully or partially renovated EMS buildings. The 4,950 beds provided by these hospitals barely met the ordinary needs of the troops then in Great Britain. The Eighth Air Force, with four bombardment groups committed to combat, relied almost entirely on RAF and EMS hospitals to care for its wounded. Hawley declared of the first six months of the hospital construction effort: "The only thing that has prevented a terrible debacle is the modification of the BOLERO plan." [33]

Although they produced only limited immediate practical results, the planning and initial construction efforts of 1942 laid the foundation of the European Theater hospital program. Through close cooperation, Hawley and his British colleagues identified the general requirements for supporting BOLERO and ROUNDUP, as well as the provisions for meeting them; selected hospital locations; and settled on building types and construction procedures. The principles they successfully worked out would govern hospital construction when the BOLERO buildup resumed in full force.

Medical Manpower and Supplies

During the summer and autumn of 1942 the BOLERO buildup rapidly gathered momentum. American troop strength in the European Theater increased from about 55,000 at the end of June to a peak of over 233,000 in October. The 1st and 29th Infantry Divisions and the II Corps headquarters augmented the ground contingent. The Services of Supply expanded from 1,900 officers and men to 41,000, as engineer, quartermaster, motor transport, signal, ordnance, chemical warfare, and medical units arrived. The SOS reinforcements were needed to handle an increasing flow of incoming cargo—over 75,000 tons in July, 186,000 in August, 240,000 in September, and 143,000 in October.

The Eighth Air Force established itself in England and went into combat. In mid-June Maj. Gen. Carl Spaatz, the Eighth's commander, arrived with his headquarters and 11,000 ground and service troops. Transatlantic ferrying of bombers, fighters, and transport aircraft began later that month. On 17 August Eighth Air Force B–17's flew their first mission over Nazi-controlled Europe, striking railroad yards in occupied France. Other raids followed, 70- to 100-bomber attacks on transportation targets, airfields, and submarine bases in France and the Low Countries. Testing the Air Force tactic of daylight high-altitude precision bombing, the B–17 and B–24 crews met increasingly heavy German

[33] Quotation from Memo, Hawley, to CG, SOS, 20 Jan 43, in Larkey "Hist," ch. 7, app. 1. See also in ibid., pp. 18–19; and Mae Mills Link and Hubert A. Coleman, *Medical Support of the Army Air Forces in World War II* (hereafter cited as *AAF Medical Support*) (Washington, D.C.: Office of the Surgeon General, U.S. Air Force, 1955), pp. 543–45. The hospitals were: 2d General Hospital, Oxford, 1,000 beds; 30th General Hospital, Mansfield, 600 beds; 298th General Hospital, Bristol, 500 beds; 67th General Hospital, Taunton, 1,000 beds; 3d Station Hospital, Tidworth, 250 beds; 152d Station Hospital, Bath, 250 beds; 38th Station Hospital, Winchester, 250 beds; 10th Station Hospital, Belfast, Northern Ireland, 350 beds; and 2d Evacuation Hospital, Diddington, 750 beds.

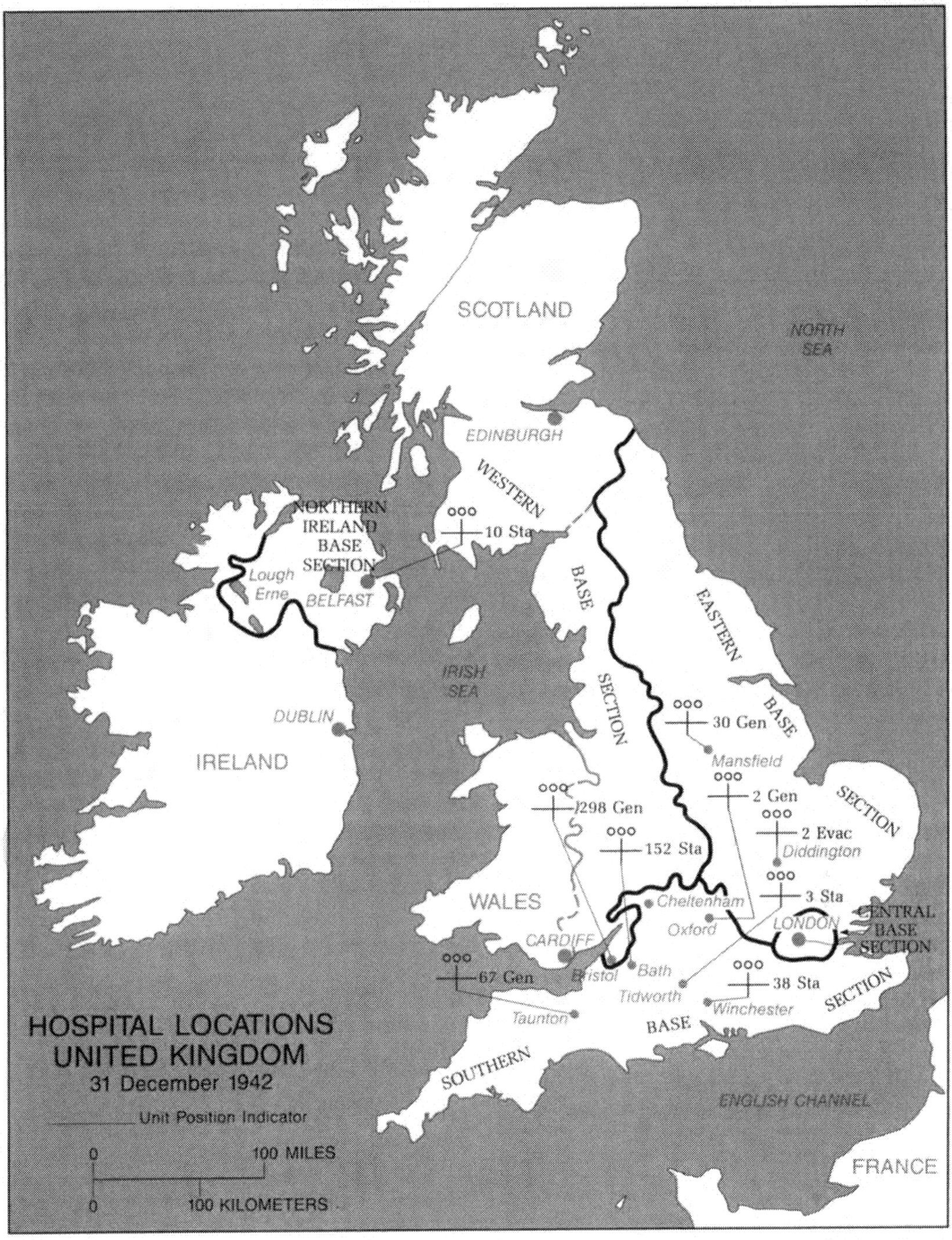

SCOTLAND
NORTH SEA
EDINBURGH
WESTERN
NORTHERN IRELAND BASE SECTION
10 Sta
Lough Erne
BELFAST
BASE
EASTERN
IRISH SEA
SECTION
30 Gen
BASE
DUBLIN
IRELAND
Mansfield
2 Gen
SECTION
298 Gen
2 Evac
152 Sta
Diddington
3 Sta
WALES
Cheltenham
CENTRAL BASE SECTION
Oxford
LONDON
CARDIFF
Bath
67 Gen
Bristol
38 Sta
Tidworth
Winchester
SECTION
Taunton
BASE
HOSPITAL LOCATIONS
UNITED KINGDOM
31 December 1942
SOUTHERN
Unit Position Indicator
ENGLISH CHANNEL
0
100 MILES
FRANCE
0
100 KILOMETERS

MAP 2

fighter and antiaircraft opposition. By the end of 1942 nearly 190 wounded officers and men of the Eighth Air Force had been evacuated to U.S. Army and RAF hospitals.[34]

As the buildup accelerated, the ETO medical service struggled to overcome a personnel shortage and a chaotic supply system. The growing responsibilities of the chief surgeon's office, combined with the requirement to staff the offices of four base section surgeons and to furnish medical planners and administrators for the Allied Force Headquarters, stretched General Hawley's small corps of capable assistants to the breaking point. Reinforcements were few. Unit medical officers were competent in their clinical fields, and the professional consultants who joined Hawley's staff were some of the best in their specialties. But most of these new arrivals lacked the experience and training for high-level planning and administration. Hawley sent repeated pleas to the surgeon general for more qualified administrators, only to be told that "we are scratching the bottom of the pot and . . . the pickings are very, very thin." Hawley had to place unqualified men in some key posts and hope they would learn on the job, and he threw ever more work on such stalwarts as Spruit, Kimbrough, Gordon, and McNinch. In September he resorted to borrowing medical officers from the V Corps for both his own and the base section surgeons offices. Later that same month he reported: "All my officers are working very hard and are accomplishing miracles. . . . If any one of my key officers—and every Regular I have is a key officer—goes sick on me, we are sunk." [35]

By the end of December Hawley's staff included fifty-one officers, fifty-six enlisted men, and sixty-two civilian employees, but the shortage of qualified administrators had not eased and some division chiefs had proven unequal to their expanding responsibilities. Hawley declared on 31 December: "I simply have to have fifteen good soldiers soon or this place is going to pot. . . . I'll stay in here and pitch but I've got to have someone who can bat in some runs." [36]

The offices of the base section surgeons, which were supposed to oversee most day-to-day medical service to the troops, suffered from even more serious manpower deficiencies in both quantity and quality. Hawley and the SOS G–1 agreed in August that each base section headquarters

[34] Ruppenthal, *Logistical Support*, 1:100 and 103; Maurice Matloff, *Strategic Planning for Coalition Warfare, 1943–1944*, United States Army in World War II (Washington, D.C.: Office of the Chief of Military History, Department of the Army, 1959), pp. 551–52; Craven and Cate, eds., *AAF*, 1:640–48; ibid., vol. 2, *Europe: TORCH to POINTBLANK, August 1942 to December 1943* (1949), pp. 209–60; Surg, Eighth Air Force, Annual Rpt, 1942, file HD 319 ETO (8thAForce) 1942.

[35] Quotations from Ltrs, TSG to Hawley, 24 Oct 42, and Hawley to TSG, 11 Sep 42, file HD 024 ETO O/SC (Hawley-SGO Corresp). In same file, see Ltrs, Hawley to TSG, 17 Jul and 7 Aug 42; Ltr, Hawley to Col George F. Lull, MC, 28 Aug 42; and Ltr, TSG to Hawley, 17 Jul 42. See also Ltrs, Hawley to Col Charles E. Brenn, MC, 4 and 18 Sep 42, and Memo, Hawley to Brig Gen Davis, 19 Oct 42, sub: Information for Gen Snyder, all in file HD 024 ETO CS (Hawley Chron); Hawley Interv, 1962, pp. 15 and 18, CMH; MFR, Conference with Gen Hawley, 18 Apr 50, and Memo, Graves H. Wilson to D. O. Wagner, 10 Nov 50, sub: Interview With Maj Gen James C. Magee, both in file HD 000.71, CMH.

[36] Quotation from Ltr, Hawley to TSG, 31 Dec 42, file HD 024 ETO O/CS (Hawley-SGO Corresp). See also "Med Svc Hist, 1942–43," p. 1, file HD 314.7-2 ETO.

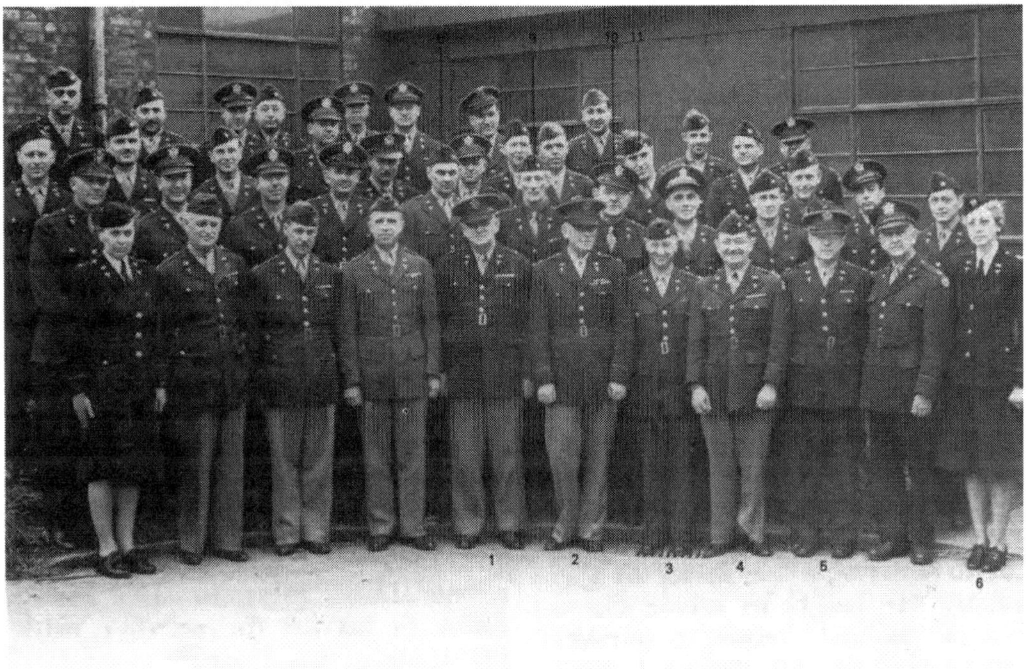

THEATER CHIEF SURGEON AND STAFF, CHELTENHAM, NOVEMBER 1942. *To oversee the medical requirements of BOLERO, General Hawley (1) relied on such able administrators as Col. Eli E. Brown (2), chief of the Hospitalization Division; Col. William S. Middleton (3), chief consultant in medicine; Colonel Mason (4), chief of the Operations Division; Lt. Col. John E. Gordon (5), chief of the Preventive Medicine Division; Capt. Margaret E. Aaron (6), chief of the Nursing Division; Lt. Col. Rex L. Diveley (7), senior consultant in orthopedic surgery; Col. Kimbrough (8), chief of the Professional Services Division; Col. Elliott C. Cutler (9), chief consultant in surgery; Lt. Col. Paul Padget (10), senior consultant in venereal disease; and Lt. Col. Joseph H. McNinch (11), chief of the Medical Records Division.*

should have at least ten medical officers. Until late in the year each actually had received no more than one or two—often borrowed from units—and a handful of enlisted men. Only the Southern Base Section reached the desired strength, with eleven medical officers and forty-one enlisted men at the end of 1942. The Western Base Section, responsible for the American ports of entry into the United Kingdom, finished the year with eight medical officers. The Eastern Base Section, which supported the Eighth Air Force, had only four. To furnish even this slim complement, Hawley perforce employed men of inferior ability, a number of whom had failed in other assignments. The Western Base Section surgeon, according to Hawley, "was recommended by his first C.O. for reclassification. I had to give him another job and Surgeon, Western Base Section, was the only place I could put him with his rank. . . . You can gauge the others by him—he is no worse than they." [37]

The original BOLERO plans called for an SOS medical establishment of about 55,000 people, in hospitals of various types, ambulance battalions, sanitary and depot companies, hospital train units, laboratories, and other organizations. These units were in addition to the medical detachments of ground, air, and service forces and to the attached medical formations of divisions, corps, and armies. Hawley had no direct responsibility for the deployment of the non-SOS medical troops, who moved with their parent commands, but he did have to secure shipping space for SOS medical units and to determine the order of their coming. He sought to assure the arrival of medical troops in numbers proportional to the overall buildup, but in the intense competition for scarce transport the Medical Department received low priority.[38]

Medical troops, accordingly, reached England at a slower rate than did those of the other SOS technical services. By late July the ETO medical service, with about 2,300 men on hand or scheduled for shipment, had fallen over 50 percent behind its projected strength for that point in the buildup, while the Services of Supply as a whole had exceeded its buildup target. Hawley attempted to limit his monthly requests for units to what he absolutely needed; he asked for hospitals, for example, only as buildings became ready for them to occupy. Nevertheless, he pointed out that "every requisition for medical troops has been cut—most of them severely." Compounding the shortage, many units arriving from the United States lacked organic medical detachments, forcing Hawley to request hundreds of nonattached doctors, nurses, and medical soldiers ("casuals") to staff temporary dispensaries, as well as to reinforce his own office and those of the base section surgeons. These requests, also, usually failed to survive the monthly battle for shipping allocations.[39]

By 1 September, when the European Theater and the Services of Supply as a whole had reached 15 percent of their planned troop strength, the ETO medical service had attained only 7 percent. Its buildup rate was the slowest of any of the technical services, lagging behind even Chemical Warfare. "In view of the fact that no chemicals have been used in this war," Hawley observed, "I cannot help considering this an eloquent fact." The autumn BOLERO force reduction, which cut planned SOS medical strength from 55,000 to 25,000, did nothing to speed the arrival of

[37] Quotation from Ltr, Hawley to TSG, 31 Dec 42; see Ltr, Hawley to Lull, 28 Aug 42. Both in file HD 024 ETO O/CS (Hawley-SGO Corresp). See also Surgs, Eastern, Western, and Southern Base Sections, Annual Rpts, 1942. Other base section staff sections had similar manpower shortages; see Collins Interv, 8 Apr 44, CMH.

[38] For the establishment of SOS medical troop strength, see Memos, Hawley to Plans Section, GS, 16 May 42, and Hawley to G–4, SOS, 21 Jul 42, in Larkey "Hist," ch. 4, apps. 1 and 3; Memo, Hawley to G–4, SOS, 29 Jul 42, sub: The Medical Situation, file 370 (Bible File of Troop Requirements, Early Planning).

[39] Quotation from Memo, Hawley to G–4, SOS, 29 Jul 42, sub: The Medical Situation, file 370 (Bible File of Troop Requirements, Early Planning). See also Larkey "Hist," ch. 4, pp. 22–25 and apps. 3–4; Ltrs, Hawley to TSG, 31 Jul and 7 Aug 42, file HD 024 ETO O/CS (Hawley-SGO Corresp); Memo, Hawley to Personnel Division, OofCS, SOS, 14 Sep 42, sub: Casuals in Troop Basis of Medical Service, SOS, file HD 024 ETO CS (Hawley Chron).

immediately needed units and troops. By early October the medical service "was relatively so weak that not only could it not furnish adequate support in any operation but it was unable to care for the routine sick and nonbattle injured in a static situation." In response to urgent pleas from General Hawley, who now faced the loss of some of his hospitals to TORCH, the ETO chief of staff on the twentieth called a special conference on medical personnel. The conferees, who included Hawley and the ETO deputy chief of staff and G-4, agreed that the medical manpower shortage was critical. As a result of the conference Hawley and the theater G-4, at the direction of the chief of staff, drew up plans for bringing the medical service to its proper relative strength by adding about 4,500 hospital beds and 3,500 people per month during November and December and 3,500 beds and 2,900 personnel a month during early 1943.[40]

This plan, while it also fell victim to the worldwide shortage of shipping, did result in deployment of more medical troops. By the end of November SOS medical strength had increased to over 7,000; enough additional reinforcements arrived in December to keep the service at 6,500 people, even after the departure of some hospitals for North Africa. Besides the one evacuation, four general, and four station hospitals in operation, SOS medical units in the United Kingdom at the end of 1942 included one general and five station hospitals, changing location or waiting for buildings; a medical supply depot company; two general dispensaries; and an auxiliary surgical group. The SOS medical buildup, nevertheless, still was proceeding more slowly than that of the organization as a whole. General Hawley estimated early in December that when the Services of Supply reached 59 percent of its projected strength, the medical service would have expanded to only 43 percent. "In the troops priorities now set up," he concluded, "the medical service becomes proportionately weaker and weaker until near the very end of the buildup, when it is suddenly built up to strength." [41]

From the start of the BOLERO buildup shortages and administrative deficiencies hampered medical supply efforts. Many of the administrative shortcomings originated in the Supply Division of General Hawley's office. Hawley, by his own admission, was "less familiar with the technique of medical supply than with other aspects of medical service" and "therefore, more dependent upon the

[40] As of 1 September, the Engineers were 86 percent of planned strength; the Signal Corps had reached 22 percent and Chemical Warfare 8.5 percent. Memos, Hawley to CG, SOS, 6 Oct 42 (source of quotation), and Hawley to G-4, ETO, 21 Oct 42, in Larkey "Hist," ch. 4, apps. 6 and 15 (see also pp. 10-11); Memos, Hawley to G-4, SOS, 10 Sep 42, and Hawley to Col Charles B. Spruit, MC, 11 Sep 42, file 370 (Bible File of Troop Requirements, Early Planning); Memos, Hawley to Gen Littlejohn, 21 Oct 42, and Hawley to G-4, ETO, 23 Oct 42, file HD 024 ETO CS (Hawley Chron).

[41] Quotation from Memo, Hawley to G-1, SOS, 2 Dec 42, sub: Troop Unit Priorities for SOS, file HD 024 ETO CS (Hawley Chron). In December another 3,400 medical personnel were in non-SOS units and detachments in Great Britain. See John H. McMinn and Max Levin, *Personnel in World War II*, Medical Department, United States Army in World War II (Washington, D.C.: Office of the Surgeon General, Department of the Army, 1963), pp. 308-09; "Med Svc Hist, 1942-43," p. 15, file HD 314.7-2 ETO.

advice and action of my supply chief than upon other chiefs of division." Unfortunately, throughout 1942, his Supply Division chiefs were among the least capable of his subordinates. Hawley's first supply officer, Col. Earle G. C. Standlee, MC, came highly recommended by the surgeon general, but in Hawley's opinion lacked the ability to do large-scale planning and could not make decisions rapidly. In August Hawley seized the opportunity to transfer Standlee to the Allied Force Headquarters, but the supply chief's successor, Lt. Col. Clarence E. Higbee, SC, was no improvement. Higbee, Hawley reported, "seems to understand how supplies get out of a depot, but hasn't the faintest idea of how they get in." The floundering division head "did the very best he could," but "the job was simply too big for him." Nevertheless, for lack of a better replacement, Hawley left Higbee in his post until late December.[42]

Neither Standlee nor Higbee had much manpower with which to work. Established in mid-June with only two officers and one enlisted man, the Supply Division included 8 officers and 13 enlisted men at the end of the year. In the field a detachment of the 8th Medical Depot Company arrived in May with the MAGNET troops and operated the medical section of the Belfast quartermaster depot. Aside from this element the only trained medical supply personnel in the European Theater were the 16 officers and 227 men of the 1st Medical Depot Company, which landed in England in July and eventually was spread among five separate depots. A second depot company reached England during the autumn, only to embark immediately for North Africa.[43]

All medical supplies from the United States destined for the European Theater passed through the New York Port of Embarkation. At New York a port medical supply officer, on the staff of the port commander, ensured that embarking medical detachments and units had full initial allowances of equipment and supplies. He and his staff, under direction from the Office of the Surgeon General, edited theater requisitions, after which the Port Overseas Supply Division called materiel forward from depots and arranged for its embarkation. Most resupply was supposed to go forward without theater requisition, in the form of medical maintenance units, each an assembly of basic supplies for 10,000 men for thirty days. On the basis of troop strength reports the port medical supply officer was responsible for requisitioning and shipping enough of these units to keep a prescribed number of days' supply always on hand in the theater.[44]

[42] Quotations from Ltrs, Hawley to Col Francis D. Tyng, MC, 7 Nov 42 and 3 Mar 43, file HD 024 ETO O/CS (Hawley-SCO Corresp). See also Ltr, Tyng to Hawley, 19 Jun 42, in same file, and Charles M. Wiltse, ed., *Medical Supply in World War II*, Medical Department, United States Army in World War II (Washington, D.C.: Office of the Surgeon General, Department of the Army, 1968), pp. 265–66.

[43] "Med Svc Hist, 1942–43," p. 5, file HD 314.7-2 ETO. The 1st Medical Depot Company was organized as a tactical unit but had to be used to operate base depots. See Ltr, Tyng to Hawley, 19 Jun 42, file HD 024 ETO O/CS (Hawley-SGO Corresp).

[44] To handle the expected huge volume of wartime supplies, the War Department in January 1942

Continued

Throughout 1942 the Port of Embarkation had only scarce medical supplies upon which to draw. The Army Medical Department possessed few reserves of the 5,000 or so items that it procured and issued. Its contractors, who had to compete with other vital industries for scarce raw materials, could not quickly fill huge war orders and often fell seven to nine months behind their delivery schedules. Indispensable items, such as surgical instruments, had been imported before the war from Germany and occupied Europe; American efforts to start domestic production took time to yield results. The Medical Department had to share what stocks were available with the voracious lend-lease program, the demands of which, given top priority by presidential directive, steadily increased. In mid-June Col. Francis C. Tyng, MC, chief of the Finance and Supply Division, Office of the Surgeon General, informed Hawley: "We have a daily shortage of some 2,000 items at all times in our depots." The Medical Department apportioned these shortages among the United States and overseas theaters by cutting all requisitions and allowances to a minimum.[45]

Availability of supplies did not guarantee their orderly arrival in the theaters, as the Medical Department learned when it attempted to provide the European Theater with complete hospital assemblies. Each deploying hospital was supposed to embark with a full allowance of furniture, instruments, and medicines; and the Medical Department sent additional outfits, tailored to various hospital types and sizes, to England in advance of units to establish a reserve. Few assemblies, however, left New York all at the same time on one vessel. For that to occur, shipments from medical and other depots throughout the eastern United States had to reach the port within at most a few days of each other. Inevitably, some materiel failed to appear on schedule. The port authorities, rather than delay a convoy, shipped out whatever partial assemblies were on hand. Making matters worse, inexperienced packers often failed to mark properly the crates belonging to a single assembly so that collecting the materiel and dispatching it to its proper destination in Great Britain were all but impossible. By early November ETO depots contained partial assemblies for one surgical, nineteen station, eleven general, and eight evacuation hospitals. To equip any one unit, the depots had to take apart two or three outfits. "Obviously," Hawley complained, "it is much better to get a few units complete than to get parts of many." [46] But the requirements for rapid port clearance and convoy movement took

had decentralized most overseas supply operations to a designated embarkation port for each theater, that for the European Theater being New York. See Ruppenthal, *Logistical Support,* 1:92–94. A medical maintenance unit contained 700–900 items, depending on the theater; weighed 15 tons; occupied 1,500 cubic feet of space; and was worth about $10,000. See Wiltse, ed., *Medical Supply,* pp. 146–47 (also pp. 143–46 and 148–53).

[45] Quotation from Ltr, Tyng to Hawley, 19 Jun 42, file HD 024 ETO O/CS (Hawley-SGO Corresp). See also Wiltse, ed., *Medical Supply,* p. 15.

[46] Quotation from Ltr, Hawley to Brig Gen W. M. Goodman, 7 Oct 42, file HD 024 ETO CS (Hawley

Continued

precedence over Medical Department convenience.

The buildup of theater supply reserves was the subject of constant disagreements between Hawley's office and that of the surgeon general. Due to confusion on the part of both Hawley and his Supply Division chiefs, the theater repeatedly sent large requisitions to the Port of New York for reserve supplies. The surgeon general's office, trying to husband scarce materiel, after review disallowed most of these requisitions as duplicating both initial unit allowances and the automatic resupply contained in the medical maintenance units. Hawley, in turn, complained that the maintenance units, which were not designed for any particular theater, failed to meet all his needs and at any event were not arriving on schedule.[47]

For the ETO medical service, as for the rest of the Services of Supply, industrialized Great Britain was a logical alternative supply source, especially as British support could reduce the burden on scarce transatlantic shipping and give the U.S. industry time to mobilize. To obtain British medical supplies, Hawley's Supply Division at Cheltenham worked through the SOS general purchasing agent, who had opened an office in London in May. The medical procurement officer on the purchasing agent's staff, Lt. Col. George W. Perkins, Chemical Warfare Service, transmitted specific ETO medical requests to the purchasing agent. That official then passed them to the British Ministry of Supply, which arranged for manufacture or purchase of the items under a reciprocal aid program known as reverse lend-lease.[48]

Procurement from the British had problems and uncertainties of its own. The British, early in the BOLERO planning, agreed to provide most nonmedical equipment for the hospitals they were to build for the Americans. Implementation of this arrangement went smoothly, aside from the overall construction delays, but unit medical equipment and medical resupply proved more difficult to secure. The British themselves were short of vital items and always had imported other key pieces of equipment, for example, X-ray tubes. They were reluctant to turn over any of their own large reserve medical stocks, which consisted in good part of lend-lease supplies, and instead preferred to manufacture new items for the Americans. The British, accordingly, while promising to meet all

Chron). See Memo, Edward Reynolds to Maj Gen LeRoy Lutes, 8 Dec 42, sub: Shipments of Incomplete Hospital Assemblages to England and Delays in Shipment of Maintenance Medical Supplies, file HD 024 ETO O/CS (Hawley-SGO Corresp). In same file, see also Ltrs, Tyng to Hawley, 18 Oct 42, and Hawley to Tyng, 7 Nov 42.

[47] Ltrs, Tyng to Hawley, 19 Jun and 18 Oct, Hawley to TSG, 31 Jul 42, and Hawley to Tyng, 7 Nov 42; Memo, Reynolds to Lutes, 8 Dec 42, sub: Shipments of Incomplete Hospital Assemblages to England and Delays in Shipment of Maintenance Medical Supplies. All in file HD 024 ETO O/CS (Hawley-SGO Corresp). See also Memo, Hawley to Maj Gen Styer, 10 Sep 42, and Ltr, Hawley to TSG, 3 Nov 42, sub: Medical Supply, both in file HD 024 ETO CS (Hawley Chron).

[48] Perkins, a pharmaceutical company executive in civilian life, initially was a member of the SOS Procurement Division. In August he was transferred to Hawley's staff, but he continued to serve as liaison officer between the chief surgeon and the general purchasing agent. See "Med Svc Hist," 1942–43, p. 56, file HD 314.7-2 ETO; Wiltse, ed., *Medical Supply*, pp. 267–68.

their Allies' needs, requested large-scale orders far in advance of the desired delivery dates, to give their plants time to plan production and tool up. Colonel Perkins had difficulty formulating such orders, as he could not obtain reliable early information on requirements from Standlee and Higbee. Changes in buildup plans forced frequent revision of what estimates he did receive. Perkins also discovered that the Americans and British used different names for many of the same items; the resulting breakdown of communication made it difficult to determine exactly what American requirements the British could fill. In an effort to resolve this problem, General Hawley put his professional consultants to work on a catalog of equivalent British and American medicines and equipment, but this catalog was not available during most of 1942.

In spite of these difficulties, the SOS Procurement Division between June and October placed several large orders for British medical supplies, including complete hospital assemblies. Colonel Perkins, whom Hawley considered "a fine gentleman and . . . unusually capable," combined tact with firmness in moving the British from general promises to particular commitments. He also ferreted out untapped commercial reserves of operating room furniture, surgical instruments, and other needed materiel. During the last months of 1942 a growing amount of British supplies flowed into American depots, in time to be of indispensable help in outfitting the TORCH forces. Even with the initial delays British medical supply deliveries during the last half of 1942 amounted to 84,000 ships' tons, far exceeding the 28,000 tons received from the United States. At the beginning of 1943 Hawley expressed confidence that he could obtain almost 90 percent of his hospital equipment and general medical supplies from his Allies—nearly everything, in fact, except field chests and other articles for mobile units. Nevertheless, due to the slow start and uncertain reliability of local procurement, the chief surgeon's Supply Division customarily sent duplicate requisitions to the United States for everything it ordered from the British, intending to cancel these requisitions if the British delivered. This practice only compounded the resupply misunderstandings between Hawley's office and that of the surgeon general.[49]

Whether American or British in origin, medical supplies, once procured, had to run a gauntlet of obstacles before reaching the troops who needed them. During the summer and early autumn the flood of BOLERO and TORCH cargo swamped the already heavily taxed western British ports through which most American goods arrived. Shipments were split up during unloading and some items smashed by unskilled stevedores. Much materiel from the United States came without bills of lading and in containers wrongly labeled, if labeled at all, and never reached the depots for which it was intended. As a result,

[49] "Med Svc Hist, 1942–43," pp. 56–58, file HD 314.7–2 ETO; Wiltse, ed., *Medical Supply*, pp. 268–70; Larkey "Hist," ch. 5, pp. 6–11. See also Ltrs, Hawley to TSG, 9 Jun 42, 6 Jul 42, and 3 Mar 43; Ltr, Hawley to Tyng, 7 Nov 42; Memo, Col Elliott C. Cutler, MC, to TSG, 26 Nov 42; Ltr, Hawley to General Purchasing Agent, ETOUSA, 15 Oct 42; Note, Hawley, 6 Nov 42. All in file HD 024 ETO CS (Hawley Chron).

General Hawley complained continually of the nonarrival of promised supplies, while the surgeon general's office and the Port of New York claimed that the stores had been shipped. British medical supplies, sent directly from a factory or warehouse to a particular depot, more often reached their intended destinations; however, due to the terminological confusion, depot staffs often failed to issue them, out of ignorance of what requirements the items could fill.

The burden of distributing supplies fell upon the 1st Medical Depot Company, which by early September was operating medical sections of five Army general depots. The company augmented its overstretched manpower with unattached (and usually untrained in supply) officers and men and eventually with British civilian employees. Its depot medical sections labored heroically to put together hospital assemblies, to sort and store supplies, and to make issues to units in their geographical areas. But inexperienced personnel and inadequate facilities hampered them, as did the failure of the Supply Division to establish a uniform inventory and stock control system.[50]

Especially as it struggled to meet the supply demands of TORCH, the European Theater medical service lived from hand to mouth, with shortages and uncertainty the rule. Hawley reported in September: "We have no way of knowing how many medical maintenance units have been shipped; but the number that has arrived is far too little for actual maintenance, not to speak of building up the prescribed reserve." Hospitals and other organizations went from depot to depot seeking supplies and equipment and usually not finding them, either because of shortages or because of the lack of reliable inventories. At least one medical officer gave up on the Army system and ordered some urgently needed items from the Red Cross without even attempting to obtain them through the ETO chief surgeon. This action drew a stinging rebuke from Hawley, who called it "the worst outrage that has been perpetrated in ETOUSA." At about the same time the chief surgeon informed the surgeon general: "The medical supply problem in this theater has been acute since 1 February 1942 and is now becoming critical." [51]

As the year ended, the first influx of British supplies into the depots enabled the medical service to meet the most pressing demands. On both sides of the Atlantic, efforts got under way to improve the supply systems. During November and December representatives of Surgeon General

[50] The five depots were located at Thatcham (G-45), Burton-on-Trent (G-20), Bristol (G-35), Liverpool (G-14), and Taunton (G-50). General depots, administered by the Quartermaster Corps, all had the "G" prefix. See Wiltse, ed., *Medical Supply*, pp. 270-74; Larkey "Hist," ch. 5, pp. 5-6 and 25-27; Ltrs, Tyng to Hawley, 18 Oct 42, and Hawley to Tyng, 7 Nov 42, filed HD 024 ETO O/CS (Hawley-SGO Corresp); Memo, Hawley to G-4, ETO, 16 Oct 42, file HD 024 ETO CS (Hawley Chron). For a description of overall ETO supply problems during this period, see Ruppenthal, *Logistical Support*, 1:91-96.

[51] First quotation from Memo, Hawley to Styer, 10 Sep 42. Second quotation from Ltr, Hawley to Surg, Northern Ireland Base Section, 6 Nov 42. Third quotation from Ltr, Hawley to TSG, 3 Nov 42, sub: Medical Supply. All in file HD 024 ETO CS (Hawley Chron). See also Larkey "Hist," ch. 5, pp. 26-27.

Magee worked out with the New York port commander a new method for shipping hospital assemblies in more nearly complete condition. In response to Hawley's reports that the medical maintenance unit did not fully meet ETO resupply requirements, the surgeon general's office arranged for the dispatch of supplementary materiel. Surgeon General Magee began a search for a better qualified supply officer for Hawley. The chief surgeon himself, in late December, replaced Higbee with Lt. Col. Howard Hogan, MC, an officer already in the European Theater. Hogan, who had previous though brief experience as a medical procurement officer, showed early signs of being more effective than his predecessors. As a result of Hogan's efforts, Hawley reported early in 1943 that

> the supply situation is greatly improved. We know what we have in depots (at least I am given figures which are said to be correct). Our units are getting medical supplies promptly. Hospitals are being equipped without delay as fast as buildings become available. Local procurement, while not completely satisfactory, is very much improved and British supplies are rolling into our depots by the car load.

"Yet," he concluded, "I am far from being completely happy with the situation." Hawley's unhappiness with his medical supply service was to continue for another year.[52]

Supporting TORCH

As the ETO medical service struggled with its personnel shortage and supply problems, it also had to furnish manpower and materiel for the invasion of North Africa. General Eisenhower and his AFHQ staff began planning for TORCH early in August, but Anglo-American disagreements over the timing, number and location of landings delayed until September publication of the overall concept of operations. Under the final plan an all-American Western Task Force, organized and equipped in the United States, was to assault Casablanca on the Atlantic coast of Morocco on or about 8 November. Simultaneously, the Anglo-American Center and Eastern Task Forces, fitted out in England, would strike from the Mediterranean respectively at Oran and Algiers. The Center and Eastern Task Forces were to draw logistics support from the United Kingdom until the Allies consolidated their position; then support responsibility for all three task forces would shift to the United States.

During September and October, under general guidance from the Allied Force Headquarters, the task forces completed their own tactical and logistics planning. In Great Britain embarkation of troops and stores of the Center and Eastern Task Forces began late in September. The loaded transports assembled in the

[52] Ltr, Hawley to Tyng, 3 Mar 43, and Memo, Reynolds to Lutes, 8 Dec 42, sub: Shipments of Incomplete Hospital Assemblages to England and Delays in Shipment of Maintenance Medical Supplies, both in file HD 024 ETO O/CS (Hawley-SGO Corresp); Memo, Brig Gen R. M. Littlejohn, QMC, to Lee, 4 Dec 42, sub: Maintenance Stocks of Medical Supplies, and Ltr, Hawley to TSG, 19 Dec 42, sub: Maintenance Stocks of Medical Supplies, both in file HD 024 ETO CS (Hawley Chron). Hogan, who relieved Perkins in Procurement on 20 November, previously had been a special assistant to the chief of Supply in the surgeon general's office. See Name-Rank file, CMH.

Firth of Clyde and, after a final landing rehearsal off the Scottish coast, departed for the Mediterranean on 22 and 26 October. On 8 November the landings took place on schedule. Follow-up convoys left England on the eighth, eleventh, and twenty-first.[53]

This simply described sequence of plans and preparations was a trying time for the ETO medical service. General Hawley, although responsible for furnishing troops and supplies, had no direct role in medical planning for the 40,800-man Center Task Force, the logistical support of which was the primary task of ETOUSA.[54] Instead, the Allied Force Headquarters, with Colonel Corby acting as deputy to a British chief surgeon, and the U.S. II Corps, of which Col. Richard T. Arnest, MC, was surgeon, prepared the plans with little coordination with ETOUSA and even less with the other task forces. Delay in completing the overall Allied operation plan further confused matters, because the task force had to start planning without a final directive, a procedure which led to repeated last-minute changes. The Allied Force Headquarters did not issue its logistics plan for the whole operation until December. Until then Hawley had to proceed without definite answers to such vital questions as the duration and extent of ETO responsibility for care of North African casualties. Hawley eventually lost patience with the chaotic procedures, as revealed in his 11 December letter to the surgeon general:

> I watched the muddled medical planning until I could stand it no longer and then went to the Chief of Staff, ETO and told him that the stage was all set for the biggest medical scandal since the Spanish-American War. That jolted them a little, and General Eisenhower told me to step in and straighten things out. I did, but within a week things were right back to where they were—each separate task force doing its own planning without the least coordination. . . .[55]

The theater Services of Supply had to provide hospitals and other medical units, primarily for the Center Task Force, as directed by the Allied Force Headquarters. While meeting these requirements, Hawley struggled successfully to retain his important operating units. An early AFHQ troop list, for instance, included the 3d and 10th Station Hospitals, both full of patients, and a detachment of the overextended 1st Medical Depot Company. The chief surgeon secured deletion of these organizations and their replacement with others due in from the United States. By the end of the year the Services of Supply had given up to TORCH five station and two general hospitals and a medical supply depot company. In addition, a medical regiment, a medical battalion,

---

[53] TORCH plans and preparations are described in Matloff and Snell, *Strategic Planning*, pp. 286–93 and 315–516; George F. Howe, *Northwest Africa: Seizing the Initiative in the West*, United States Army in World War II (Washington, D.C.: Office of the Chief of Military History, Department of the Army, 1957), pp. 46–47, 70–72, app. A.

[54] The Eastern Task Force, British in composition except for two American regimental combat teams, received medical and other logistical support almost entirely from the British Army.

[55] Quotation from Ltr, Hawley to Hillman, 11 Dec 42, file HD 024 ETO O/CS (Hawley-SGO Corresp). Wiltse, *Mediterranean*, pp. 105–08, summarizes TORCH medical planning. See also Howe, *Northwest Africa*, pp. 32–33 and 63–67; MFR, McNinch and Lewison, 24 May 49, sub: Interview With Col James B. Mason, MC (Ret.) file HD 000.71, CMH.

and one surgical and three evacuation hospitals passed through the United Kingdom on their way to North Africa. The II Corps, the 1st Armored Division, and the 1st and 34th Infantry Divisions took away their own organic medical units and detachments. From his own office Hawley lost seven officers and eighteen enlisted men; SOS and non-SOS medical units that stayed in Great Britain also surrendered personnel to fill up TORCH organizations. In spite of these losses increased arrivals from the United States kept total SOS medical strength at between 6,000 and 6,500 through early 1943; nevertheless, the departure of experienced key people and temporary personnel shortages hindered the work of hospitals and other units.[56]

The supply demands of TORCH on the ETO medical service were more extensive and crippling than those for personnel. The Services of Supply was required to equip all North Africa-bound ETO units and medical detachments, as well as furnish a sixty-day reserve of supplies. Difficulties abounded. Many hospital and other units designated for TORCH arrived in Great Britain with 25 percent or less of their basic allowances, a fact of which Hawley received no advance warning. As each command tried to remedy its own shortages, requisitions poured into the chief surgeon's office from a variety of sources. At one point the Supply Division was receiving requisitions, many of them duplicates, from three separate TORCH headquarters—AFHQ, the II Corps, and the Twelfth Air Force (which was being formed out of the Eighth for North African service). Hawley, lacking authority to coordinate TORCH supply, could do no more than suggest that all commands channel their requisitions through Colonel Corby at the Allied Force Headquarters "so that he may detect these duplications and establish appropriate priorities." Units at times made almost impossible demands. The 16th Medical Regiment, alerted on 7 October for embarkation in a November convoy, failed to requisition needed equipment until 1 November and then complained of delays in delivery.[57]

In an attempt to coordinate TORCH supply, the theater G-4 set up a committee of representatives from each of the technical services. Maj. Clark B. Meador, MC, the most active ETO medical service member of this committee, "practically unaided, undertook the whole calculation of medical requirements, of shipping requirements, of phasing of supply and the checking of unit shortages against T/E allowances." Meador formed special teams to inspect all medical units designated for TORCH and determine exactly what they had and what they needed. Because much materiel for filling shortages would come

[56] Memo, Hawley to Larkin, 7 Sep 42, in Larkey "Hist," ch. 4, app. 5 (see also ch. 4, pp. 4, 8, 11, and app. 7; and ch. 5, p. 35); Ltr. Hawley to Col J. F. Corby, MC, 6 Oct 42, box 2, Hawley Papers, MHI; "Med Svc Hist, 1942-43," p. 53, HD 314.7-2 ETO; Administration Division, OofCSurg, HQ, ETOUSA, Annual Rpt, 1942, p. 6

[57] Ltrs, Hawley to Col A. L. Hamblen, 26 Sep 42, and Hawley to TSG, 3 Nov 42, sub: Medical Supply; Memo, Hawley to CO, 16th Medical Regt, 4 Nov 42, sub: Requisition No. MR-114-3(F); and Ltr, Hawley to Corby, 5 Nov 42. All in file 024 ETO CS (Hawley Chron). See also Wiltse, ed., *Medical Supply*, pp. 204-05.

from the British and no catalog of Anglo-American equivalents and substitutes yet was available, Meador improvised his own. Through his efforts and those of others, the medical service managed to outfit the units embarking for TORCH. Equipment for some organizations arrived in time from the United States. For others, the medical service transferred articles from non-TORCH units or used British supplies.[58]

To assemble equipment for the eleven hospitals dispatched from Britain to North Africa, the depot medical sections broke up most of the thirty-odd partial outfits that had arrived from the United States and, where necessary, added British materiel. Until TORCH preparations began, only the medical section of Depot G–45 at Thatcham had assembled hospitals. As demands increased and time ran short, the Supply Division shifted some assembly work to the other four depot medical sections, which until then had only stored and issued supplies. The short-handed, inexperienced staffs learned rapidly on the job. A warrant officer at Depot G–35 in Bristol, tasked with putting together a 1,000-bed general, a 750-bed evacuation, and a 250-bed station hospital, recalled: "The only things I had to help me was one Basic Equipment List and a prayer. . . . I needed both of them, as no one in the Medical Section at that time had any idea of the procedure used in assembling a hospital, and no one even knew what an assembled hospital looked like." [59]

In the course of mounting TORCH the ETO medical service assembled and shipped five station, three evacuation, one surgical, and two general hospitals. It completed the equipment of all embarking organizations and sent out twenty-two medical maintenance units. Hawley reported: "We . . . got the North Africa units out fully equipped and, in that show, were probably the best of the services." The cost to the European Theater, however, was substantial. TORCH stripped the depots of supplies and left many medical units short of equipment. Replenishment was slow in coming, as the North African campaign received priority in shipping. Viewing the aftermath, Hawley declared: "The mess that is left will take months to straighten out." His chief of Preventive Medicine, Colonel Gordon, observed that the theater "had much the appearance of a plucked fowl. . . ." [60]

The shift of forces and attention to North Africa reduced the European Theater of Operations temporarily to a backwater and made uncertain the

[58] Quotation from Memo, Hawley to CG, ETOUSA, 11 May 44, sub: Recommendation for the Award of the Legion of Merit, file HD 024 ETO CS (Hawley Chron). See also Memos, Hawley to CofS, SOS, 14 Sep 42, and Hawley to Lee, 19 Sep 42, in same file, and Wiltse, ed., *Medical Supply*, pp. 266–67.

[59] WO(jg) Lewis H. Williams is quoted in Wiltse, ed., *Medical Supply*, p. 274. See Larkey "Hist," ch. 5, pp. 35–37; Memo, Hawley to Lt Col C. E. Higbee, SC, 9 Oct 42, file HD 024 ETO CS (Hawley Chron); Ltr, Hawley to Tyng, 7 Nov 42, file HD 024 ETO O/CS (Hawley-SGO Corresp).

[60] First and second quotation from Ltrs, Hawley to Tyng, 7 Nov 42, and Hawley to Hillman, 5 Feb 43, file HD 024 ETO O/CS (Hawley-SGO Corresp). Third quotation from John E. Gordon, "History of Preventive Medicine in the European Theater of Operations, USA, 1941–1945" (hereafter cited as Gordon "Hist"), vol. 1, pt. 10, p. 10, CMH. See also "Med Svc Hist, 1942–43," pp. 57–58, file HD 314. 7-2 ETO. For the general difficulties of TORCH supply, see Ruppenthal, *Logistical Support*, 1:96–99.

future of BOLERO. TORCH took out of England all but one combat unit, the 29th Division. The Eighth Air Force lost four fighter and two bombardment groups, much equipment, and 25,000 officers and men. In all, over 150,000 troops left England for North Africa. Total ETO strength, even with reinforcements from the United States, dropped to 105,000 and would remain at that level until well into 1943. Monthly cargo deliveries declined from 240,000 long tons in September 1942 to only 20,000 in February 1943. ETO headquarters and the BOLERO Combined Committee suspended most of their buildup and cross-Channel assault planning. After a year-end visit to medical installations in Great Britain, Surgeon General Magee observed: "One could not escape the feeling that service there represented a back-eddy since the opening of activities in Africa." [61]

For the medical service, as for the rest of ETOUSA, 1942 proved to be a year of large plans and false starts, culminating in a convulsive flurry of improvisation that left the theater impoverished and temporarily outside the mainstream of wartime events. Yet in spite of these vicissitudes, the theater medical service succeeded in completing its basic organization and implementing medical programs, some with systemic problems. The chief surgeon, with the cooperation of the British, organized a comprehensive American hospital system and saw construction begin, however haltingly. U.S. Army hospitals, once in operation, furnished medical care that the surgeon general described as "adequate and in some instances superior." [62] The supply system still needed to be overhauled. Supply shortages remained severe, causing the Allies to meet most medical supply requirements from sources within the United Kingdom. In mounting TORCH the ETO medical service gained valuable, if often painful, administrative and logistics experience, readying it for continued growth with the European Theater when the latter resumed its place as the focal point of the American war effort in the new year.

---

[61] Memo, Magee to CG, SOS, 12 Jan 43, file HU: Experience in Medical Matters F/Overseas Force. For the impact of TORCH on the European Theater, see Harrison, *Cross-Channel*, pp. 46–47; Ruppenthal, *Logistical Support*, 1:99–104, 110; and Craven and Cate, eds., *AAF*, 2:50–52, 231–32, 235.

[62] Memo, Magee to CG, SOS, 12 Jan 43, file HU: Experience in Medical Matters F/Overseas Force.

CHAPTER III

Theater Chief Surgeon

During 1943 strategic initiative in Europe and the Mediterranean passed to the Allies. After the surrender of 250,000 Germans and Italians in Tunisia in May, the Americans and British followed up their North African victory with a successful invasion of Sicily that precipitated the collapse of Mussolini's government. Italy, under new rules, deserted the Axis early in September, as United States and British Empire troops landed on its mainland. German divisions, however, poured into Italy to continue the battle. By the end of the year the Allies were pushing slowly and painfully toward Rome, against tenacious Nazi resistance. Meanwhile, the Allied bombing of Germany expanded in scale and destructiveness. At sea U.S. and British naval forces gradually secured the upper hand over the U-boats. On the eastern front the Russians, after major victories at Stalingrad and Kursk, began a counteroffensive that would end only in the rubble of Berlin.

While the Mediterranean offensive continued, the Americans during 1943 maneuvered the initially reluctant British, step by step, toward a firm commitment to a cross-Channel invasion aimed at the liberation of France and the conquest of Germany. At the Casablanca conference in January President Roosevelt, Prime Minister Churchill, and their Combined Chiefs of Staff agreed in principle to launch a full-scale cross-Channel attack in 1944. They created the Anglo-American staff known as COSSAC to draft detailed plans for the operation, as well as for small-scale raids and a limited attack in 1943. The conference also decided to enlarge the bombing offensive and to resume the full million-man BOLERO buildup. In May, at the TRIDENT conference in Washington, the Allied leaders set 1 May 1944 as the target date for the invasion, initially code-named ROUNDHAMMER but soon given its permanent and historic title: OVERLORD. In August, at the QUADRANT conference in Quebec, the president, the prime minister, and their military staffs approved COSSAC's outline OVERLORD plan and directed COSSAC to proceed with detailed planning and preparations. They accorded OVERLORD first priority for 1944 among European and Mediterranean operations. Finally, at the combined Cairo and Teheran conferences (22 November–7 December 1943), Soviet Premier Josef Stalin declared his support for OVERLORD; and the British and Americans decided to undertake an invasion of southern France with forces from the Mediterranean to supplement the main blow on the Normandy coast.[1]

For the European Theater of Operations the year's developments in strategy led to boundary and command changes. On 4 February 1943, as the result of agreements reached at Casablanca, the U.S. Joint Chiefs of Staff created a new North African Theater of Operations (NATOUSA), encompassing the former Mediterranean and North African portions of ETOUSA. The latter theater now consisted of Iceland, the United Kingdom, Scandinavia, France, the Low Countries, Germany, and most of Central and Eastern Europe; and it gradually ended its logistical support of North African operations. Also in February General Eisenhower, who had moved his headquarters to Algiers late in 1942, assumed command of the North African Theater. He was succeeded as ETO commander first by Lt. Gen. Frank M. Andrews, former commander of U.S. forces in the Middle East, and then, after Andrew's death in an airplane crash on 3 May, by Lt. Gen. Jacob L. Devers. Devers remained at the head of ETOUSA until 16 January 1944, when Eisenhower returned to London to take over the Supreme Headquarters, Allied Expeditionary Force (SHAEF), an Anglo-American organization built on COSSAC to conduct OVERLORD under direction of the Combined Chiefs of Staff. Eisenhower had under him Allied air, naval, and ground commands. At the same time he functioned as commanding general of ETOUSA, responsible for administrative and logistical purposes to the U.S. War Department.[2]

By the time General Eisenhower returned to London, the renewed BOLERO buildup, initiated at Casablanca, was approaching its climax. The buildup had gotten off to a slow start. Although the Casablanca conferees called for deployment of 1.1 million Americans, including fifteen–nineteen divisions, in the United Kingdom by the end of 1943, the manpower, supply, and shipping requirements of the North African campaign, continuing U-boat depredations, and the persistent tentativeness of the Allied commitment to the cross-Channel assault curtailed the movement of men and materiel to Britain during the first five months of the year. ETO strength remained at less than 150,000. The floodgates opened after the TRIDENT conference set the OVERLORD target date and directed the establishment of a U.S. force of 1.3 million in Great Britain by that time. By mid-1943 the Allies were winning the Battle of the Atlantic, and the combination of declining losses and rising production alleviated the shipping shortage that for so long had crippled BOLERO. The buildup

---

[1] This account of Anglo-American strategic deliberations is based on Matloff, *Strategic Planning*, chs. I, V, VI, VIII, X, XV, and XVI; Harrison, *Cross-Channel*, chs. I, II, and III. COSSAC means Chief of Staff to the Supreme Allied Commander (Designate). TRIDENT and QUADRANT were code names for the Allied summit conferences.

[2] Matloff, *Strategic Planning*, pp. 60–63 and 403–04; Ruppenthal, *Logistical Support*, 1:111–13 and 193–95; and Harrison, *Cross-Channel*, ch. III, cover in detail the evolution of the complex OVERLORD command structure. The European Theater relinquished jurisdiction over southern France to NATOUSA on 6 February 1944; responsibility for Iceland passed to the Eastern Defense Command on 30 July 1944.

rate now depended more on British port capacity than on availability of bottoms.

Accordingly, during the last quarter of 1943, over 100,000 American troops per month disembarked in Britain, bringing ETO strength at the end of the year to over 770,000, including eleven divisions. Cargo flow increased in proportion, from 348,900 measurement tons in June to over 1 million tons in December. Between January and May 1944 the buildup further accelerated. American troop strength doubled to over 1.5 million men, with an average of two divisions, plus supporting units, arriving each month, along with almost 1.5 million measurement tons of freight. By the end of May 1944 BOLERO substantially had reached its targets. In the process large tracts of the English countryside were transformed into American cantonments, vehicle parks, and storage depots.[3]

Command Problems Solved

During the decisive months of strategy-making and mobilization in 1943 General Hawley's position in the theater chain of command remained ill-defined. The chief surgeon and the other service chiefs continued to be under the Services of Supply and physically separated from theater headquarters. They could issue technical directions to their subordinate elements operating outside the Services of Supply only through the cumbersome process of drafting instructions for review and endorsement first by SOS and then by ETO headquarters. Hawley, attempting to explain the system to his staff, indicated the operating difficulties:

> In all technical directions, directives and functions this office deals directly with the surgeons of all echelons in the theater as a whole . . . [but directives affecting the theater as a whole] must be published by the theater headquarters and go to them for publication. Now, occasionally, to expedite getting something started, we have had a command directive published in S.O.S. and sent the same directive to ETO to be published for the entire theater and that was merely to get things going in the theater. . . . Any paper that comes up, weigh it carefully—is this a theater matter or is this a S.O.S. matter . . . and having decided that, it is very simple.[4]

The other service chiefs and, more importantly, General Lee recognized the inadequacy of the existing structure. When General Andrews became ETO commander, Lee pressed upon him the desirability of giving the Services of Supply clear-cut theater-wide logistical and administrative authority. He won his point. On 21 March 1943, in a general order and accompanying letters of instruction, Andrews designated the headquarters as "the Commanding General's agency for administrative service and supply of the theater." Andrews gave General Lee authority, within his area of delegated responsibility, to issue instructions to non-SOS elements by order of the theater commander. Hawley and the other technical service chiefs re-

[3] Matloff, *Strategic Planning*, pp. 53–54 and 407; Ruppenthal, *Logistical Support*, 1:115 and 118–22.

[4] Notes of Conference Held in Chief Surgeon's Room, 0830 Hours, 25 January 1943, prepared by Col O. H. Stanley, MC, 29 Jan 43, file 323.362 Power and Duties (Office of the Chief Surgeon), ETOUSA. For a general discussion of this problem in the Services of Supply, see Ruppenthal, *Logistical Support*, 1:160–61.

mained under the Services of Supply "for coordination, supervision, operational control, and direction," but they were to move back to London so as to function more effectively as theater staff officers.[5]

The 21 March redefinition of SOS authority benefited the chief surgeon. Hawley transferred himself and a portion of his staff to London in May, while the bulk of his office stayed at Cheltenham. Return to the capital solved most of the chief surgeon's difficulties in liaison with the British and improved his access to the ETO staff. The increase of General Lee's authority—which Andrews' successor, General Devers, further expanded in May by assigning Lee to additional duty as the ETO G-4—enlarged the effective powers of Hawley and the other technical chiefs. Hawley, for example, now could shift medical personnel within the ground and air forces by means of directives from General Lee acting for the theater commander.[6]

Andrews' restructuring of theater command relations, while favorable from the SOS viewpoint, still did not definitively settle the question of SOS authority over the ground and air forces. In July, as a result of protests from the Eighth Air Force, General Devers revoked Lee's authority to issue orders outside the Services of Supply. Hawley and other service chiefs continued to plead for "an unbroken chain of technical control through all the echelons" of the European Theater. Over and above this long-standing issue, the shift of tactical control of ground forces—and of most operational planning—to newly established U.S. army group and army headquarters and to SHAEF left ETOUSA with little to do but duplicate the administrative and logistical functions of the Services of Supply.[7]

General Devers recognized that he had one command echelon too many in the theater. During late 1943 his staff, in consultation with representatives of General Eisenhower, developed a plan for merging ETO and SOS headquarters. Following this plan Eisenhower, as commander of both SHAEF and ETOUSA, on 17 January 1944 issued an order consolidating the theater headquarters and staff with those of the Services of Supply. Eisenhower appointed his SHAEF chief of staff, Maj. Gen. Walter Bedell Smith, also chief of staff of the new headquarters, which continued to be known as the European Theater of Operations. At the same time Eisenhower made General Lee deputy theater commander for supply and administration, with authority to "act, in all appropriate cases, for the Theater Commander,"

[5] GO No. 16, HQ, ETOUSA, 21 Mar 43; ETO LOI to CG, SOS, ETOUSA, 21 Mar 43; Staff Memo No. 29, HQ, ETOUSA, 8 Apr 43, sub: Organization of HQ, ETOUSA, and HQ, SOS, ETOUSA. All in file HD 024 ETO O/CS (Spruit Policy Notebook). See also Ruppenthal, *Logistical Support*, 1:161–63.

[6] Col Charles B. Spruit, MC, Diary, January–August 1943 (hereafter cited as Spruit Diary), 1 Apr 43; Administration Division, OofCSurg, HQ, ETOUSA, Annual Rpt, 1943. For the question of authority over personnel transfers, see Memos, CSurg to G–1, SOS, 22 Apr 43; G–1, SOS, to CSurg, 24 Apr 43; CSurg to CofS, SOS, 27 Apr 43; and CofS, SOS, to CSurg, via G–1, 3 May 43. All in file HD 008 ETO O/CS (Policy Book).

[7] The overall development of SOS authority is recounted in Ruppenthal, *Logistical Support*, 1:163–68. Hawley's continuing concern is expressed in SOS Minutes of Command and Staff Conference, 29 Nov 43 (Supplement), pp. 6–7, file HD 337 (Command and Staff Conferences), and in Ltr, Hawley to TSG, 6 Jan 44, file HD 024 ETO O/CS (Hawley-SGO Corresp).

and with direct control over all SOS forces. Lee now clearly outranked ground and air component commanders and could give directives to them; the heads of his special staff sections possessed confirmed theater-wide technical authority over their services.[8]

The January 1944 reorganization, which remained in effect until V–E Day, at last placed General Hawley in what he considered a satisfactory position in the chain of command. Hawley, who had had differences with General Smith during the TORCH preparations, at first feared that Eisenhower would bring in a new theater chief surgeon. This apprehension proved groundless. The entire SOS staff continued in placed in the revamped ETO–SOS headquarters. Writing in early February to Brig. Gen. Norman T. Kirk, the surgeon general as of May 1943, Hawley explained that

> our organization here seems to have been completely cooked and has now jelled. . . . All Chiefs of Services, including myself, are Chiefs of Services of ETO and, in addition to their other duties, are Chiefs of Services of SOS. This is an exact reversal of the previous organization in which the Chiefs of Services were assigned to the SOS and, in addition to their other duties, were Chiefs of Services of the ETO. This is, of course, a small point but [it] is proving to be a most important point.[9]

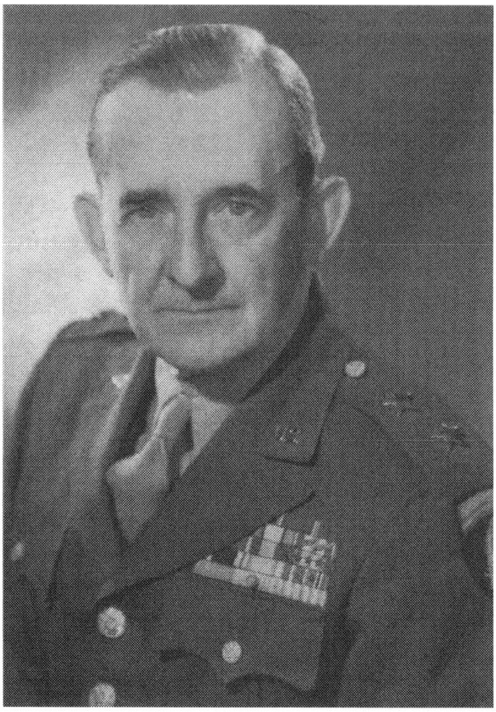

MAJ. GEN. ALBERT W. KENNER

Hawley, who received his second star on 27 February 1944, needed this reinforcement of his authority to maintain ascendancy amid the proliferation of high-level American staffs that accompanied the BOLERO buildup. His most formidable potential rival for theater medical predominance was Maj. Gen. Albert W.

[8] Quotation from GO No. 5, HQ, ETOUSA, 17 Jan 44. See also Ruppenthal, *Logistical Support*, 1:198–201. Eisenhower, as Allied Supreme Commander, directed operations of air, ground, and naval forces of all nationalities and in this capacity was responsible to the Anglo-American Combined Chiefs of Staff. His SHAEF staff included British and other Allied officers as well as Americans. The various national forces under Eisenhower looked to their own national authorities for supply and administration. As ETO commander Eisenhower was responsible to the War Department for performing those functions for U.S. forces. In fact, he delegated most of the task to General Lee and the combined ETO-SOS headquarters.

[9] Quotation from Ltr, Hawley to TSG, 4 Feb 44, file HD 024 ETO O/CS (Hawley-SGO Corresp); in same file, see Ltr, TSG to Hawley, 12 Feb 44. For the threat to Hawley's position, see Interv, OSG with Brig Gen Charles B. Spruit, MC (Ret.), 20 May 49 (hereafter cited as Spruit Interv, 1949), file HD 000.71, CMH; Ltrs, Hawley to Brig Gen Fred W. Rankin, 26 Nov 43, and Hawley to TSG, 4 Dec 43, file HD 024 ETO O/CS (Hawley-SGO Corresp).

Kenner, MC, SHAEF's chief medical officer, who took up his duties in London in February. Kenner, a Regular Army medical officer and close acquaintance of Marshall, Eisenhower, and Lt. Gen. George S. Patton, Jr., had accompanied the latter to North Africa in November 1942 as surgeon of the Western Task Force. As the African campaign developed, Kenner advanced to the dual position of AFHQ chief surgeon and NATOUSA chief surgeon. He served Eisenhower as a personal front-line inspector and emissary, as well as a medical staff officer. Returning to the United States early in 1943, Kenner narrowly missed becoming surgeon general to replace the retiring General Magee. His relationship with Eisenhower, seniority in rank, and military medical experience brought Kenner the SHAEF assignment.[10]

As SHAEF's chief medical officer Kenner reported directly to Eisenhower, and thus was higher in the chain of command than Hawley. He advised the "Supreme Commander and the Staff of Supreme Headquarters, on all matters pertaining to the Medical Service within the areas under the command of the Supreme Commander, Allied Expeditionary Force," and coordinated "medical policy on an inter-allied basis." He also had the right to inspect medical installations and units and to investigate and report on any aspect of the medical service that he chose. The exact boundary between Kenner's sphere of interest and that of General Hawley—and indeed the overall demarcation line between the activities of the American staff of SHAEF and the ETO staff—never was very clear.[11]

Kenner and Hawley, nevertheless, maintained a harmonious working relationship. In the preinvasion months Kenner and his four-man Anglo-American staff concentrated on reviewing and coordinating British and American OVERLORD medical plans, especially those for cross-Channel evacuation. Kenner declared that his relationship to the U.S. Army medical service was "policy-making and inspectional, never operational. . . . I never interfered with Hawley's work; I never issued Hawley any orders." Participants later differed in their recollections of the extent to which Kenner, directly or indirectly, influenced ETO medical policies and operations. Most of the time the chief medical officer appears to have left Hawley to his own devices. If nothing else, the small size of Kenner's staff, and his resulting dependence on Hawley's much larger office for information and the execution of directives, would have limited his ability to intervene. When Kenner did choose to step in, he had the authority to

[10] Name-Rank file, Special History Branch, CMH; Kenner Interv, 1952, file HD 000.71, CMH. General Marshall strongly supported Kenner for the position of surgeon general because of Kenner's administrative ability and combat theater experience, and for a while his appointment seemed assured. President Roosevelt, however, insisted on someone more eminent in the estimation of the civilian medical profession, and General Kirk, also an able administrator, received the appointment. See Armfield, *Organization and Administration*, pp. 200–202.

[11] Kenner's duties are established in Memo, CMedOff, SHAEF, to ACofS, G–3, via ACofS, G–4, 1 Mar 44, sub: Functional Chart of Medical Division, and Admin Memo No. 3, SHAEF, 24 Apr 44, both in Medical Division, COSSAC/SHAEF, War Diary, March–April 1944. See the same source, January–June 1944, for a running account of the chief medical officer's activities.

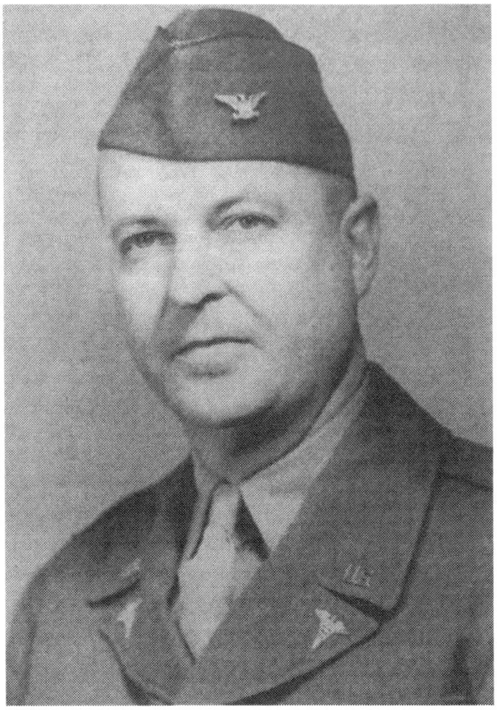

COL. ALVIN L. GORBY

make his wishes prevail, but he used this power sparingly. Such restraint, combined with frequent conferences and exchanges of views with the ETO chief surgeon, and with the maintenance on both sides of an atmosphere of mutual respect, prevented what could have been a disruptive conflict of authority.[12]

[12] Quotations from Kenner Interv, 1952, file HD 000.71, CMH. For views of the Kenner-Hawley relationship, see Spruit Interv, 1949, and Interv, OSG with Col Alvin L. Gorby, MC, 10 Nov 49 (hereafter cited as Gorby Interv, 1949), both in file HD 000.71, CMH; Interv, OSG with Col John K. Davis, MC (hereafter cited as Davis Interv), 19 Jun 45, box 222, RG 112, NARA; and Interv, NLM with William S. Middleton, July and November 1968, February 1969 (hereafter cited as Middleton Interv, 1968–69), vol. 1, p. 261, NLM. Ruppenthal, *Logistical Support,* 1:200–201, outlines the continuing SHAEF-ETO problem of staff jurisdiction.

During late 1943 and the first months of 1944 the U.S. Army ground forces completed their organization for OVERLORD. As invasion preparations intensified, the War Department in October 1943 established headquarters of the U.S. 1st Army Group at London and the U.S. First Army at Bristol, both initially under Lt. Gen. Omar N. Bradley, to act in planning as opposite numbers of the British 21 Army Group and its two subordinate field armies. On the twenty-third the First Army assumed operational control of all American ground combat elements in Great Britain, superseding the V Corps, which until then had been the senior ground command. In January of the following year the European Theater set up another U.S. army, the Third, under General Patton. This headquarters helped administer the divisions now pouring into the United Kingdom and began planning for continental operations after establishment of the initial lodgement.

The surgeons of these headquarters meshed their activities smoothly with those of Hawley and his staff. Col. Alvin L. Gorby, MC, arrived in England in January 1944 for duty in Hawley's office, but then was reassigned as the 1st Army Group surgeon. He had to develop his own charter of responsibility. "We'd never had a group in the U.S. Army before," he recalled, "and the concept of what the Group Surgeon's office would do, and what its organization should be, we just had to pull it out of the air and set it in." Gorby decided early that his role would be analogous to that of a corps or division surgeon, "a tactical setup, rather than administrative, and that we ought to . . . just ride herd, and only take over and jump in when it seemed like there was some need." To this end, he limited the size of his staff to eight or ten officers and about the same number of enlisted men. Until D-Day Gorby and his assistants concentrated on OVERLORD planning; they worked closely with 21 Army Group, with Kenner and Hawley, and with the First Army that was preparing the detailed assault plans for the American landings. "All we did," the army group surgeon declared, "was go down and pat them on the back and ask them if we could be of aid." [13]

The army surgeons, Col. John A. Rogers, MC, of the First and Col. Thomas D. Hurley, MC, of the Third, came out from the United States with the cadres of their respective headquarters. Under the Army Ground Forces organization then prevailing, a field army performed most logistical and administrative services for its component units, leaving corps and divisions a strictly tactical role. Each army surgeon, accordingly, had a staff about twice as large as Colonel Gorby's, with specialized divisions covering roughly the same range of functions as those of the theater chief surgeon's office. During the buildup the army surgeons devoted much attention to invasion and operations planning. They directed the training of the medical units and personnel assigned to their armies, supervised supply, and conducted active preventive medicine programs. Especially in the latter two functions, they worked closely with the SOS base section surgeons. The army surgeons were under Hawley's technical direction and generally deferred to him on matters of policy. Hawley declared of Colonel Rogers: "With all these new heresies of staff control that have suddenly burst upon our Army, it is refreshing to have a surgeon in a subordinate echelon who adheres to the old and tried doctrine of technical control through staff channels as dis-

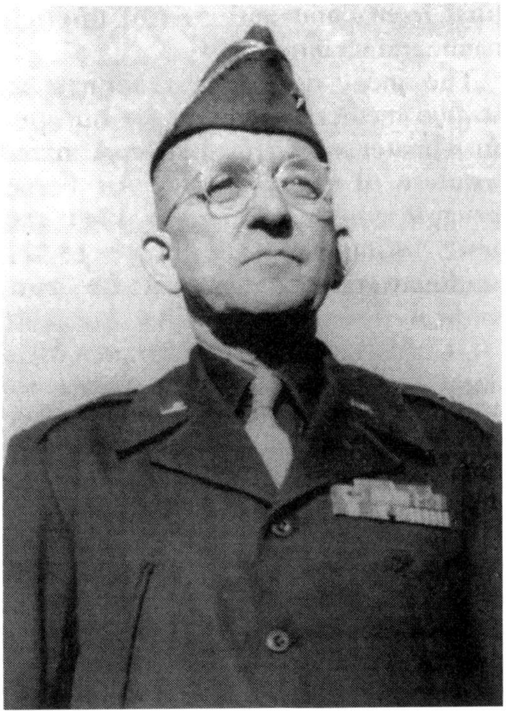

BRIG. GEN. THOMAS D. HURLEY
(Rank as of 20 March 1945)

[13] Quotations from Historical Unit, U.S. Army Medical Service, Advisory Editorial Board for the History of Medical Service in the European Theater in World War II, Minutes of Sessions, 9-10 October 1962 (hereafter cited as Editorial Advisory Board, 1962), pp. 75-77. See also 12th Army Group Report of Operations, vol. XIII (Medical Section), pp. 7-8 and 15-20; in CMH, both Gorby Interv, 1949, file HD 000.71, and Interv, OSG with Maj Gen Alvin L. Gorby, MC, 8 Oct 62 (hereafter cited as Gorby Interv, 1962), pp. 2-3.

tinct from command control through command channels." [14]

The most significant challenge to unified medical service in the European Theater was a theater-level manifestation of the worldwide Air Force struggle for autonomy. In 1941 the newly formed Army Air Forces (AAF) headquarters had secured its own medical division under Air Surgeon Lt. Col. David N. W. Grant, MC. Grant was nominally subordinate to the surgeon general, but he waged a series of increasingly bitter bureaucratic conflicts and gradually won effective independence. To justify this drive for autonomy, Grant and his colleagues argued that the unique clinical and technical problems of air warfare could be dealt with only by a specialized aviation medical service. In 1943 the surgeon general disagreed, insisting that treatment of air crew casualties in most respects involved the same medical and surgical practice as treatment of any other casualties. Step by step the air surgeon gained ground. By the end of the year Grant, now a major general, controlled what amounted to an independent personnel procurement system and a separate supply service. In the United States the Air Force had its own convalescent centers and station and general hospitals, and the air surgeon had begun pushing for similar hospitals in the overseas theaters.[15]

In the European Theater the Air Force expanded rapidly under the impact of the Casablanca decision to intensify the bombing offensive against Germany. By mid-1944 AAF strength in the United Kingdom had reached almost 427,000 officers and men of the Eighth (strategic) and Ninth (tactical) Air Forces and various support and service commands, under the overall control of Headquarters, United States Strategic Air Forces (USSTAF). Of these troops almost 13,000 were members of the Army Medical Department, headed by USSTAF surgeon, Brig. Gen. Malcolm C. Grow, MC.[16]

From the early days of the buildup, when the Eighth Air Force, with Colonel Grow as surgeon, was the senior air headquarters in the theater, the air service waged a running battle with

[14] Quotation from Ltr, Hawley to TSG, 4 Dec 43, file HD 024 ETO O/CS (Hawley-SGO Corresp). See also First U.S. Army Report of Operations, 20 Oct 43–1 Aug 44, bk. I, pp. 13–15, and bk. VIII, an. 16 (Medical Section); Surg, Third U.S. Army, Annual Rpt, 1944; Editorial Advisory Board, 1962, pp. 85–86.

[15] For the general development of the AAF medical service, see Armfield, *Organization and Administration*, pp. 47–48 and 79–82, and Link and Coleman, *AAF Medical Support*, passim. See also Ltr, TSG to Hawley, 7 Aug 43, file HD 024 ETO O/CS (Hawley–SGO Corresp).

[16] Air command arrangements were complicated by the fact that the Combined Chiefs of Staff retained direct control over the strategic bombing offensive until the final months before OVERLORD, while General Eisenhower, through SHAEF, controlled British and American tactical air. Hence, USSTAF had both operational and administrative control of the Eighth Air Force in England, operational control of the Fifteenth in the Mediterranean, and administrative control of the Ninth, formed in Britain early in 1944 to furnish tactical air support to the American armies. Eisenhower had operational control of the Ninth through the Allied Expeditionary Air Forces, a division of SHAEF. For the air buildup and command relations, see Ruppenthal, *Logistical Support*, 1:192–93 and 202–03; Craven and Cates, eds., *AAF*, 2:639; and ibid., vol. 3, *Europe: ARGUMENT to V–E Day, January 1944 to May 1945* (1951), pp. 107–19. See also Link and Coleman, *AAF Medical Support*, pp. 558–59 and 580.

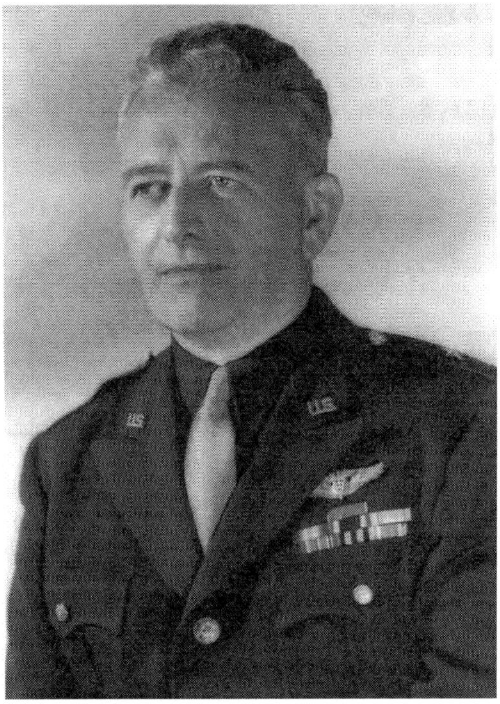

BRIG. GEN. MALCOLM C. GROW

the Services of Supply for administrative and logistical independence. In the medical sphere the issues were hospitalization and supply. Under agreements reached early in 1942, SOS station and general hospitals were to treat all Air Force sick and wounded who required more than short-term care. The Air Force was to have no hospitals of its own except 25-bed unit dispensaries. The Services of Supply was to furnish all medical supplies except items used exclusively by air surgeons, which would come from the United States through Air Force channels. Grow and his staff steadily undermined these arrangements, taking advantage of early SOS delays in hospital construction and slow supply deliveries to justify independent action. Before the end of 1942 Grow, over strenuous objections from Hawley, had obtained theater authorization for separate Air Force convalescent centers and an Air Force medical service school, although the Eighth Air Force surgeon lost a battle to set up 50-bed air base hospitals. Grow also managed to open his own supply pipeline from the United States for common items as well as for those peculiar to the Air Force. To Hawley's continuing irritation, the Air Force as a result always seemed able to obtain materiel when the chief surgeon could not. Hawley repeatedly demanded a halt to "this pernicious practice." But he never could shut off the flow, and the continuing ineffectiveness of his own Supply Division afforded the Air Force an excuse for its irregularities.[17]

General Hawley consistently opposed the setting up of an independent Air Force medical service, and especially the establishment of separate Air Force–controlled station and general hospitals. While he recognized

[17] For overviews of the AAF–SOS jurisdictional conflict, see Ruppenthal, *Logistical Support*, 1:170–71; Craven and Cates, eds., *AAF*, 1:648–49; Armfield, *Organization and Administration*, pp. 331–32; and Link and Coleman, *AAF Medical Support*, pp. 555–71. On rest homes and schools, see Ltrs, Hawley to Brig Gen David N. W. Grant, 30 Mar 43, and Hawley to TSG, 8 Jul 43, both in file HD 024 ETO O/CS (Hawley-SGO Corresp); Items 47 and 55, file HU 312.3 (Corresp File, ETO Chief Surgeon). On the dispensary fight, see file 320.2 ETO (T/O Medical Dispensary). On supply, see Ltrs, Hawley to Tyng, 7 Oct 42, Hawley to G–4, SOS, 14 Oct 42, and 1st End, Hawley to CG, SOS, 9 Nov 42, file HD 024 ETO CS (Hawley Chron); see also Ltrs, Tyng to Hawley, 18 Oct 42, Hawley to Tyng, 7 Nov 42, and Hawley to TSG, 19 Aug, 9 Sep, and 14 Oct 43, file HD 024 ETO O/CS (Hawley-SGO Corresp). The AAF in the United States had secured a supply of common medical items, held in its own depots, from which it filled Grow's requisitions.

the "special medical problems" of air crew care, he insisted: "There is not the slightest technical difference between an air soldier wounded by fragments of a 20mm cannon shell and an infantryman wounded by fragments of an 88mm artillery shell." A hospital capable of treating one also could treat the other. ETO station and general hospitals, Hawley pointed out, cared for all American patients from a given area, so if the Air Force took over any existing fixed hospitals, its flight surgeons would spend most of their time working on ground and service troops. Establishment of additional hospitals solely for Air Force casualties would result in diversion of scarce manpower and materiel to underused specialist institutions. Hawley summed up:

> If we turn over any hospitals in this Theater to the Air Force, it will result either in the Air Force being required to care for thousands of sick and injured in the Ground Forces or in constructing at least $10,000,000 worth of new hospitals. . . . Regardless of such a waste of money, this additional construction cannot be accomplished in this Theater because both labor and materials for hospital construction have now been exhausted.[18]

While adamant in principle against separate Air Force medical facilities, Hawley tried to make the SOS medical service as responsive as possible to Air Force requirements. He added aviation medicine specialists to the staffs of station and general hospitals that treated large numbers of airmen, and he pressed the British hard for early completion of hospital plants near the major AAF bases and troop concentrations. He badgered his Supply Division for prompt response to Air Force requisitions. In his unsuccessful campaign to block creation of a separate AAF medical service school, Hawley went so far as to offer command of the SOS medical school to an Air Force medical officer. Hawley kept up a friendly relationship with General Grow and worked hard to win over Air Surgeon Grant when the latter visited England in September 1943. Other members of Hawley's staff were less conciliatory. Colonel Spruit, the chief surgeon's representative in London until Hawley's move from Cheltenham in May 1943, always abrasive, irritated Eighth Air Force officers to the point where they unsuccessfully tried to have him relieved. Nevertheless, Hawley's approach paid dividends. Grow made no real attempt to press for independent Air Force station or general hospitals and repeatedly expressed to Grant his satisfaction with SOS medical support.[19]

The Air Force hospital issue came to a head early in 1944. By that time Eighth Air Force bombers were flying daily missions deep into Germany, suffering a heavy toll of air crew fatalities, wounds, and mental and physical exhaustion. The confrontation in

[18] Quotations from Ltr, Hawley to TSG, 10 Aug 43, file HD 024 ETO O/CS (Hawley-SGO Corresp); see other letters in same file. See also Ltr, Hawley to Brig Gen Ray W. Barker, 5 Mar 43, box 2, Hawley Papers, MHI; Ltr, Hawley to G–1, ETO, 15 Oct 42, file HD 024 ETO CS (Hawley Chron).

[19] Link and Coleman, *AAF Medical Support*, pp. 566–67, summarize Grow's reports to Grant. Hawley's relationship with Grant and Grow and Spruit's feud with the Eighth Air Force are reflected in many letters for 1943–44 in file HD 024 ETO O/CS (Hawley-Corresp) and in MFR, Conference with Gen Hawley, 18 Apr 50, file HD 000.71. Hawley Operational Directive No. 13, 25 Jun 43, box 2, Hawley Papers, MHI, shows his concern for Air Force supply; in the collection, see Ltr, Hawley to Barker, 5 Mar 43, and Operational Directive No. 34, 18 Aug 43.

this instance originated in Washington, where acquaintances hinted privately to President Roosevelt—whose son Elliot was an Air Force officer—that aviator casualties in the European Theater were receiving medical care inferior to that given British fliers in RAF hospitals. Roosevelt directed Surgeon General Kirk, Air Surgeon Grant, and Dr. Edward A. Strecker, a civilian consultant to the Navy and Air Force, to go to England and investigate the problem.

During February and March the three men toured Army and RAF hospitals in the United Kingdom. They conferred with USSTAF and Eighth Air Force commanders and with Hawley, Grow, and other medical officers. Their unanimous report, issued on 20 March, amounted to a ringing vindication for General Hawley. Kirk, Grant, and Strecker concluded that Air Force patients—and all other U.S. troops—were receiving "superior" medical and surgical care and that RAF hospitals were inferior in most respects to American ones. SOS station and general hospitals were sufficient in number and properly located to meet Air Force requirements, according to the investigators, and the professional staffs "very definitely realized Air Forces problems and met them effectively." The board noted with approval the "close cooperation" prevailing between the staffs of the USSTAF and ETO surgeons. Kirk, Grant, and Strecker did criticize delays in returning recovered airmen to duty through the SOS replacement system, a long-standing Air Force grievance, and they recommended adding flight surgeons to the disposition boards of general hospitals treating Air Force patients. Hawley and Grow quickly implemented this suggestion. In the face of Air Force commanders' expressions of preference for totally Air Force–run hospitals, the board concluded: "In view of the long established system of hospitalization in the ETO and contemplated new operations, . . . any change in the general principle of hospitalization . . . at this time should not be recommended." Although the air surgeon continued to agitate for his own overseas hospitals, the Kirk-Grant-Strecker report effectively closed the question in the European Theater. SOS hospitals continued to care for Air Force patients until the end of the war. The Air Force theater medical establishment, in this important respect at least, remained firmly within Hawley's control.[20]

Within the Services of Supply the chief surgeon had to define his relationship to the base section headquarters, which steadily expanded in number, size, and administrative importance. At the beginning of 1943 the United Kingdom was divided into three base sections—the Southern, Eastern, and Western (which included Northern Ireland). During the year the SOS headquarters added two more sections: a Central Base Sec-

[20] Quotations from Memo, Maj Gen N. T. Kirk, Maj Gen D. N. W. Grant, and Dr. E. A. Strecker to CofS, via DepTheaterCdr, ETOUSA, 20 Mar 44, copy in file HD 024 ETO O/CS (Hawley-SGO Corresp). For background of this investigation, see Link and Coleman, *AAF Medical Support*, pp. 88–91, 563–66, 568, and Hawley Interv, 1962, p. 32, CMH. The question of returning AAF patients to duty involved both reducing the time during which they were lost to their parent units and determining accurately fitness to resume flying. For the role of the air surgeons in disposition boards, see Mins, 23d Meeting of Base Section Surgeons, 5 Jun 44, p. 5, file HD 337.

tion, encompassing the London area, and a revived Northern Ireland Base Section.[21]

General Lee, in a directive issued on 24 August, resolved the long-standing special staff-base section conflict over control of the technical services in favor of the base section commanders. Each base section commander, Lee declared, was responsible for "all SOS operations" within his area and had "the authority of command . . . over all SOS individuals, units and installations . . . in his base section." A base section was to provide most logistical services for all American forces within its boundaries, including hospitalization and evacuation. Under this order General Hawley lost all formal control over SOS medical units and installations, including general hospitals. Even the right to transfer medical personnel within a base section, hitherto a prerogative of the chief surgeon's Personnel Division, now belonged to the base section commanders, although the chief surgeon still controlled assignments of new medical units to base sections and could transfer officers and men between sections.[22]

As a result of Lee's policy, which he called centralized control and decentralized operation, most day-to-day direction of SOS medical service rested with the base section surgeons and their staffs. Initially undermanned and lacking qualified administrators, the offices of the base section surgeons by late 1943 possessed at least adequate manpower and had established a divisional organization that corresponded closely to that of the chief surgeon's office. Each base section surgeon acted as both a staff officer of the section commander, informing his superior of the health of the command and administering the medical service under his direction, and as the technical representative of the chief surgeon. In the latter capacity a base section surgeon collected information and disseminated technical directives, policies, and procedures. By early 1944 each base section surgeon had under his purview an establishment that was larger than the entire ETO medical service scarcely a year before. The Western Base Section alone contained almost 10,500 medical troops in eighty-five units and had seven station and six general hospitals in operation.[23]

To maintain uniformity of medical policy and practice in the base sections, General Hawley in August 1943 instituted twice-monthly conferences of section surgeons and his office division heads. Individual divisions held their own regular meetings with base section counterparts and helped train and indoctrinate base section medical staffs. The Hospitalization Division, for example, instructed base section

[21] The original Northern Ireland Base Section was reduced to a district of the Western Base Section on 9 December 1942, for lack of troops, but was revived again with the buildup of forces in Northern Ireland. See Ruppenthal, *Logistical Support,* 1:168–70.

[22] Cir No. 49, HQ, SOS, 24 Aug 43, and Cir No. 1, HQ, SOS, 8 Jan 44, define base section authority and functions. See also Memo, Lee to CG, ETOUSA, 15 Jun 43, sub: Report on Structural Organization of the SOS, file 129 Admin (ETO). For the question of medical personnel transfers, see Spruit Diary, 20 Apr 43; Personnel Division, OofCSurg, HQ, ETOUSA, Annual Rpt, 1943; Notes of Base Section Surgeons Conference, 2 Aug 43.

[23] Mins, 14th Meeting of Base Section Surgeons, 31 Jan 44, p. 14, file HD 337. For base section surgeon's office organization and activities, see Eastern, Western, Southern, Central, and Northern Ireland Base Sections Annual Rpts, 1943 and 1944.

hospital inspectors in standard procedures. Although Lee's 24 August order formally placed general hospitals under the base sections, General Hawley managed to retain effective control over them. He and members of his staff regularly visited—in effect, inspected—these hospitals. When necessary, Hawley used his personal influence with General Lee to pressure base section commanders to improve substandard hospitals or to block detrimental base section interference. "For all practical purposes," Hawley recalled, "even though the base section commanders commanded the general hospitals . . . , we got pretty much what we wanted." [24]

Office Expansion

As other headquarters multiplied, the chief surgeon's office expanded in both manpower and number of functional divisions. Between May 1943, when BOLERO resumed in full force, and the eve of invasion the office force grew from 64 officers, 63 enlisted men, and 81 civilian employees to 135 officers, 335 enlisted men, and 122 civilians. Most of the additional officers entered the theater as casuals, and the vast majority were non-Regulars. Until late 1943 General Hawley continued to complain about a shortage of administrators. But the increasing number of qualified men available, and a more determined effort by the surgeon general's office to send the best to the European Theater, assured the arrival of sufficient managerial talent. By early 1944 only the Supply Division still lacked adequate staff. [25]

Hawley's office at the beginning of 1943 contained eleven divisions—Administration, Hospitalization, Supply, Personnel, Preventive Medicine, Professional Services, Operations and Training, Medical Records, Nursing, Dental, and Veterinary, all located at Cheltenham. During the next year and a half these divisions multiplied, combined, recombined, and gravitated toward London. The geographical movements resulted in part from an effort to place in the capital those divisions most involved in theater-wide planning and operations, and in part from the fact that the shift of any one division created almost irresistible pressure for other closely associated divisions to follow.

On 13 May 1943, when General Hawley returned to the capital, he formally divided his office into London and Cheltenham echelons. The London office at 9 North Audley Street, headed in person by the chief surgeon, had responsibility for "formulation of policy and broad planning" and for "administration and technical supervision of the medical

[24] Quotation from Editorial Advisory Board, 1962, pp. 38–40. For an example of his pressure on a base section commander, see Ltr, Hawley to Brig Gen C. O. Thrasher, CG, Southern Base Section, 16 May 44, and Memo, Hawley to Lee, 16 May 44, both in file HD 024 ETO CS (Hawley Chron). See also MFR, OofCSurg, ETOUSA, 26 Jul 43, sub: Notes From the Chief Surgeon, file HD 024 ETO O/CS (Spruit Policy Notebook); Mins, 1st Meeting of Base Section Surgeons, 2 Aug 43, file HD 337; Ltr, Col Liston to Col Abner Zehm, General Board, USFET, 14 Aug 45.

[25] Personnel Division, OofCSurg, HQ, ETOUSA, Annual Rpts, 1943 and 1944. For the gradual resolution of the administrative personnel shortage, see January–December 1943 correspondence in file HD 024 ETO O/CS (Hawley-SGO Corresp). The problems of the Supply Division are covered in Chapter VI of this volume.

service of the theater as a whole." The Cheltenham office, under the acerbic but able Colonel Spruit, who thus was removed from hostile contact with the Air Force, consisted of the bulk of the staff and supervised the SOS medical service; it also collected the information required for theater medical planning. In July Hawley created two new London-based divisions. The Planning Division, set up in conformity to general SOS policy, took over from Operations and Training the tasks of coordinating medical planning and of keeping abreast of overall theater planning. At the same time the new Evacuation Division assumed charge of that function, hitherto overseen by Operations and Training. Earlier, the chief surgeon had organized a Gas Casualty Division at Cheltenham to direct medical preparations for defense against and care of casualties from chemical warfare, then still considered a significant threat.[26]

Additional changes and moves occurred during early 1944, aimed mostly at improving medical planning and coordination as D-Day approached. In February the Operations and Training Division transferred to London. Renamed the Operations Division, it absorbed Planning, the functions of which it overlapped, as a branch and at the same time again took over Evacuation. Preventive Medicine, now concerned with preparing for continental operations as well as protecting the health of troops in England, moved to the capital in February, followed in March by Hospitalization, which also had to plan for post-invasion activities. Early in June a Rehabilitation Division, headquartered in London, split off from Hospitalization to direct an increasingly elaborate convalescent reconditioning program. Meanwhile, a Historical Division had begun operations at 9 North Audley Street, overseeing public relations and the medical photographic laboratory as well as undertaking the work that led ultimately to the present volume. On D-Day the chief surgeon's office (*Chart 3*) consisted of fourteen divisions, five of which were located in London and nine in Cheltenham.[27]

The Professional Services Division, which included the theater medical and surgical consultants, played a crucial role in tying together the entire medical establishment. General Hawley, following the Army's precedent in the use of consultants in World War I, as well as the example of the British, had activated this division on 19 June 1942. The division chief was Colonel Kimbrough, formerly the head of the Urology Section at Walter Reed Army Medical Center. By early 1944 Kimbrough, promoted to full colonel, headed the division's Cheltenham office, consist-

---

[26] For an example of the considerations governing division moves, see Ltr, Hawley to Spruit, 1 Oct 43, file HD 024 ETO O/CS (Spruit Policy Notebook); Office Order No. 1 (source of quotations), OofCSurg, HQ, ETOUSA, 13 May 43, and Planning Directive No. 8, 10 Jul 43, encls. 1 and 2 to Planning Division, OofCSurg, HQ, ETOUSA, Annual Rpt, 1943. See also annual reports, 1943, for the Administration, Evacuation, Operations, Hospitalization, and Gas Casualty Divisions. Evacuation had been under the Hospitalization Division until October 1942, when Operations and Training took it over.

[27] Administration and Preventive Medicine Divisions, OofCSurg, HQ, ETOUSA, Annual Rpts, 1944; Larkey "Hist," ch. 8, pp. 2-5 and app. 2.

CHART 3—ORGANIZATION OF THE OFFICE OF THE CHIEF SURGEON, ETOUSA, JUNE 1944

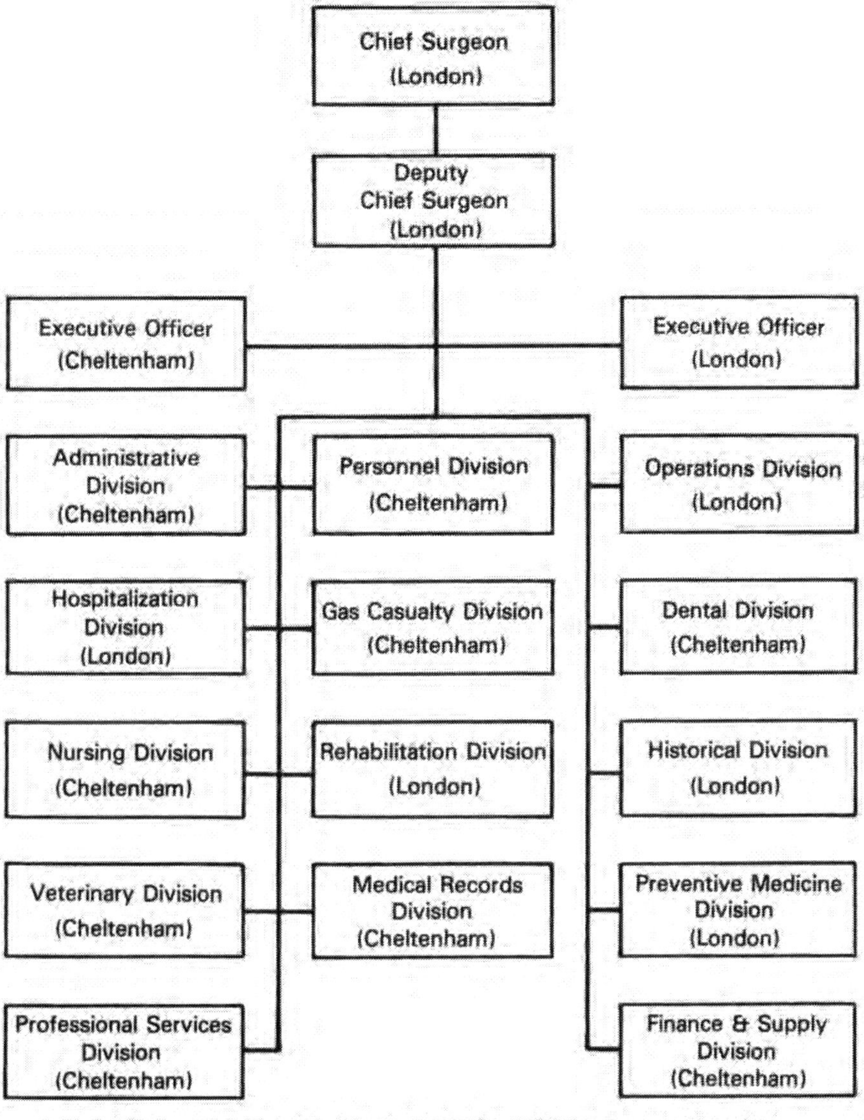

Source: Encl. 1, Personnel Division, OofCS, HQ, ETOUSA, Annual Rpt, 1944.

ing of seventeen officers, six enlisted men, and ten civilian employees.[28]

Kimbrough's immediate subordinates were Chief Consultant in Surgery Col. Elliott C. Cutler and Chief Consultant in Medicine Col. William S. Middleton. Arriving in the European Theater in mid-1942, both had served in the Army Medical Department in the previous war before attaining civilian professional eminence—Cutler as Moseley professor of surgery at Harvard and Middleton as dean of the University of Wisconsin Medical School. Each chief consultant had under him a number of senior consultants in particular surgical or medical specialties. Cutler kept most of his senior consultants on duty in his own office, using them as a personal staff. Middleton, who thought that consulting in most fields did not require the full time of scarce experts, maintained only his dermatology and neuropsychiatry consultants at Cheltenham. For other specialties he relied on general hospital chiefs of service assigned to additional duty. Regardless of how organized, the senior consultants, authorities in the civilian profession and mostly new to the Army, required careful handling. Kimbrough, according to Middleton, had to employ "unusual talents" in managing his "prima donnas." In moments of crisis "he would first cajole them. Then he would quote Shakespeare and then the Scripture. Finally he'd burst out into the vilest profanity you have ever heard." [29]

The consultants' primary task was to ensure uniformity and high quality in theater surgical and medical practice, but General Hawley used them for much more than that. He made them his personal advisers, agents, and inspectors and involved them in most aspects of ETO medical policy and administration. The Professional Services Division, Hawley declared, "was an operating division. And probably, except for the Operations and Training Divison, was the really controlling division in the office." At the consultants' first general meeting, in October 1942, Hawley told them:

> I expect advice from this group, not only when I ask for it, but when any member of this group thinks that I need it. . . . You people, within your specialties, are to represent me and act with my complete authority. . . . You have technical control of the practice of your specialties in this Theater. . . . I do want you to correct things I spot. . . . You have my complete authority to make corrections in technical procedures right on the spot. . . .[30]

[28] Professional Services Division, OofCSurg, HQ, ETOUSA, Annual Rpt, 1944. For the origins and World War I background of the consultant system, see W. Paul Havens, Jr., ed., *Activities of Medical Consultants*, Medical Department, United States Army in World War II (Washington, D.C.: Office of the Surgeon General, Department of the Army, 1961), pp. 1-4 and 231-32, and B. Noland Carter, ed., *Activities of Surgical Consultants*, Medical Department, United States Army in World War II, 2 vols. (Washington, D.C.: Office of the Surgeon General, Department of the Army, 1962-64), 2:1-5. For British consultants, see Crew, *AMS, Administration*, 1:136-45.

[29] Quotations from Middleton Interv, 1968-69, vol. 1, pp. 195-96, NLM. See also ibid., pp. 197-98 and 228-30; Havens, ed., *Medical Consultants*, pp. 232-34; Carter, ed., *Surgical Consultants*, 2:5-9, 19-21, 28; Larkey "Hist," ch. 3, pp. 54-59.

[30] First quotation from Hawley Interv, 1962, pp. 24-26, CMH. Second quotation from Verbatim Report of First Meeting of the Chief Surgeon's Consultants Committee, 16 Oct 42, in Professional Services Division, OofCSurg, HQ, ETOUSA, Annual Rpt. 1942. See also Carter, ed., *Surgical Consultants*, 2:6-8, 13-14, 22; Ltrs, Hawley to Hillman, 5 Feb 43, and Hawley to TSG, 28 Sep and 14 Oct 43, file HD 024 ETO O/CS (Hawley-SGO Corresp). The position of the consultants in the European Theater contrasted sharply with that in the Pacific. See Armfield, *Organization and Administration*, pp. 421-23.

The theater consultants involved themselves in most aspects of the medical service. Colonel Cutler's surgical consultants, free of other duty, were especially active. They visited each arriving medical unit; evaluated the professional qualifications of the staff; and recommended to the Personnel Division assignments and transfers, to make the best use of talents and to assure balanced strength in each hospital. Cutler and his staff reviewed the medical supply tables, eliminating superfluous or obsolete drugs and instruments, and put together a catalog of British and American supply equivalents. Late in 1942 Cutler discovered severe deficiencies in division surgical equipment and recommended supplementary issues, all of which could be made with items obtainable in England. The consultants performed research on surgical problems and oversaw the development of specialized treatment facilities and convalescent rehabilitation programs. They supervised professional training in the hospitals and advised and assisted in general medical unit training. They helped organize a theater blood collection and transfusion system, directed the introduction of penicillin into ETO medical practice, and devised a simplified patient record. Before the invasion the surgical consultants designed prototypes of a truck-mounted field surgical unit and a mobile X-ray unit. The medical consultants also evaluated personnel, inspected hospitals, and advised other divisions of the chief surgeon's office. Colonel Middleton held periodic conferences for the chiefs of medical service from all operating hospitals "in the interest of the coordination and consolidation of medical practice." [31]

As the ETO medical service expanded and the Services of Supply delegated operating responsibility to the base sections, General Hawley established a system of base section consultants in general surgery and medicine. He also arranged for the appointment of regional and later hospital center or group consultants in various special fields. Many of the base section consultants were theater senior consultants on additional duty; regional and center consultants usually were general hospital chiefs of service. These consultants, who worked under the base section surgeons but sent copies of all reports to the Professional Services Division, took on much of the task of supervising clinical practice in their areas of responsibility. The base section consultants also evaluated unit personnel and oversaw hospital operations and evaucation. In addition to these SOS consultants each field army headquarters had consultants in surgery, medicine, and neuropsychiatry, often personally selected by the army commander. The higher AAF headquarters also maintained its own group of consultants.[32]

---

[31] Professional Services Division, OofCS, HQ, ETOUSA, Annual Rpt, 1944, especially Medical Consultation Service sec.; Carter, ed., *Surgical Consultants*, 2:11–17 and 38–40; Havens, ed., *Medical Consultants*, pp. 241–45 and 266–70; Middleton Interv, 1968–69, vol. 1, p. 208, NLM.

[32] Base section surgeons selected their consultants, under guidance from the chief surgeon. Initially, the chief surgeon's office designated all regional consultants, but this procedure became too cumbersome and General Hawley in February 1944 delegated this task to the base section surgeons. See Professional Services Division, OofCSurg, HQ,

Continued

The Professional Services Division bound all these experts into a unified network (*Chart 4*). The division conducted weekly meetings for theater, base section, army, and air force consultants, at which the participants exchanged information and reached consensus on professional matters. General Hawley held similar monthly conferences with consultants from all commands. The chief surgeon encouraged consultants at every level to deal directly with each other on "purely professional" subjects, outside regular command and technical channels. Because "professional" matters were broadly defined in the ETO medical service, and because civilian reputation lent great weight among doctors to even informal suggestions from the senior consultants, these experts constituted, in effect, a separate medical line of communications into every major headquarters. According to Colonel Middleton, "You could, in a period of minutes by telephone . . . carry out any professional policy. One did not have to communicate through chains of military command. . . ." The effect, Middleton noted, "was centripetal . . . since General Hawley's office, through this medium, was constantly in touch with all medical echelons of the theater." [33]

In the two and a half years before D-Day General Hawley established effective central control over the potentially fragmented ETO medical service. His ascendency resulted in part from the success of General Lee's efforts to secure theater-wide logistics authority for the Services of Supply, but it also depended heavily on intangible personal elements. Longevity worked in Hawley's favor. Having been in England since late 1941, Hawley knew the country and its medical facilities better than any other senior American medical officer except possibly Grow; he had unmatched British official and professional contacts. Hawley worked hard at his job. He kept thoroughly informed about even minor details of his service's operations, and he spent as much time as he could visiting medical units and installations, especially favoring unannounced descents on hospitals. At the same time Hawley readily delegated responsibility to subordinates and won their firm personal loyalty even as he drove them hard. His consultants, and former members of his staff at other headquarters, provided him with an informal communication network covering most of the theater.[34]

ETOUSA, Annual Rpt, 1944, especially Chief Consultant in Surgery and Medical Consultation Service secs.; Carter, ed., *Surgical Consultants*, 2:118–21; Havens, ed., *Medical Consultants*, pp. 238–39. Col. J. B. Coates, in Editorial Advisory Board, 1962, pp. 85-90, describes the personality problems attending General Patton's choice of a Third Army surgical consultant.

[33] First quotation from Middleton Interv, 1968–69, vol. 1, pp. 197–98, NLM. Second quotation from Havens, ed., *Medical Consultants*, pp. 239-40. See also Professional Services Division, OofCSurg, HQ ETOUSA, Annual Rpts, 1943 and 1944.

[34] On Hawley's grasp of detail, see file Hawley Planning Directives, box 2, Hawley Papers, MHI, and Ltr, Hawley to Col Mack M. Green, MC, 11 May 44, file HD 024 ETO CS (Hawley Chron). For an example of an officer who went from Hawley's staff to SHAEF, see Davis Interv, 19 Jun 45, box 222, RG 112, NARA. For Hawley's effect on subordinates, see Middleton Interv, 1968–69, vol. 1, pp. 193–95, NLM, and Interv, Medical History Branch, CMH, with Brig Gen Sam F. Seeley, MC, 14 Aug 79 (hereafter cited as Seeley Interv, 1979), sess. 2, cassette 4, p. 2, HSF (Seeley–1979), Medics' War Ms, Accession no. 319–88–055, RG 319, NARA.

Always skilled in political maneuver, Hawley maintained profitable contacts with those above him in the chain of command. He kept on good terms with his imperious immediate superior, General Lee. "We gave on small things," he recalled, including agreement to Lee's pet project of using osteopaths in patient rehabilitation, "and always won our point on the large issues." Through correspondence and a brief Washington visit early in 1944, Hawley maintained close ties to Surgeon General Kirk. A more forceful administrator than his predecessor, Kirk gave Hawley all the support he could, although he noted: "This office doesn't have much to say about what happens in these theaters. We are told." Effective medical planning and control depended in the end on the theater chief surgeon. Hawley was equal to the task.[35]

[35] First and second quotations from copy of Ltr, Hawley to Col E. C. Cutler, 5 Jun 46, Misc Notes–ETO file, CMH. Third quotation from Ltr, TSG to Hawley, 3 Dec 43, file HD 024 ETO O/CS (Hawley-SGO Corresp); in same file, see Ltrs, Hawley to TSG, 4 Dec 43 and 20 Apr 44.

CHAPTER IV

Hospitalization and Evacuation

The ETO chief surgeon's largest, most complex task during the buildup was the establishment of a system of hospitals and a chain of evacuation in Great Britain. The system had to be capable both of supporting the expanding American Army in the British Isles and of receiving and treating mass casualties from the European battlefront. In a steadily more crowded island General Hawley, competing for manpower and materiel with other equally urgent projects, secured construction of more than 100 large hospital plants and moved staffs, furniture, and equipment into them. He worked through and alongside the military chain of command to link these plants into a unified, mutually supporting network of general and specialized patient care, and he sought to maintain within his hospitals the highest possible standards of military discipline and professional practice. At the same time Hawley forged hospitals and transportation—air, road, and rail—into an evacuation chain able to handle swiftly, yet gently, a steadily increasing flow of sick and wounded soldiers. He established a theater evacuation policy that attempted to balance patient welfare against ETO manpower needs and the availability of intratheater and transatlantic transportation.

Hospital Construction: The Final Drive

In early 1943 hospital construction was very nearly at a standstill. Initial BOLERO plans for establishment of over 90,000 beds in the United Kingdom to support a force of 1 million or more men had given way, under the impact of TORCH, to a program of about 40,000 beds, for a total theater strength of 427,000. Implementation of even this reduced program scarcely had begun. Only 4,900 of the projected beds were in operation; construction of the rest by the British Ministry of Works lagged far behind schedule. Hawley's pleas and exhortations to his sluggish Allies, as well as his suggestion that the available labor and materials be concentrated at a few of the most urgently needed plants instead of spread over all the projects, had produced few visible results. Fortunately, the theater troop buildup had fallen equally short of objectives, preventing a critical shortage of hospitals.[1]

[1] Hospitalization Division, OofCSurg, HQ, ETOUSA, Annual Rpt, 1943, p. 7; Larkey "Hist," ch. 7, pp. 17-18 and app. 1. Hawley's efforts to

Continued

British and American BOLERO planning resumed after the Casablanca conference. General Lee, even before that conference, ordered his SOS staff to start preparing supply and accommodation estimates for an army of 1.1 million. On 5 February he directed all staff sections to develop complete plans for this larger force. At about the same time, the London Combined Committee and its subcommittees reopened their discussions, which TORCH had interrupted. Work intensified in May, after TRIDENT, and culminated on 12 July with publication of a complete Fourth Key Plan. This plan, issued by the British War Office, provided for accommodation of 1.34 million American troops (later increased to over 1.4 million) in Great Britain by 30 April 1944. It governed the final buildup for invasion.[2]

The chief surgeon and his staff began hospital planning for the expanded force in January 1943. As he received each new projection of final ETO troop strength, Hawley calculated the number of hospital beds needed to support it, using a slightly modified version of his 1942 planning formula: 4 percent of the total strength, plus an additional 2 percent of black troops for sick and nonbattle injured; 1.5 percent of the air forces for aircrew wounded; and 7 percent of the ground forces for their battle casualties. Under this formula 1.1 million troops required about 90,600 fixed beds. As estimates of ultimate theater strength steadily increased during the first half of 1943, so did bed requirements, rising to 103,690 for the 1.34 million troops of the Fourth Key Plan. Early in June Hawley, in order to give the British definite goals for their construction planning, put a ceiling of 95,000 on the number of fixed beds to be procured in the United Kingdom. These, the chief surgeon estimated, would be enough to support the buildup and the first weeks of combat, after which additional hospitals could be established on the Continent.[3]

To provide the 95,000 required beds, Hawley and his staff revived their original BOLERO plan. They arranged to resume construction of the facilities—twelve 834-bed station hospitals, five 1,084-bed general hospitals, and thirty convertible troop camps—for which the Americans and British already had agreed on sites and plans but which had been deleted from the program in the late-1942 reduction. In general, the plant sizes and locations earlier specified required few alterations beyond adding a few station and general hospitals to serve the enlarged air force in East Anglia and new troop concentrations in Wales and extreme western England. During July, at the insistence of Surgeon General Kirk, Hawley substi-

---

speed British construction can be followed in Hospitalization Division O/CS Hospital Construction Correspondence, 18 May 42–31 May 43 (hereafter cited as HospDivConstCorresp, 1942–43), file HD 600.1 ETO (Construction). For a discussion of initial BOLERO plans, see Chapter II of this volume.

[2] For details of the renewed BOLERO planning, see Ruppenthal, *Logistical Support*, 1:115–17, 122–23, 240–43. The Fourth Key Plan essentially brought up to date the earlier plans.

[3] For the start of planning, see Memo, Col R. B. Lord to CQM, COrdOff, CSigOff, CSurg, CTransOff, 4 Feb 43, HospDivConstCorresp, 1942–43, file HD 600.1 ETO (Construction); Spruit Diary, 12 Feb 43; Hospitalization Division, OofCSurg, HQ, ETOUSA, Annual Rpt, 1943, pp. 7–8 and 13; Larkey "Hist," ch. 2, pp. 48–49; Hawley Planning Directive No. 1, 11 Jun 43, box 2, Hawley Papers, MHI.

tuted general hospital units for a number of station hospitals requisitioned for the theater. This change entailed no major alteration in construction because a British-built 834-bed plant, with minor additions to wards and staff quarters, could accommodate a 1,000-bed general hospital. To reduce his demands on scarce British construction labor and material, Hawley tried to secure existing EMS buildings, but to no avail. The Emergency Medical Services, hard-pressed to support British invasion forces, insisted on retaining thousands of empty beds for possible air raid casualties and offered only a few hospitals large enough or well-enough equipped for American use. It also tendered blocks of beds in hospitals it would continue to operate, but these Hawley summarily rejected. Except in the direst emergencies, he wanted only beds in plants entirely under U.S. control.[4]

Reflecting these negotiations and rearrangements, the Fourth Key Plan provided for 94,108 beds—14,896 of them in former British and EMS hospitals; 51,220 in newly constructed plants, mostly 834- and 1,084-bed; and 27,992 in convertible troop camps. The exact number, location, and types of hospitals continued to change almost until D-Day, in response to alterations in troop deployment and to delays and difficulties in construction. As the head of the Hospitalization Division, Col. Joseph R. Darnall, MC, put it, "The constant shuffling of work priorities, and of plans, made it necessary to build and rebuild our . . . program in a recurring administrative fog and on the shifting sands of uncertainty." Nevertheless, the broad outlines established in mid-1942 and reaffirmed in the Fourth Key Plan remained generally intact.[5]

Most of the over 100 plants eventually built or acquired under this program represented a few standard types. Commonest were the new 834-bed station and 1,084-bed general hospitals. Almost invariably consisting of semicylindrical metal Nissen huts on concrete foundations, each such installation sprawled over up to fifty acres of ground, often in the park of a country estate where the bleak military construction incongruously adjoined a medieval manor house or Georgian mansion. Convertible troop cantonments included British militia camps and dual-purpose camps. The militia camps consisted of hut barracks arranged in spider-like clusters radiating from a central core, as well as operating rooms, laboratories, and administration buildings constructed by the Ministry of Works on the parade grounds; the dual-purpose

[4] Ltrs, Hawley to Brig Gen H. McC. Snyder, 21 Jul 43, and Hawley to TSG, 21 Jul 43, file HD 024 ETO O/CS (Hawley-SGO Corresp); correspondence in HospDivConstCorresp, 1942–43, file HD 600.1 ETO (Construction); Memos, Hospitalization Division to Chief, Installations Branch, G–4, SOS, 24 May 43, and Hospitalization Division to DepCSurg, 14 Oct 43, Hospitalization Division O/CS General Correspondence file, 1943 (hereafter cited as HospDivGenCorresp, 1943), file HD 312 ETO; Hospitalization Division, OofCSurg, HQ, ETOUSA, Annual Rpt, 1943, p. 3; Larkey "Hist," ch. 2, pp. 50–51, and ch. 7, p. 20.

[5] Quotation from Joseph R. Darnall, "Hospitalization in the European Theater of Operations, U.S. Army, World War II," *The Military Surgeon* 103 (December 1948): 427–28. Colonel Darnall, a Regular Army medical officer since 1919, relieved Col. Eli E. Brown as head of the Hospitalization Division on 1 July 1943. The Fourth Key Plan is reproduced in Larkey "Hist," ch. 2, pp. 49–50.

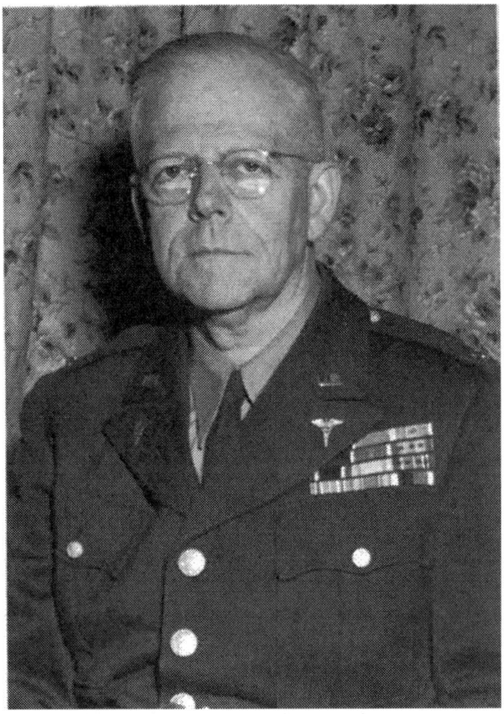

COL. JOSEPH R. DARNALL

camps, built of brick and cinder-block, contained all structures needed for general hospitals but doubled as housing for the troops until D-Day. In fact, none of the latter were completed before the invasion and only hospital units ever occupied them. Conversion camps, of Nissen-hut construction, were designed primarily as barracks and required the addition of operating rooms, clinics, and laboratories to become 750-bed station hospitals. Five American general hospitals occupied former EMS plants and used Nissen-hut additions to expand each permanent brick structure to a 1,000-bed capacity. Other American units took over British Army hospitals of various sizes, as well as converted barracks and schools, modern municipal hospitals in Bath and Liverpool, and the cavernous old Royal Victoria Hospital at Southampton, later turned over to the U.S. Navy. Many general and station hospitals were widely scattered to cover troop concentrations, ports, and airfields; other newly built general hospitals were grouped in previously planned centers around Cirencester, Great Malvern, and Whitchurch in the west of England.[6]

The layout and facilities of these Army hospitals, whether newly constructed or taken over from the British and remodeled, incorporated a series of compromises between American and British standards of design. General Hawley in May 1942 had agreed to allow the British to build his hospitals to their plans and specifications, with changes to meet particular American requirements. Because British standards of hospital accommodation were lower in many respects than American, and the Ministry of Works resisted alterations calling for additional labor and materials, each modification became the subject of hard bargaining. Results were mixed. The Americans won out on floor space per patient (72 square feet as opposed to the British 60), on enlarged bathing facilities, and on operating room design and equipment, among other issues. The British had their way on kitchens, on the omission of central heating, and on the location of nurses quarters. The Ameri-

[6] Hospitalization Division, OofCSurg, HQ, ETOUSA, Annual Rpt, 1943, pp. 2-3; Larkey "Hist," ch. 7, pp. 1-2, 5, 7; Darnall, "Hospitalization," pp. 427-30; Memo, Col J. H. McNinch to Surgs, Eastern and Southern Base Sections, 16 Nov 43, sub: Militia Camp Conversion, HospDivGenCorresp, 1943, file HD 312 ETO.

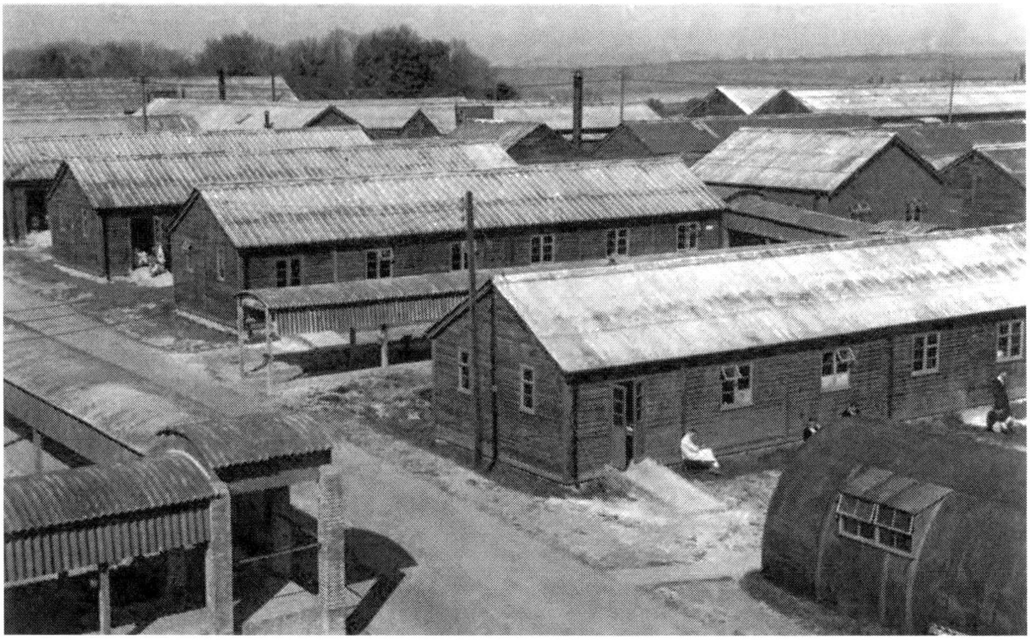

FOURTH KEY PLAN MEDICAL FACILITIES. *The British militia camp is typical of those converted into hospitals. One wing of the British Royal Victoria Hospital housed a U.S. Army general hospital.*

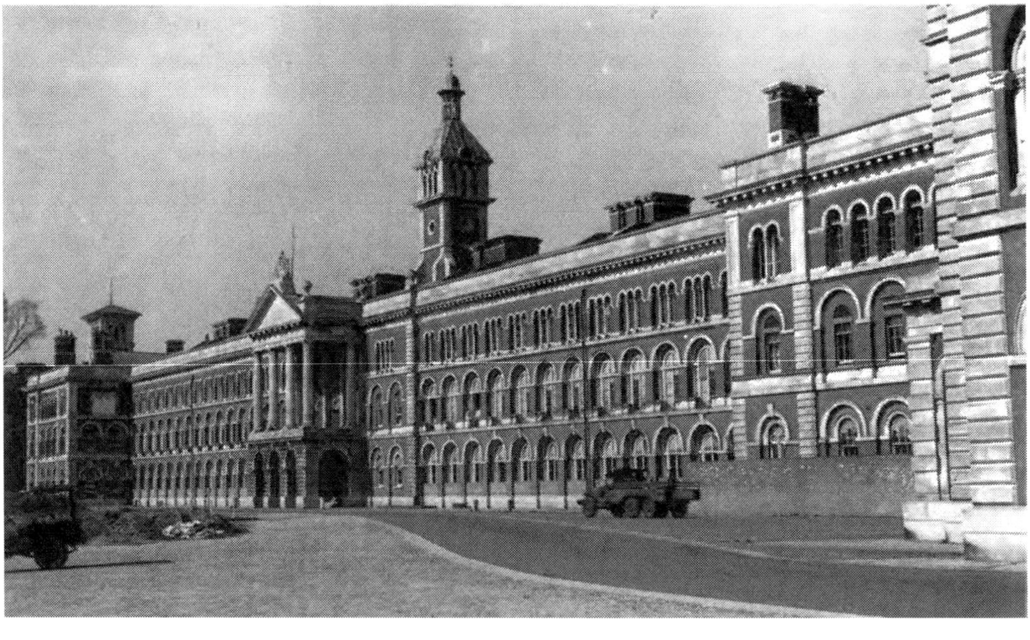

cans insisted upon and obtained dual 110- and 230-volt wiring systems, to accommodate both U.S. and British electrical equipment. They also secured flush toilets and sewage treatment plants. Hawley and his staff took pains to ensure ample, pure water for each hospital, either from a nearby municipal system or from a carefully tested and inspected stream. In spite of these improvements American hospital staffs still found their new facilities austere and in some ways primitive. They had to learn to use soft coal-burning stoves for heat and to adapt to what seemed to them scanty and spartan toilets and showers.[7]

The Hospitalization Division of General Hawley's office bore the main burden of securing plants of all types. As the division head, Colonel Darnall, put it, the process was "dubious—and often devious." All requests for new hospitals, after approval by General Lee and the ETO commander, went to the theater Engineers chief, who had charge of construction and quartering. The Engineers, in consultation with the British War Office and other ministries, the Hospitalization Division, and the appropriate base section surgeon, selected sites and arranged with the War Office for construction. The War Office then passed the project on to the Ministry of Works, which let the actual contract and supervised the job. Darnall's division, in close cooperation with the base sections, kept track of construction progress and notified the British, through the Engineers, which plants should have the highest priority. The entire process entailed almost daily conferences at Cheltenham and London, involving Hawley; Darnall; other division heads; the Engineers, both American and British; the theater G-4; and Ministry of Works representatives. "Conferences were not always in accord," Darnall recalled. "Confusion, in some degree, was seldom lacking and disagreement . . . was apt to be just around the corner." [8]

Most of the disagreements concerned construction delays, as the British failed to meet deadline after deadline. As had been the case since the start of the buildup, shortages of labor and materials caused the majority of these delays. Hospital construction, in contrast to any other type of BOLERO project, required not only a large number of workers (as many as 1,200 to finish an 834-bed station hospital in reasonable time) but also a higher proportion who were skilled artisans. These men, essential to build a hospital's many vital and complicated systems, were few and in high demand. Reports of delays in hospital completion repeatedly carried the notations "shortage of

[7] Interv, ETO with Maj Gen P. R. Hawley, 23 Mar 44 (hereafter cited as Hawley Interv, 1944), CMH; Larkey "Hist," ch. 7, pp. 3-6; Memo, Capt I. A. Marshall, MC, to Surg, Southern Base Section, 22 Feb 43, HospDivGenCorresp, 1943, file HD 312 ETO; Middleton Interv, 1968-69, vol. 1, p. 221, NLM.

[8] Quotations from Joseph R. Darnall, "Sidelights on the Hospital Program, European Theater of Operations," *The Military Surgeon* 104 (January 1949): 22. See also Hospitalization Division, OofCSurg, HQ, ETOUSA, Annual Rpt, 1943, pp. 2 and 19-20; Memo, Hospitalization Division to DepCSurg (Cheltenham), 28 Jun 43, HospDivGenCorresp, 1943, file HD 312 ETO; Hawley Planning Memo No. 1, 7 Feb 43, HospDivConstCorresp, 1942-43, file HD 600.1 ETO (Construction). The latter file contains examples of notifications of which plants should have priority.

plumbers and electricians" or "shortage of skilled labor." In competition for building material, whether furnished locally or shipped from the United States, hospitals had a low priority when compared, for example, to airfields. As construction went on, the Americans discovered innumerable small omissions or defects in British plans and demanded corrections. These corrections entailed use of more labor and material, and hence still more delay. Then, too, the other agencies, both British and American, through which the medical service had to work all faced conflicting demands on their own resources and had to set their own priorities, in which hospitals seldom ranked first. At times, only the personal intervention by Hawley—and, on occasion, Lee—kept the hospital program moving at all.[9]

Once a hospital was completed the British Army area command in which the plant was located appointed a "Taking Over Board" for it. This board, which included representatives of the War Office, the Ministry of Works, the theater chief surgeon's office, and the base section surgeon's office, examined the plant to ensure that it met plans and specifications and then either recommended acceptance or ordered the additional work needed to correct any deficiencies. After the base section surgeon, who had authority in the matter under the SOS decentralization plan, accepted the facility, the chief surgeon's office arranged for its occupation by a medical advance party of one officer and fifteen enlisted men. These troops guarded the plant until arrival of the hospital unit assigned to it. With the advance party on the premises, the British Army, as part of the reverse lend-lease supply arrangement, furnished and equipped the new hospital up to the standard for a comparable British unit. Hawley's Supply Division sent in additional material to bring the facility up to the higher American standard. In an effort to speed up this process Hawley, in August 1943, authorized the dispatch of advance parties and supplies to still incomplete hospitals where essential construction could be finished within three weeks of the initial party's arrival. At the same time he insisted that no hospital be formally accepted as complete until the facility was actually ready for a unit to occupy.[10]

After a similar inspection and approval process, American units took over existing British military hospi-

[9] Ltr, Brig R. A. Riddell to Hawley, 16 Jan 43; OofCEngr, ETOUSA, Constuction and Quartering Division Monthly Rpt, 31 Jan 43; Hawley Planning Memo No. 1, 7 Feb 43; Ltr (synopsis), Lee to CG, ETOUSA, 3 Mar 43, sub: Sites—VIII Air Force; Memo, Col E. E. Brown to CEngr, SOS, 10 Mar 43. All in HospDivConstCorresp, 1942–43, file HD 600.1 ETO (Construction). See also Darnall, "Hospitalization," p. 429; Hospitalization Division, OofCSurg, HQ, ETOUSA, Annual Rpts, 1943, p. 22, and 1944, encl. 4; Hawley Interv, 1944, CMH; Ruppenthal, *Logistical Support,* 1:246–47.

[10] Memo, Brown to CSurg, SOS, 22 May 43, sub: Current Policies and Procedures of the Hospitalization Division, in Hospitalization Division, OofCSurg, HQ, ETOUSA, Annual Rpt, 1943; Memos, Brown to DQMG(L), 12 May 43, sub: Advance Guards for Hospitals, Hospitalization Division to DepCSurg (Cheltenham), 28 Jun 43, Col P. D. Berrigan to Engrs of Southern, Western, and Eastern Base Sections, 14 Aug 43, sub: Minimum Hospital Facilities, all in HospDivGenCorresp, 1943, file HD 312 ETO; Memo, Hawley to Hospitalization Division, 1 Jun 43, and Ltr, Hawley to Col E. G. Plank, 2 Jan 43, both in HospDivConstCorresp, 1942–43, file 600.1 ETO (Construction). The latter file contains many examples of requests for advance parties and British supplies for new plants.

tals, complete with patients and equipment, by gradual infiltration. U.S. doctors and nurses, a few at a time, relieved British counterparts; the soldiers being treated remained, under American care, until recovery and discharge. New EMS plants, although usually empty of staff and patients, required complicated turnover transactions, because the Emergency Medical Services legally handed the facilities over, not to the Americans, but to the War Office. The latter, as an EMS tenant, then in effect sublet the plants to the U.S. Army. Three ministries—Health, Works, and the War Office—provided portions of the furnishings and equipment, creating bewildering accountability requirements.[11]

In spite of these elaborate turnover procedures, defects in design and workmanship in many of the hastily built hospitals annoyed staffs; hindered operations; and required expensive, time-consuming corrections. Many hospital units had to repaint poorly painted buildings. Most had to use their own personnel to complete roofs over outside walkways. Floors were a perpetual source of irritation. The Allies initially had planned to cover all hospital floors with linoleum to ensure a hard, smooth, easily cleaned surface—required both for good appearance and proper sanitation. Linoleum was in short supply, however, leaving many new plants with bare floors of poor-quality concrete, which the British contractors had put in in anticipation of another covering being laid on top of it. Often rough and not level, these floors crumbled under foot, creating large amounts of dust. They were impossible to keep clean, and the irregular surfaces damaged delicate equipment that was wheeled over them. Hawley pressed the British hard for suitable floor coverings. After unsuccessful experiments with various coatings, the Ministry of Works settled on pitch mastic, a synthetic black material, spread in liquid form, which congealed into a hard, smooth, waxable surface. While adequate, floors of this substance showed every scratch and dust particle, softened around hot stoves, and would not support heavy furniture unless it had wide pads under each leg. American doctors and nurses learned to live with pitch mastic floors but not to like them.[12]

Still other defects appeared. The new EMS hospital at Odstock, near Salisbury, one of the first turned over, had "tremendous difficulties" with roof leaks and water seepage. The 5th General Hospital, which moved from Belfast to Odstock in late 1942, found that the facility had neither heat nor running electricity and

[11] Memo, Brown to CSurg, SOS, 22 May 43, sub: Current Policies and Procedures of the Hospitalization Division, in Hospitalization Division, OofCSurg, HQ, ETOUSA, Annual Rpt, 1943. For an example of takeover arrangements, see Memo, Brown to Operations and Training Division, OofCSurg, 12 Feb 43, HospDivGenCorresp, 1943, file HD 312 ETO. Crew, *AMS, Administration*, 1:406–07, gives the British view of hospital turnovers.

[12] Hawley Operational Directives No. 16, 29 Jun 43, and No. 32, 6 Aug 43, box 2; Ltr, Hawley to Surg, Southern Base Section, 20 Sep 42, and Memo, Hawley to CEngr, SOS, 24 Jul 43, sub: Effects of Poor Walks in New Hospital Construction, box 3. All in Hawley Papers, MHI. HospDivGenCorresp, 1943, file HD 312 ETO, contains exhaustive coverage of floor and other problems. See also Darnall, "Sidelights," p. 22; Hawley Interv, 1962, p. 31, CMH; Col Lee D. Cady, MC, USAR, "Notes on the 21st General Hospital (AUS)," p. 570, Lee D. Cady Papers, MHI.

that the grounds were "just a mass of mounds and hummocks of building material and excavated dirt. . . ." At another EMS hospital the brick buildings began to settle and threatened to collapse on the 1,100 patients. Investigating, Colonel Darnall discovered that a coal mine had caved in 800 feet under the plant. Heavy shoring saved the building, allowing continued use of a badly needed facility. General Lee, inspecting a new 834-bed hospital near Cheltenham, smelled feces around one of the grease traps. An investigation revealed that the builders mistakenly had connected the sewer line to both the grease traps and the water pipes, contaminating the entire plumbing system.[13]

For all the delays and deficiencies, the construction program made impressive progress during 1943. By the end of the year the European Theater had fifty-eight fixed hospital plants open, with 41,131 beds in operation, about 20,000 of them occupied. Of the projected new construction, plants containing roughly half of the general hospital beds and all but 3,800 of the station hospital beds were completed.[14]

While the hospitals in service by the end of 1943 more than sufficed to care for the nonbattle sick and injured of the entire BOLERO force, the prospects for finishing by D-Day the additional 50,000 beds needed for battle casualties appeared much less promising. Shortages of construction labor and materials persisted and British authorities continued to relegate hospital construction to the lowest priority. As a result, ETO medical officers seriously doubted that the remaining station and general hospitals, not to mention the convertible troop camps, would be completed, as planned, by mid-May. Early in March 1944 the newly appointed SHAEF chief medical officer, General Kenner, estimated that, at the existing rate of progress, the theater would have only 61,000 of its projected 94,000 beds ready on D-Day.[15]

General Hawley, supported at SHAEF by Kenner, resorted to a number of expedients to bring more beds into service by the invasion deadline. The chief surgeon arranged for earlier removal of troops form militia and conversion camps to make way for constuction. He authorized base section surgeons to accept and open any hospital plant capable of functioning at any fraction of capacity. Hospital personnel and engineer troops augmented the overextended British labor force at most construction sites. Medical troops roofed outdoor walkways, poured concrete foundations, painted, laid brick, and even installed wiring and plumbing.[16]

[13] Quotations from Keeler Interv, 17 Jul 45, box 223, RG 112, NARA. See also Darnall, "Sidelights," pp. 23–24.

[14] Hospitalization Division, OofCSurg, HQ ETOUSA, Annual Rpt, 1943, pp. 1, 10–13, 15, 22; Hospitalization Division Bed Status Rpt, as of 31 Dec 43, HospDivGenCorresp, 1943, file HD 312 ETO.

[15] Memos, Kenner to CAdminOff, via ACofS, G–4, SHAEF, 8 Mar 44, and Kenner to ACofS, G–4, SHAEF, 13 Apr 44, in Medical Division, COSSAC/SHAEF, War Diary, March–April 1944. Kenner conferred frequently with Hawley on hospital construction problems. See ibid., February, March, and April 1944.

[16] Hospitalization Division, OofCSurg, HQ ETOUSA, Annual Rpt, 1944, p. 5 and encl. 4; Memo, Hawley to Gen Crawford, 4 Mar 44, file HD 024 ETO CS (Hawley Chron); Mins, 14th Meeting of Base Section Surgeons, 31 Jan 44, p. 10.

Continued

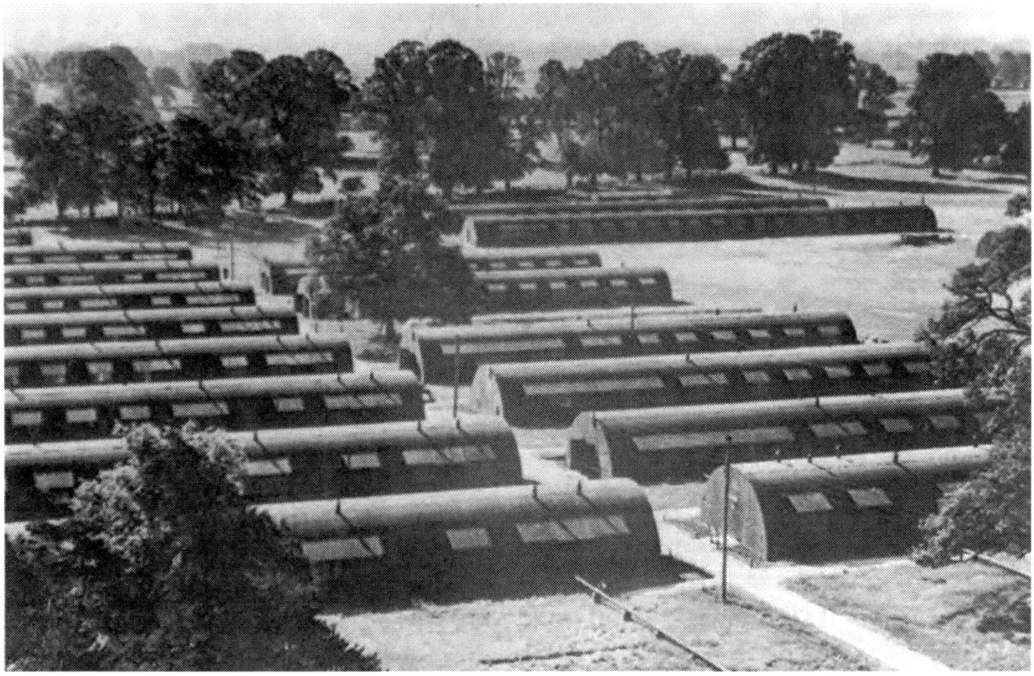

Nissen-Hut 834-Bed Station Hospital *and one of its medical wards*

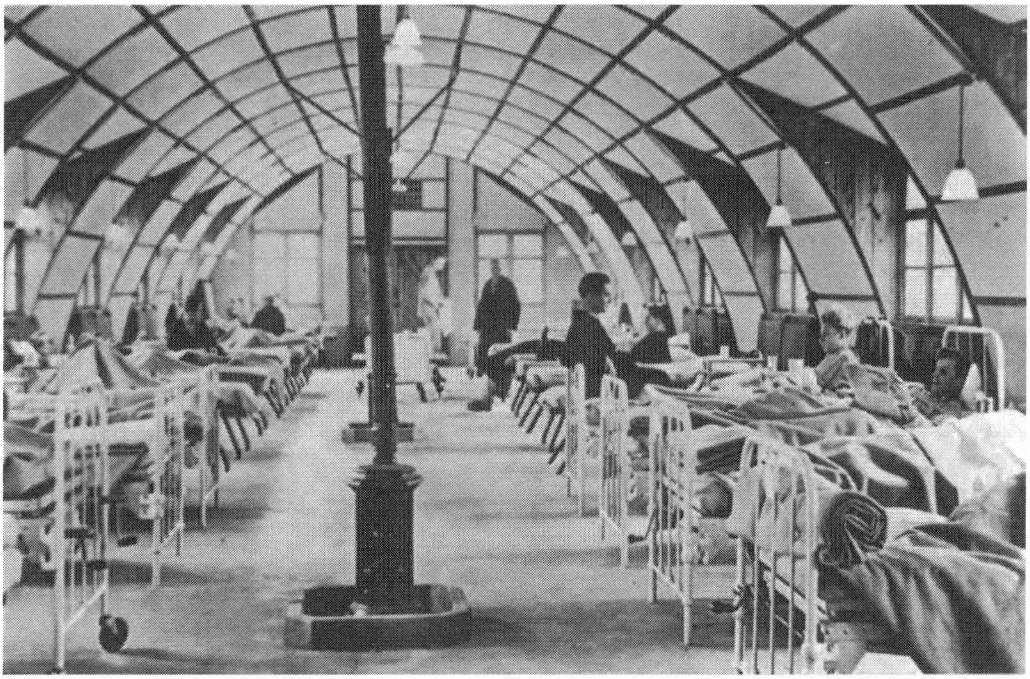

Abandoning his earlier opposition to fixed hospitals under canvas, Hawley directed the addition of tented expansion wards to most station and general hospitals. The chief surgeon had begun planning for this measure as early as July 1943, surveying each hospital to find out how many beds over its table-of-organization (T/O) capacity it could add without overtaxing its operating rooms, messes, and lavatories. The tents, preferably erected at the rear of each hut ward, were to have concrete floors, stoves, and insulation against winter cold. To protect the overall BOLERO program, Hawley secured British concurrence that such enlargements were a supplement to—not a replacement for—the planned beds in semipermanent buildings. Construction of the tented additions began in December and continued through the eve of the invasion, with the British War Office and the U.S. Army Engineers furnishing material and the hospitals providing labor. Despite delays in securing British consent for the necessary grading at the sites and the slow arrival of supplies, hospital units put almost 25,000 expansion beds into operation before D-Day, in annexes to hutted wards and in three complete tented 750-bed station hospitals. By this means, most 1,084-bed general hospitals in the United Kingdom increased their capacity to between 1,100 and 1,500 beds; many 834-bed station hospitals (often occupied by 1,000-bed general hospital units) made room for up to 1,300 patients.[17]

On 6 June 1944, as a result of this accelerated effort, the European Theater of Operations had over 84,000 fixed hospital beds ready to receive patients, only 26,000 of them in use. These beds included about 59,000 in regular BOLERO installations plus the 25,000 in tented expansions. The first militia, conversion, and dual-purpose camps became available for occupancy in mid-May, with the rest following in June and July. With these, and the gradual completion of other planned installations, Generals Kenner and Hawley could count on having enough hospital space for the casualties of each stage of the projected campaign. Although by a narrow margin, the BOLERO hospital construction program had reached its goal.[18]

and 19th Meeting of Base Section Surgeons, 10 Apr 44, p. 1, file HD 337; Surg, Western Base Section, Rpt, 1 Jan–31 Aug 44, p. 10.

[17] Larkey "Hist," ch. 7, pp. 25 and 27–29; Hospitalization Division, OofCSurg, HQ, ETOUSA, Annual Rpt, 1944, pp. 5–6; Ltr, Hawley to TSG, 13 Dec 43, HD 024 ETO O/CS (Hawley-SGO Corresp); Ltrs, Hawley to Base Section Surgs, 5 Jan 44, sub: Preparation for Expansion of Hospitals, and Hawley to CO, Eastern Base Section, 23 Feb 44, HD 024 ETO CS (Hawley Chron); Memo, McNinch to Base Section Cdrs, 6 Jul 43, sub: Expansion of Existing Hospitals, and Ltr, McNinch to Surgs, Eastern, Western, and Southern Base Sections, 2 Dec 43, sub: Preparation for Tented Expansion, both in HospDivGenCorresp, 1943, file HD 312 ETO; Mins, 16th, 17th, 18th, 20th, and 22d Meetings of Base Section Surgeons, respectively 28 Feb, 13 Mar, 27 Mar, 24 Apr, and 22 May 44, file HD 337.

[18] Larkey "Hist," ch. 7, pp. 27–29; Memo, Kenner to ACofS, G–4, SHAEF, 5 Jun 44, in Medical Division, COSSAC/SHAEF, War Diary, June 1944; Mins, 23d Meeting of Base Section Surgeons, 5 Jun 44, pp. 1–2 and 4, file HD 337. In addition to these fixed beds, large numbers of beds in tactical units were available as transit, holding, and other special-purpose hospitals. See Chapter VI of this volume for details of their activities.

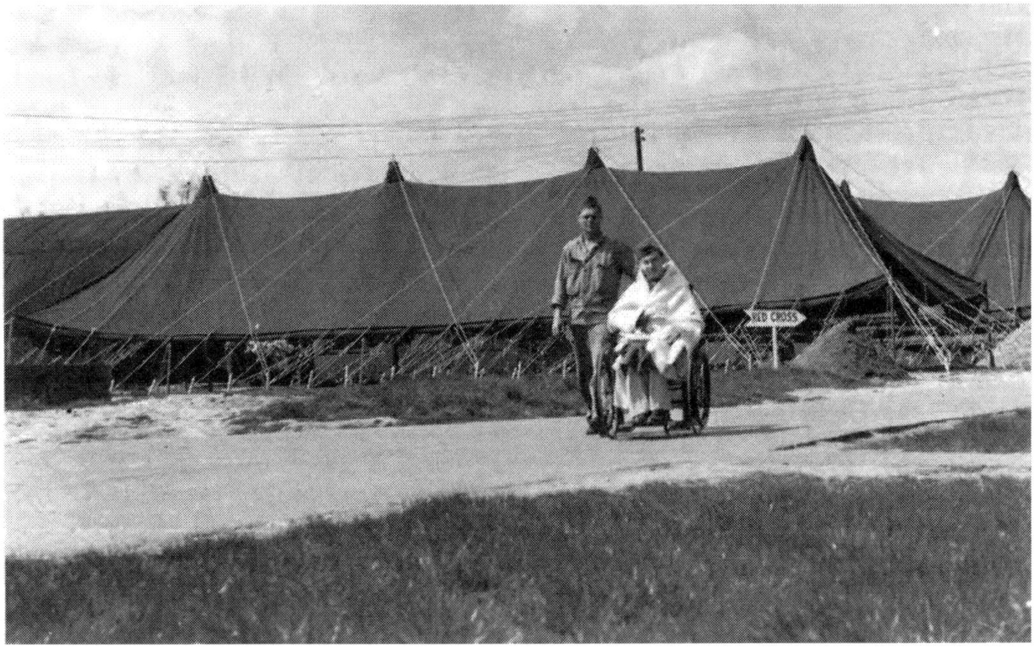

TENTED EXPANSION WARDS. *Note the adjoining Nissen hut (far left).*

Organizing a Hospital System

In the months before D-Day the ETO medical service organized its separate plants into a unified hospital system that could enforce uniform professional standards and ensure efficient handling of casualties. In cooperation with the base sections, it refined the hospitals' military and technical chains of command; redistributed both personnel and functions among hospitals so as to employ most effectively scarce medical and surgical specialists; concentrated patients requiring difficult, long-term care at selected specialized facilities; and, to free beds for the more severely ill and injured as well as to facilitate the recovery of soldiers on the mend, established a network of convalescent rehabilitation and reconditioning camps.

The seventy-five fixed SOS hospitals in operation on D-Day answered to a number of authorities. They were under the military command of the base sections. At the same time they received technical direction—which in fact covered most of their activities—from the Hospitalization and Professional Services Divisions of the chief surgeon's office. The Hospitalization Division issued instructions on all nonclinical aspects of hospital operations. Its directives, enforced by quarterly and, for delinquent units, monthly inspections, dealt with supply, general administration, staff military training and discipline, and disaster plans, among many other matters. The divisions' inspectors, reflecting General Hawley's soldierly approach to military medicine, emphasized the minutia of military courtesy and appearance. To hospital staffs, especially veteran ones from the Mediterranean Theater, the frequent inspections and many spit-and-polish requirements seemed like "unnecessary show and 'play-war' procedures." Medical people searching in haste for shined shoes, with an inspector at the gate, coined a new name for the ETO: "European Theater of Inspections."[19]

To regulate medical and surgical practice, the Professional Services Division drafted and enforced directives on treatment procedures and on the use of drugs and surgical techniques. Its network of senior, base section, and regional consultants, besides advising hospital staffs on particular cases, also supervised the general conduct of their specialties and saw to it that deficiencies were corrected. Colonel Cutler, the chief surgical consultant, enjoined his base section surgical consultants to "keep familiar with the level of professional work . . . at all hospitals in your base section. This means constant personal visits. Written directions . . . can never take the part of the influence of a real surgeon at the bedside of the patient." Cutler's medical counterpart, Colonel Middleton, declared that he "made medical rounds each time I went into a hospital and that was with my stethoscope and not with the white gloves and towel. So that I knew what medicine was doing." Supplementing the efforts of his consultants, General Hawley kept in close touch with hospital operations through informal contacts, as well as his own often unannounced visits, and through reports. He exhorted, and occasionally threatened, his base section surgeons and individual hospital commanders in an effort to enforce his principle that "there is nothing satisfactory in a hospital here except 'superior.' "[20]

To simplify control of the largest geographical clusters of general hospitals, the chief surgeon in 1944 activated three hospital centers (*Map 3*). These were regular T/O medical units,[21] each designed to coordinate and assist the work of a variable number of general hospitals. Two of these units, the 12th and 15th Hospital Centers, arrived in Britain during March. General Hawley in early June

[19]The base section surgeons actually did the inspecting, using men trained by the Hospitalization Division and working under its guidelines. See Darnall, "Hospitalization," p. 431; Hospitalization Division, OofCSurg, HQ, ETOUSA, Annual Rpts, 1943, pp. 1 and 14–17, and 1944, pp. 1–2; Cir Ltr No. 80, OofCSurg, HQ, ETOUSA, 10 Jun 44, sub: Policies and Procedures Governing Care of Patients in ETO, ex. M, which digests earlier policy directives; Ltrs, McNinch to Surgs, Eastern, Western, and Southern Base Sections, 6 Sep 43, sub: Inspection Reports of Fixed Hospitals and General Dispensaries, and McNinch to Surg, Western Base Section, 22 Sep 43, same sub, HospDivGenCorresp, 1943, file HD 312 ETO. For complaints about spit-and-polish, see Max S. Allen, ed., *Medicine Under Canvas: A War Journal of the 77th Evacuation Hospital* (Kansas City, Mo., 1949), pp. 96–97. Quotation from latter source.

[20]Cutler quotation from Professional Services Division, OofCSurg, HQ, ETOUSA, Annual Rpt, 1944, Chief Consultant in Surgery sec., pp. 1–2. Middleton quotation from Middleton Interv, 1968–69, vol. 2, p. 209, NLM. Hawley's remark from Mins, 21st Meeting of Base Section Surgeons, 8 May 44, p. 10, file HD 337. See also Professional Services Division, OofCSurg, HQ, ETOUSA, Annual Rpt, 1943. General Hawley's relationship to his hospitals can be followed in file HD 024 ETO CS (Hawley Chron), file HD 024 ETO O/CS (Hawley-SGO Corresp), file HD 024 ETO O/CS (Spruit Policy Notebook), and Hawley Operational and Planning Directives, box 2, Hawley Papers, MHI.

[21]Each included some 30 medical officers and 230 enlisted men in a headquarters and service company, a convalescent camp, and a laboratory.

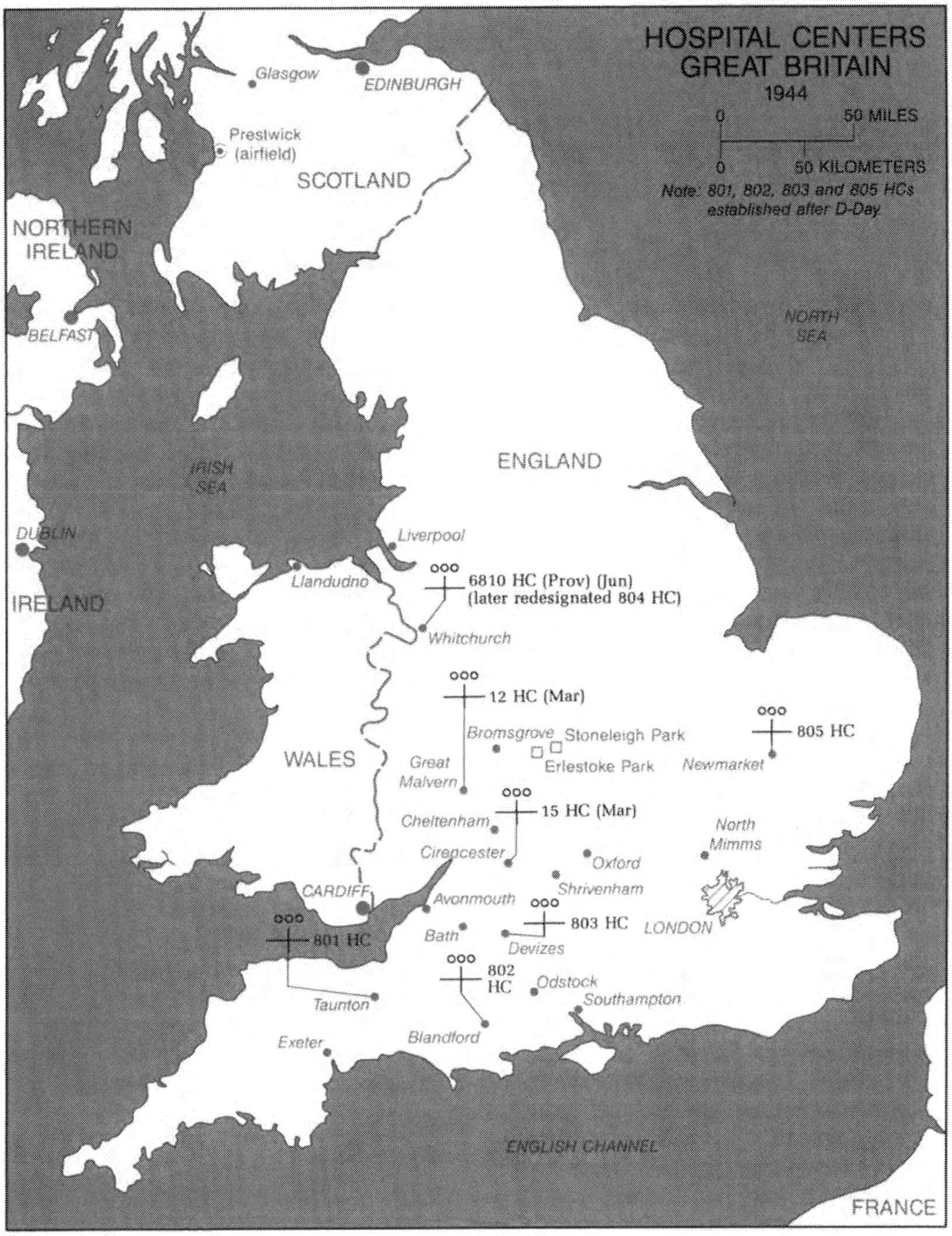
HOSPITAL CENTERS
GREAT BRITAIN
1944
0
50 MILES
0
50 KILOMETERS
Note: 801, 802, 803 and 805 HCs established after D-Day.
Glasgow
EDINBURGH
Prestwick (airfield)
SCOTLAND
NORTHERN IRELAND
BELFAST
NORTH SEA
IRISH SEA
ENGLAND
DUBLIN
IRELAND
Liverpool
Llandudno
6810 HC (Prov) (Jun) (later redesignated 804 HC)
Whitchurch
12 HC (Mar)
Bromsgrove
Stoneleigh Park
805 HC
WALES
Great Malvern
Erlestoke Park
Newmarket
15 HC (Mar)
Cheltenham
North Mimms
Cirencester
Oxford
Shrivenham
CARDIFF
Avonmouth
803 HC
LONDON
801 HC
Bath
Devizes
802 HC
Odstock
Southampton
Taunton
Exeter
Blandford
ENGLISH CHANNEL
FRANCE

MAP 3

activated a third, the 6810th Hospital Center (Provisional), from personnel in the theater. The 12th and 15th Hospital Centers established themselves respectively at Great Malvern and Cirencester in the Western Base Section, to control the hospitals, clustered around those two places. The 6810th set up at Whitchurch, also in western Britain, the center of a third group of general hospitals.

At the outset the exact functions of these centers were uncertain. Hospital centers had existed in the American Expeditionary Forces in World War I, but few ETO medical officers had had any experience with their operations. The table of organization provided only that each center was to coordinate hospital administration and to establish a supply depot and convalescent camp. When the 12th and 15th Hospital Centers began setting up in May, after a period of orientation, they found no plans or standard operating procedures (SOP) to guide them. Col. Asa M. Lehman, MC, the 12th Hospital Center commander, drafted an SOP of his own, which General Hawley adopted and published on 5 May as an SOS directive. Under this directive a hospital center would "act as Headquarters for a group of general hospitals; to correlate and coordinate their activities, to relieve them insofar as possible from administrative details and supply problems; to supervise evacuation and reception of patients[;] and by frequent inspections, [to] aid and assist them in maintaining the highest possible degree of professional, administrative and training excellence." Each center would maintain a central supply depot upon which its hospitals could draw, thereby eliminating the need for the individual hospital to deal with base sections and SOS depots. Center receiving and evacuation officers would oversee all movement of patients into and out of the attached hospitals, as well as select patients for evacuation to the United States. Center commanders would monitor professional activities in their hospitals, and they could designate hospitals to specialize in particular types of cases. Beyond these prescribed functions, Hawley's directive encouraged center commanders to adopt any expedient for pooling hospital resources and for freeing the operating units from administrative chores. Hospital centers constituted an intermediate headquarters between the base section and the individual hospital. Hawley told base section surgeons: "You can use these center commanders and it will cut down your work." [22]

By mid-June the 12th and 15th Hospital Centers each had seven general hospitals attached, and each center controlled (with tented expansion of many plants) about 9,500 beds. For the most part, the centers performed the administration, supply, and evacuation functions specified in the 5 May directive. Center commanders tried to keep out of the internal administration and practices of their hospitals, playing the role of helpers rather than inspectors, but

[22] First quotation from Admin Memo No. 63, OofCSurg, HQ, ETOUSA, 5 May 44, sub: Operation of Hospital Centers, ETO, in Hospitalization Division, OofCSurg, HQ, ETOUSA, Annual Rpt, 1944. Second quotation from Mins, 21st Meeting of Base Section Surgeons, 8 May 44, pp. 3-4, file HD 337. See also 12th and 15th Hospital Centers Annual Rpts, 1944.

they gradually established many uniform procedures. They also became involved in efforts to balance professional staffs. According to Colonel Lehman of the 12th, most of his general hospitals displayed a "tendency toward internal specialization." One hospital "might have a surplus of capable surgeons, but be entirely wanting of an officer . . . competent . . . as chief of medical service. In contrast, another hospital would be overstaffed with exceptional medical service personnel, the surplus being used in positions for which they had no special qualifications." To build up weak services, Lehman transferred doctors temporarily between hospitals; he arranged with the base sections and the chief surgeon's office for permanent reassignments if the changes proved beneficial. The center headquarters soon found that they needed less than one-third of their assigned personnel for administration; they used their extra medical and dental officers to reinforce hospital staffs and their extra enlisted men to aid in patient rehabilitation. Even before the invasion, hospital centers were proving effective in simplifying control over the many plants. Their value in coordinating evacuation would become apparent as soon as trainloads of wounded from France began moving inland from the Channel ports.[23]

A network of specialized hospitals took shape. During 1943 General Hawley designated certain general and station hospitals to receive severe cases of particular types from other hospitals. The 36th Station Hospital at Exeter, for example, became the theater's treatment center of psychotics and men with other noncombat-related mental disorders; the 5th General Hospital, in addition to its normal functions, established special facilities for care of soldiers suffering from combat fatigue. Other general hospitals set up facilities for burns and cold injury. Under an arrangement with the ETO medical service, a British facility, Saint Dunstan's Institute for the Blind, began the retraining and rehabilitation process for American servicemen who had lost their sight prior to evacuation to the United States. In 1944 each hospital center arranged to concentrate burn treatment, neurosurgery, and thoracic, urological, plastic, and maxillofacial surgery at one or two of its attached hospitals. At the same time General Hawley, on the advice of his senior consultants, designated nine hospitals not attached to centers as specialized neurosurgical facilities and seven hospitals for plastic and maxillofacial surgery and burns. Station and general hospitals were to transfer to these installations any patient whose condition, in the hospital commander's judgment, required unusually complicated or lengthy treatment. Specialized-care hospitals made efficient use of scarce medical and surgical talent and eased the burden of difficult cases upon general-care hospitals. The consultants, however, constantly had to combat the tendency of hospital commanders to treat those patients who would fare better if dis-

[23] Quotations from 12th Hospital Center Annual Rpt, 1944, p. 29 (see pp. 1, 27–32, 40). See also 15th Hospital Center Annual Rpt, 1944; Interv, OSG with Maj Oliver J. Irish, SC, 13 Oct 44, box 220, RG 112, NARA.

patched immediately for specialized care.[24]

The medical service specialized institutions included a growing number dedicated to rehabilitating and reconditioning convalescents. Creation of these facilities owed much to the work of Col. Rex L. Diveley, MC, senior consultant in orthopedic surgery. In the early days of the buildup Diveley was impressed by the effectiveness of the convalescent rehabilitation system the British Army, Royal Air Force, and Royal Navy had established as a result of their wartime experience. British medical officers learned early in the conflict that carefully controlled and gradually intensified mental and physical training, begun while the patient was still in bed and culminating in hiking, drill, and general military instruction at special reconditioning camps, would speed a soldier's recovery from wounds or illness. Such training also reduced the formerly high rate of hospital readmissions among casualties newly returned to duty.

Diveley persuaded General Hawley to organize a similar program for the European Theater. Hawley, in turn, secured the support of General Lee, although at the cost of including in the program osteopaths and manipulative therapy, in which Lee had great faith but the chief surgeon did not. While the employment of osteopaths was still under discussion, Diveley, on 19 April 1943, opened Rehabilitation Center Number 1 at All Saints' Hospital, Bromsgrove, Worcestershire. The 150-bed 16th Station Hospital constituted the medical staff of this institution, reinforced by five medical officers and six enlisted men trained in British convalescent depots. The Bromsgrove facility received ambulatory convalescents from station and general hospitals and put them through remedial exercises and general physical conditioning. It contained over 400 patients by 1 September.[25]

With Diveley informally in charge in addition to his consultant duties, rehabilitation expanded rapidly during late 1943 and early 1944. As activities rapidly outgrew the Bromsgrove plant, Diveley acquired a general hospital site at Stoneleigh Park, Warwickshire, for a second and larger branch of Rehabilitation Center Number 1. Opened on 5 October, this facility housed over 1,700 officer and enlisted trainees by the end of the year. In February 1944 the medi-

[24] Cir Ltr No. 113, OofCSurg, HQ, ETOUSA, 24 Jul 43, sub: Hospitalization and Disposition of Neuropsychiatric Patients, file HD 024 ETO O/CS (Operational and Planning Directives); Hospitalization Division, OofCSurg, HQ, ETOUSA, Annual Rpt, 1942, p. 6; Operations Division, OofCSurg, HQ, ETOUSA, Annual Rpt, 1943; Memo, Col O. H. Stanley, MC, to General Hospitals, 3 Dec 42, file ETO 700.1 (MiscMedSvc); Ltr, Hillman to Hawley, 26 Jan 43, file HD 024 ETO O/CS (Hawley-SGO Corresp); Memo, Hawley to DepCSurg (Cheltenham), 16 Dec 43, file HD 024 ETO O/CS (Spruit Policy Notebook); Professional Services Division, OofCSurg, HQ, ETOUSA, Annual Rpt, 1944, pp. 7–8 and Chief Consultant in Neurosurgery sec., pp. 1–2, which comments on the tendency of general-care hospitals to retain patients needing specialized-care facilities.

[25] For the British program, see Crew, *AMS, Administration,* 1:433–38; Rehabilitation Division, OofCSurg, HQ, ETOUSA, Annual Rpt, 1944, pp. 1–2; Mins, 3d Conference of Chiefs of Medical Services, HQ, SOS, 26 Jan and 4 Feb 44, ex. A, Medical Consultation Service sec., Professional Services Division, OofCSurg, HQ, ETOUSA, Annual Rpt, 1944. For the osteopath issue, see file HD 024 ETO O/CS (Hawley-SGO Corresp) and file HD 024 ETO CS (Hawley Chron) for 1943–44. For a description of the program, see Interv, OSG with Capt. F. E. LeBaron, MC, 4 Sep 44, box 220, RG 112, NARA.

cal service designated Bromsgrove as a separate rehabilitation facility for officers, using Stoneleigh exclusively for enlisted men, and also established a new camp at Erlestoke Park, Wiltshire, a general hospital site, for convalescents who required only ordinary exercise and military training—reconditioning—to make them fit for duty. Patients needing special remedial exercise as well continued to go to Bromsgrove, if officers, or to Stoneleigh. To staff these facilities, the chief surgeon assigned 750-bed station hospitals reinforced with officer and enlisted casuals. By D-Day two station hospitals were so employed, the 307th at Stoneleigh and the 77th, split between Bromsgrove and Erlestoke. The chief surgeon extended convalescent reconditioning into station and general hospitals. He instructed the commander of each to appoint a rehabilitation officer and set up a training program, similar to those in the centers, for patients who needed only a short recovery period before return to duty. In spite of extensive promotional and training efforts by Hawley and his staff, however, implementation of this part of the program went slowly before D-Day, due to the unfamiliarity of medical officers with this approach to convalescent care and to the skepticism of many about its value.[26]

Although slow to take hold in the hospitals, the new rehabilitation methods were proving their effectiveness by the end of 1943. By that time over 3,000 officers and men had been admitted to Bromsgrove and Stoneleigh, about 80 percent of them orthopedic patients and the rest evenly divided between general surgical and medical. Of 1,800 men discharged from the centers, 83 percent went back to duty, while 17 percent had to return to hospitals for additional treatment. Surgeon General Kirk, when informed about the program, questioned whether the medical service should be involved in an effort some phases of which looked like basic infantry training, but General Hawley strongly defended rehabilitation and expressed satisfaction with its results. He pointed out that the program reduced patients' hospital convalescence by an average of two or three weeks and that it revived the self-confidence and military spirit of men long confined to bed. In recognition of the value and importance of the program, Hawley on 3 June 1944 established the Rehabilitation Division in his office under Colonel Diveley, now relieved of duty as orthopedic consultant. Diveley and a small staff at once began negotiating for still more facilities and planning for post-invasion expansion.[27]

[26] Rehabilitation Division, OofCSurg, HQ, ETOUSA, Annual Rpt, 1944, pp. 2–9, and, in ibid., Admin Memo No. 68, OofCSurg, HQ, ETOUSA, 12 May 44; Operations Division, OofCSurg, HQ, ETOUSA, Annual Rpt, 1943, pp. 17 and 20–21; Mins, 13th, 14th, and 22d Meetings of Base Section Surgeons, respectively 17 Jan, 31 Jan, and 22 May 44, file HD 337. The 16th Station Hospital left Bromsgrove for London in September 1943 and was replaced temporarily by the 8th Convalescent Hospital, a field army unit, which in turn was replaced in December by the 307th Station Hospital. In each change, most of the personnel at Bromsgrove remained there.

[27] Statistics from Carter, ed., *Surgical Consultants*, 2:495. For different figures, but in roughly the same proportions, see Mins, 3d Conference of Chiefs of Medical Services, HQ, SOS, 26 Jan and 4 Feb 44, ex. A, Medical Consultation Service sec., Professional Services Division, OofCSurg, HQ, ETOUSA,

Continued

The Flow of Patients

Besides establishing hospitals, the chief surgeon laid down policies governing the flow of sick and wounded men from units and their movement through the medical system to ultimate return to duty or departure from the theater. Within his office responsibility for evacuation shifted repeatedly among the Hospitalization and Operations Divisions and a short-lived Evacuation Division. Eventually, in February 1944, the latter organization became a branch of the Operations Division, which oversaw evacuation throughout the remaining life of the theater. Throughout these alterations the same people, for the most part, remained on the job; for example, the Evacuation Division chief, Lt. Col. Fred H. Mowrey, MC, continued in office when his division became a branch. Actual conduct of evacuation was divided between the base section surgeons and General Hawley's office. The section surgeons, under Hawley's technical guidance, controlled all patient movement within their sections. The chief surgeon's office directly managed all transfers to general hospitals and between base sections, as well as all evacuation to the United States.[28]

For the sick and injured of units in garrison and training, and for wounded Eighth Air Force bomber crewmen, hospitalization and evacuation followed the outlines established by the first SPOBS medical officer, Major Welsh. In all air, ground, and SOS commands, sick and injured men who required less than 4 days of hospitalization went to dispensaries operated by unit medical personnel. Patterned after those of the British Army, the dispensaries provided practical training for doctors and aidmen and, by keeping minor casualties out of the hospitals and replacement system, reduced the length of time men were lost to their organizations. Unit surgeons sent more serious cases to station hospitals, each of which served all troops in its geographical area and could keep patients for up to 30 days. Typically, a division would evacuate to a single station hospital. General hospitals were supposed to receive from station hospitals patients who required more than 30 days of treatment or specialized care. In fact, during the buildup, many general hospitals acted as station hospitals for neighboring units, while at times station hospitals performed general hospital work. Early in 1944, to free general hospital beds for battle casualties, General Hawley authorized station hospitals to hold patients for up to 60 days. He also authorized five specially

Annual Rpt, 1944. General Kirk's concern resulted from seeing a color film produced by Diveley's staff. See Ltrs, Kirk and Hawley, 3 Nov 43, and Hawley to Kirk, 13 and 26 Nov 43, file HD 024 ETO O/CS (Hawley-SGO Corresp). See also Rehabilitation Division, OofCSurg, HQ, ETOUSA, Annual Rpt, 1944, pp. 8–9. In addition to the rehabilitation system, there was a separate set of convalescent homes, one each for officers, nurses, and enlisted men, run by the Hospitalization Division in cooperation with the Red Cross. Designed for people who required only short periods of rest before returning to duty, these homes were not part of the rehabilitation/reconditioning system and provided no systematic physical training. See Hospitalization Division, OofCSurg, HQ, ETOUSA, Annual Rpt, 1944.

[28] Evacuation Division, OofCSurg, HQ, ETOUSA, Annual Rpt, 1943, p. 1 and an. A; Surg, Eastern Base Section, Annual Rpt, 1943, p. 3; Surg, Southern Base Section, Annual Rpt, 1943, p. 11; Surg, Northern Ireland Base Section, Annual Rpt, 1943, p. 2.

reinforced and equipped station hospitals, which treated Eighth Air Force sick and wounded, to retain men for 180 days—in effect to function as general hospitals.[29]

During 1942, with few U.S. hospitals in operation, ETO units often evacuated sick and injured troops to nearby British Army, Royal Navy, Royal Air Force, or EMS institutions, in that order of preference. These British hospitals treated Americans under agreements made early in 1942 by Major Welsh and reconfirmed by Hawley. The sending of American patients to Allied hospitals gradually ceased during 1943, as more U.S. Army facilities opened. Periodically, the Office of the Chief Surgeon informed base section surgeons how many Americans were in British hospitals in their areas and directed transfer of these men, as soon as their condition allowed, to U.S. Army installations.[30]

[29] Admin Order No. 1, HQ, SOS, August 1942, an. E, file ETO 700.1 (MiscMedSvc); Memo, Lt Col G. D. Newton to CSurg, SOS, ETO, 9 Dec 42, sub: Policies Affecting Hospitalization, file HD 312 (HospDivChronCorresp, 1942); Ltr, Hawley to TSG, 29 Apr 42, file HD 024 ETO O/CS (Hawley-SGO Corresp); Cir Ltr No. 70, OofCSurg, HQ, ETOUSA, 15 May 44. For examples of overlapping hospital functions, see 5th General Hospital Annual Rpt, 1944, p. 2; 168th Station Hospital Annual Rpt, 1944, p. 4; Interv, OSG with Maj Ralph Soto-Hall, MC, 30th General Hospital, 24 Apr 44, box 219, RG 112, NARA.

[30] Memo, Brown to Surgs of All Units . . . , 26 Jul 42, sub: Tentative Instructions Regarding Hospitalization of U.S. Forces in Great Britain, in Hospitalization Division, OofCSurg, HQ, ETOUSA, Annual Rpt, 1942. For examples of transfer directives, see Ltrs, Brown to Surg, Southern Base Section, copy to Surg, Eastern Base Section, 25 Jan 43, and Brown to Surgs, Eastern and Southern Base Sections, 10 Mar 43, sub: Hospitalization in Other Than U.S. Hospitals, in HospDivGenCorresp, 1943, file HD 312 ETO.

The 700-square mile London metropolitan area, organized in April 1943 as the Central Base Section, posed special hospitalization and evacuation problems with its numerous headquarters and service units, many of which lacked organic medical personnel, and with its constantly large transient population of soldiers on leave or temporary assignment. During 1943 and 1944 two general dispensaries—the 7th and 10th—provided outpatient care for casuals and people from units lacking medical detachments and dispensaries. The general and unit dispensaries evacuated all enlisted men who needed hospital treatment directly to the 1st General Hospital at North Mimms, an hour away from London by ambulance. Officer patients went from the dispensaries to the 16th Station Hospital, a 150-bed unit installed in a former British civilian plant and reinforced with extra staff and equipment to make it a "show-place" for its patients, many of whom were of high rank. The 16th evacuated officers needing long-term or specialized care to the 91st General Hospital at Oxford, a three-hour ambulance ride from the capital.[31]

During late 1942 and early 1943 the ETO medical service temporarily formed part of the evacuation chain from North Africa. Under the TORCH plan patients from the Western Task Force in Morocco went directly back to the United States on returning transports. The Central and Eastern Task Forces, in the first stages of the campaign, evacuated their sick and

[31] Surg, Central Base Section, History of Medical Section, January–July 1944.

wounded, American and British alike, to the United Kingdom in British hospital ships. Under an agreement between General Hawley and the War Office to divide the labor of unloading these vessels, American Army medical units handled casualties of both nations at the Bristol Channel ports. Between 17 December 1942 and 8 April 1943 Company C, 53d Medical Battalion, working under the supervision of the Bristol port surgeon, discharged seven hospital ships from North Africa at Avonmouth. The company moved over 2,100 casualties, about 660 of them Americans, to the nearby 298th General Hospital for triage and initial treatment. The British Army then collected its troops from the 298th for evacuation to its own as well as EMS hospitals. American casualties ceased arriving from the Mediterranean in early April, as NATOUSA fixed hospitals went into operation. American medical units continued to unload British hospital ships at Bristol, however, and the 298th treated those few disembarked patients who could not be moved immediately to Allied facilities.[32]

General Hawley's office had responsibility for securing the means of evacuation by road and rail. In this, as in so many other areas of BOLERO preparations, the Americans initially had to depend heavily on the British. The British, for example, provided the American Army with many of its ambulances. In June 1942 they turned over to the chief surgeon 600 four-litter Austins for issue to his units and hospitals. These two-wheel-drive vehicles were well suited to the road travel involved in most evacuation within the United Kingdom. Their availability permitted Hawley to redeploy his relatively scarce four-wheel-drive U.S. Dodge ambulances, designed for cross-country work, at hospitals and depots to equip units going into the field and also at air stations for removing wounded from aircraft that crashed in the vicinity of the airfields. The supply of American-built ambulances expanded rapidly, as organizations brought their allowances with them and the War Department shipped extra ambulances, as well as other vehicles, to outfit later-arriving units and to replace combat losses. With this inflow from the United States and the Austins supplied by the British, the theater maintained a comfortable ambulance surplus at all times and by D-Day had accumulated a reserve of over 1,200.[33]

Besides the small Austin ambulances, the British supplied the Americans with passenger buses converted for carrying patients. The Emergency Medical Services, anticipating a need to move many casualties quickly during air raids, had refitted 300 London Green Line commuter buses

[32] The British Army similarly unloaded patients at Clyde- and Merseyside ports. See Operations and Training Division, OofCSurg, HQ, ETOUSA, Annual Rpt, 1942; Evacuation Division, OofCSurg, HQ, ETOUSA, Annual Rpt, 1943; "Med Svc Hist, 1942–43," pp. 19–20 and 107, file HD 314.7-2 ETO. For termination of U.S. evacuation to Great Britain, see messages in Evacuation From Europe and North Africa file, CMH.

[33] Troop Movements and Training Branch, Operations Division, OofCSurg, HQ, ETOUSA, Annual Rpt, 1944, p. 43; Memo, Hawley to AG, SOS, via G–4, 7 Nov 42, sub: Exchange of Field Ambulances for British-Made Ambulances, file HD ETO 451.8 (Amb), 1942–44. See also other correspondence in same file.

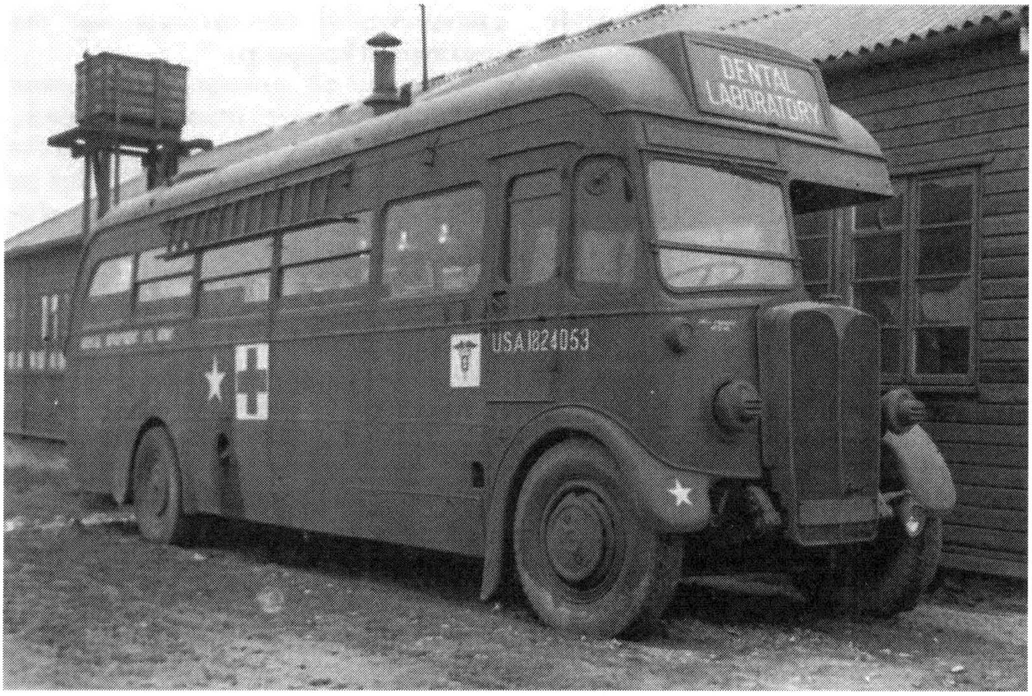

BRITISH-SUPPLIED AMBULANCE BUS, *converted into a mobile dental laboratory*

to accommodate nine or ten litters to a vehicle. In June 1942 Sir Francis Fraser, the EMS medical director, offered 100 of these buses to Hawley for handling ROUNDUP casualties. Hawley accepted only 30 at the outset. He did not yet need the rest, and the buses required specially trained drivers who would have to come from the scanty ETO pool of casuals or from hospital enlisted detachments. The Americans soon discovered that the buses were unsatisfactory for moving stretcher cases, as it was difficult to maneuver litters in and out of them. However, when equipped with seats, each bus could carry comfortably twenty-two ambulatory patients. Accordingly, the medical service arranged with the Ordnance Department to have 28 of the first 30 buses refitted with seats, taking a few at a time out of service for this purpose. The Dental Corps appropriated the remaining two buses for a mobile laboratory and clinic. By D-Day the medical service had procured 35 more buses, all for moving ambulatory patients. General Hawley assigned some of these vehicles to hospitals and pooled others under control of the base surgeons.[34]

General Hawley turned to the British again for hospital trains, his

[34]For EMS conversion of buses, see Col R. W. Bliss, MC, Emergency Medical Services, With Particular Reference to Hospitalization, 9 Dec 40, Bliss Rpts, file ETO 7/1; Ltr, Hawley to TSG, 9 Jul 42, file HD 024 ETO O/CS (Hawley-SGO Corresp); Correspondence, June 1942-June 1944, in file HD ETO 451.8 (Amb), 1942-44.

principal reliance for large-scale, long-distance patient movement, both in Britain and in projected continental operations. At the chief surgeon's request the Ministry of War Transport agreed to assemble, from its own rolling stock, a total of 39 trains for American use in Britain and eventually across the Channel. Medical equipment for these trains came partly from British and partly from American stocks. U.S. Army hospital train units constituted the on-board medical staff. The trains came in two versions: "home" trains designed to run in the United Kingdom; and "overseas" trains, with a different braking system, for use in France. Both types included kitchen, surgery, pharmacy, and staff accommodation cars, as well as 36-litter ward cars, coaches for ambulatory patients, and their own diesel heating and power plants. General Hawley considered the trains, of standard British design with American-specified alterations, "the finest that our Army has ever had." The problem, as usual in dealing with the hard-pressed British, was obtaining delivery on time. By the end of 1943 the Ministry of Transport had turned over to the Americans 6 out of a promised 15 home trains and 1 out of a promised 24 overseas models, along with 7 separate ward cars (designed by a U.S. Army Transportation Corps officer) for attachment to ordinary freight and passenger trains. Receipt of the remaining trains was delayed, and the issue became the subject of much negotiation and pressure by Hawley and his staff in the weeks before D-Day. With some improvisation, the Allies had enough of them ready in time to meet the initial requirements of the invasion and the continental campaign.[35]

As soon as enough trains were available to meet immediate needs, General Hawley began using them for all patient movements of 25 miles or more. He thus saved patients the discomfort of long ambulance rides, as well as conserving rationed tires and gasoline. The chief surgeon's office centrally controlled all rail movement, arranging with the theater chief of transportation to schedule trips at the request of base sections or to collect patients for evacuation to the United States. Each hospital train had a home siding, or "stable," close to a station or general hospital. The fixed installation housed and fed the train's medical complement and kept the cars supplied with food, linens, and other rapidly consumed items. Hospital train and car operations proceeded with few difficulties, despite occasional complaints of poor food and dirty cars as well as failures by hospitals to load the numbers and classes of patients planned on in scheduling a run.[36]

---

[35]Quotation from Ltr, Hawley to TSG, 8 Jul 43, file HD 024 ETO O/CS (Hawley-SGO Corresp). See also Evacuation Division, OofCSurg, HQ, ETOUSA, Annual Rpt, 1943; Operations Division, OofCSurg, HQ, ETOUSA, Annual Rpt, 1943, p. 18; Evacuation Branch, Operations Division, OofCSurg, HQ, ETOUSA, Annual Rpt, 1944, pp. 2–3; Hawley Interv, 1944, CMH. A hospital train unit included 4 officers, 6 nurses, and 33 enlisted men.

[36]Essential Technical Medical Data Rpt, HQ, ETOUSA, June 1944, encl. 4, pp. 6–7; Mins, 2d Meeting of Base Section Surgeons, 16 Aug 43, p. 13, and 20th Meeting of Base Section Surgeons, 24 Apr 44, pp. 2–5, file HD 337; Surg, Southern Base Section, Annual Rpt, 1943, p. 11; Surg, Eastern Base Section, Annual Rpt, 1943, p. 3. For loading problems, see Memo, Col F. H. Mowrey, MC, to Surgs, Western and Southern Base Sections, 18 May 44, sub: Evacuation of Patients, in Evacuation

Continued

The medical service made limited use of air evacuation within the United Kingdom, primarily to move patients from the Northern Ireland Base Section to England. Troop strength in this base section increased from 3,000 men to 78,000 in the last three months of 1943, overburdening the section's hospitals. General Hawley, therefore, set aside 1,500 beds elsewhere in the United Kingdom for Northern Ireland patients and arranged with the Ninth Air Force's IX Troop Carrier Command for periodic evacuation airlifts. In Northern Ireland the 79th General Hospital at Waringfield, near Belfast, acted as holding and transit unit for all air evacuees, including men destined for return to the United States as well as overflow patients. C–47s of the IX Troop Carrier Command picked up their first patients on 16 December and by the end of the month had transported 217 men. Inclement weather often forced cancellation of scheduled flights, necessitating the return to their original hospitals of patients who had been moved as far as 40 miles to meet airplanes. When the system worked, however, it took only four hours to transfer a sick or injured soldier from his bed in Northern Ireland to a new bed in a general hospital in England.[37]

Branch, Operations Division, O/CS Correspondence re Evacuation, February 1944–February 1945 (hereafter cited as EvacCorresp, 1944–45), file HD 370.05 ETO.

[37] Surgeon, Northern Ireland Base Section, Annual Rpt, 1943, p. 2, and Final Rpt, January–15 Jun 44, pp. 1 and 3; "Med Svc Hist, 1942–43," p. 22, file HD 314.7-2 ETO. For delays, see Mins, 3d Conference of Chiefs of Medical Services, 26 Jan and 2 Feb 44, p. 30, in Medical Consultation Service

Transatlantic Evacuation

Evacuation from the United Kingdom back to the United States was a controversial, unresolved issue in the months before D-Day. The controversy involved both policy and ways and means. From mid-1942 on, General Hawley advocated a 180-day evacuation policy, meaning that the theater would send home only those patients deemed unlikely to return to duty within that time period. Hawley pressed his case in spite of the preference of Surgeons General Magee and Kirk for a 120-day policy for overseas theaters. He argued that a 180-day policy reduced losses to the theater of experienced personnel and required less shipping for both evacuees and replacements. The chief surgeon also realized, although he did not mention this consideration in discussions with Magee and Kirk, that adoption of a 120-day policy might lead to attempts to reduce his large BOLERO hospital construction requirement, which was based on 180 days. Col. Eli E. Brown, Darnall's predecessor as the Hospitalization Division chief, warned Hawley in May 1943: "If the 120-day policy does become effective it is very desirable that it not be [instituted] until our present hospital program is approved and completed." The War Department, in the end, accepted the chief surgeon's arguments about lack of shipping and the need to retain manpower. In August 1943 it formally authorized a 180-day evacuation policy for the European Theater.[38]

sec., Professional Services Division, OofCSurg, HQ, ETOUSA, Annual Rpt, 1944.

[38] Quotation from Memo, Brown to CSurg, ETOUSA, 29 May 43, HospDivGenCorresp, 1943,

Continued

Until well afer D-Day, the European Theater and the War Department disagreed on whether mentally ill patients requiring restraint and nonambulatory cases should be evacuated on returning troopships.[39] In contrast to specially designed hospital ships, which were protected by the Geneva and Hague Conventions, troop transports were legitimate targets for U-boats. For this reason, General Hawley insisted from the start of BOLERO planning that "no officer or soldier who is unable to care for himself in the event of enemy attack upon the vessel in which he is a passenger, be evacuated on any but a plainly marked and regularly operated hospital ship." The theater adopted this principle as official policy in June 1942. At the same time the London Combined Committee endorsed Hawley's request for ten U.S. hospital ships for the European Theater.[40]

Those hospital ships, however, did not exist in mid-1942 and were still lacking two years later, due to vacillating War Department policy. In June 1942, after an Army-Navy dispute over how many hospital ships should be obtained and which service should build and operate them, the Joint Chiefs of Staff decided to procure only three Army hospital ships, none for the European Theater. At the same time the Joint Chiefs, through General Somervell, instructed ETOUSA and the other theaters to evacuate their sick and wounded whenever possible on returning transports. The transports would be equipped with beds for mental and nonambulatory patients up to 5 percent of their passenger capacity and for ambulatory patients up to 20 percent, as well as with surgical, laboratory, pharmacy, and other supporting facilities, and the ports of embarkation would furnish hospital ship platoons to reinforce the transports' own medical complements. This policy prevailed for less than a year. As the general shipping shortage eased, and in response to pleas from the surgeon general and the theaters, the Joint Chiefs on 11 June 1943 reversed themselves and ordered evacuation of nonambulatory men on hospital ships. The Chiefs now authorized the Army to develop its own fleet of twenty-four such craft, most of them converted from other passenger and cargo types. Refitting of the vessels went slowly so that the first U.S. Army hos-

file HD 312 ETO. At this time, in its first effort to set an official evacuation policy for each theater, the War Department, with the surgeon general's assent, authorized 120 days for all theaters but the ETO and the Pacific, both of which were allowed 180 days. See Smith, *Hospitalization and Evacuation*, pp. 215-16. The ETO rationale is summarized in Memo, Lt Col R. P. Fisk, to CG, ASF, 5 Jul 43, sub: Evacuation Policy for Overseas Commands, file 008 (Policy re Evac for Overseas Cmds).

[39] The Army Service Forces in August 1942 established four patient classes for evacuation: Class I (mental patients requiring locked wards or other restraints); Class II (bed patients who could not move about or care for themselves); Class III (ambulatory but requiring much medical and nursing care, e.g. the blind, amputees, men with heavy casts, and patients needing special diets); and Class IV (ambulatory patients needing minimal medical attention and able to travel in ordinary troop accommodations). See Smith, *Hospitalization and Evacuation*, pp. 331-32.

[40] Quotation from Larkey "Hist," ch. 2, pp. 52-54. See also Ltr, Hawley to TSG, 25 Apr 42, sub: Hospital Ships, file HD 024 ETO O/CS (Hawley-SGO Corresp); Msgs, Lee to AGWAR, 11 Aug 42, and ETO to AGWAR, 16 Aug 42, Evacuation From Europe and North Africa file, CMH. The ETO authorities emphasized that hospital ships also could carry medical supplies and personnel outbound from the U.S. without violating international conventions.

pital ship reached British waters only a short time before D-Day.[41]

During most of the time that the evacuate-on-transports policy was in effect, the European Theater managed to avoid following it. Between August 1942 and December 1943 the theater sent only 7,800 patients to the United States. With this relatively small number of evacuees, and with hospital space in Great Britain for long retention of patients, the medical service embarked almost all the mental and nonambulatory patients it did evacuate—some 1,600—on British and Canadian hospital ships and ambulatory casualties on U.S. and British transports. In March 1944, as the number of transatlantic evacuees increased due to the expansion of American forces and the drive to clear hospital beds before D-Day, General Hawley—now going against both his own preference and Army-wide policy—obtained temporary War Department permission to embark bed patients on troop transports. Hawley regarded this as strictly a temporary expedient. He held to the principle that helpless evacuees should be restricted to hospital ships and, in the absence of enough such vessels, was willing to keep patients longer in his own hospitals. The entire question of using transports to move casualties remained unresolved and would arise again in late 1944, as part of a general review of ETO hospitalization and evacuation policies.[42]

The actual conduct of transatlantic sea evacuation was the joint responsibility of the European Theater and its supporting New York Port of Embarkation. The port provided vessels, and also medical hosptial ship platoons to care for patients on the voyage. The theater selected men to be evacuated, under the 180-day policy, and moved them to British ports for embarkation. In each hospital center and separate general hospital a disposition board, made up of the chiefs of surgery and medicine and the ward officer of the patient concerned, decided which cases merited being sent home. If the casualties were Air Force troops, Eighth or Ninth Air Force flight surgeons usually sat with the boards to advise on the patients' suitability for further aviation duty. Hospital commanders had final authority to approve or reject disposition board findings, and the Professional Services Division of Hawley's office periodically reviewed selected proceedings to ensure technical competence and promptness of decision. The consultants also enforced General Hawley's preference for holding soldiers in the theater if they were likely to be fit for even lim-

[41] For the twists and turns of hospital ship policy, see Smith, *Hospitalization and Evacuation*, pp. 394–411; Msgs, Somervell to CG, U.S. Forces, London, 15 and 24 Aug 42, Evacuation From Europe and North Africa file, CMH. See also Memo, TAG, WD, to CGs of Departments, Theater of Operations, Base Commands, and Task Forces . . . , 25 Jan 43, sub: Sea Evacuation Operations; Msg, SECWAR, 25 Jan 43, sub: Sea Evacuation; Memo, Col D. E. Liston, MC, to G–4, ETO, 27 Mar 44. All in Evacuation Branch, Operations Division, O/CS Correspondence re Evacuation, 1942–44 (hereafter cited as EvacCorresp, 1942–44), file HD 024 ETO. The War Department at the outbreak of war was uncertain whether the Axis powers would respect the provisions of the Geneva and Hague Conventions on hospital ships. Increasing evidence that the Axis powers were doing so strengthened the case for more hospital ships.

[42] "Med Svc Hist, 1942–43," pp. 18–20 and 108, file HD 314.7-2 ETO; Memo, Liston to G–4, ETO, 27 Mar 44, with endorsements, EvacCorresp, 1942–44, file HD 024 ETO.

ited duty, so as to conserve all possible manpower.[43]

Most transatlantic evacuees, whether on transports or hospital ships, sailed under the British flag because relatively few U.S. troopships, and initially no hospital ships, operated in the Atlantic. On British transports the American patients and their attending hospital ship platoon constituted a subordinate command under a British senior medical officer who had overall control of the vessel's medical facilities. General Hawley, who wanted to keep evacuation of American patients entirely under American authority, accepted this arrangement with reluctance, and only with the proviso that the evacuees and medical personnel be under the "immediate control" of a U.S. Army medical officer. By American standards British troopships, even the large converted luxury liners *Queen Mary* and *Queen Elizabeth*, afforded only barely adequate evacuation accommodations. On one voyage of the *Queen Elizabeth*, for example, fifty-eight U.S. and Canadian Class I mental patients were quartered in three separate parts of the ship, an arrangement which, according to the New York port commander, "handicapped medical supervision to the extent that there were fights among some of the . . . patients." Such incidents merely strengthened Hawley's determination to move seriously ill and wounded men only on hospital ships.[44]

A small but growing number of medical evacuees crossed the Atlantic by air. Under a War Department policy announced in September 1942 the AAF's Air Transport Command (ATC) was to fly casualties back to the United States at the request of theater chief surgeons, who could call for air evacuation of three categories of patients: emergency cases for whom essential treatment was not locally available, men whose air evacuation the chief surgeons deemed a "military necessity," and men who required prolonged hospital and convalescent care. The ETO medical service considered blinded patients; those with severe burns and head, face, or jaw injuries; and some orthopedic patients as priority candidates for air movement. When spaces on planes were available, the Evacuation Division transferred patients in these categories from general hospitals to the transatlantic military air terminal at Prestwick, Scotland, where Air Force and SOS medical people loaded the evacuees on four-engined C-54s for the flight to the United States. During late 1942 general and station hospitals in the United Kingdom had to detach nurses and enlisted men to attend patients on the aircraft, but in 1943 AAF medical air evacuation transport squadrons began

[43] Smith *Hospitalization and Evacuation*, pp. 331-36; Memo, HQ, SOS, 3 Jun 44, sub: Transfer of Patients to General Hospitals, Zone of the Interior, in EvacCorresp, 1942-44, file HD 024 ETO; Memo, Professional Services Division, OofCSurg, to CSurg, ETOUSA, 8 Sep 43, sub: Review of Disposition Board Proceeding, file HD 024 ETO O/CS (Spruit Policy Notebook); Mins, 16th Meeting of Base Section Surgeons, 28 Feb 44, p. 5, and 22d Meeting of Base Section Surgeons, 22 May 44, pp. 7-8, file HD 337; Medical Bulletin No. 16, OofCSurg, HQ, ETOUSA, 1 Mar 44, pp. 2-3

[44] First quotation from Ltr, Hawley to Maj Gen C. P. Gross, CofTrans, SOS, WD, 30 Jun 43, EvacCorresp, 1942-44, file HD 024 ETO. Second quotation from Msg, New York Port of Embarkation to CG, SOS, ETO, 1 Mar 44, file HD 024 O/CS (Hawley-SGO Corresp).

arriving in the theater and took over this task. Ten of these units had reached Britain by D-Day.[45]

During the first year and a half of the buildup very few sick and wounded were evacuated by plane. The War Department, in its air evacuation instructions of September 1942, enjoined that requests be kept to a minimum, and the ETO medical service complied. Furthermore, the Air Transport Command, primarily concerned with carrying troops and supplies, gave medical evacuees a low priority, and the European Theater had a constant backlog of higher-priority westbound passengers. Up to the end of 1943 only 116 patients, many of them ambulatory convalescents, left the United Kingdom by air.[46]

Air evacuation expanded in scale and increased in tempo in early 1944. By this time aircraft had proved their worth in carrying patients in the Mediterranean and Pacific, both for bringing casualties the benefits of early care and for reducing the number of medical personnel needed to attend them in transit. In the European Theater the Air Transport Command had more planes and aviation medical people available. It also had improved its equipment; a new stretcher bracket for cargo aircraft, for example, increased the carrying capacity of the C-54 from 10 litter patients to 18. In March 1944, as part of the final invasion preparations, the command began enlarging medical facilities at intermediate stations on its transatlantic routes, a necessary preliminary to mass patient movements. The following month gave the theaters more latitude in establishing priorities for loading U.S.-bound flights. In May the European Wing, Air Transport Command, began making long-term commitments to the ETO medical service of space for air evacuation, allowing more ambitious planning by the chief surgeon. About 1,600 patients left England by plane between 1 January and 31 May. The Evacuation Branch looked forward to flying out 6,000 to 10,000 casualties each month after the campaign began.[47]

As air evacuation expanded, the geographical defects of Prestwick, for medical pruposes, became apparent. The ATC terminal was located far from most general and station hospitals and had no facilities to house and care for patients awaiting planes. In mid-1943 the medical service acquired the 750-bed Cowglen Hospital, an EMS facility in Glasgow, and installed there the 2d Evacuation Hospital, later replaced by the 50th General Hospital, to operate an air

[45] For the general development of air evacuation, see Smith, *Hospitalization and Evacuation*, pp. 337-40; Link and Coleman, *AAF Medical Support*, pp. 384-90. See also Msg, AGWAR to USSOS, ETO, 26 Sep 42; Air Priorities Instruction No. 4 (source of quotation), Air Priorities Division, HQ, Air Transport Command, AAF, 26 Feb 43; Memo, 1st Lt D. J. Twohig, MC, to Medical Field Service School, American School Center, 21 Apr 43, sub: Air Evacuation; Memo, Fisk to CG, SOS, ETOUSA, 13 Sep 43, sub: Delegation of Authority To Authorize Patients To Travel by Air. All in Evacuation Branch, Operations Division, O/CS file on Air Evacuation (hereafter cited as AirEvacCorresp), file HD 580 ETO.

[46] Operations and Training Division, OofCSurg, HQ, ETOUSA, Annual Rpt, 1942; "Med Svc Hist, 1942-43," pp. 19-20, file HD 314.7-2 ETO.

[47] Link and Coleman, *AAF Medical Support*, pp. 391-95; Evacuation Branch, Operations Division, OofCSurg, HQ, ETOUSA, Annual Rpt, 1944, pp. 14-15 and encl. 11; Evacuation Branch, Operations Division, OofCSurg, HQ, ETOUSA, Daily Diary, 16 May 44, file HD 024 ETO.

evacuee holding unit that eventually expanded to 1,000 beds. Cowglen, however, was 32 miles from Prestwick, and the chief surgeon wanted a holding point closer to the airfield. Accordingly, the Hospitalization Division and the Evacuation Branch, after an extensive search and much negotiation with the British, in May 1944 took over Westfield House, an estate near Prestwick, as a 90-bed facility for ambulatory patients. At the same time the medical service secured an abandoned laborers camp, located near the Prestwick runways, as a 125-bed holding unit for litter cases. The Western Base Section provided the 1st Platoon, 29th Field Hospital, to operate Westfield House; the 18th Hospital Train, reinforced with people from the 811th Medical Air Evacuation Transport Squadron, manned the airfield unit. Both facilities opened a few weeks after D-Day, barely in time for the flood of battle casualties.[48]

[48] Cowglen initially was acquired as an ordinary 750-bed station hospital. See Memos, OofCEngr, ETOUSA, to AG, ETOUSA, via CSurg, 10 Apr 43, and CSurg, ETO, to AG, ETO, 15 Apr 43, file HospDivGenCorresp, 1943, file HD 312 ETO. See also Evacuation Branch, Operations Division, OofCSurg, HQ, ETOUSA, Daily Diary, 17 May 44, pp. 1, 3, and 17 Jun 44, file HD 024 ETO.

By mid-1944 the theater medical service had put in place the rearmost elements of its system for handling casualties from the future European battlefields. It constructed and organized a large and complex hospital network spread over much of Great Britain; assembled the means for removing casualties from its camps and installations in the island nation, as well as the reserves for transporting the massive flow of sick and wounded soon to come from the Continent; and grasped the potentialties of air evacuation by preparing and employing aircraft for both intratheater and transatlantic movement of casualties. Nevertheless, the combination of a 180-day theater evacuation policy, General Hawley's insistence on moving helpless patients only on hospital ships, and a shortage of such vessels threatened to make the theater hospitalization and evacuation system a rapidly filling tub with only a very small outlet. As casualties arrived from the Continent, the system at some point would reach the limits of its capacity for evacuation and treatment. That condition, when reached, would be a most difficult time for the ETO medical service and General Hawley.

CHAPTER V

Medics in Britain

During the BOLERO buildup U.S. Army medics in the United Kingdom lived and worked on the margin between war and peace.[1] Food rationing, blackouts, occasional air raids, and the arrival of wounded men from Eighth Air Force fields reminded them that they were at war, as did the constantly expanding number of American troops, the invasion preparations, and the growing tension as D-Day approached. Yet embattled Great Britain still offered many of the amenities of urban-industrial civilization, and in areas outside the blitzed cities war at times could seem far away. Colonel Middleton, the theater chief medical consultant, lived in a room in a small Cheltenham hotel that overlooked a garden, "always well kept up even during war . . . as a British garden would be." He and his colleagues, in their infrequent spare time, attended concerts in the nearby town hall and took weekend walks in the Cotswolds. Lower-ranking officers and enlisted medics subsisted under less comfortable conditions. Still, they resided among hospitable people who spoke more or less the same language; they could enjoy the society of British professional counterparts; and they had access to a wide range of amusements, wholesome and otherwise.[2]

ETO medics also had work to do. Besides completing their hospitalization and evacuation system, they conducted their own portion of the BOLERO personnel buildup. They furnished day-to-day medical service to the growing American Army in the United Kingdom. They conducted militarily and scientifically significant research, exchanged information and ideas with British colleagues, trained for their wartime missions, and sought to preserve the health of the fighting forces.

[1]The term *medics* is used in this volume as shorthand for "the men and women of the U.S. Army Medical Department." Enlisted medics are identified either by this term or as aidmen, litterbearers, etc.

[2]Quotation from Middleton Interv, 1968–69, vol. 1, pp. 201–04, NLM. For recollections of the experience of other medics, see Interv, Medical History Branch, CMH, with Col Virginia Brown, ANC, 5 and 13 Jul 79 (hereafter cited as Brown Interv, 1979), CMH; Interv, Medical History Branch, CMH, with Maj Gen Collin F. Vorder Bruegge, MC (Ret.) (hereafter cited as Vorder Bruegge Interv), 29 Jan 80, tape 1, side 1, pp. 7–8, CMH. See also reminiscences of Mrs. Jane A. Lee, a former nurse, in Interv, Medical History Branch, CMH, with Lee, June 1981 (hereafter cited as Lee Interv, 1981), CMH.

The Personnel Buildup

Of the major BOLERO tasks facing the Office of the Chief Surgeon, securing medical units and personnel entailed the fewest difficulties. General Hawley and his staff largely determined the number of people and units required for the theater medical establishment—what was known as the troop basis. Certain portions of the troop basis, such as the medical detachments of most air, ground, and SOS units and the medical establishments of the infantry and armored divisions, were prescribed by tables of organization and automatically deployed with their parent formations. These, however, accounted for a relatively small proportion of theater medical manpower. Hawley, as the ETO and SOS chief surgeon, had an almost completely free hand in establishing medical unit requirements for the Services of Supply and for the ground force echelons above corps, subject only to the BOLERO plans and to a War Department ceiling on fixed and mobile hospital beds as a percentage of troop strength. This manpower planning was, at best, an inexact science. The chief surgeon and his staff had to work from incomplete and constantly changing theater buildup and operational plans. Hence, they relied heavily on rules of thumb derived from past experience, especially that of World War I.[3]

At the end of 1942 the planned SOS medical component, designed for a theater of 427,000 troops, included about 25,000 officers and men, barely a fourth of whom actually were in Great Britain. In January 1943, during and after the Casablanca conference, the medical and other technical services, at General Lee's direction, began working out new troop bases for supporting an army of 1.1 million. The operational plan that this army was to carry out did not yet exist; nevertheless, the theater needed at least a tentative troop basis to guide the BOLERO buildup. In the absence of a tactical plan the supply services drew on World War I precedents and tried to comply with repeated War Department and ETO directives to minimize the number of support troops.

On 8 February General Hawley presented to General Lee a request for SOS medical units with a total strength of 74,109 officers and men. His Operations Division, which drew up this proposal, based its estimate of general and station hospital unit requirements on the number of beds called for in the theater hospitalization plan; [4] it requested other organi-

[3] McMinn and Levin, *Personnel*, p. 384–97; First Army Report of Operations, 20 Oct 43–1 Aug 44, bk. VII, p. 61. Until August 1943 each theater established its own hospital bed requirement, which largely determined its medical manpower requirement, usually working from World War I casualty statistics. In August 1943 the Office of the Surgeon General and the General Staff, using the lower casualty rates thus far incurred in World War II, set a ceiling of fixed and mobile beds for each theater; those for the European Theater were, respectively, 8 and 4 percent of total troop strength. These limitations had little effect on ETO medical troop planning, since Hawley from the beginning had kept his requests within them. See Smith, *Hospitalization and Evacuation*, pp. 216–18; Memo, Lt Col C. B. Meador, MC, to DepCSurg (Cheltenham), 27 Sep 43, sub: Theater Troop Basis, file ETO 320.2 (Strength).

[4] At Hawley's instructions, force planners ignored the 95,000-bed ceiling eventually set on hospital construction (see Chapter IV) and based unit requests on the full 100,000-plus beds required to meet the percentage-of-strength hospitalization formula. See Hawley Planning Directive No. 1, 11 Jun 43, box 2, Hawley Papers, MHI.

zations in proportion to overall ETO troop numbers. In all, the chief surgeon called for fifty-three general, sixty-one station (mostly 750 beds), three convalescent, and ten field hospitals; eleven medical sanitary, six depot, and two ambulance companies; twenty-eight hospital train crews; two medical gas treatment battalions; and four general dispensaries, as well as hospital centers, an auxiliary surgical group, and a medical general laboratory.

Defending this troop basis to General Lee and the ETO staff, Hawley emphasized that it was the result of careful study of American Expeditionary Forces (AEF) medical operations in World War I and of British practice in the current war. He noted that the number of medical troops asked for was a smaller percentage of the strength of both the total theater and the Services of Supply than the AEF medical service had required in 1917–18. Hawley asked that shipping priority during 1943 be given to the station and general hospitals needed to care for sick and nonbattle injured. Other units should be sent as space permitted, preferably in proportion to the troop buildup.[5]

On 19 February Colonel Spruit, then Hawley's representative in London, issued a medical troop basis for the then projected ground force of 591,000 men in two field armies and eight corps. Assuming that divisions and smaller formations would deploy with their organic medical units and detachments, Spruit called for an additional 33,000 corps and army medical troops. This initial list, which included such soon to be abolished units as medical regiments and surgical hospitals, would require extensive revision to take into account the general 1943 reorganization of Army Ground Forces units, including medical ones.[6]

As the TRIDENT and QUADRANT conferences set firm invasion dates and COSSAC developed an outline operational plan, ETO troop basis discussions became more detailed and definite. In early July the theater's air, ground, and service components began working out a definitive two-phase list of manpower and unit requirements. Phase One of this new troop basis set preinvasion buildup goals; Phase Two specified the forces needed to break out of the beachhead and advance across the continent. This planning process was lengthy and complex, as the theater tried to adapt to changing invasion plans and varying War Department estimates of what forces would be available. At the same time, the theater had to achieve a balance between the often exhorbitant demands of each of its components.

General Hawley, like the other technical service chiefs, repeatedly revised his troop lists. Besides respond-

[5] Operations Division, OofCSurg, HQ, ETOUSA, Annual Rpt, 1944, pp. 5–6; Larkey "Hist," ch. 4, pp. 11–13 and apps. 8–9; Memo, Lt Col J. B. Mason, MC, to ACofS, G–1, SOS, 22 Jan 43, sub: Medical Troops for "B" Plan (Revised), file ETO 320.2 (Strength); Memo, Lt Col J. B. Mason, MC, to ACofS, G–1, SOS, 6 Feb 43, file HD 024 ETO O/CS (Planning, Hawley) 1943; Memo, Hawley to CG, SOS, 8 Feb 43, sub: Medical Troop Basis, SOS, file 370 (Bible File of Troop Requirements, Early Planning). For overall SOS troop planning, see Ruppenthal, *Logistical Support*, 1:117–20.

[6] Memo, Col C. B. Spruit, MC, to ACofS, G–3, ETO, 19 Feb 43, sub: Tentative Troop Basis, Ground Forces, file ETO 024 (Spruit File re Policy).

ing to ETO and War Department directives, usually to cut service forces, the chief surgeon followed General Kirk's instructions to use more general and fewer station hospitals. He and his staff also adapted ground force and SOS troop bases to changes in medical unit tables of organization, replacing fixed-T/O medical regiments and battalions with the new flexible group and battalion headquarters detachments and separate collecting, clearing, and ambulance companies. Profiting from experience in North Africa and Italy, Hawley increased the number of field hospitals with the ground forces, to provide forward surgical support for division clearing stations.[7]

By late November the European Theater and the War Department had settled on a total force of nearly 2.8 million troops and had developed a month-by-month unit deployment schedule for reaching this strength by 1 February 1945. Of these forces about 1.42 million men—417,000 Air Force, 626,000 ground forces, and 375,000 SOS—were to be in the United Kingdom before D-Day. The medical service, which would amount to 7.5 percent of theater strength, was to include about 43,600 officers and men in units attached to the armies and 127,500 in the Services of Supply. About half of these troops were scheduled to reach Great Britain before the invasion. By mid-December Hawley's Operations Division had made up detailed lists of the number and types of units in the ground force and SOS medical complements *(Table 2)* and had established a monthly schedule of arrivals. Among ground force units 400-bed evacuation hospitals, field hospitals, and collecting, clearing and ambulance companies accounted for most of the manpower. In the SOS troop list 1,000-bed general hospitals—141 of them—made up the largest single block of personnel. Only 45 station hospitals remained on the list, reflecting the surgeon general's directive to minimize use of that type of unit. In response to pleas from General Hawley, 22 of the 46 field hospitals called for, which were intended for service with the armies, were counted against ground force strength rather than that of the Services of Supply, even though field hospitals were not Army Ground Forces units. In the months remaining until the assault the exact mixture of units altered repeatedly, in response to changing availability in the United States and to new requirements of the armies and Services of Supply. Nevertheless, the basic list of unit types, and the general proportion of medical manpower absorbed by each, stayed more or less stable throughout the buildup and the invasion.[8]

[7] For the overall establishment of the troop basis, see Ruppenthal, *Logistical Support,* 1:123–29; Smith, *Hospitalization and Evacuation,* pp. 218–19 and 451–52; Operations Division, OofCSurg, HQ, ETOUSA, Annual Rpt, 1944, pp. 6–7; Larkey "Hist," ch. 4, pp. 16–17 and app. 17; Hawley Planning Directive No. 9, 13 Jul 43, box 2, Hawley Papers, MHI. For an example of adjustment to new T/Os, see Memo, CSurg to CofOpns, SOS, 21 Oct 43, file ETO 320.0 (Strength). File HD 024 ETO O/CS (Hawley-SGO Corresp), July–November 1943, includes his negotiations with the surgeon general.

[8] Ground Forces and SOS Medical Troop Bases, 13 Dec 43; MFR, Brig Gen James B. Mason, MC, 4 Aug 67. Both in box 1, James B. Mason Papers, MHI. See also Troop Movements and Training Branch, Operations Division, OofCSurg, HQ,

Continued

TABLE 2—CHIEF SURGEON'S RECOMMENDED TROOP BASIS, JANUARY 1944

Unit	Strength Per Unit	Theater Total	
		SOS	Ground Forces
Headquarters and Headquarters Detachment, Medical Battalion (Separate)	29	8	53
Medical Sanitary Company	117	16	
Medical Gas Treatment Battalion	502	1	4
Medical Ambulance Company (Motorized, Separate)	93	24	63
Field Hospital (400 beds)	227	24	22
Hospital Train	50	45	
Hospital Center	289	2	
General Hospital (1,000 beds)	662	141	
Station Hospital (150 beds)	125	1	
Station Hospital (250 beds)	201	13	
Station Hospital (500 beds)	364	1	
Station Hospital (750 beds)	508	30	
Auxiliary Surgical Group	378	1	4
Headquarters, Medical Department, Concentration Center	27	1	
Medical General Laboratory	99	1	
General Dispensary	41	8	
Medical Depot Company	178	6	6
Medical Detachment, Museum & Medical Arts	7	1	
Attached Medical Sections	11	75	
Headquarters and Headquarters Detachment, Medical Group	30		12
Collecting Company (Motorized)	105		72
Clearing Company (Motorized)	117		36
Medical Laboratory (Army)	58		4
Evacuation Hospital (750 beds)	409		2
Evacuation Hospital (400 beds)	296		46
Convalescent Hospital	223		4
Medical Battalion (Motorized)	465		3

Source: Adapted by authors from Troop Movements and Training Branch, Operations Division, OofCSurg, HQ, ETOUSA, Annual Rpt, 1944, chart A.

By the time ETOUSA completed its final troop lists, the buildup already was under way, guided by the earlier tentative statements of requirements. The number of American soldiers in Great Britain increased from 122,000 in January 1943 to 773,000 at the end of the year. Initially Air Force units predominated in the transatlantic flow; later in the year SOS organizations received precedence. The ground forces, which would be needed last, built up more slowly, with only five divisions arriving in 1943. Medical troop strength increased at about the same rate as that of the theater as a whole, from 10,000 officers and men (6,700 of them in the SOS) in January to over 65,000 (31,000 in the SOS) in December. Medical forces continued to build up rapidly during the first half of 1944, with the arrival of large numbers of

ETOUSA, Annual Rpt, 1944, pp. 6–9 and charts A, B, C; Larkey "Hist," ch. 4, pp. 18–20. For the questions of field hospitals, see file HD 024 ETO O/CS (Hawley-SGO Corresp), November-December 1943.

field units paralleling the now rapid influx of ground combat troops.[9]

Medical units arriving from the United States came under the oversight of the Troop Movements and Training Branch of Hawley's Operations Division. This branch requested orders from the theater G-3 assigning each new unit to a major command, and, in the case of SOS units, to a base section. Non-SOS medical units received their final duty assignments from Air Force or 1st Army Group headquarters. The Troop Movements and Training Branch also proposed changes in the unit shipment schedule when necessary, for example, to advance the arrival of urgently needed depot companies for the Supply Division; and it kept the base sections, which were responsible for moving and housing debarking units, informed of the organizations they could expect to receive.[10]

Typically, European Theater medical units disembarked at Scottish, western English, or Welsh ports and then moved by train to their assigned locations. Until the final inrush of units before D-Day most general and station hospitals spent time in temporary billets awaiting either completion of their plants or instructions to take over an already operating hospital. The Western Base Section, which received most newly arrived hospitals, quartered them in towns and cantonments around Llandudno, Wales. Here, the units underwent orientation to the theater and preliminary professional evaluation of their staffs, under supervision of the Western Base Section surgeon. While awaiting permanent assignments, medical officers, nurses, and enlisted men lived in hutted camps or were billeted with British families. A nurse who entered Britain early in 1944 with the 48th General Hospital recalled: "The policeman took a group of you and walked down the street and said, 'One goes here and two goes there,' and you walked into a stranger's house and that's where you stayed for about a month." [11]

Since the beginning of mobilization in 1940, the Office of the Surgeon General had fought, in the main successfully, for the activation of enough medical units of all types for the expanding Army. As a result of these efforts, the units required for the ETO medical troop basis became available in the United States at about the same rate as the forces they were to support.[12] Nevertheless, as the buildup proceeded, General Hawley had to cope with several persistent manpower problems. By D-Day, shortages of key personnel had begun to develop, most resulting from Army-wide—even

[9] For strength, see McMinn and Levin, *Personnel*, pp. 308–11; slightly different figures are given in Personnel Division, OofCSurg, HQ, ETOUSA, Annual Rpt, 1943, p. 11. For general progress of the buildup, see Ruppenthal, *Logistical Support*, 1:130–32 and 231–40, and Matloff, *Strategic Planning*, pp. 551–52. Encl. 8 of Troop Movements and Training Branch, Operations Division, OofCSurg, HQ, ETOUSA, Annual Rpt, 1944, details the unit types arriving in 1944.

[10] Troop Movements and Training Branch, Operations Division, OofCSurg, HQ, ETOUSA, Annual Rpt, 1944, pp. 9, 11, 13. Memos, Lt Col J. B. Mason, MC, to Surgs, Western and Southern Base Sections, 10 Aug 43, file 320.2 (Strength), are examples of advance information to base sections.

[11] Quotation from Brown Interv, 1979, CMH. See also Surg, Western Base Section, Rpt, 1 Jan–31 Aug 44, pp. 2–3.

[12] For development of the overall Army medical troop basis, see Smith, *Hospitalization and Evacuation*, pp. 38–39 and 149–51.

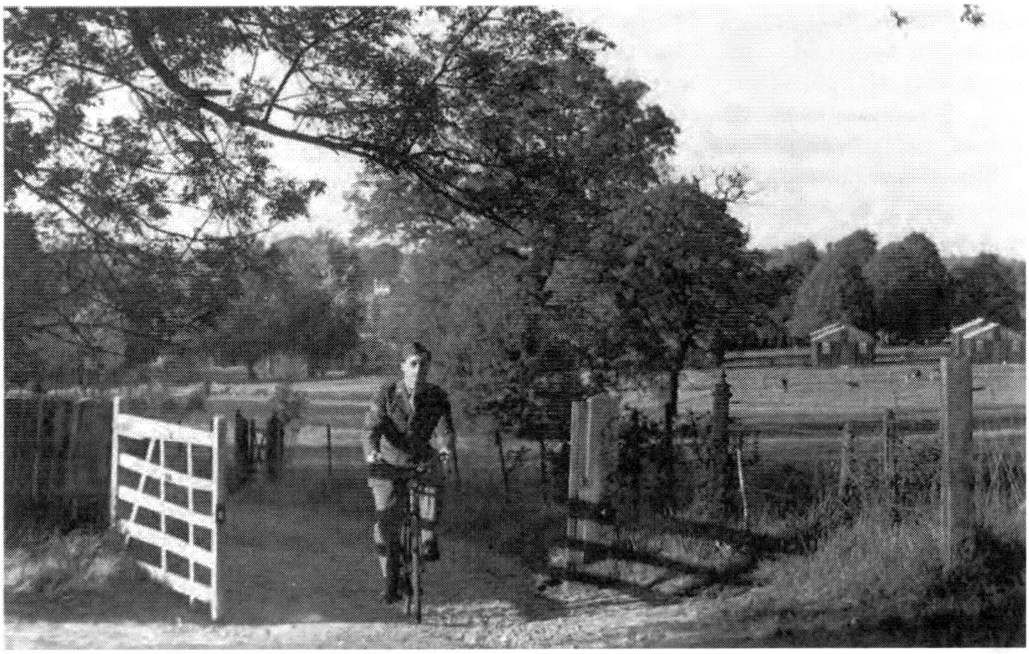

Medical Personnel Enjoying the Amenities of British Life.
A soldier bicycles through the countryside and nurses take tea in a garden.

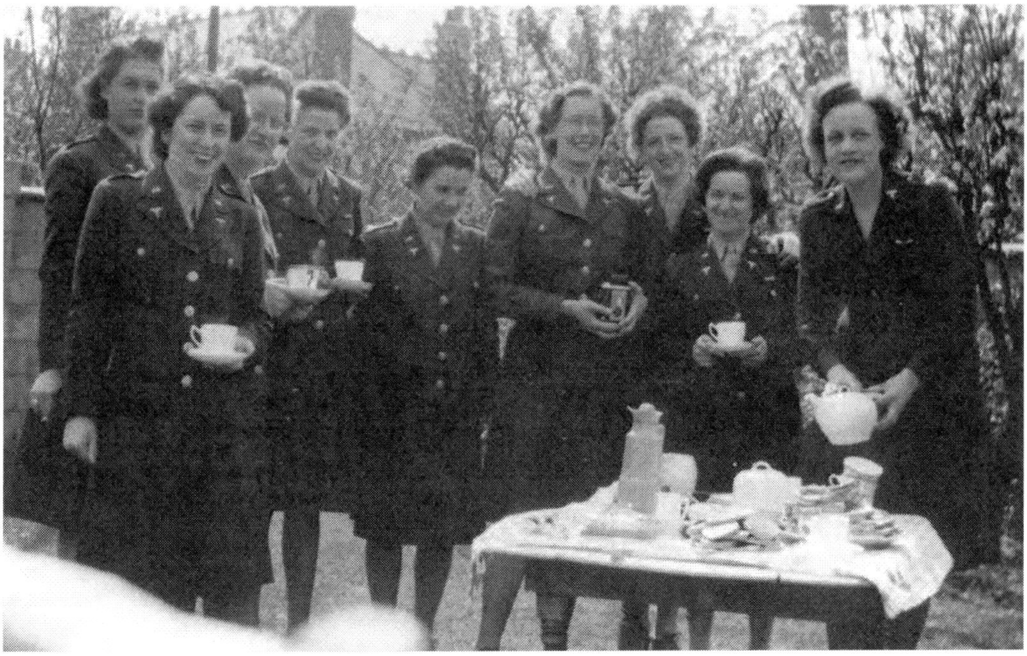

nationwide—conditions. While these shortages had little effect on invasion preparations, they were warning signals of greater difficulties to come as the campaign progressed.

The chief surgeon labored with only partial success to meet apparently limitless demands for medical officers and enlisted men not attached to T/O units. He needed these casuals to staff his own office and those of the base section surgeons; to operate convalescent facilities and the central dental laboratory and blood bank; to staff various theater schools; and to reinforce hospital units whose bed capacities were being expanded. In addition, many nonmedical units, especially of the other technical services, arrived without T/O medical detachments and had to be provided with first-echelon support. Finally, in early 1944, General Hawley had to find still more personnel for new Communications Zone staffs being formed to complete logistics plans for the invasion. To meet these requirements, Hawley continually pressed theater headquarters and the Office of the Surgeon General for larger allotments of casuals. By 1 April 1944 his allowance of such personnel had grown to 362 officers and 1,348 enlisted men—still not enough for all the jobs to be filled. Hawley also asked for 100 eleven-man medical sections, to be attached to organizations that lacked their own doctors and aidmen. He eventually received only 75, added to the SOS medical troop basis. Requirements continually outstripped the supply of both individual casuals and organized detachments, forcing constant borrowing of people from hospitals and other units. The chief of the Personnel Division observed late in 1943: "Peter must necessarily be robbed to pay Paul, Peter in each instance being a T/O unit." [13]

Compounding the shortage of non-T/O casuals, the ETO medical service had difficulty obtaining sufficient replacements, especially of doctors, from the United States. In January 1943 the SOS G–1 put into effect the supply service's first system for requisitioning replacements. Under it, each chief of a technical service submitted a monthly request for people to fill existing shortages in both T/O and non-T/O organizations. This system produced few people from the United States before the theater terminated it in June, along with all manpower requisitioning, in an effort to stabilize the personnel situation. Early in August the Services of Supply transferred to the base sections responsibility for securing replacements for their subordinate units. At the same time it began calling in advance for people from the United States on the basis of a standard attrition rate for each technical service, derived from expected troop strength and from World War I loss rates.

This method, like the earlier one, produced few medical officer replacements. Of 130 Medical Corps (MC) officer requests for the Services of

[13] Quotation from Personnel Division, OofCSurg, HQ, ETOUSA, Annual Rpt, 1943, pp. 9–10. See also ibid., pp. 5–6, 21, app. B (4); ibid., 1944, p. 12; Operations Division, OofCSurg, HQ, ETOUSA, Annual Rpt, 1943, pp. 19–20; Troop Movements and Training Branch, Operations Division, OofCSurg, HQ, ETOUSA, Annual Rpt, 1944, p. 39; Hawley Planning Directive No. 15, 22 July 43; and Memo, Hawley to CofAdmin, SOS, 3 Aug 43, both in file HD 024 ETO O/CS (Operational and Planning Directives); McMinn and Levin, *Personnel*, p. 103. For discussion of the problem of detachments, see file 320.2 (Strength).

Supply during October, November, and December 1943, none had arrived or was under orders to the European Theater as the year ended. Replacements for Dental Corps and Sanitary Corps officers, nurses, and enlisted men came in at a better rate, but still in smaller numbers than were needed. The situation improved not at all in the following year, especially for medical officers. Shipments of doctors, as a percentage of their numbers in the theater, actually declined during 1944 from the already inadequate 1943 level. Losses, in static service in Great Britain, fortunately were far below the rates on which replacement requisitions were calculated, but the diminishing trickle in the pipeline meant that the theater would have to rely primarily on its own resources to fill in for combat casualties.[14]

The dearth of medical officer replacements was only one manifestation of a general shortage of doctors throughout the Army. By late 1943 the Army Medical Department claimed to need about 9,000 more doctors than were available to it, with the most severe shortages in surgical and other specialists. Surgeon General Kirk resorted to a variety of expedients to stretch the available trained professional manpower. During early 1944, for example, the War Department began sending hospitals overseas with general practitioners in place of some specialists called for by the tables of organization, on the assumption that the theaters could balance these staffs through transfers from other better-manned units.

In the case of the European Theater this assumption was correct. General Hawley possessed a rich pool of talent in his many affiliated hospitals and had begun raiding these units during 1943 to obtain chiefs of service for weaker hospitals. He enlarged upon this practice in the spring of 1944, as the new, inadequately staffed units began to arrive. Hawley's Personnel Division and consultants facilitated the process by developing a file of machine-readable records detailing the training and qualifications of each MC officer. The chief surgeon overcame the affiliated units' objection to the breakup of their close-knit staffs by ensuring that transfer meant promotion for every affected officer. Eventually, professionally well-endowed affiliated hospitals, such as Harvard's 5th General Hospital took pride in the number of executive officers and chiefs of service they furnished to other organizations.[15]

In late 1943, at Surgeon General Kirk's suggestions, the War Department began assigning Medical Administrative Corps (MAC) officers, of whom there was an ample supply, to

[14]Personnel Division, OofCSurg, HQ, ETOUSA, Annual Rpt, 1943, pp. 6–7, app. G, pp. 1–2 and encl. 3; ibid., 1944, p. 6; McMinn and Levin, *Personnel*, pp. 297–98 and 303–05.

[15]For dimensions of the physician shortage and expedients for overcoming it, see Maj Gen Albert W. Kenner, MC, et al., Report of Medical Department Personnel Board, 25 Oct 43, file HD 334; McMinn and Levin, *Personnel*, p. 316; Ltr, Hawley to TSG, 29 Jul 43, file HD 024 ETO O/CS (Hawley-SGO Corresp), and other letters in same collection, November 1943–May 1944; Personnel Division, OofCSurg, HQ, ETOUSA, Annual Rpt, 1944, pp. 1–2, 7–8, app. D, p. 1; Mins, 17th and 21st Meetings of Base Section Surgeons, 13 Mar 44, p. 2, and 8 May 44, p. 7, file HD 337. Middleton Interv, 1968–69, vol. 1, pp. 209–13, NLM, describes the reaction of the 5th General Hospital to transfers. See also Hawley Interv, 1962, pp. 26–28, CMH.

replace one surgeon in each battalion and fill as many other former MC slots as did not absolutely require doctors. General Hawley welcomed this policy and hoped to use the MC officers thereby released as a general theater reserve and replacement pool. The number of MAC officers in the European Theater grew from under 900 in November 1943—when the substitution policy went into effect—to over 2,400 by D-Day, but most of them arrived too late to be integrated into units before the invasion. When they finally entered service, the MC officers they relieved barely sufficed to replace current combat losses.[16]

As D-Day approached, a nurse shortage was in prospect, the result, like the doctor shortage, of recruiting difficulties in the United States. The Army Medical Department, anticipating a worldwide lack of nurses, reduced the T/O complements of its fixed hospitals and announced plans to send units overseas without nurses to absorb the paper surpluses thereby created in the theaters. Accordingly, under instructions from theater headquarters, General Hawley in May 1944 began cutting the nursing force of each of his general hospitals from 100 to 83 in order to staff twelve general hospitals coming over with no nurses. Base section chief nurses prepared lists of women for transfer to the new units, except for key specialties selecting them by lot to prevent hospitals from dumping their undesirables. Nurses from units long in the theater and earmarked for early movement to France bitterly resented these transfers, but the process went inexorably forward. The 10,500 nurses on hand at D-Day were enough to meet immediate requirements, but General Hawley had to anticipate strains on a limited force and further T/O reductions as the campaign developed.[17]

As the troop buildup accelerated, one category of theater medical manpower diminished in relative importance if not in absolute numbers. During the TORCH preparations General Hawley had encouraged Army hospitals to employ British civilians to replace military personnel detached for North African service. By mid-1943 over 500 British laborers, secretaries, and telephone operators were working in American hospitals, as were a few medical professionals, including 4 women contract doctors. While useful as a temporary expedient, this policy was military undesirable, because a hospital heavily staffed with local employees would lose much of its labor force whenever it moved. The British, at the same time, objected to the Americans' removal from their economy of scarce, vitally needed workers. With military personnel now available to replace many of the civilians, Hawley's Personnel Division, in conjunction with the British Ministry of Labor and War Office, issued on 11 September 1943

[16]Ltrs, TSG to Hawley, 3 Nov and 3 Dec 43, and Hawley to TSG, 13 Dec 43, file HD 024 ETO O/CS (Hawley-SGO Corresp); Personnel Division, OofCSurg, HQ, ETOUSA, Annual Rpt, 1944, pp. 8–9; War Department, *Strength of the Army*, 30 Nov 43, 30 Jun 44.

[17]Ltr, Lt Gen Eisenhower to CGs and Base Section Cdrs, 19 May 44, sub: Release of Nurses From General Hospitals, file HD 024 ETO CS (Hawley Chron); Mins, 23d Meeting of Base Section Surgeons, 5 Jun 44, p. 3, file HD 337; Hawley Speech on Nurse Shortage, 4 Jan 45, file HD 024 ETO O/CS (Medical Organization in ETO).

new guidelines that sharply restricted the number of local workers in each type of American Army hospitals. A 1,000-bed general hospital, for example, could hire no more than 32 Englishmen. In all hospitals civilians could perform only nonmedical tasks, such as manning telephone switchboards and operating sewage treatment and boiler plants. In response to this directive Army hospitals rapidly reduced their civilian labor components. In May 1943 the theater medical service included 1 hired civilian for every 7.5 enlisted men; by December, although the total number of British employees had risen to 986, their share of the work force had declined to 1 per 22 medical soldiers.[18]

By 31 May 1944, in spite of imminent shortages of doctors and nurses, nagging demands for casuals, and the unsatisfactory replacement flow, the medical service, like the rest of ETOUSA, substantially had met its first-phase buildup goals. About 133,000 medical officers, nurses, and enlisted men were in Great Britain, preparing for their multifarious D-Day tasks. Of these personnel some 71,000 belonged to SOS units, another 49,000 were with the ground armies, and the remainder supported the air forces. The theater still fell short (by 35) of its authorized Medical Corps officer strength. The Dental Corps also lacked its full complement, while the Veterinary Corps, Sanitary Corps, and Medical Administrative Corps were over strength, as was the Army Nurse Corps (by virtue of the reduction in general hospital staffs).[19]

The Status of Nurses

The morale and welfare of ETO nurses received considerable command attention during the BOLERO personnel buildup. According to Lt. Col. Margaret E. Aaron, the Army Nurse Corps (ANC) representative in General Hawley's office, ANC officers "were not a very happy group" at the outset of theater operations. Mostly young and new to the Army, the women found themselves bewildered and homesick in a strange country. Wearing uniforms and work dresses ill-adapted to the cold, damp climate, and minimally heated buildings, they suffered a high rate of colds, flu, and pneumonia. Many nurses, lacking enough work to keep them occupied in the partially filled hospitals, applied for transfer to Mediterranean bound units in search of more interesting and professionally useful activity.[20]

Lieutenant Colonel Aaron and her successor as chief of the Nursing Division, Lt. Col. Ida W. Danielson, labored to improve nurses' morale and professional performance, assisted by a gradually expanding number of base section, army, and hospital center chiefs of nursing. Training, in

[18]Personnel Division, OofCSurg, HQ, ETOUSA, Annual Rpt, 1943, p. 4 and app. E. The 11 September 1943 directive emphasized use of British workers in maintenance and plant operation because they were familiar with the intricacies and idiosyncracies of the largely British-built hospitals. In the same manner, it was thought British telephone operators had a better chance of placing calls successfully in their own country's telephone system.

[19]Personnel Division, OofCSurg, HQ, ETOUSA, Annual Rpt, 1944, app. D, pp. 1–2; Larkey "Hist," ch. 8, pp. 27–28; McMinn and Levin, *Personnel,* pp. 105–07.

[20]"Med Svc Hist, 1942–43," p. 60, file HD 314.7-2 ETO.

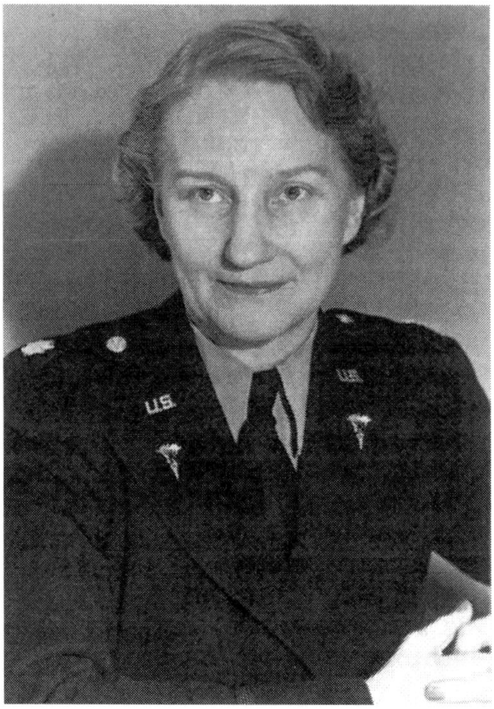

LT. COL. IDA W. DANIELSON

hospitals and at the theater Army Nurse Corps School,[21] filled idle time and acquainted nurses with their military duties. Both the theater medical service and the Red Cross furnished recreational facilities. The Red Cross, for example, set up a commodious London club for nurses on leave. The arrival of warmer weather and gradual adjustment to the climate helped reduce the nurses' sick rate, as did the issue of more serviceable uniforms. Shortages and inadequacies in clothing, however, plagued ETO nurses throughout the war. Over half the nurses did not receive the olive-drab general service uniform, introduced early in 1943 to replace the prewar blue in which most of them arrived in the theater, until well into 1944. The campaign in France was long under way before the Quartermaster Department could provide an adequate nurses field uniform.[22]

The chief surgeon, at the urging of Surgeon General Kirk, tried to give his nurses more rank. This was possible as the result of congressional action in 1942, which, besides substantially equalizing the pay and allowances of nurses and male officers in the same grades, for the first time allowed advancement of significant numbers of nurses to ranks higher than that of first lieutenant.[23] Hawley welcomed the opportunity to promote his nurses, as a way of recognizing the importance of their services and

[21] The theater Army Nurse Corps School is discussed later in this chapter.

[22] "Med Svc Hist, 1942-43," pp. 59-63, file HD 314.7-2 ETO; Pauline E. Maxwell, "History of the Army Nurse Corps, 1775-1948" (hereafter cited as "ANC Hist"), ch. XI, pp. 11-13 and 83-86, CMH. For continuing clothing problems, see Ltr, Lt Col M. G. Phillips, ANC, to Lt Col Danielson, 2 Feb 45 and Memo, Maj Gen Littlejohn to TSG, 21 Mar 45, sub: Purchase of Nurses' Clothing in United Kingdom, both in March 1945 Reading File, Robert M. Littlejohn Papers, MHI.

[23] Nurses since the end of World War I had possessed "relative rank," which meant that they had military titles, the right to wear officer insignia, and limited command authority; however, until 1942 they were not entitled to pay and allowances equal to those of male officers. Congress acted in 1942 under pressure from the Army Medical Department and civilian nursing organizations. It authorized promotion of nurses to the relative ranks of major and lieutenant colonel, whereas previously advancement—except for the War Department superintendent of nurses and her assistant—had been limited to captain. With well over 90 percent of all nurses in 1942 holding the rank of second lieutenant, the surgeon general, under political pressure to accelerate promotion, increased the number of higher nurse grades in hospital tables of organization, urged the theaters to fill these vacancies rapidly, and set quotas for increasing the total number of nurses above the rank of second lieutenant. See McMinn and Levin, *Personnel*, pp. 462-64, and Maxwell, "ANC Hist," ch. VIII, pp. 47-65, CMH.

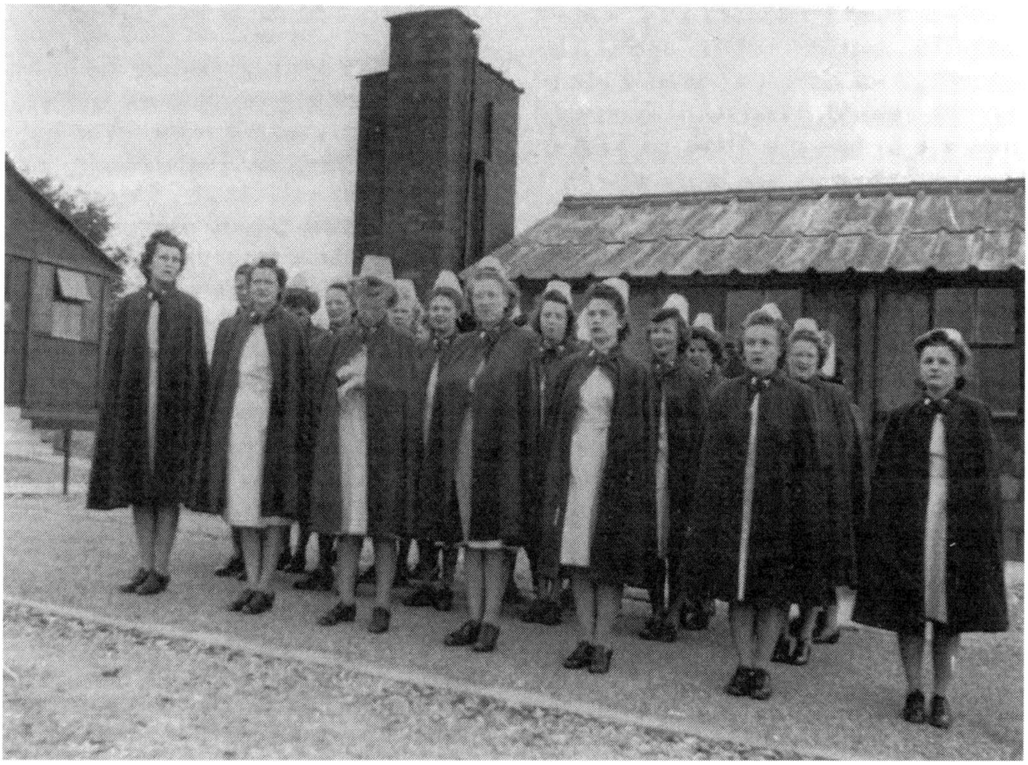

NURSES OF THE 250TH STATION HOSPITAL

responsibilities. Furthermore, the new policy would place U.S. Army nurses on a more nearly equal footing with their British counterparts of Queen Alexandra's Imperial Military Nursing Service, who held full commissioned officer status, generally at higher grades than those of American nurses in comparable positions. However, in line with his overall approach to officer promotions, Hawley resisted the indiscriminate bestowal of higher rank. He declared: "T/O vacancy is no excuse for promotion. I think of nurses the same as I think of an officer. They must be very good to reach the grade of lieutenant colonel. I am going to disapprove all wholesale promotions." In response to continued prodding from the surgeon general and from Colonel Danielson, Hawley encouraged hospital commanders to recommend for promotion to first lieutenant all properly qualified nurses who met a theater minimum requirement of seven months in grade and three months in a single position with a performance rating of Excellent. He also used some of the additional hospital field-grade slots to give his base section chief nurses rank commensurate with their responsibilities.[24]

[24] Quotation from Mins, 10th Meeting of Base Section Surgeons, 6 Dec 43, p. 5, file HD 337. See

Continued

Under these guidelines ETO nurses gradually acquired more rank. The percentage of nurses in grades above that of second lieutenant increased from 4.4 in January 1944 to 11.6 in June, including in the latter month 1 lieutenant colonel, 14 majors, 133 captains, and 1,067 first lieutenants. By the end of the year 21 percent of all nurses were above second lieutenant, a proportion still short of the surgeon general's suggested maximum of 30 percent. In most units, nevertheless, nurse ranks remained low. A general hospital nurse remembered: "Our chief nurse was a captain. . . . Most were second lieutenants, a few were first. And our unit was overseas about a year before anybody got promoted." In spite of relatively slow promotions the Nursing Division chief expressed satisfaction with the military position of ETO nurses. After Congress, in July 1944, granted nurses full officer status for the duration, Colonel Danielson commented: "The change in official status has had no material effect upon the actual status of nurses in this theater. They have been treated as officers and have been expected to act and behave as officers." [25]

Black Medics in the ETO

The ETO medical service included a modest contingent of black officers, nurses, and enlisted men. Although the Army Medical Department, following general War Department policy, enlisted blacks in rough proportion to their total numbers mobilized,[26] General Hawley was less than forthcoming about employing blacks, especially medical professionals, in his theater. He considered such personnel too few to remedy significantly any of his manpower shortages. In addition, the presence of commissioned black doctors and nurses—given the white racial attitudes of the time which Hawley showed no inclination to challenge—would create uncomfortable social and administrative problems. Hence, from the beginning of BOLERO in mid-1942 Hawley rejected the surgeon general's offer of all-black hospital units, arguing that they could not care efficiently for the ETO's widely dispersed black troops and could not be employed for any other purpose. As a result of Hawley's policy, most of the 150 black medical officers and 5,300 enlisted men who eventually arrived in the theater served either in the medical

also ibid. for 14th, 15th, and 19th, respectively 31 Jan, 14 Feb, and 10 Apr 44, same file; Ltr, Hawley to TSG, 16 Jun 44, file HD 024 ETO O/CS (Hawley-SGO Corresp). For Hawley's general promotion policy, see Notes of Speech Made by General Hawley at Command and Staff Conference, 1 Feb 44, in Hawley Papers, MHI; in same collection, see Ltr, Hawley to Brig Gen W. B. Smith, 14 Nov 42, box 2. Crew, *AMS, Administration,* 2:15, details the position of British Army nurses.

[25] First quotation from Brown Interv, 1979, CMH. Second quotation from Nursing Division, OofCSurg, HQ, ETOUSA, Annual Rpt, 1944, p. 22; for promotion statistics, see p. 20 and encl. 13.

[26] The Medical Department employed its limited complement of black doctors and nurses in a few all-black hospitals and in black wards of white station hospitals. The majority of Medical Department blacks went into ambulance and sanitary companies, the latter units functioning essentially as labor troops. All-black hospital units were deployed overseas during the war, in Liberia, the Southwest Pacific, and the China-Burma-India Theater. See Ulysses Lee, *The Employment of Negro Troops,* U.S. Army in World War II (Washington, D.C.: Office of the Chief of Military History, Department of the Army, 1966), ch. XX and pp. 130–31 and 196–97; and McMinn and Levin, *Personnel,* pp. 317–24 and 411–12.

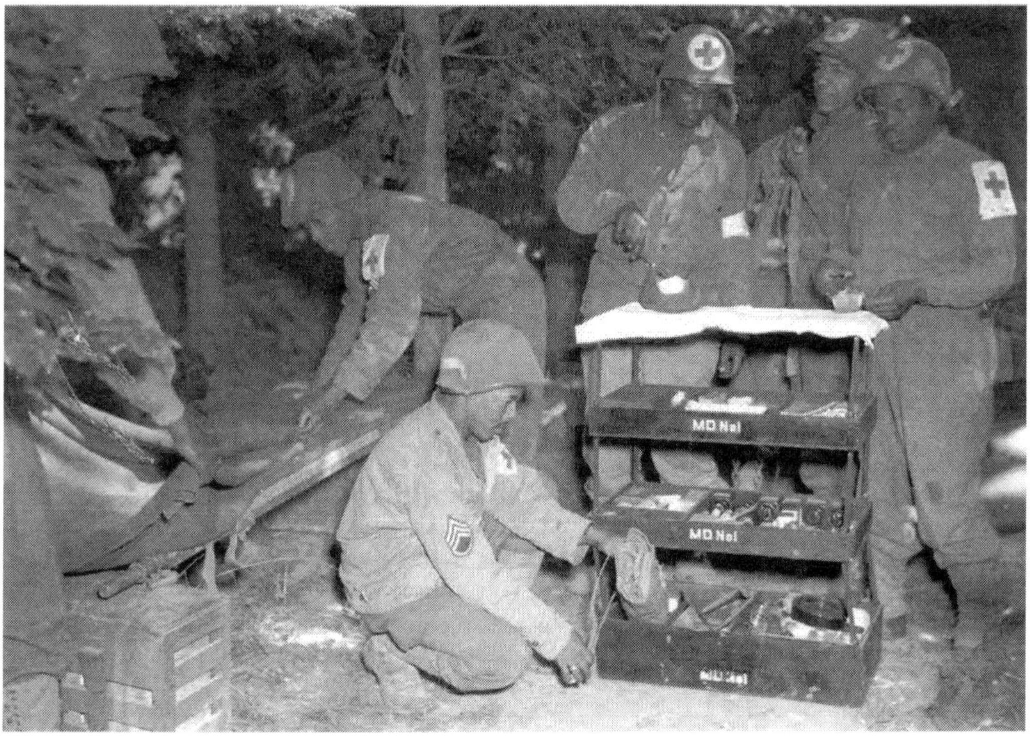

BLACK MEDICS PREPARE FOR EVACUATING CASUALTIES

detachments of segregated combat and support units or in the ten black ambulance and seventeen sanitary companies.

The one major exception to this rule was a group of 63 black nurses. General Hawley accepted these women in May 1944, at the personal request of General Kirk who was under political pressure to send more blacks overseas. The nurses reached Great Britain in July. After training at the theater ANC school, they began work in September at the 168th Station Hospital, a 1,700-bed facility near Manchester, then caring for wounded German prisoners. The nurses performed satisfactorily in the white-officered 168th, but their experience was far from happy. The officers complained that the women were less efficient and required more supervision than a comparable number of white nurses. Conducting an official inspection, a black officer found that the black nurses "feel that they are a separate group, set apart for a particular type of service, and have little hope for advancement or any variation in the type of service they are performing." Sadly, that was in fact the case, not only for the nurses of the 168th but for the theater's other black medics as well.[27]

[27] Quotation from Memo, Brig Gen B. O. Davis to Maj Gen C. H. Bonesteel, 21 Feb 45, sub: Special

Continued

Hospitals at Work

Until mid-1944 station and general hospitals in the United Kingdom, according to Colonel Darnall, the Hospitalization Division chief, were "operating in a rather inactive theater." They treated the diseases and accidental injuries of troops in garrison and training camp and carried on a large outpatient service for neighboring units. Especially in the Eastern Base Section, hospitals received a modest but steady flow of Eighth Air Force combat casualties—bomber crewmen with burns and bullet-and-shell fragment wounds. These casualties arrived at an average rate of about 90 a month during 1943 and then rose to some 800 a month in the first half of 1944, as Air Force strength increased and aerial combat intensified. Under an agreement between General Hawley and the director of the Emergency Medical Services, station and general hospitals organized emergency surgical teams to assist nearby British military and EMS hospitals in air raids and other disasters and made plans for receiving mass civilian casualties. The hospitals never had to carry out these plans. German bombing continued sporadically throughout the buildup, but British resources more than sufficed to care for the injured.[28]

U.S. Army hospitals themselves underwent only two German bombings, both of them in 1944. At 0100 on 19 April a 2,400-pound bomb fell on the 121st Station Hospital, a 834-bed unit near Braintree. The explosion destroyed or damaged fifteen Nissen huts, slightly injured twenty-five staff and patients, and temporarily put 280 beds out of service; but the hospital remained in operation. In the second incident, on 29 July, a pilotless V-1 exploded in a field close to the 1st General Hospital at North Mimms, wrecking thirty-five huts in the enlisted men's living area. Fortunately, the bomb hit during the work day when the area was almost deserted; only twelve medical soldiers suffered minor injuries. This hospital, also, kept on with its normal activities during repairs. In both cases medical officers attributed the limited casualties and damage to the sturdiness of the Nissen hut. The Americans regarded these bombings as accidental. German pilots generally seemed to avoid hospitals, which were not cam-

Inspection 168th Station Hospital, file ETO 322.15. For additional information on the black nurses, see 168th Station Hospital Annual Rpt, 1944, and Interv, ETO with 1st Lt Dorothy Smith, ANC (hereafter cited as Smith Interv), 12 Dec 44, box 220, RG 112, NARA. For black numbers, see War Department, *Strength of the Army*, 1 May 45, p. 50. Hawley's suggested answer to AGWAR cable on 4 Jan 44 is in file HD 024 ETO CS (Hawley Chron). See also Ltr, TSG to Hawley, 16 May 44, file 291.2 ETO (Negro Personnel, ANC).

[28] Quotation from Hospitalization Division, OofCSurg, HQ, ETOUSA, Annual Rpt, 1944, p. 21. For outpatient services, see Professional Services Division, OofCSurg, HQ, ETOUSA, Annual Rpt, 1944, Otolaryngology Consultant sec., p. 2; and Mins, 15th Meeting of Base Section Surgeons, 14 Feb 44, p. 2, file HD 337. For AAF casualties, see Link and Coleman, *AAF Medical Support*, pp. 692 and 699, and Interv, OSG with Maj Ralph Soto-Hall, MC (hereafter cited as Soto-Hall Interv), 29 Jun 44, box 219, RG 112, NARA. On plans to aid the British, see Ltr, Hawley to Prof F. R. Fraser, 3 Nov 42; and Memo, Col J. H. McNinch, MC, to All Base Section Surgs and Cdrs, U.S. Army Hospitals, 14 Sep 43, sub: Emergency Medical Assistance to EMS and British Military Hospitals, both in file ETO 700.1 (Misc Medical Service).

ouflaged and by their distinctive layout were easy to spot from the air even though the British did not permit them to display Red Cross markers.[29]

With their light patient load, hospitals in the United Kingdom devoted much attention to research. Staff doctors, in close cooperation with General Hawley's consultants, studied the prevention and treatment of militarily important diseases, the surgical repair of wounds, and the properties and effects of new drugs. Often, they collaborated with British colleagues or drew upon British research and war experience. General Hawley regularly incorporated the results of his people's research directly into clinical and administrative policies.[30]

The interaction between research, policy, and administration was especially evident in the case of penicillin, in 1942 a scarce antibiotic of unexplored but probably great potency. ETO penicillin investigations centered at the 2d General Hospital, located near the Oxford laboratory of Professor Howard Florey. Florey during the late 1930s had developed a method for producing penicillin in substantial quantities and had pioneered in clinical trials of the drug. In mid-1942 Lt. Col. Rudolph N. Schullinger, chief of Surgical Service at the 2d General Hospital, met Professor Florey at an Oxford University reception. This acquaintanceship led to visits by Schullinger, and later Chief Consultant in Medicine Colonel Middleton, to Florey's laboratory and also to research collaboration between Schullinger and the British scientist. As part of Florey's team Schullinger observed and reported to Professional Services on British military and civilian use of penicillin. The ETO medics began their own penicillin tests after General Hawley, in May 1943, procured from the United States the theater's first 18 million units of the drug, early fruits of a recently undertaken mass-production effort. Hawley sent all but 2 million units—given to the Soviet Union as a medical goodwill gesture—to the 2d General Hospital for use in clinical investigations.

To direct experiments, and to oversee administration of the drug to the first American patients, Hawley appointed a board that included Chief Consultant in Surgery Colonel Cutler; Colonels Middleton and Schullinger; and the chiefs of Medical and Laboratory Service at the 2d General Hospital. Under a policy worked out by Hawley and Cutler, hospitals used penicillin to treat American soldiers with gas gangrene and other life-threatening infections, and the board carefully observed the results. As additional penicillin arrived from the United States, Cutler in September began experimenting with local application of the antibiotic during initial surgical treatment of the wounds of Eighth Air Force battle casualties, to determine if such use in front-line

[29] Hospitalization Division, OofCSurg, HQ ETOUSA, Annual Rpt, 1944, p. 13; Darnall, "Hospitalization," p. 435; Memo, Hospitalization Division to DepCSurg (Cheltenham), 22 Jul 43, HospDiv-GenCorresp, 1943, file HD 312 ETO. The British forbade display of the Red Cross markers to prevent the Germans from using them to orient themselves in attacking nearby legitimate military targets. U.S. Army hospitals on the Continent would suffer much greater damage from enemy action. See Chapters XII and XIV of this volume.

[30] For a summary of research efforts, see Professional Services Division, OofCSurg, HQ ETOUSA, Annual Rpts, 1943 and 1944.

surgery would prevent or reduce infection. Besides supervising these clinical trials, the board trained officers form Army general hospitals in what was then known about the use and storage of penicillin, so as to have in each installation at least one doctor acquainted with the new antibiotic.[31]

In late 1943 Surgeon General Kirk was able to promise the European Theater regular penicillin shipments of 100 million or more units per month from the expanding American production. With a steady supply thus assured, General Hawley on 7 December authorized the issue of penicillin to all general and two station hospitals. General hospitals, the staffs of which had been trained in penicillin therapy at the 2d General Hospital, now were to instruct the surgical, medical, and laboratory chiefs of neighboring hospitals in preservation and administration of the drug. While he distributed penicillin widely, the chief surgeon restricted its use to patients with life-threatening or persistent infections and to those with sulfa-resistant venereal diseases—priorities suggested by the surgeon general for all theaters. Hawley threatened disciplinary action against any doctor who diverted the antibiotic to unauthorized treatments or experiments, declaring that "even as we widen its use, we must control its use. Otherwise, some damn fools are going to waste it trying it on ingrowing toenails so that they can write a paper on it." Colonel Cutler in April 1944 completed plans for using penicillin as a prophylactic in forward surgery, although he expressed his "firm conviction . . . that surgery will be responsible for 95 per cent of the success or failure in battle casualties." [32]

Professional societies and meetings, strongly encouraged by the chief surgeon as a means of keeping up morale and disseminating useful knowledge, proliferated among ETO doctors during the months of the buildup. Much of this activity was international in character. For example, in mid-1942, Colonel Cutler helped start the Inter-Allied Conference on War Medicine and Surgery,

[31] U.S. penicillin research and mass production began after a 1941 visit of Professor Florey to America. See Wesley W. Spink, *Infectious Diseases: Prevention and Treatment in the Nineteenth and Twentieth Centuries* (Minneapolis, Minn.: University of Minnesota Press, 1978), pp 89–100; Carter, ed., *Surgical Consultants*, 2:68–69 and 133–46; Havens, ed., *Medical Consultants*, 1:265–66; Professional Services Division, OofCSurg, HQ, ETOUSA, Annual Rpt, 1943, p. 7; Col E. C. Cutler, Lt Col P. C. Morton, and Maj J. W. Sandusky, "Observations on the Prophylactic Use of Penicillin in the Wounds of Aerial Warfare," ex. H, Chief Consultant in Surgery sec., Professional Services Division, OofCSurg, HQ, ETOUSA, Annual Rpt, 1944; Middleton Interv, 1968–69, vol. 1, pp. 218–20, NLM.

[32] First quotation from Ltr, Hawley to Brig Gen Fred W. Rankin, 16 Feb 44. Second quotation from Ltr, Cutler to Rankin, 25 Apr 44. Both in file HD 024 ETO O/CS (Hawley-SGO Corresp). See this source, September–December 1943, for a running account of the development of penicillin supplies and policy. See also Memo, Col Kimbrough to DepCSurg (Cheltenham), 13 Nov 43, file HD 024 ETO O/CS (Spruit Policy Notebook); Professional Services Division, OofCSurg, HQ, ETOUSA, Annual Rpts, 1943, p. 7, and 1944, pp. 6 and 8; Carter, ed., *Surgical Consultants*, 2:142–45; Mins, 13th, 14th, and 15th Meetings of Base Section Surgeons, respectively, 17 Jan, 31 Jan, and 14 Feb 44, file HD 337. Before the advent of sulfa drugs, treatment of gonorrhea and other venereal diseases had been lengthy and painful for the patient, keeping men away from duty for long periods and requiring much hospital space, staff, and equipment. The use of sulfa and penicillin for a faster, simpler cure greatly reduced both the logistics burden on the theater medical service and the Army's noneffective rate. See Haven, ed., *Medical Consultants*, 1:24–25;

which brought American doctors together with British colleagues and with the exiled medical elite of occupied Europe. At least 100 American medical officers attended each of the society's conferences, held in London under sponsorship of the Royal Society of Medicine, to hear papers and enjoy cocktail hours and dinners. British medical associations accepted Americans into membership. They opened their meetings and their libraries to their American colleagues. Hawley's senior consultants met regularly with their British counterparts, and the chief surgeon hosted occasional dinners at which American officers mingled with distinguished British medical men.[33]

In July 1943, at General Hawley's suggestion, U.S. Army doctors formed their own European Theater of Operations Medical Society, of which all Army MC officers were autmatically members. At first, the entire membership met once a month at a particular general hospital for papers, ward rounds, and lunch. As the theater expanded in late 1943, the organization perforce broke down into base section branches, each of which carried on its own social and professional program. Dentists and veterinarians established similar theater and base section associations. Local activities abounded. Station and general hospitals, for example, organized frequent clinical and pathological conferences open to medical officers of neighboring hospitals and units. The contribution to the war effort of this constant round of professional conferences and socializing was difficult to measure, but it promoted the sharing of knowledge and experiences and fostered acquaintanceships that eased working relationships among Army medical officers and between the latter and their British colleagues.[34]

ETO hospitals made the most of the time and relative leisure afforded them by the long wait for the beginning of full-scale combat. In March 1944 Surgeon General Kirk, after touring theater hospitals in the course of the presidentally directed review of Air Force patient care, expressed high praise for what he had seen. Patients in the European Theater, he told Hawley,

> are receiving superb treatment as a result of professional efficiency and individual care. . . . Surgical pavillions are well planned, the wards bright, cheerful and immaculate in cleanliness. Your General Medical Laboratory, dental clinic and laboratories, both fixed and mobile, are ideal. The research work that is being carried on is outstanding. . . . We are assured that the Medical Department will be ready to do its job on D-Day.[35]

Organizing the Dental Service

In hospitals and unit medical detachments the ETO dental service conducted its own buildup, coped with its own problems, and contribut-

---

[33] Maj Gen Sir H. L. Tidy, ed., *Inter-Allied Conference on War Medicine, 1942–1945* (London: Staples Press, 1947), pp. 12–15 and passim; Middleton Interv, 1968–69, vol. 1, pp. 199–201, 225–27, 231, NLM; Professional Services Division, OofCSurg, HQ, ETOUSA, Annual Rpt, 1943, pp. 12–13; Hawley Papers, MHI, passim.

[34] American Medical Society, ETO, memoranda and meeting programs, various dates, box 3, Hawley Papers, MHI; Hawley Interv, 1962, p. 49, CMH; Surg, Northern Ireland Base Section, Annual Rpt, 1944, p. 4; Surg, XIX Corps, Annual Rpt, 1944, p. 2.

[35] Ltr, TSG to Hawley, 19 Mar 44, file HD 024 ETO O/CS (Hawley-SGO Corresp).

ed its own technical innovations. Throughout BOLERO the Dental Corps labored under a shortage of officers, especially in unit detachments. The corps was still about 10 percent understrength in late 1944, although the bulk of vacant positions now were in general hospitals. In the early month of BOLERO dentists often reached Britain without their basic field chest. Dental equipment for hospitals arrived only slowly and in small amounts, due to procurement delays and difficulties on the other side of the Atlantic. The first American units in England, therefore, sent troops needing dental work to neighboring British forces for treatment, and American dentists had prostheses made in British laboratories. They also borrowed what supplies they could from their Allies, whose own stocks were limited. Dental field and laboratory chests arrived in adequate numbers during 1943, but hospital equipment remained difficult to procure until late in the year, forcing the Supply Division to outfit newly opened hospitals by breaking up field chests. In spite of these obstacles ETO dentists did a substantial amount of work. Between November 1942 and November 1943 they held over 650,000 patient sittings, made 250,000 restorations, extracted more than 62,000 teeth, and fitted about 15,000 full and partial dentures.[36]

Besides overseeing the training and professional work of dentists, the Dental Division of the chief surgeon's office improvised central dental laboratories for the theater. The War Department did not establish a T/O unit of this type for overseas service, even though the theaters would need laboratories for large-scale fabrication of prostheses and repair of instruments. Instead, each theater was to develop a laboratory organization tailored to its own needs and requisition men and equipment from the United States for it.

The ETO Dental Division, accordingly, in July 1942 prepared a table of organization that the Services of Supply and the theater approved and transmitted to the New York Port of Embarkation. In the next fifteen months none of the requested people and only a few items of equipment reached Great Britain. The Dental Division nevertheless managed to assemble two central dental laboratories during 1943, one at London and the other at Cheltenham. Each had a staff of four officers and forty enlisted men drawn from hospitals, dispensaries, and other SOS medical organizations. Equipment came from hospitals, from the British, and from laboratory field chests. Each central laboratory had attached to it a mobile section with a clinic, mounted on a bus ambulance converted by the Ordnance Department. The Dental Division employed these mobile laboratories to bring service to organizations in the United Kingdom that needed large amounts of extra dental work—for example, the 9th Infantry Division, redeployed to England after fourteen months in the field in North Africa and Sicily.

[36] George F. Jeffcott, *United States Army Dental Service in World War II*, Medical Department, United States Army in World War II (Washington, D.C.: Office of the Surgeon General, Department of the Army, 1955), pp. 166–68 and 180–85; "Med Svc Hist, 1942–43," pp. 46–48 and 52, file HD 314.7-2 ETO; Dental Division, OofCSurg, HQ, ETOUSA, Annual Rpts, 1942, pp. 4–5, and 1944, pp. 3 and 8.

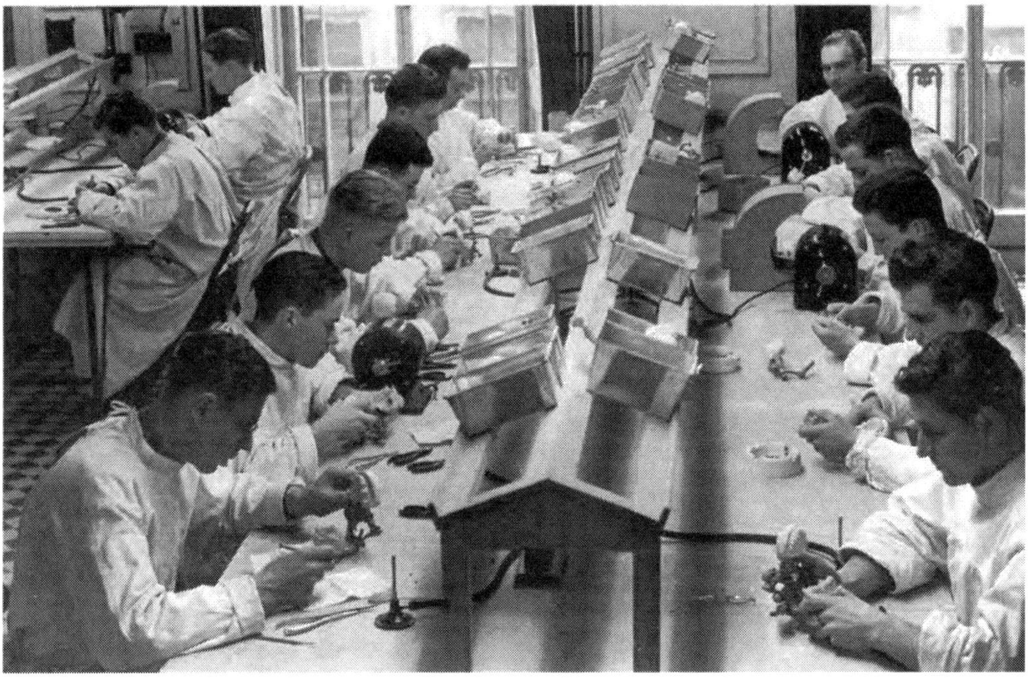

London Central Dental Laboratory *(top)* and Mobile Clinic *(bottom)*

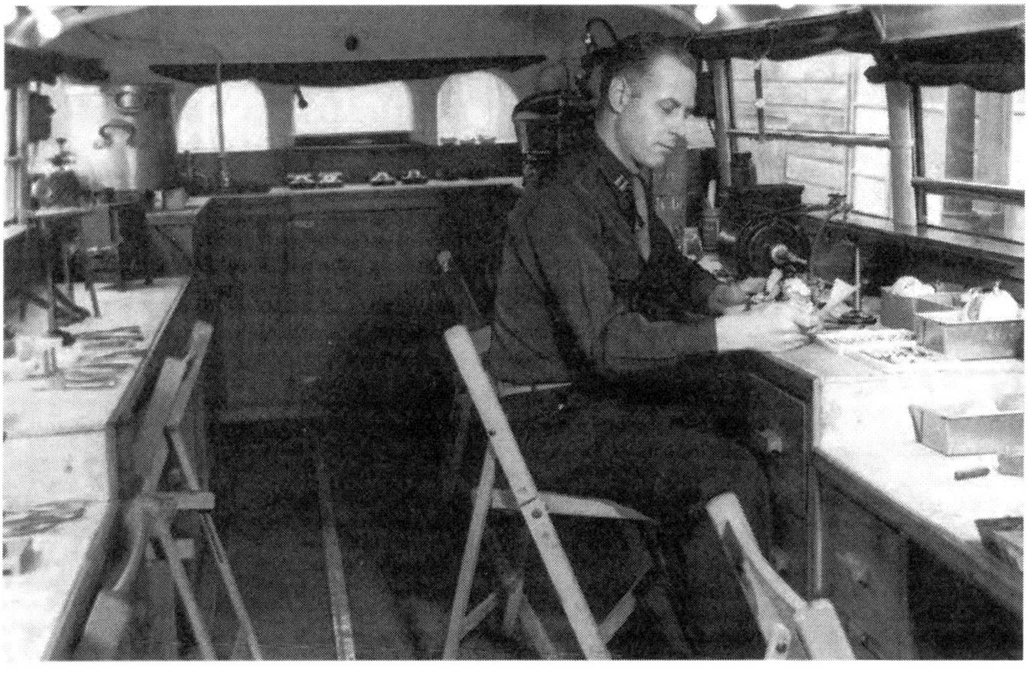

The laboratories were to serve a similar purpose on the Continent for combat units resting behind the front.[37]

As a result of the initiative of one Dental Corps officer, Capt. Stanley F. Erpf of the 30th General Hospital, the European Theater developed a new type of artificial eye, thereby helping to solve an Army-wide problem of supply and patient welfare. The Army by 1943 faced a growing demand for glass eyes, both for men with empty sockets resulting from accidental and combat injuries and for one-eyed recruits being inducted under lowered physical standards. However, material for glass eyes, previously imported from Europe, was in short supply. The eyes themselves took up to two months to make and fit to the individual and also broke easily. In September 1943, at the request of a staff opthalmologist whose patient had broken his glass eye, Captain Erpf devised an artificial eye made of the clear acrylic resin used in dentures. Erpf's type of eye, which he began producing for other patients on an experimental basis, could be moulded and fitted to an individual, using standard dental tools, in no more than four days. Properly colored and painted, an acrylic eye could match exactly the patient's good eye, a feature of great psychological benefit. Further, acrylic eyes irritated socket tissues less than did glass ones and were almost indestructable.

Late in 1943, after reviewing Erpf's initial reports and results, the chief surgeon, on the advice of the Dental Division and of his senior opthalmology consultant, adopted the acrylic eye for theater-wide use. In January 1944 the medical service set up a two-week course at the 30th General Hospital, taught by Erpf, to train both U.S. Army and British Army dental officers in fabricating and fitting the eyes. By the time the course closed down for the invasion in late May thirty-three dentists had graduated from it. The acrylic eye school later reopened at the two central dental laboratories. On the strength of reports from the European Theater, the War Department adopted the acrylic eye as a substitute for glass throughout the Army and brought Erpf back to the United States in June to help organize production and employment of his invention.[38]

Training

ETO medics put many hours into training. Training, besides filling time, was in fact much needed, because few doctors, nurses, or aidmen arrived in the theater fully instructed in their military tasks. Even Regular Army medical officers, as Hawley had pointed out ever since the establishment of the European Theater, lacked administrative and command experi-

[37] All the theaters had difficulty obtaining men and equipment for the central dental laboratories; see Jeffcott, *Dental Service*, pp. 327–29; "Med Svc Hist, 1942–43," pp. 48–50, file HD 314.7-2 ETO; Dental Service, OofCSurg, HQ, ETOUSA, Annual Rpt, 1944, p. 10; Surg, 9th Infantry Division, Annual Rpt, 1944, p. 4.

[38] The idea of using dental acrylic for artificial eyes evidently occurred to a number of medical and dental officers more or less at the same time, but Erpf probably was the first to complete a satisfactory eye. See Jeffcott, *Dental Service*, pp. 235–37; Dental Division, OofCSurg, HQ, ETOUSA, Annual Rpt, 1944, pp. 7–8; Soto-Hall Interv, 29 Jun 44, box 219, RG 112, NARA; Mins, 16th Meeting of Base Section Surgeons, 28 Feb 44, pp. 3–4, file HD 337.

ence. The reservists and civilians in uniform who staffed most medical units were even more deficient in these fields. In addition, Hawley pointed out, "few physicians ever see, in civil practice, injuries of the type that are incurred in war. They do not know how to care for such injuries properly; and, unless given special training, will care for them improperly." Newly enlisted nurses had come directly to Army hospitals with no military orientation, even in such basics as saluting and proper wear of the uniform. Enlisted technicians included a mixture of backgrounds and qualifications. In one general hospital the chief of Laboratory Service recalled, "The chief of the bacteriology section had been superintendent of schools in Albuquerque and the chief of hematology . . . had been an orchestra leader in Georgetown." Units going overseas usually received their full personnel complements only shortly before embarkation so that they had little opportunity to train their own people or to develop a sense of group cohesion.[39]

General Hawley, as both theater and SOS chief surgeon, established training objectives and standards of proficiency for ground force and SOS medical units, while army and base section commanders supervised the conduct of instruction. The Air Force independently trained its unit and base dispensary medical personnel. For the organizations under his purview General Hawley laid down both military and professional training requirements. On the military side, medical units were to make sure that their people mastered basic service customs and wore the correct uniform. Both male and female personnel were to engage in close-order drill, calisthenics, and cross-country marching. They were to learn to read maps, use compasses, and interpret aerial photographs, as well as how to protect their patients and themselves under air and gas attack. Hospitals and collecting and clearing companies were to practice setting up, taking down, and moving their equipment. The chief surgeon directed that professional instruction of doctors and nurses concentrate on practical elements of war medicine and surgery. He opposed efforts to train people in specialties for which they had not been qualified before entering the Army, although he provided extensive refresher courses for doctors already proficient in various fields. Enlisted medics were to be well versed in basic anatomy and physiology, medical nomenclature, first aid, and ward management. Hawley also wanted them to be able to speak and write clear Eng-

[39] First quotation from Memo, Hawley to G–3, ETO, 1 Jul 43, file HD 024 ETO O/CS (Operational and Planning Directives); in the same file, see Memo, Col. J. H. McNinch, MC, to CSurg 12 Jul 43, and Hawley Operational Directive No. 24, 1 Jul 43. Second quotation from Vorder Bruegge Interv, 29 Jan 80, tape 1, side 1, p. 6, CMH. See also Maj Gen Paul R. Hawley, Brig Gen James B. Mason, and Col Robert E. Peyton, "Training in the European Theater in World War II" (hereafter cited as "ETO Training"), p. 30; Operations Division, OofCSurg, HQ, ETOUSA, Annual Rpt, 1943, p. 14; Study No. 88, General Board, USFET, sub: Training Status of Medical Units and Medical Department Personnel Upon Arrival in the European Theater of Operations, pp. 1–4, file 353/2. Smith Interv, 12 Dec 44, box 220, RG 112, NARA, comments on the nurses' lack of training.

lish so as to make themselves understood to patients and doctors alike.[40]

In providing medical training facilities General Hawley made every effort to expose his personnel to the professional and operational expertise of their British colleagues. Beginning in mid-1942, under agreements made by Colonel Kimbrough with the Royal armed services and Ministry of Health, British military and civilian medical schools allocated places in their courses for Americans. Hawley's office distributed these openings among air, ground, and service commands. U.S. Army doctors took five-day war medicine and surgery courses at the British Post-Graduate Medical School. They studied tropical medicine and parasitology at the London School of Hygiene, and they attended a transfusion and shock course at the British Army blood supply depot in Bristol. Surgeons and dentists went to the Queen Victoria Hospital in Sussex for training in plastic surgery and repair of jaw injuries. Other surgeons studied treatment of chest wounds with Mr. A. Tudor Edwards, the EMS thoracic surgery consultant, who was one of the country's leaders in that field. Groups of medical officers each week visited the major London teaching hospitals for ward rounds, discussions, and lunch with the professional staffs.

EMS and military hospitals trained American operating room nurses to assist in maxillofacial surgery and neurosurgery. RAF hospitals gave nurses two weeks' intensive training in care of burn patients. The British Army School of Hygiene at Aldershot taught field sanitation to enlisted medics. Under an Anglo-American exchange program, American doctors and nurses went to British military hospitals for thirty-day duty tours. Staff from inactive U.S. hospitals also worked in British wards. The hundreds of American officers, nurses, and medical soldiers who attended these British courses or labored in British hospitals benefited from the medical lessons of three years of combat, as well as learned their British counterpart's methods of operation.[41]

The ETO medical service lost no time in setting up its own training facilities. On 8 March 1943 General Hawley formally opened the European Theater Medical Field Service School at Shrivenham, in a former British officer candidates school. Su-

[40] Hawley et al., "ETO Training," pp. 8 and 10–14; Mins, 14th Meeting of Base Section Surgeons, 31 Jan 44, pp. 4–5, file HD 337; Operations and Training Division, OofCSurg, HQ ETOUSA, Annual Rpt, 1942, p. 15. See also Cir Ltr No. 45 (Training Ltr No. 1), OofCSurg, HQ ETOUSA, 12 Oct 42; Troop Movements and Training Branch, Operations Division, OofCSurg, HQ ETOUSA, Annual Rpt, 1944, pp. 23, 27, 36, and encl. 18. Ltr, Hawley to Brig Gen Charles C. Hillman, 17 Mar 43, file HD 024 ETO O/CS (Hawley-SGO Corresp), expresses the chief surgeon's opposition to training people in specialities. For a general view of the Medical Department's role in training, see Robert J. Parks, ed., *Medical Training in World War II*, Medical Department, United States Army in World War II (Washington, D.C.: Office of the Surgeon General, Department of the Army, 1974), pp. 247–51.

[41] Hawley et al., "ETO Training," pp. 44–47; Operations and Training Division, OofCSurg, HQ ETOUSA, Annual Rpt, 1942, pp. 15–16; Operations Division, OofCSurg, HQ ETOUSA, Annual Rpt, 1943, pp. 13–17; Troop Movements and Training Branch, Operations Division, OofCSurg, HQ ETOUSA, Annual Rpt, 1944, pp. 21–23; Maxwell, "ANC Hist," ch. XI, pp. 73–74, CMH. Brown Interv, 1979, CMH, includes impressions of work in a British hospital.

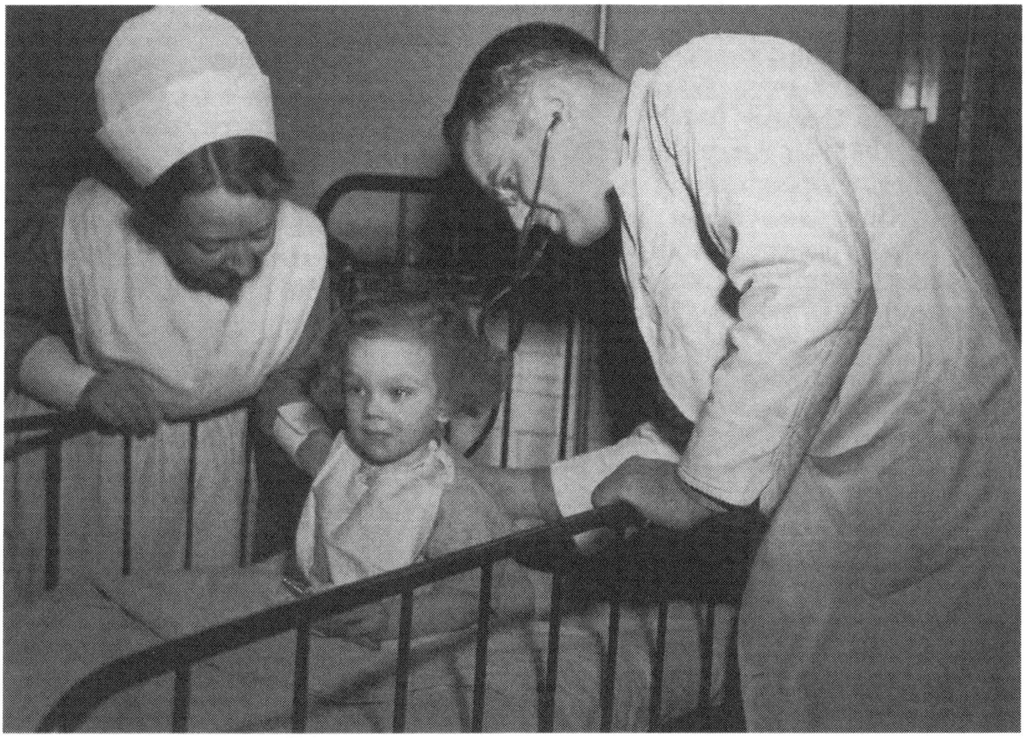

U.S. Army Medical Officer on Temporary Duty at a British Civilian Hospital

pervised by the Operations Division of Hawley's office, this institution was part of the ETO's American School Center. It had the mission of instructing medical officers, particularly those serving with field units, in "aspects of military medical practice not ordinarily familiar to civilian physicians." Under the teaching of a small faculty, assisted by the senior consultants and other outside lecturers, forty- and fifty-man classes of medical officers learned the fundamentals of field hygiene and sanitation, care of casualties under combat conditions, motor vehicle maintenance, medical record-keeping, and chemical warfare defense. As D-Day approached, the school added transportation of sick and wounded and principles of medical support for and amphibious assault; it brought in doctors who had campaigned in North Africa and Sicily to impart battlefield experiences. Besides receiving classroom instruction, students took part in field maneuvers with other departments of the school, establishing and displacing aid stations and evacuating simulated casualties. After one such overnight exercise, acording to the school history, the "exhausted appearing group of officers . . . had a better understanding of what Medical Department soldiers undergo to bring sick and wounded to the rear . . . for treatment." Over 1,300 air, ground, and service force medical officers, most of them captains and first lieutenants, graduated from this course before the Medical Field Service School ceased operations in October 1944.[42]

In May 1943, an Army Nurse Corps School began operations at Shrivenham in close association with the Medical Field Service School and with an almost identical charter. Chief nurses and potential chief nurses took an intensive three-week course designed to remedy their lack of basic military training, as well as improve their preparation for professional duties. The women lived udner strict discipline, receiving demerits for minor deficiencies in military courtesy and appearance. They spent so much time in drill and physical conditioning that they nicknamed the program "Commando School for Nurses." They studied first aid, field sanitation, chemical warfare defense, Medical Department and hospital organization and administration, the types and care of battle wounds, and major diseases of military importance. During 1944, as nurses who had undergone basic training in the United States began arriving, the school reduced or eliminated its bootcamp features and emphasized instead advanced military and professional instruction, concentrating on ETO policies and problems. Almost 800 nurses passed through the school before it closed in October 1944. They went back to their units to help train other nurses and to set a more military tone among their colleagues.[43]

In September 1943, at General Hawley's request, the European Theater activated the 1st Medical Demonstration Platoon, attached for quarters and administration to the Shrivenham school center. The 2 officers and 30 enlisted men of this unit spent two weeks in each base section in rotation, showing other organizations how to train medical soldiers. Between trips, the platoon acted as school troops for the Medical Field Service School. Early in 1944 the medical service partially transferred control of the demonstration platoon to the Field Force Replacement System, which began using it to train medical troop replacements. This arrangement led to disputes between the chief surgeon's staff and that of the school center commander, Col. Walter G. Layman (who also headed the replacement system), over scheduling of the platoon's activities and, as a result, substantially reduced its usefulness to the medical service. In May 1944, as part of the preparations for receiving D-Day casualties, the European Theater turned the platoon over to the Southern Base Section,

[42] Quotations from Medical Field Service School, American School Center, "Medical Field Service School History," pp. 1 and 156, file HD 353 ETO. See also ibid., pp. 2 and 47–48, same file; Hawley et al., "ETO Training," pp. 33–35; Operations Division, OofCSurg, HQ, ETOUSA, Annual Rpt, 1943, pp. 14–15; Troop Movements and Training Branch, Operations Division, OofCSurg, HQ, ETOUSA, Annual Rpt, 1944, p. 17. For a general history of the American School Center, set up to remedy training deficiencies of a number of ETO elements, see Ruppenthal, *Logistical Support*, 1:335–36.

[43] Hawley et al., "ETO Training," p. 35; Operations Division, OofCSurg, HQ, ETOUSA, Annual Rpt, 1943 p. 15; Nursing Division, OofCSurg, HQ, ETOUSA, Annual Rpt, 1944, pp. 7–8. In July 1943 the Army Service Forces established ANC basic training centers in the United States similar in purpose and curriculum to the ETO school. See Parks, ed., *Medical Training*, pp. 127–32. For the effect of the school upon hospitals, see Maxwell, "ANC Hist," ch. XI, pp. 59–61 and 71, CMH.

which reorganized it as a provisional ambulance company.[44]

As it expanded in numbers and facilities, the theater medical service introduced numerous short specialized courses and training programs. Five days to two weeks in duration, these classes met at the Medical Field Service School, or, more often, at general and station hospitals; they supplemented and in some instances replaced courses in British institutions. Officers and nurses took instruction in anesthesiology, to remedy a theater-wide shortage of people in this field, as well as studied the latest theories and techniques in treatment of combat exhaustion and other neuropsychiatric illnesses. They learned how to perform blood transfusions in the field and how to apply plaster of Paris bandages. Dental Corps officers received additional training in maxillofacial surgery. Enlisted medics took courses that would qualify them as laboratory and surgical technicians and went to depots for practice in equipment maintenance and repair. Some short courses, for example, Detachment Training in the Treatment of Neuropsychiatric Patients, taught at the 312th Station Hospital, were designed for teams of officers, nurses, and enlisted medics from evacuation or other types of hospitals. Most working general hospitals functioned to some degree as teaching institutions, offering specialized instruction, usually in the form of individual practice with an authority in a particular field.[45]

Medical units developed and implemented their own training schedules under the supervision and inspection of base section surgeons in the Services of Supply and of field army and corps surgeons in the ground forces. Each unit sent its quota of people to the various ETO schools and courses and tailored its own activities to its particular mission. General and station hospitals, for example, held exercises in which they practiced receiving and caring for hundreds of simulated casualties. Staffs of general hospitals expecting early orders to move to France after D-Day practiced pitching and striking tents and devoted time to physical conditioning, often by cross country marches. Officers and enlisted medics of the 298th General Hospital, by the time of the invasion, were in good enough shape to cover 12 miles of hilly terrain, carrying full packs, in three and one-half hours. Nurses in the same hospital could go 7 miles in two and one-half hours, wearing combat clothing and laden with canteens, helmets, and gas masks.[46]

---

[44] Hawley et al., "ETO Training," pp. 39–40; Operations Division, OofCSurg, HQ, ETOUSA, Annual Rpt, 1943, p. 16; Troop Movements and Training Branch, Operations Division, OofCSurg, HQ, ETOUSA, Annual Rpt, 1944, p. 32; Memo, Anon. to CSurg, 20 Jul 43, file HD 024 ETO O/CS (Operational Planning Directives).

[45] Hawley et al., "ETO Training," pp. 40–43; Operations and Training Division, OofCSurg, HQ, ETOUSA, Annual Rpt, 1942, p. 17; Operations Division, OofCSurg, HQ, ETOUSA, Annual Rpt, 1943, pp. 15–16; Troop Movements and Training Branch, Operations Division, OofCSurg, HQ, ETOUSA, Annual Rpt, 1944, pp. 18–21; Keeler Interv, 17 Jul 45, box 223, RG 112, NARA; Memo, HQ, SOS, to CGs, Northern Ireland, Southern, and Western Base Sections, 18 Jan 44, sub: Technical Training of Medical Department Enlisted Men of Field Force Units, HD 024 ETO O/CS (Operational Planning Directives).

[46] 298th General Hospital Annual Rpt, 1944, pp. 284–50. For the role of base sections in training, see Surg, Western Base Section, Rpt, 1 Jan–31 Aug 44, pp. 2–3; Surg, Northern Ireland Base Section, Annual Rpt, 1944, p. 4

Medical units and detachments in the armies concentrated heavily on preparations for moving and living in the field. Evacuation and field hospitals, which usually were not caring for patients before D-Day, repeatedly packed up their full equipment, transported it to new locations, set it up, and took it down again. Collecting and clearing companies also emphasized mobility and gained practical experience by supporting divisions in maneuvers and amphibious exercises. In the First Army two veteran evacuation hospitals from the Mediterranean Theater provided instructors and acted as demonstration units for organizations fresh from the United States, passing on techniques and improvisations proven effective in North Africa and Sicily. Company aidmen with the infantry regiments received much the same tactical training as riflemen, including familiarization firing of weapons. They accompanied the troops on all exercises. In field units gas defense received much attention. An aidman in the army's 120th Infantry recalled that whenever the troops gathered for a lecture or demonstration "there would be men sneaking around with tear gas grenades. These would be thrown at unexpected intervals so that we would be trained in sudden . . . application of our gas masks." [47]

A shortage of instructional materials and inadequate inspection and testing hindered the training effort. The theater medical service never obtained enough War Department field and technical manuals, motion pictures, and filmstrips to meet unit requirements; troops often had to improvise such simple but vital teaching aids as blackboards. Key materials arrived too late to be useful. The training film "Amputations of the Lower Extremities" did not reach the theater until after D-Day, by which time the field and evacuation hospital surgeons who performed most such amputations already were in or staging for combat. A film on combat exhaustion, produced in the European Theater and intended for first- and second-echelon personnel, had similarly delayed distribution. The chief surgeon's office, the base sections, and the armies all prescribed proficiency standards and attempted to enforce them by frequent inspection and testing; but shortages of staff, especially in base section surgeons' offices, often reduced these efforts to sketchy formalities. In operating units the pressure of other duties inevitably cut into training schedules. Col. Angwald Vickoren, in charge of training in Hawley's office, complained early in 1944 that hospital commanders "have been very busy getting hospitals organized and they have forgotten about . . . training." Hawley himself, as late as a month before D-Day, still found many units deficient in first aid instruction.[48]

[47] Quotation from Robert B. Bradley, *Aid Man* (New York: Vantage Press, 1970), p. 38. See also ibid., pp. 29–37; First Army Report of Operations, 20 Oct 43–1 Aug 44, bk. VII, p. 61; Surg, Third U.S. Army, Annual Rpt, 1944, pp. 15–18, 99, 111, and ex. V; 91st Evacuation Hospital Annual Rpt, 1944, 2–3; 128th Evacuation Hospital Annual Rpt, 1944, pp. 1–2. Typical training programs are described in Surg, XIX Corps, Annual Rpt, 1944, pp. 1–4 and encls. 9–10, and in Surg, 1st Infantry Division, Annual Rpt, 1944, pp. 1–2.

[48] Quote from Mins, 14th Meeting of Base Section Surgeons, 31 Jan 44, pp. 4–5, file HD 337. See also ibid. for 21st, 8 May 44, p. 8, same file; Troop

Continued

In spite of these shortcomings, by the time General Hawley suspended most instruction in April 1944 the theater medical service had achieved its major training objectives. It remedied the lack of military orientation among medical personnel new to the Army and acquainted them with the problems and techniques of war medicine. Constant training helped standardize medical and surgical practice; it maintained the professional interest and sharpened the skills of temporarily idle or underemployed staffs; and above all, it contributed to transforming hastily assembled collections of medical personnel into units ready to function as close-knit teams within a larger whole.[49]

Preventive Medicine

During the prolonged buildup ETO medics guarded the health of the expanding American force. To carry out this mission, the chief surgeon established the Preventive Medicine Division and in June 1942 selected the newly commissioned Lt. Col. John E. Gordon as division chief. Gordon, an epidemiologist, had been working in public health in the United Kingdom since 1940, when he arrived with the Red Cross-Harvard Field Hospital Unit, and had become a respected member of the British medical establishment. A U.S. Army colleague considered him "the most efficient civilian turned military I've ever seen." Gordon, subsequently promoted to full colonel, headed the division until V-E Day. The branches—Sanitation, Nutrition, Epidemiology, and Venereal Disease Control—also benefited from continuity of leadership; the same branch chief remained in office for all or most of the war and, consequently, was able to keep the junior staff for long periods. Length of service, and the resulting chance to learn on the job, in part compensated for a theater shortage of medical officers with public health experience. Of thirty officers in key preventive medicine positions, Gordon estimated, only fifteen had worked in the field before joining the European Theater; the rest were trained in other specialties, many as internists or pediatricians.[50]

Besides the staff at Cheltenham, the Preventive Medicine Division included the ETO's central medical laboratory at Salisbury. The theater, in July 1942, acquired a central laboratory by the simple expedient of taking over Gordon's Red Cross-Harvard Unit, complete with facilities and staff, as the provisional Medical General Laboratory A. During late 1942 and early 1943 the medical service enlarged the Salisbury plant to accommodate a T/O central laboratory unit. This unit, the 1st Medical General Laboratory, arrived from the United States in June 1943. Medical General Laboratory A then disbanded, part of its staff remaining with the new organization and the rest going to other ETO assignments. From then until

Movements and Training Branch, Operations Divisions, OofCSurg, HQ, ETOUSA, Annual Rpt, 1944, pp. 24, 27–28, 32–35.

[49] Troop Movements and Training Branch, Operations Division, OofCSurg, HQ, ETOUSA, Annual Rpt, 1944, pp. 23–24 and 28, evaluates the effectiveness and deficiencies of the training effort.

[50] Quotation from Editorial Advisory Board, 1962, p. 47. See also Gordon "Hist," vol. 1, pt. 1, pp. 7–8, and pt. 2, pp. 3–4 and 6, CMH.

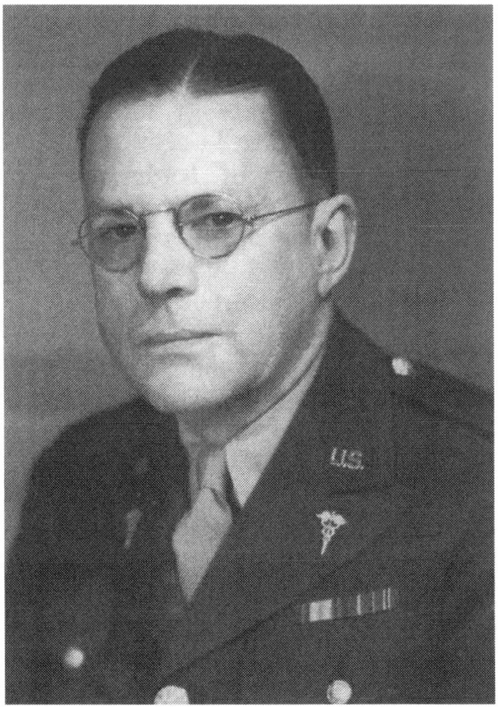

COL. JOHN E. GORDON

the end of hostilities the 1st Medical General Laboratory served as the central theater facility for pathology, epidemiological investigations, and food quality control, as well as assisted hospital laboratories with difficult or specialized problems and trained laboratory and sanitation technicians.[51]

During 1943 each base section surgeon's office established its own Preventive Medicine Division, with branches for epidemiology, nutrition, sanitation, and venereal disease control. The base sections directed most preventive medicine operations, with Gordon's office setting general policy, advising, and assisting. The ground armies and air forces also developed preventive medicine staffs. Until the invasion, army preventive medicine officers concentrated largely on planning for the European campaign. Air force staffs specialized in the health problems of flying. Both ground and air forces relied on the SOS base sections for such functions as water quality control and supervision of garbage and sewage disposal.[52]

Housing and water supply, on which the preventive medicine staffs at various headquarters worked closely with the Corps of Engineers, posed few health-related problems. The British Army barracks and cantonments, new hutted camps, converted civilian buildings, and billets in private homes in which most troops lived were adequate by American standards of comfort and cleanliness, although usually crowded and less well heated than most Americans would have liked. Poor ventilation, caused by troops closing windows and ventilators to comply with blackout regulations or to keep in what heat small stoves and rationed fuel provided, constituted the most severe health hazard. Water from municipal systems and wells, which generally met American requirements for purity, was rationed to conform to planned action by the medical service, the Engineers, and the British War Office to conserve limited natural supplies, further reduced by two years of drought. To protect water quality, the medical service arranged for added chlorination at most installations, rebuilt stor-

[51] Gordon "Hist," vol. 2, pt. 7, pp. 3–5, CMH.

[52] Gordon "Hist," vol. 1, pt. 1, pp. 11 and 13–14, and pt. 2, pp. 7 and 11–12. For details of base section activities, see Surgs, Southern, Eastern, Western, Central, and Northern Ireland Base Sections, Annual Rpts, 1943 and 1944.

age tanks in many buildings used for quarters, and required all commands to send water samples to station or general hospital laboratories each month for bacteriological analysis.[53]

At all levels of command preventive medicine officers closely supervised garbage and sewage disposal. Garbage removal entailed few difficulties. Following British law and practice, American units sold their edible refuse to local contractors for animal food; they separately salvaged grease and bones for turnover to their Allies. Sewage disposal proved to be more difficult. At hospitals and other large installations British-built waste treatment plants lacked adequate provision for drying out and disposing of sludge. Engineers and medical officers had to engage in much rebuilding and improvisation to keep them sanitary. Units in smaller camps, forbidden to dig pit latrines because of British fears of ground water contamination, learned the unsavory details of using and emptying latrine buckets, the latter a noisome task seldom satisfactorily performed by either troop details or civilian contractors. Some units tried burning their feces in incinerators, in the process subjecting themselves to foul odors. Where possible, the Americans copied a British expedient called the Otway pit—a hole in the ground, 10 feet on each side and 10 feet deep, lined with canvas or sheet metal and with a flyproof timber cover. A single such pit, properly maintained, could accommodate the waste of 100 men for a long period. Medical officers considered Otway pits more practical and less offensive than other disposal means, but they were at best the least of evils.[54]

General Hawley, in setting up his office, placed nutrition under Preventive Medicine in order to emphasize the importance of diet in maintaining troop health. Officers of the Nutrition Branch cooperated with those of the Subsistence Branch of the chief quartermaster's office in planning menus and overseeing food procurement and preparation. During the buildup most units in Great Britain lived on a garrison ("A") ration, modified to take account of shipping limitations and make use of locally procured foodstuffs. The first troops to arrive in early 1942 ate the standard British Army ration. Neither they nor their medical officers liked it, because it contained too little meat, milk products, tomatoes, fruit, and coffee; furnished too few calories; and did not include the amounts of calcium, riboflavin, and ascorbic acid considered necessary by American nutritionists. During late 1942, as American supply depots went into operation, most commands shifted to a ration jointly planned by representatives of Preventive Medicine and the chief quartermaster. This ration met American vitamin and calorie requirements, although it included canned milk and powdered eggs; incorporated British

[53] Gordon "Hist," vol. 2, pt. 9, pp. 4–8, and pt. 10, pp. 2–6, CMH. Mins, 22d Meeting of Base Section Surgeons, 22 May 44, p. 5, file HD 337, is an example of many exhortations to conserve water.

[54] Gordon "Hist," vol. 2, pt 9, pp. 16–18, CMH. For technical deficiencies of sewage treatment plants, see Ralph S. Cleland, "Sanitary Engineering in the European Theater of Operations," *The Military Surgeon* 101 (July 1947): 36–40, and 168th Station Hospital Annual Rpt, 1944, p. 14. Crew, *AMS, Administration,* 2:100–101, describes the Otway pit.

flour, bread, cereals, condiments, and vegetables; and was short of fresh fruits and salad ingredients. Hospital patients received the standard ration, supplemented with extra chicken, fruit, and eggs and with British-produced fresh milk, which General Hawley refused to have issued to all troops in order not to aggravate local shortages and because most British processing plants did not conform to American hygenic standards.

The resulting diet more than sufficed to nourish the troops, provided that they ate all the prescribed items. To ensure that they did so, the Nutrition Branch, and nutrition officers in the base sections, worked closely with commands to educate men in proper eating habits and to train cooks to make nourishing foods appealing. Officers from the Preventive Medicine Division attended Quartermaster mess management conferences, made nutritional inspections and surveys of units, and furnished educational posters and material to messes and to the soldiers newspaper, *Stars and Stripes*. In the Western Base Section the surgeon, trying to increase consumption of canned milk and powdered eggs, distributed recipes for using these items in scrambled eggs, lemon cream pie filling, baked custard, and other delicacies he hoped would be enticing.[55]

[55] Gordon "Hist," vol. 1, pt. 2, p. 5, and pt. 4, passim, CMH; Preventive Medicine Division, OofCSurg, HQ, ETOUSA, Annual Rpt, 1944, p. 26; Surg, Western Base Section, Annual Rpt, 1943. For the evolution of the ETO ration, see William F. Ross and Charles F. Romanus, *The Quartermaster Corps: Operations in the War Against Germany*, United States Army in World War II (Washington, D.C.: Office of the Chief of Military History, Department of the Army, 1965), pp. 290–92.

ETO veterinarians assisted the Preventive Medicine Division in ensuring food quality. The personnel of the Veterinary Division, who numbered 118 officers and 282 enlisted men by D-Day, were parceled out among base sections, general and Quartermaster depots, ports of embarkation, the 1st Medical General Laboratory, and ground and air forces headquarters. With no animals for which to care except a few pigeons and sentry dogs, veterinarians concentrated on their other primary task of inspecting food and supervising its storage and transportation. Although their mission normally encompassed only foods of animal origin, veterinarians in July 1943, under an agreement with the theater chief quartermaster, also began examining fresh fruit and vegetables and canned and packaged products. Veterinarians in the ports functioned as perishable freight officers, supervising the unloading of refrigerator ships. The inspecting officers found few deficiencies in Army foodstuffs, but the equipment and sanitary practices of British commercial carriers fell short of American standards and caused much spoilage. At the suggestion of the Veterinary Division, the theater transportation chief ordered 800 refrigerator cars from the United States and by the end of 1943 had 45 of them running on British railways moving highly perishable items.[56]

[56] Veterinary Division, OofCSurg, HQ, ETOUSA, Annual Rpts, 1943 and 1944; "Med Svc Hist, 1942–43," pp. 6 and 68–69, file HD 314.7-2 ETO; Everett B. Miller, *United States Army Veterinary Service in World War II*, Medical Department, United States Army in World War II (Washington, D.C.: Office of the Surgeon General, Department of the Army, 1961), pp. 271–72.

Suppression of disease outbreaks involved every level of command. Unit surgeons, assisted by base section, army, and air force staff epidemiologists, had primary responsibility for spotting health problems early and taking corrective action. In the chief surgeon's office the Epidemiology Branch of the Preventive Medicine Division established general policies for controlling particular diseases, distributed information, and sent doctors to help meet particularly severe emergencies. Colonel Gordon received periodical formal reports on the health of the Army from the Medical Records Division and the base sections, and he maintained informal contact with other divisions of the chief surgeon's office that were concerned with treatment and prevention of disease. Colonel Middleton, the chief consultant in medicine, recalled: "Virtually daily interchanges occurred between [Gordon] and me or some members of our staff, so that there was a ready communication from the clinical standpoint to preventive medicine." As a result of Gordon's rapport with the British, Preventive Medicine obtained weekly reports from the Ministry of Health and the War Office on outbreaks of infectious disease in the British civilian population and armed forces.[57]

For U.S. Army forces in the United Kingdom sickness was more a nuisance than a menace. The troops lived and worked in a temperate—if damp and chilly—climate and in a developed industrial country which understood basic sanitation and either never had had, or long ago had eradicated, most of the deadliest communicable diseases. Insects and vermin were limited in numbers and constituted no major threat to the health of the Army. Not only was the environment relatively favorable, most soldiers arrived in Great Britain with their required immunizations against smallpox, typhoid, paratyphoid, typhus, and tetanus. The Preventive Medicine Division supervised a continuing program of reimmunization and was prepared to provide additional immunization, as required for military missions, against a variety of other disease threats.[58]

Epidemics did occur, the first being the serum hepatitis outbreak of mid-1942.[59] The climate, and the often poorly heated and ventilated living quarters, produced a high continuing incidence, especially in winter, of influenza and other respiratory infections, which accounted regularly for about 30 percent of all disease among ETO troops. To control these infections, medical officers and unit commanders emphasized personal cleanliness among their men, tried to improve barracks heat and ventilation, and provided extra facilities for drying clothing. Scattered outbreaks of diarrhea—sixty between January and October 1943—and less frequently of dysentery and food poisoning plagued the Army. The medical service traced most of these to unsanitary mess practices, typically efforts

[57] Quotation from Middleton Interv, 1968–69, vol. 1, pp. 206–07, NLM. See also Gordon "Hist," vol. 1, pt. 2, pp. 2–3, and pt. 3, sec. 1, pp. 5–6, CMH.

[58] Medical Bulletin No. 6, OofCSurg, HQ, ETOUSA, 15 Jun 43, pp. 7–9; Mins, 15th and 19th Meetings of Base Section Surgeons, 14 Feb and 10 Apr 44, file HD 337; Gordon "Hist," vol. 2, pt. 3, sec. 7, pp. 4–5, CMH.

[59] For details, see Chapter 1 of this volume.

to store food too long without adequate refrigeration. Epidemics of a mild form of hepatitis constantly recurred, especially during the winter of 1943–44, when divisions redeploying from the Mediterranean for OVERLORD brought the disease with them. Medical officers never determined definitely the mode of transmission of this infection, and the Army would suffer from occasional hepatitis epidemics until V–E Day.[60]

The four divisions and an engineer special brigade that entered the United Kingdom from the Mediterranean in November 1943 carried with them a clinically more severe, and militarily a more potentially disruptive, disease than hepatitis: They brought malaria. By the beginning of the twentieth century indigenous malaria very nearly had disappeared from the British Isles. However, at least one species of mosquitoes—Anopheles—lived there, and the troops from the Mediterranean, as well as aircraft crews who picked up the infection at African stopovers on transatlantic flights, provided a new reservoir of the parasite, creating conditions for further spread of the disease. As men in the newly arrived units stopped taking suppressive Atabrine, the European Theater's rate of hospital admissions for malaria began rising. All cases, of the vivax variety, were benign and all, as judged by medical officers, resulted from infection outside the United Kingdom.

To check the spread of the disease to the rest of the Army and the British people, hospitals kept malaria patients isolated under mosquito netting or in screened rooms until treatment cleared their bloodstreams of the parasite. Preventive medicine officers in the base sections started or intensified mosquito eradication efforts around hospitals and camps. Unit medical officers tested the blood of all men who had served in malarial regions to detect carriers of the parasite. To prepare for the invasion, affected units transferred out the men most debilitated by malaria, and two weeks before D-Day they put all soldiers who had had malaria within the past twelve months back on daily doses of Atabrine. These measures prevented the occurrence of new cases among troops and civilians, but already infected men in the veteran units would continue to be incapacitated by the disease during the assault on continental Europe.[61]

Venereal disease, in spite of rapid and effective treatment with sulfa drugs and penicillin, cost the Army heavily in lost time from duty and diversion of medical resources, as well as being a source of political and social tension between the Americans and their British hosts. Recognizing the importance of this health prob-

[60] Gordon "Hist," vol. 1, pt. 3, sec. 2, no. 1, pp. 8–9, and sec. 3, no. 1, pp. 1–2, 12–15, and vol. 2, pt. 3, sec. 6, pp. 9–16, 22–25, CMH; Essential Technical Medical Data Rpt, HQ, ETOUSA, October 1943, p. 2. HQ, Eastern Base Section, Directive, 19 Dec 42, sub: Common Respiratory Diseases, in Surg, Eastern Base Section, Annual Rpt, 1942, is typical of measures against respiratory diseases.

[61] The affected units were the 1st and 9th Infantry, the 2d Armored, and the 82d Airborne Divisions and the 1st Engineer Special Brigade. See also Gordon "Hist," vol. 1, pt. 3, sec. 5, no. 2, pp. 1–11, CMH. On malaria in the Mediterranean, see Ebbe C. Hoff, ed., *Communicable Diseases: Malaria*, Medical Department, United States Army in World War II (Washington, D.C.: Office of the Surgeon General, Department of the Army, 1963), pp. 262–64.

lem, General Hawley in September 1942 organized a separate Venereal Disease Control Branch in the Preventive Medicine Division. Headed by Lt. Col. Paul Padget, a venereal disease specialist from John Hopkins University, this branch had responsibility for control and prevention, while the Professional Services Division supervised treatment. As the medical service expanded, base sections, air forces, armies, and lower-echelon headquarters acquired their own venereal disease control officers. Padget and his small staff made general policies, gave advice, and held periodic meetings of control officers from other commands to exchange ideas and experiences.[62]

Padget and his colleagues, as well as troop commanders at every echelon, employed the standard Army methods of controlling venereal disease. Commands worked with the Red Cross and Special Services to provide wholesome recreation for their troops and (rarely) took disciplinary action against men who became infected. Units emphasized education. Line officers, surgeons, chaplains, and specially trained NCOs lectured on the dangers of venereal disease and the methods of preventing it. Films and posters, the latter often drawn by enlisted men in contests, graphically presented the same themes. All media urged men on grounds of patriotism, unit pride, faithfulness to loved ones at home, and personal self-interest to avoid illicit sexual contact, which, it was emphasized, almost invariably led to infection. If the soldiers were unable to comply, the education program urged them to be careful by using correctly the mechanical and chemical prophylactics the Army provided. Getting down to basic details, the Northern Ireland Base Section surgeon suggested that venereal disease lecturers "secure a model penis and show the men the exact method of putting on and taking off a condom."[63]

The medical service furnished prophylaxis in abundance and in a variety of forms. It issued condoms without charge at a rate of six per man per month and individual chemical prophylactic kits ("V-Packettes") at a rate of two per man per week. Because many units, especially in the Air Force and Services of Supply, were located some distance away from the hospitals and dispensaries that served them, the Preventive Medicine Division arranged for the Quartermaster Department to distribute individual prophylactics along with its other supplies so that, as Padget put it, organizations "drew their condoms at the same time they drew their soap and

[62] Gordon "Hist," vol. 1, pt. 2, pp. 5–6, and vol. 2, pt. 5, pp. 1–2 and 8, CMH; Interv, OSG with Lt Col Paul Padget, MC (hereafter cited as Padget Interv), 1 Aug 45, box 223, RG 112, NARA. Padget later assumed the additional duty of senior consultant in venereal disease.

[63] Quotation from "Suggestions for Venereal Disease Control Program," encl. 6, Surg, Northern Ireland Base Section, Rpt, 1 Jan–15 Jun 44; see encl. 7 for training of NCOs as lecturers. See also Memo, Col Kimbrough to Brig Gen Hillman, 27 Nov 42, HD 024 ETO O/CS (Hawley-SGO Corresp); Padget Interv, 1 Aug 45, box 223, RG 112, NARA; Interv, OSG with Capt P. B. Pulman (hereafter cited as Pulman Interv), 9 Mar 44, box 219, RG 112, NARA; Gordon "Hist," vol. 2, pt. 5, pp. 8–9, CMH. James P. Pappas, "The Venereal Disease Problem, United States Army," *The Military Surgeon* 93 (August 1943): 172–83, sums up then-current Army doctrine. For typical programs, see Surg, Southern Base Section, Annual Rpt, 1943, p. 8; Surg, 9th Infantry Division, Annual Rpt, 1944, pp. 3–4; and Surg, 29th Infantry Division, Annual Rpt, 1944, p. 3.

brushes." Prophylactics for women soldiers became the subject of delicate negotiations between General Hawley, General Lee, and the senior officer of the Women's Army Auxiliary Corps (WAAC). The fact that such equipment had contraceptive as well as hygienic uses was, Hawley declared, "political dynamite." Nevertheless, all concerned decided that the women's health had to receive priority. The medical service issued equipment for douches to WAAC organizations while taking pains to emphasize the hygienic purpose and ruling out measures "primarily contraceptive in nature." [64]

Besides furnishing individual equipment, base sections and other commands set up prophylactic stations in cantonments and, after much haggling with the British—and, according to Gordon, "relentless" pressure upon them—in towns and cities frequented by men on pass. The Red Cross allowed the Army to place prophylactic stations in its clubs, where most soldiers on leave stayed. Many potentially infected men, as a result, "found a prophylactic station right in their path when they returned to quarters." Units posted the locations of prophylactic stations in neighboring towns on their bulletin boards and stamped them on passes. The Central Base Section made free condoms and V-Packettes available at every London railroad station and at billeting and transportation offices and operated sixteen prophylactic stations, many in Red Cross clubs. Reflecting the continued prevalence of racial segregation, these stations included two especially for black soldiers, staffed with black medical personnel. By arrangement with the provost marshal, every soldier confined in the Central Base Section guardhouse, unless arrested on duty, received a prophylactic treatment during booking. During the first half of 1944 the Central Base Section by these methods distributed over 10,000 V-Packettes and 33,500 condoms and gave over 30,000 station prophylactic treatments.[65]

The usual Army procedure for combating venereal disease included close cooperation with civilian authorities to stamp out prostitution in areas frequented by troops and to trace civilian sexual partners of infected soldiers. In Great Britain, law and social custom stood in the way of both these efforts. Brothels were rare, but individual streetwalkers abounded in London and other large cities. Under laws that treated even commercial sexual arrangements between individuals as entirely private, the police could not interfere with such women unless they caused public disorder. Compounding the problem, most soldiers had their sexual contacts with nonprofessional "pickups." These "enthusiastic amateurs" were totally out of reach of the police, and

[64] First quotation from Padget Interv, 1 Aug 45, box 223, RG 112, NARA. Second and third quotations from Memo, Hawley to General Lee, undated but ca. July 1943, box 1, Hawley Papers, MHI. See also Medical Bulletins Nos. 4 and 7, OofCSurg, HQ ETOUSA, 15 May 43, p. 7, and 1 Jun 43, p. 14; Gordon "Hist," vol. 2, pt. 5, p. 10, CMH; Hawley Operational Directive No. 24, 1 Jul 43, with Supply Division endorsement, 9 Jul 43, box 2, Hawley Papers, MHI.

[65] Quotations from Gordon "Hist," vol. 2, pt. 5, pp. 4–5 and 9–10, CMH. See also Surg, Central Base Section, History of Medical Section, January–July 1944, pp. 2–3 and 8–9; Pulman Interv, 9 Mar 44, box 219, RG 112, NARA.

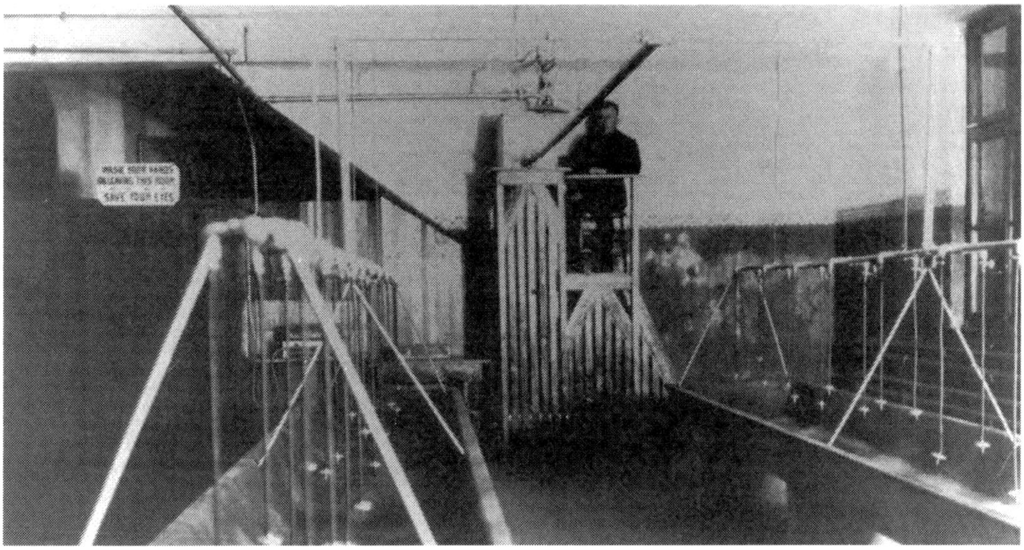

PROPHYLACTIC STATION AND PROCEDURE

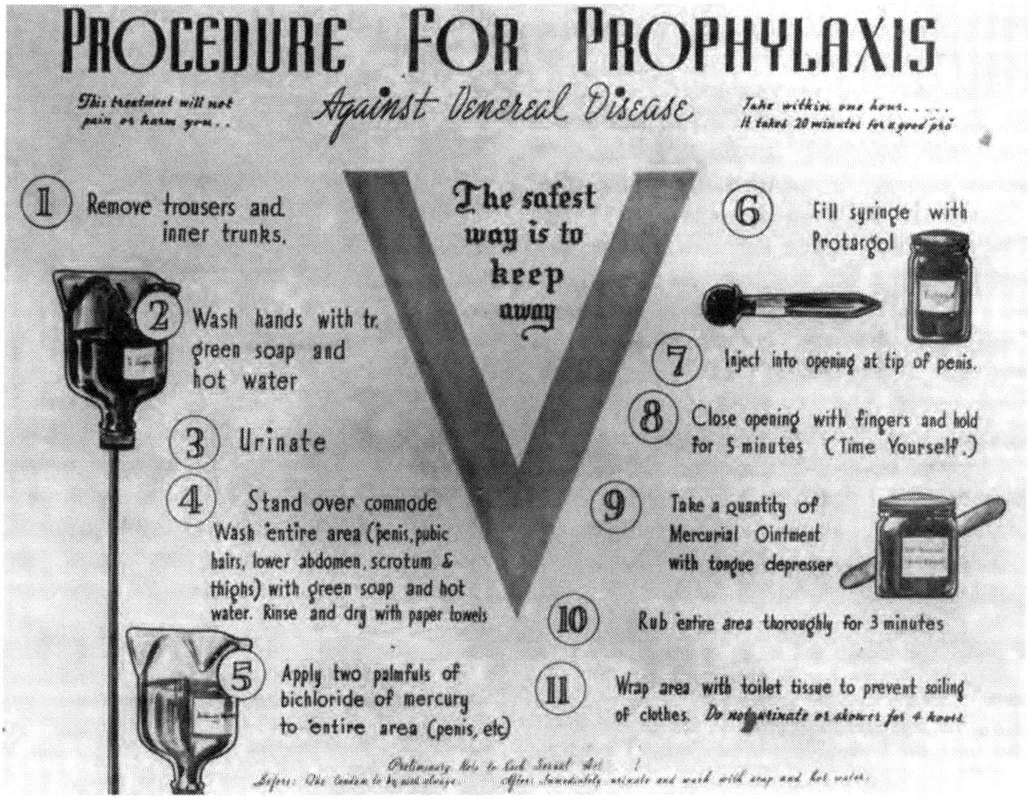

the Venereal Disease Control Act of 1916, which permitted libel action against a person who implied that someone else was infected, effectively barred British social agencies from helping the Americans trace them. The Privy Council, in Defense Regulation 33B, issued in December 1942, permitted a venereal disease patient privately to name his or her partner to a physician, who then could pass on the information to the appropriate local public health officer. After two separate identifications of the same person as the "source of infection," the public health officer could compel the individual to report for examination and treatment. This regulation was of little direct use to the theater medical service, because two soldiers rarely identified the same woman definitively enough to meet the evidentiary requirements.[66]

The medical service could do little to check prostitution, except make occasional informal arrangements with local police. In London, for example, American MPs and officers of the Metropolitan force rigorously restricted loitering by soldiers and civilians in Piccadilly Circus and Leicester Square, making pickups at least harder to arrange. The Americans had more success with contact tracing, using Regulation 33B as their opening wedge. Exploiting to the full his cordial relations with the Ministry of Health, Colonel Gordon prevailed on the reluctant British to allow U.S. Army nurses to take names of partners from infected soldiers and then visit the women, warn them they might be infected, and suggest they go to a British clinic for treatment. Because the entire action was confidential and informal and the contacts' responses were voluntary, the Americans by this means could get around the rigid rules of Regulation 33B. Colonel Padget launched the program in February 1943 in six counties in East Anglia, employing four Army nurses experienced in public health work. Much to the surprise of the sceptical British, the program provoked almost no civilian resentment and had substantial results. Of the first 500 women approached, only one—a professional prostitute—took offense, and over 75 percent eventually sought medical assistance. The Preventive Medicine Division expanded the effort throughout the United Kingdom, doubling the number of nurses assigned, and in February 1944 transferred administration of it to the base sections. British county health officers, impressed with the U.S. Army's success, organized similar contact teams and gradually began exchanging information with their Allies.[67]

In reciprocity for British acquiescence in this benign invasion of their cherished privacy, General Hawley tried to respond to Ministry of Health and Army Medical Services protests against the introduction into the United Kingdom of American soldiers

[66] Gordon "Hist," vol. 2, pt. 5, pp. 5–7 and 12–13, CMH; Padget Interv, 1 Aug 45, box 223, RG 112, NARA. For an account of antiprostitution measures and contract-tracing in the United States, see Hoff, ed., *Diseases Transmitted Through Contact*, pp. 179–81.

[67] Gordon "Hist," vol. 2, pt. 5, pp. 6, 13–14, 16, CMH; Padget Interv, 1 Aug 45, box 223, RG 112, NARA; Medical Bulletin No. 7, OofCSurg, HQ ETOUSA, 1 Jul 43, pp. 6–9; Mins, 14th and 15th Meetings of Base Section Surgeons, 31 Jan and 14 Feb 44, file HD 337.

already infected with venereal disease. He repeatedly called to Surgeon General Kirk's attention the fact that transports from the United States regularly made port with scores of new syphilis and gonorrhea cases on board, and he warned that apparent American nonchalance on this question jeopardized hard-won British cooperation with his control measures. The chief surgeon arranged to detect and hold for treatment all infected soldiers on arriving vessels. On the other side of the Atlantic the New York Port of Embarkation inspected troops carefully before embarkation and either kept infected men back for treatment or provided treatment on shipboard. Surgeon General Kirk, however, was reluctant to stop altogether shipment of men with venereal disease, lest he create a new medical way for malingerers to avoid overseas duty. Further, many troops became infected during their last preembarkation leaves, twenty-four to forty-eight hours before sailing, and their symptoms did not appear in time to be noted in boarding inspections or to be treated and cured on the voyage. The Army, as a result, continued to import venereal disease into the British Isles, and its doing so remained an unresolved irritant in Anglo-American medical relations.[68]

The medical service's broad-fronted attack on venereal disease produced encouraging results. The rate of new cases per 1,000 troops per year, which stood at 58 at the end of 1942, dropped to 21 by late 1943 and to about 20 in mid-1944. Colonel Padget attributed part of this decline to what he called a "dilution factor" resulting from the rapid influx of new troops who had not yet had time to find female company. Nevertheless, he was "reasonably certain that the lowering of the rate . . . was an actuality and not just an artifact brought about by troop movements." As was true throughout the Army, black soldiers in the European Theater had a venereal disease rate about four and one-half times that of white troops, the result of complex causes largely not correctable by the theater medical service. The black rate did respond, however, to education and prevention efforts, falling from 127 cases per 1,000 troops per year in February 1944 to 83 in June. Its general rise and decline paralleled those for other troops, only at a higher level. Among overseas theaters, which normally had higher venereal disease rates than the continental United States, the European Theater during 1942–44 ranked lower than all other theaters but the Southwest Pacific and Pacific Ocean.[69]

Between the start of BOLERO in mid-1942 and the end of May 1944 the European Theater of Operations recorded about 433,000 cases of disease admitted to hospitals and quarters, about 64,000 cases of nonbattle

[68] Ltrs, Hawley to TSG, 19 Aug and 14 Oct 43, and TSG to Hawley, 25 Aug and 2 Oct 43, file HD 024 ETO O/CS (Hawley-SGO Corresp); Ltrs, Hawley to CG, New York Port of Embarkation, 3 Feb 44, and to DepCdr, ETO, 27 Mar 44, file HD 024 ETO C/S (Hawley Chron). For the U.S. end of the problem, see Hoff, ed., *Diseases Transmitted Through Contact*, pp. 148 and 155.

[69] Quotation from Padget Interv, 1 Aug 45, box 223, RG 112, NARA. See also Hoff, ed., *Diseases Transmitted Through Contact*, p. 266; Mins, 23d Meeting of Base Section Surgeons, 5 Jun 44, p. 4, file HD 337; Gordon "Hist," vol. 2, pt. 5, pp. 28–33, fig. 18, table 7, CMH. For the venereal disease problem among black soldiers and its causes, see Lee, *Employment of Negro Troops*, pp. 277–78.

injury, and 4,300 of combat wounds. Throughout the buildup, the theater had fewer sick per 1,000 troops per year than any other overseas theater but the North American and Latin American. The ETO sick rate declined month by month, except for temporary winter upsurges reflecting the prevalence of respiratory infections, from 1,087 admissions per 1,000 in February 1942 to 245 in June 1944. Deaths from disease per 1,000 men remained consistently below 0.500 during the preinvasion period, a rate lower even than that in the United States and half what the Army suffered in the tropical Asian and Pacific areas of operations, with their greater incidence of deadly sickness. The ETO's daily average noneffective rate for all causes remained below that in the United States until the invasion. Clearly, as it awaited the invasion of Europe, the medical service was carrying out its mandate to conserve the fighting strength of the Army.[70]

[70] These figures are drawn from Frank A. Reister, ed., *Medical Statistics in World War II*, Medical Department, United States Army in World War II (Washington, D.C.: Office of the Surgeon General, Department of the Army, 1975), pp. 72–79, 608–09, 630–31. See also tables in Gordon "Hist," vol. 2, pt. 12, CMH.

CHAPTER VI

Preparations for Invasion

Medics in Britain performed their many and complex BOLERO tasks as preliminaries to their principal and most urgent mission: support of the amphibious assault on continental Europe. In the early period of the buildup, planning and preparation for that assault engaged the attention of only a few members of the chief surgeon's staff. Then, as 1943 gave way to 1944, the pace of assault planning intensified. Medical personnel of all ranks and in all units were swept up in invasion preparations. By late spring of 1944 ETO medics, like everyone else in the theater, were tensely awaiting the rapidly approaching D-Day.

Early Planning Efforts

Medical planning for a cross-Channel assault started in April 1942, after tentative approval of the American ROUNDUP invasion concept, and ran concurrently with the BOLERO buildup. The British and U.S. ground, naval, and air commands in London set up, among other committees on the ROUNDUP operation, an administrative planning staff to deal with logistical matters. The staff, in turn, was divided into lettered sections specializing in particular aspects of logistics. Section C, which did most of the medical planning, included members of the British War Office, Admiralty, Air Ministry, Combined Operations Staff, and Ministry of Health, with the theater chief surgeon and, more often, Colonel Spruit, Hawley's London representative, speaking for the American forces.[1]

Section C, in common with the other logistics planning groups, worked within uncertain parameters. By mid-June the ROUNDUP tactical planners had developed a general concept for simultaneous landings on a front stretching from the Pas-de-Calais to Cherbourg, with perhaps six divisions in the initial assault; beyond that the outlines of the operation remained unclear, clouded with doubt as to its feasibility. At the same time Section C had little amphibious warfare experience to guide it. The U.S. Navy and Marine Corps before the war had outlined a tentative amphibious doctrine, also adopted by the Army, but the resulting manuals had little useful to say about medical op-

[1] For general ROUNDUP planning, see Harrison, *Cross-Channel*, pp. 5–8 and 21–23; Ruppenthal, *Logistical Support*, 1:175–76; Larkey "Hist," ch. 2, pp. 57–59. For Spruit's role, see Hawley's recommendation for award, in file HD 024 ETO CS (Hawley Chron), April–June 1944.

erations. Wartime British Commando raids, and even the August 1942 attack on Dieppe, offered few medical lessons but confirmed that heavy casualties were to be expected. In the face of these uncertainties and areas of ignorance, Hawley, Spruit, and their British colleagues plowed ahead as best they could.[2]

From the start of their deliberations the medical planners confronted a problem that would remain a central preoccupation until D-Day: treatment and evacuation of the anticipated many casualties of the first days of the invasion. The dilemma was simple. The assault force would suffer its largest proportion of wounded at precisely the time when the fewest medical troops would be on shore to care for them. Section C, on the basis of informed guesswork, assumed that there would be 22,500 Allied wounded, almost half of them stretcher cases, during the first two days of ROUNDUP. Hawley, Spruit, and their British counterparts quickly ruled out any attempt to treat these injured on the French shore (designated in plans as the "far shore" to distinguish it from the British "nearshore"), concluding that treatment would require more medics, hospitals, and equipment than could possibly be landed in the assault and early buildup and more space than would be available in the crowded beachhead.

If the wounded were not to be cared for on the far shore, they would have to be evacuated directly from the beaches to hospitals in Great Britain, but evacuated in what? Few British and no United States hospital ships were available in the theater, and in any event these large oceangoing vessels could embark patients conveniently only at ports. Besides, such scarce ships should not be risked under enemy air attack and shore battery fire. The British had developed a smaller type of hospital ship, the hospital carrier. Converted from shallow-draft coastal steamers, these vessels, each able to accommodate 100 litter and 150 ambulatory patients, could lie close to the beaches and load by means of water ambulances—motor boats carried on board the mother craft. Hospital carriers, however, also were vulnerable to hostile air and artillery and they took hours to fill to capacity. The four that would be available in England in late 1942 could not begin to evacuate all the expected casualties.

Tactical landing craft that returned to England after unloading obviously were the only means for taking many wounded off the beaches quickly, although the types of such craft in service during ROUNDUP planning were small and not well adapted to handling men on stretchers. Nevertheless, in late 1942, for lack of any real alternative, the ROUNDUP administrative planning staff, at Section C's recommendation, established in principle a policy of maximum evacuation during the initial assault and use of returning landing craft as the main

[2] For the ROUNDUP plan, see Harrison, *Cross-Channel*, pp. 22–23 and 54–55. Ruppenthal, *Logistical Support*, 1:328–30, discusses early U.S. experiments with the logistics of amphibious assault. At Dieppe, Canadian forces—the bulk of the assault group—suffered 3,367 casualties out of 4,963 troops engaged. Of the 1,154 wounded, the withdrawing Canadians had to leave 568 behind as prisoners. See C. F. Stacey, *Six Years of War: The Army in Canada, Britain, and the Pacific*, Official History of the Canadian Army in the Second World War (Ottawa: E. Cloutier, 1955), pp. 384–89.

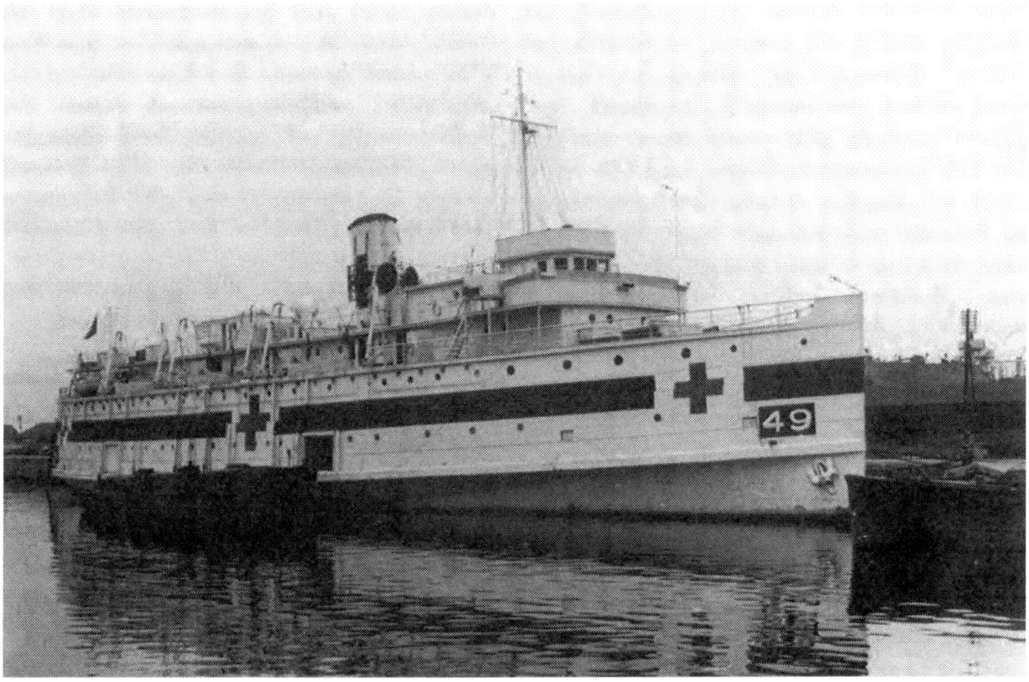

BRITISH HOSPITAL CARRIER *NAUSHON, a converted American ferryboat*

casualty carrier. What types of landing craft to employ for this purpose, how many could be made available for medical use (indeed, how many would be available at all), and whether any could be earmarked exclusively for evacuation and protected by the Red Cross—these facts the committee could not determine. The principle it adopted, however, would remain in force throughout the rest of the lengthy invasion planning process.[3]

Besides struggling with the problem of beachhead evacuation, the ROUNDUP medical planners arrived at basic decisions on a number of other important questions. They established an army-navy division of cross-Channel evacuation responsibilities that applied to both British and American forces. Under it, the armies were to collect all wounded on the far shore and move them to the beaches; the navies would load evacuation craft and care for patients on the voyage to England; the armies then would have charge of unloading the wounded and removing them to hospitals. General Hawley, Colonel Grow of the Eighth Air Force, and British medical and RAF authorities agreed on similar plans for air evacuation from the Continent to the United Kingdom.

[3] Larkey "Hist," ch. 2, pp. 56–58. For memoranda detailing the reasoning behind these decisions, see file HD 024 ETO O/CS (Spruit File re Policy); Recommendations of a Sub-Committee held in . . . the Admiralty, London, 16 Jul 42, in EvacCorresp, 1942–45, file HD 024 ETO; F. A. E. Crew, *The Army Medical Services* (hereafter cited as AMS), History of the Second World War, United Kingdom Medical Series, 5 vols. (London: Her Majesty's Stationery Office, 1956–66), vol. 4, *Campaigns: North-West Europe* (1962), pp. 45–49.

The ground forces and Services of Supply were to collect evacuees at French airstrips for pickup by transport planes returning to England. Air Force medical personnel were to care for the patients in flight, and the Services of Supply would deplane them in Britain and transfer them to hospitals. For their own forces the American planners began outlining the complicated sequence in which field army and then SOS medical units would land in France. They also roughed out a system for receiving water-evacuated casualties in England, using field hospitals and clearing stations at the ports for triage and emergency surgery and distributing transportable patients at once to selected hospitals inland.[4]

Medical invasion planning, in this period of limited theater resources, at times took on an air of unreality. During July, for example, in a last effort to avoid the diversion to North Africa, General Marshall ordered the European Theater and Services of Supply to report on the feasibility of launching a small-scale cross-Channel attack, code-named SLEDGEHAMMER, on 15 September. Hawley, in response, informed General Lee that, if the buildup continued at its present pace, the medical service would be short 8,900 beds and 8,616 officers and men on the projected attack date and would have no hospital train units, ambulance battalions, or boats for water evacuation. Pressed by Lee to report positively on how he could support the operation, the chief surgeon reiterated his previous assessment, with the qualification that he would be able to support the landing if he could borrow field medical units, hospitals, and equipment from the British, who, of course, had none to spare. Reports such as this helped scuttle SLEDGEHAMMER and ROUNDUP and paved the way for the commitment to TORCH.[5]

Cross-Channel assault planning of all sorts came to a stop in late 1942, as TORCH plans and preparations monopolized the attention of British and American staffs. Yet the ROUNDUP studies and conclusions—preserved in memoranda, data books, and individual memories—would constitute a starting point for the next round of invasion planning. Many of the principles and concepts of operation first sketchily outlined in ROUNDUP would be the foundation of the much more elaborate plans to follow.[6]

OVERLORD: The Planning Process

The decision of the Allied leaders at Casablanca, in January 1943, to revive the cross-Channel attack project for execution sometime in 1944 set in motion a lengthy, complex planning process. It began with a small Anglo-American staff, eventually drew in most British and American headquarters, and ended in the final test of strength in the west with Nazi Germany.

In March 1943, to give organizational substance to the Casablanca de-

[4] Larkey "Hist," ch. 2, pp. 68–72; Miscellaneous SPOBS/ROUNDUP Papers file, CMH.

[5] An account of this incident, with documents, is in Larkey "Hist," ch. 4, pp. 2–6 and apps. 2 and 3.

[6] Harrison, *Cross-Channel*, pp. 31–32; Larkey "Hist," ch. 2, p. 73; Memo, CG, SOS, to ACofS, G–4, and CsofSupSvcs, SOS, 1 Apr 43, sub: Administrative Planning, file HD 024 ETO O/CS (Spruit File re Policy).

cision, the Combined Chiefs of Staff established the Anglo-American staff known as COSSAC to plan the invasion and superintend preparations for it. Under the guidance of British Lt. Gen. Sir Frederick E. Morgan, COSSAC drafted the outline plan for the invasion, Operation OVERLORD, which Roosevelt, Churchill, and the Combined Chiefs approved at the Quebec conference in August. The Allies then put together the Anglo-American combined ground, naval, and air headquarters that were to fill in the details of OVERLORD and undertake its execution. In mid-January 1944 the arrival of General Eisenhower in London and the activation of SHAEF around the nucleus of COSSAC capped the invasion command structure. Eisenhower, after refining and expanding the COSSAC plan, set 1 June as the attack date. To obtain more landing craft for the enlarged assault, the Combined Chiefs canceled the originally contemplated simultaneous landing in southern France. On 1 February SHAEF published its outline plan for NEPTUNE, the code-name for 1944 operations within OVERLORD. SHAEF's ground, naval, and air headquarters followed with their outline plans and various national forces then got to work on the details of tactics and logistics.

The final plan, developed by COSSAC and expanded upon by SHAEF, selected Normandy as the point of attack because it possessed more suitable invasion beaches, was located within easier reach of major ports, and was less strongly defended than the previously favored Pas-de-Calais. In contrast to the broad front contemplated for ROUNDUP, the OVERLORD plan called for a single concentrated amphibious assault. Three British Commonwealth and two American divisions were to land north and northwest of Caen, with one of the American divisions going in on the east coast of the Cotentin Peninsula to gain position for a drive on the key port of Cherbourg. Three airborne divisions—one British and two American—were to drop to secure the flanks of the beachhead and open routes inland. This force, and follow-up troops, was to secure a compact lodgement area in which the Allies could mass men and supplies and from which they could advance methodically, first to capture additional Norman and Breton ports, then to clear the region between the Seine and the Loire, and finally to take Paris and go on to the Rhine, in the process destroying as much of the German Army as possible (*see Map 4*).[7]

With the formation of COSSAC, medical support planning paralleled every stage of OVERLORD's development. The COSSAC medical section began work in June 1943, under Chief Medical Officer Lt. Col. G. M. Denning of the Royal Army Medical Corps. Besides Denning, the small, informal section included a Royal Navy representative and Lt. Col. Thomas J. Hartford, MC, Hawley's executive officer. In September, after Hartford went to 21 Army Group to keep in touch with ground forces medical planning, Lt. Col. John K. Davis, MC, from the ETO Hospitalization Division, assumed the

---

[7] This account of the OVERLORD plan and its evolution is based on Harrison, *Cross-Channel*, pp. 47–59, 63–79, 98–127, 158–73; text of the outline plan is in Appendix A.

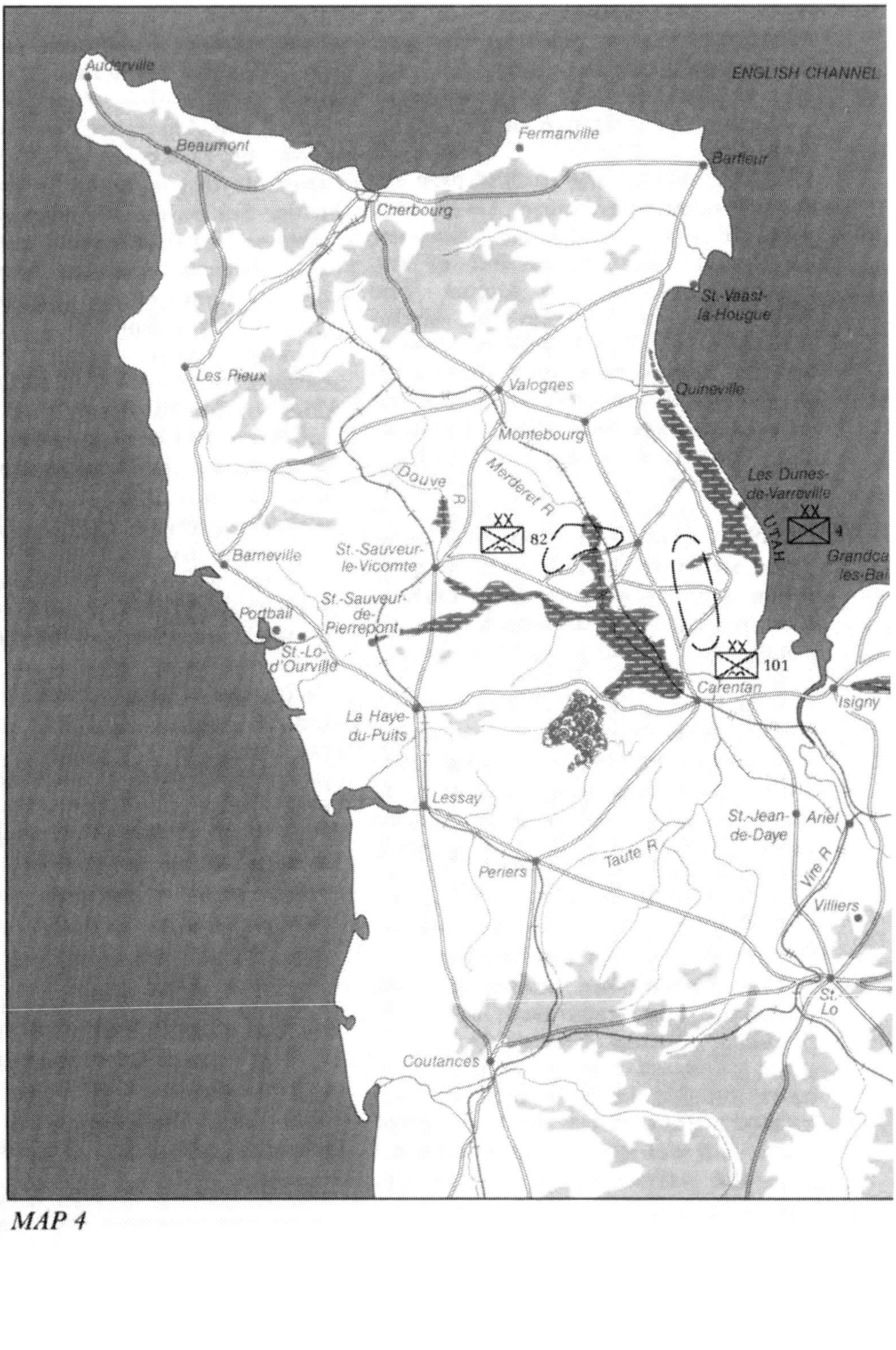
ENGLISH CHANNEL
Auderville
Beaumont
Fermanville
Barfleur
Cherbourg
St.-Vaast-
la-Hougue
Les Pieux
Valognes
Quineville
Montebourg
Douve R
Merderet R
Les Dunes-
de-Varreville
UTAH
4
82
Barneville
St.-Sauveur-
le-Vicomte
St.-Sauveur-
de-
Pierrepont
Portbail
St.-Lo-
d'Ourville
101
Carentan
Isigny
La Haye-
du-Puits
Lessay
St.-Jean-
de-Daye
Ariel
Taute R
Periers
Vire R
Villiers
St.-
Lo
Coutances

MAP 4

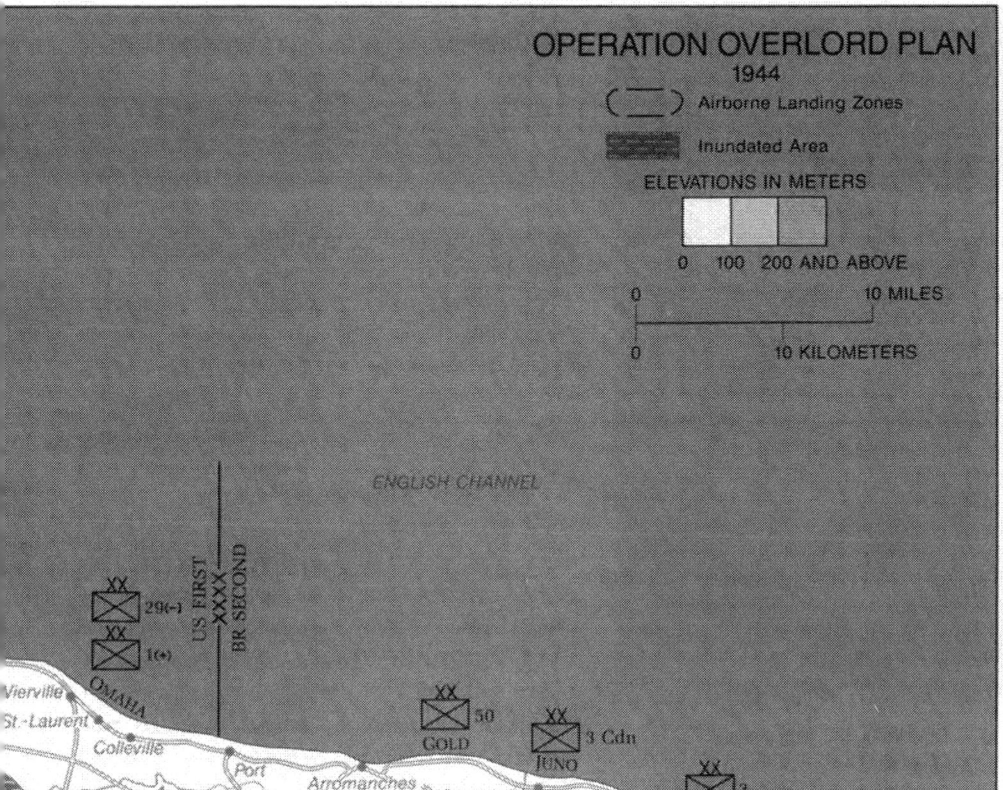
OPERATION OVERLORD PLAN
1944
Airborne Landing Zones
Inundated Area
ELEVATIONS IN METERS
0 100 200 AND ABOVE
0 10 MILES
0 10 KILOMETERS
ENGLISH CHANNEL
US FIRST
XXXX
BR SECOND
29(-)
1(+)
OMAHA
50
GOLD
3 Cdn
JUNO
3
SWORD
Vierville
St.-Laurent
Colleville
Port
Arromanches
Courseulles
Aure R
Bayeux
Seulles R
Lion
Cabourg
Ouistre-
ham
Orne R
Drome R
Balleroy
St.-Manvieu
Tilly
Troran
Dives R
Caen
Bourguebus
Esquay
Avenay
Bully
Vimont
Amaye
Caumont
Villers
Odon R
Bretteville
361

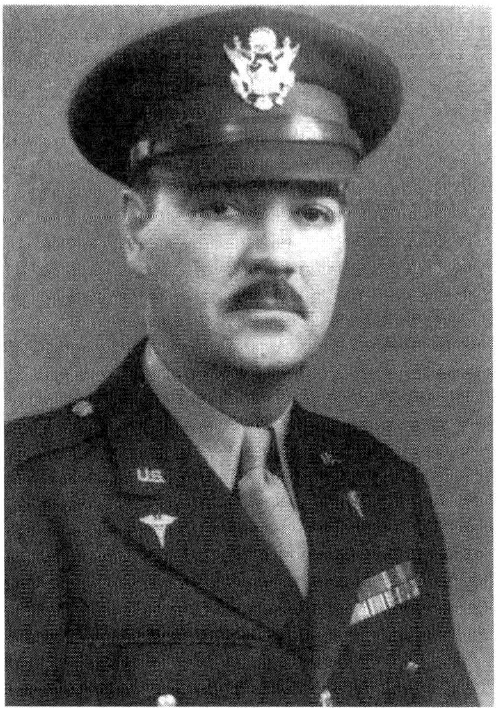

COL. THOMAS J. HARTFORD
(Rank as of October 1943)

COSSAC post. Denning and Davis remained in the medical section when it became part of SHAEF, with General Kenner as chief medical officer. The section stayed small under Kenner, never including more than four officers, evenly divided between British and Americans.

Under both COSSAC and SHAEF, the medical section made no comprehensive plans for supporting the invasion. Instead, it drafted administrative directives on certain inter-Allied and interservice problems. The section established, for example, uniform casualty-estimation formulas for use by all Allied planners, and it set basic evacuation policy and decided upon the principal means for cross-Channel transport of wounded. As part of SHAEF the section reviewed and reconciled the proliferating plans of subordinate headquarters. Most COSSAC and SHAEF medical decisions in fact represented a consensus between the chiefs of the British and American medical services, reached at frequent formal and informal conferences. Throughout the invasion planning the American medics at COSSAC and SHAEF drew upon General Hawley's office for advice and information, with the staff preparing most of their studies and position papers.[8]

Detailed American medical planning for NEPTUNE, covering the invasion and the first ninety days of the battle for France, began early in February 1944, after publication of the SHAEF outline plans. Planning took place within a complex logistics organization created to accommodate national control of supply to overall British direction of NEPTUNE ground operations. General Sir Bernard L. Montgomery's 21 Army Group functioned as both tactical and administrative ground force headquarters for the invasion. Subordinate to it, the U.S. 1st Army Group and First Army had logistical, as well as tactical, responsibility for the American troops under them, but these commands did not represent and could not control the ETO Services of Supply. To give the latter a voice in invasion planning, as well as to form the skeleton of a

[8] For medical section activities, see Medical Division, COSSAC/SHAEF, War Diary, June 1943–May 1944; Interv, Medical History Branch, CMH, with Maj. Gen. T. J. Hartford, MC, USA (Ret.) (hereafter cited as Hartford Interv), 7–8 Oct 80, tape 1, side 1, CMH; Davis Interv, 19 Jun 45, box 222, RG 112, NARA.

continental logistics system, General Eisenhower, as ETO commander, early in February activated two new headquarters: Advance Section, Communications Zone (ADSEC), and Forward Echelon, Communications Zone (FECOMZ).

Each of these new headquarters possessed immediate planning and future operational functions. The Advance Section was attached to the First Army, which had charge of all tactical planning for the American part of the amphibious assault and also did logistics planning for the first fifteen day on shore. Besides assisting with army planning, ADSEC worked out the details of SOS operations for the period from the sixteenth through the fortieth day after D-Day (D+16 through D+40). The Forward Echelon, at the outset an element of 21 Army Group headquarters, supervised ADSEC planning and itself made SOS plans for D+41 through D+90.

Operationally, ADSEC was to act as the supply element of the First Army until D+15, organizing the beach behind the advancing troops. From D+15 through D+40, after the army established its rear boundary, ADSEC would constitute the communications zone under the supervision of 21 Army Group, exercised through the Forward Echelon. FECOMZ itself was to become active on D+41, when a second U.S. army went into operation and the 1st Army Group, hitherto subordinate to 21 Army Group, became a separate command directly under SHAEF (*see Chart 5*). The Forward Echelon then would take command of the entire American support area behind the armies (whether under the U.S. army group or coordinate with it was never entirely settled). ADSEC at this point was to revert to the status of a movable base section under FECOMZ. The section would follow close behind the armies and link them to the Services of Supply, relinquishing supply activities nearer the shore to other base sections that would be formed as the campaign progressed. Around D+90 SHAEF and ETOUSA were expected to move to France, whereupon FECOMZ would merge back into the ETO-SOS headquarters and General Lee, as Eisenhower's deputy for logistics, would assume direct control of all elements of the Services of Supply—to be redesignated the Communications Zone (COMZ).[9]

Under this administrative arrangement the First Army surgeon, Colonel Rogers, and his staff, working closely with the surgeons of the two assault corps, the V and VII, drew up medical support plans for the initial landing and the first two weeks of combat. The ADSEC surgeon, Col. Charles H. Beasley, MC, and the FECOMZ surgeon, Colonel Spruit, prepared plans for establishing the medical portion of the continental Communications

[9] The SOS underwent formal redesignation as Communications Zone, ETOUSA, in GO No. 60, HQ, ETOUSA, 7 Jun 44, but the term came into increasing use from the end of February, even on SOS letterheads. COMZ will be used in this chapter in discussing logistical and medical planning, but SOS will be used in reference to operations until the narrative reaches the actual activation of COMZ. For a description of the convoluted logistics command system, see Ruppenthal, *Logistical Support*, 1:203–15 and 219–27. See also First U.S. Army Report of Operations, 20 Oct 43–1 Aug 44, bk. I, pp. 25–27; HQ, Forward Echelon, COMZ, ETOUSA, Communications Zone Plan (hereafter cited as FECOMZ Plan), 14 May 44, pp. 2–5, file HD 370 ETO.

Chart 5—Planned Command Arrangements for Overlord

AFTER U.S. 1st ARMY GROUP BECAME OPERATIONAL

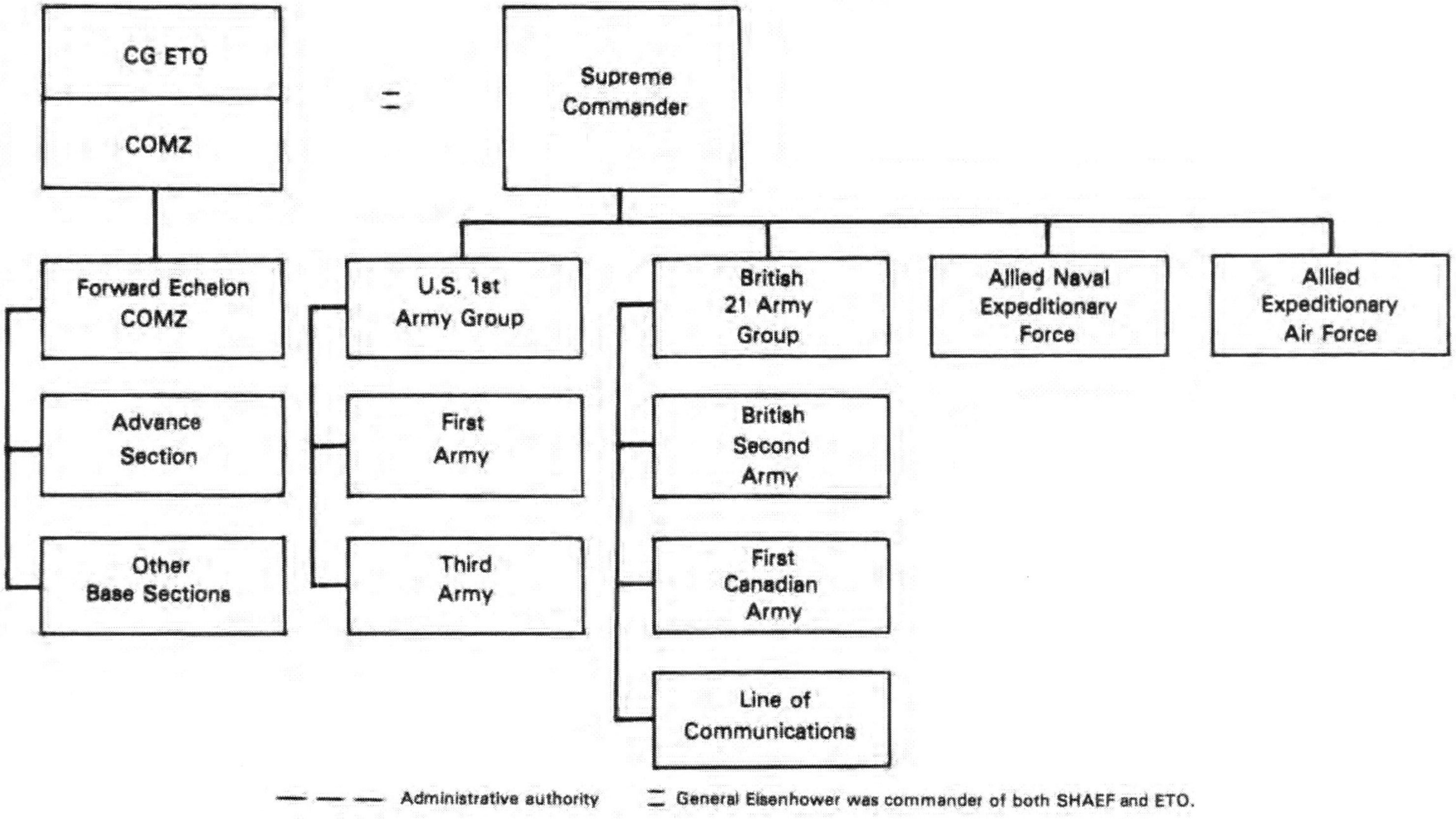

EARLY PHASES

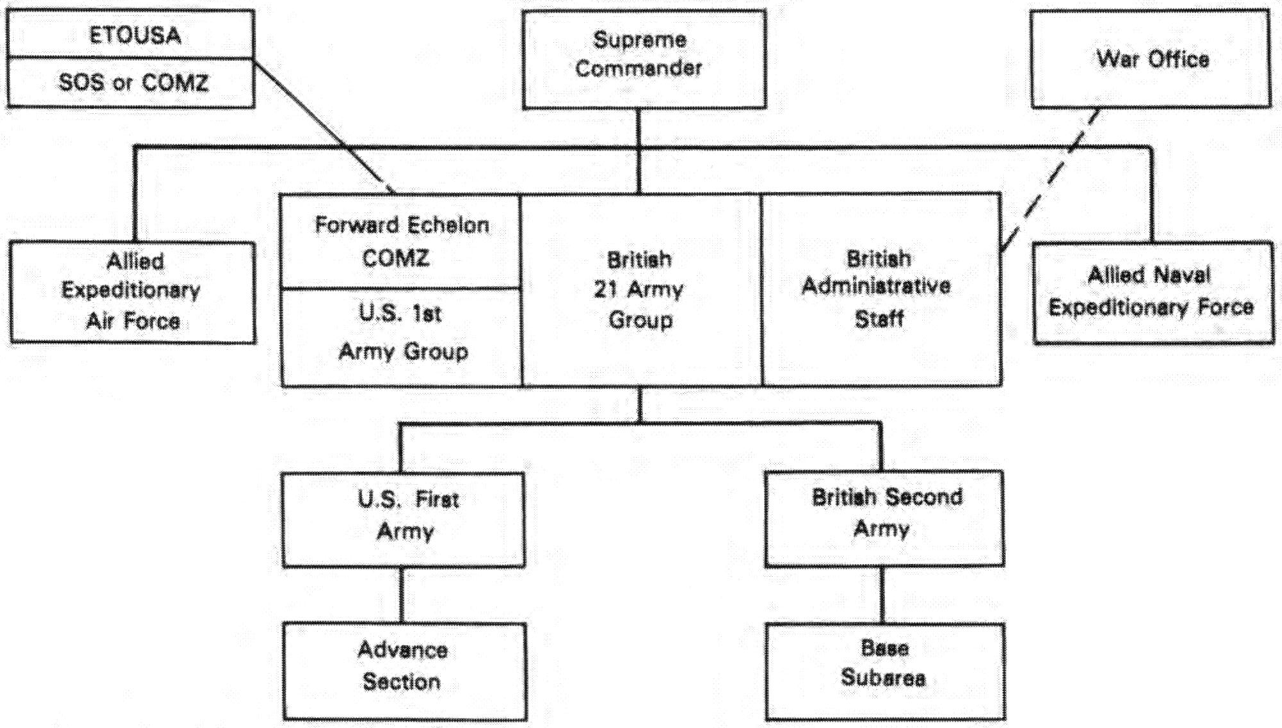

Source: Ruppenthal, *Logistical Support,* 1:225.

Zone. Roger's First Army medical section had come over from the United States with its parent headquarters and had been in operation in London and Bristol since October 1943, but the ADSEC and FECOMZ surgeons' staffs had to be improvised in haste (*see Charts 6 and 7*). Of substantial size—the ADSEC surgeon's office eventually included forty-three officers and fifty-six enlisted men—these organizations drew manpower from casuals, base section headquarters, and General Hawley's office. Colonel Beasley, for example, had been surgeon of the Eastern Base Section; his deputy, Col. James B. Mason, MC, had served as Hawley's chief of operations; and Colonel Spruit had come over to FECOMZ from running the Cheltenham branch of the chief surgeon's establishment. Each of the COMZ surgeons organized his office into divisions paralleling those under the chief surgeon. Spruit's office, indeed, was for practical purposes an advance echelon of Hawley's.[10]

While the First Army, ADSEC, and FECOMZ surgeons drafted the NEPTUNE plans, many of the decisions incorporated in them came from other headquarters. General Hawley, charged with supervising all theater medical planning, took part in establishing most major policies. His staff furnished information to the army and COMZ surgeons and wrote key portions of their plans, including, for instance, the basic army-navy agreement on division of cross-Channel evacuation responsibility. Hawley's office published its own standard operating procedure for medical service on the Continent and oversaw base section planning for support of the embarking invasion forces and for receiving casualties from the far shore. At SHAEF General Kenner kept in close touch with ETO medical planning and intervened in selected aspects of it. Of the higher-level ETO surgeons, Colonel Gorby of the 1st Army Group, in accord with the group's inactive role at this stage, had the least to do with NEPTUNE planning. He confined himself to keeping informed of First Army activities, assembling the medical portion of the troop buildup schedule, and participating in SHAEF medical policy discussions.[11]

The NEPTUNE medical planners made use of the data collected by their ROUNDUP predecessors and adopted many principles worked out for the projected earlier invasion. They also availed themselves of the medical lessons learned in amphibious operations in North Africa, Sicily, and Italy. The Fifth Army late in 1943 assembled many of these lessons into

[10]An. 9, COMZ Medical Plan (hereafter cited as An. 9—Medical), p. 1, to FECOMZ Plan, 14 May 44, file HD 370 ETO; An. 8—Medical, p. 4, to HQ, ADSEC, COMZ, NEPTUNE Operation Plan D to D+41 (hereafter cited as ADSEC Plan), 30 Apr 44, file HD 370 ETO; Surg, ADSEC, COMZ, Annual Rpt, 1944, pp. 1–5; Larkey "Hist," ch. 8, pp. 5–9; Personnel Division, OofCSurg, HQ, ETOUSA, Annual Rpt, 1944, p. 12.

[11]OofCSurg, HQ, ETOUSA, Standard Operating Procedure for Medical Service in Continental Operations (hereafter cited as O/CS Continental SOP), 4 Apr 44, file 370.02. For activities of Hawley's office, see annual reports of the Operations Division—especially Planning Branch, Evacuation Branch, Medical Intelligence Branch, Statistics and Requirements Branch—and of the Hospitalization Division for 1944, as well as Middleton Interv, 1968–69, vol. 1, p. 218, NLM. On Kenner's activities, see Medical Division, COSSAC/SHAEF, War Diary, February–May 1944. On Gorby, see 12th Army Group Report of Operations, vol. XIII (Medical Section), p. 7.

a manual for amphibious medical support, upon which the ETO planners drew extensively. Besides using the manual and other written reports, some ETO medical officers visited the neighboring theater for firsthand observation and conferences with army and SOS surgeons. During the early 1944 planning period, Colonel Hartford of 21 Army Group, Colonel Davis of SHAEF, Colonel Beasley of ADSEC, and Colonel Darnall of Hawley's Hospitalization Division made Mediterranean tours. Their visits, besides affording a change of climate, produced useful information. Hartford, for example, confirmed from Fifth Army experience the practicability of evacuating wounded over the beaches early in amphibious assault and brought back up-to-date estimates of whole blood transfusion requirements in combat surgery.[12]

NEPTUNE medical planning extended over about four months, with the First Army plan appearing in late February and those of ADSEC and FECOMZ respectively on 30 April and 14 May. These plans, while published separately, issued from a seamless process of discussion and negotiation so complex as to defy narration. The three principal medical planning staffs worked in constant consultation with each other, with nonmedical planners at their own headquarters, and with the surgeons' staffs of higher- and lower-command echelons. They kept in close touch with Navy and Air Force medical staffs and with those of their British colleagues. The ADSEC medical section had British officers attached to it for planning. In the end, as a result of this method of working, the evolution of each plan was shaped by the evolution of each of the others. Together, the major medical plans constituted a comprehensive blueprint for the NEPTUNE campaign.[13]

The NEPTUNE Campaign

The NEPTUNE plans covered the development of a continental medical service from the time the first wave of infantry hit the beaches through the securing of the French lodgement area. Essentially, the plans addressed two problems: provision of support for a strongly opposed amphibious landing, and development of an army and then a COMZ medical establishment—all to be done from a crowded British base, across a narrow but

[12]For general contact between the theaters, see Ruppenthal, *Logistical Support*, 1:331–35; Wiltse, *Mediterranean*, pp. 120–21, 142–43, 147–50, 223–26, and 267–68; 2d Lt Glen Clift, MAC, "Field Operations of the Medical Department in the Mediterranean Theater of Operations, U.S. Army" (Office of the Surgeon, MTOUSA, 1945), pp. 146–74, file HD 314.7-2, which reproduces the Fifth Army manual; Hartford Interv, 7–8 Oct 80, tape 1, side 1, CMH; Memo, Col J. K. Davis, MC, to CMedOff, SHAEF, sub: Abstract of Report on Visit to AFHQ, in Medical Division, COSSAC/SHAEF, War Diary, April 1944; HQ, ADSEC, Operations History of the Advance Section, COMZ, ETOUSA . . . , August 1945 (hereafter cited as ADSEC Hist), p. 4; Hospitalization Division, OofCSurg, HQ, ETOUSA, Annual Rpt, 1944, p. 2-3.

[13]For chronology of planning, see Ruppenthal, *Logistical Support*, 1:215–16 and 269; First U.S. Army Report of Operations, 23 Oct 43–1 Aug 44, bk. VII, p. 62; Surg, VII Corps, Annual Rpt, 1944, p. 12; ADSEC Hist, pp. 13–14 and 23; Surg, ADSEC, COMZ, Annual Rpt, 1944, pp. 1–6, 13, 15, 25, 31; Capt G. B. Dowling, MC, USN, Special Report to the Chief of the Bureau of Medicine and Surgery, USN, of U.S. Naval Medicine Service in the Invasion of Normandy . . . (hereafter cited as Normandy Rpt), 11 Jan 45, pp. 2–4, which gives the Navy view of medical planning.

CHART 6—ORGANIZATION OF THE OFFICE OF THE SURGEON, ADSEC, COMZ, ETOUSA, MAY 1944

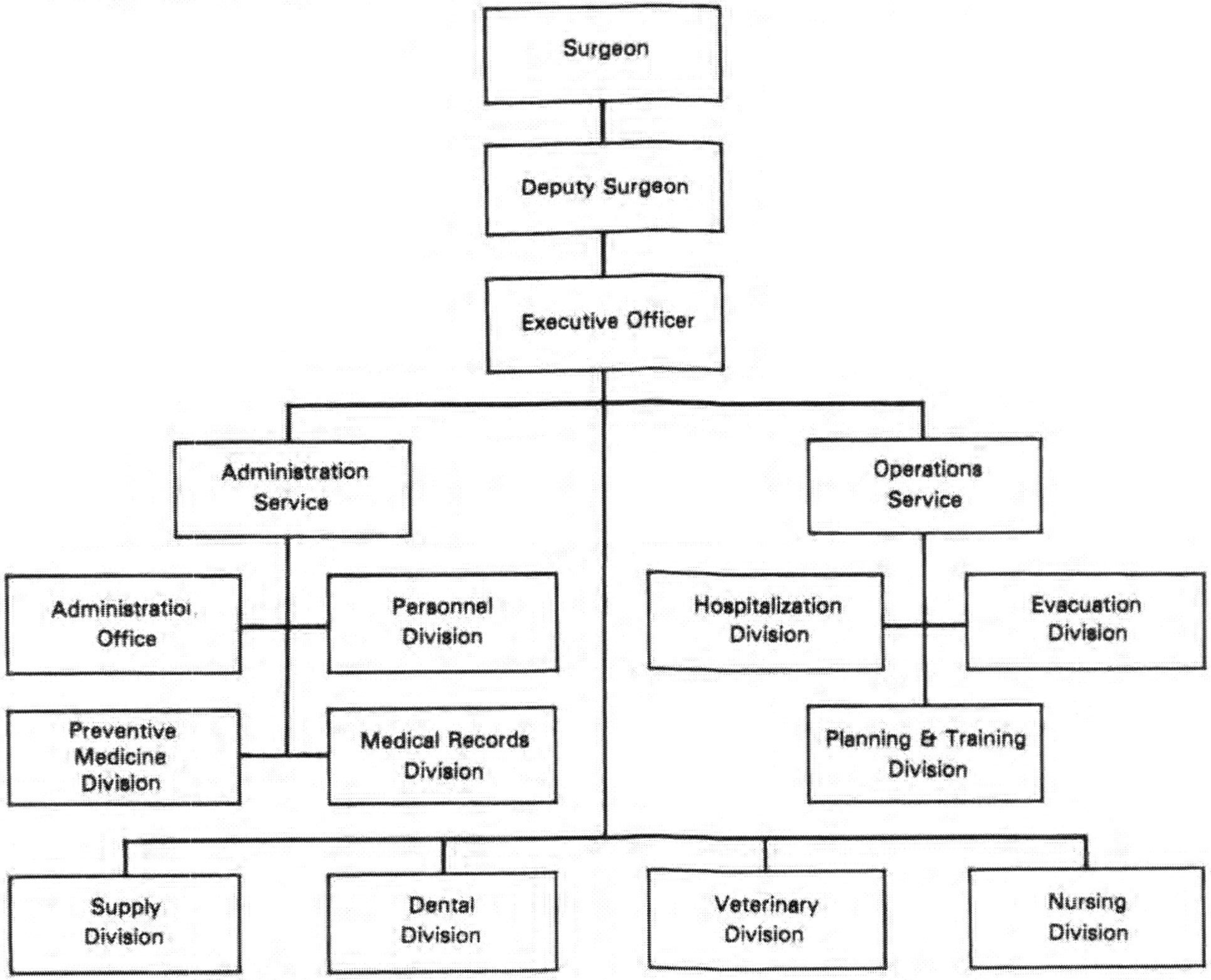

Source: Surg, ADSEC, COMZ, Annual Rpt, 1944.

CHART 7—ORGANIZATION OF THE OFFICE OF THE SURGEON, FECOMZ, ETOUSA, JUNE 1944

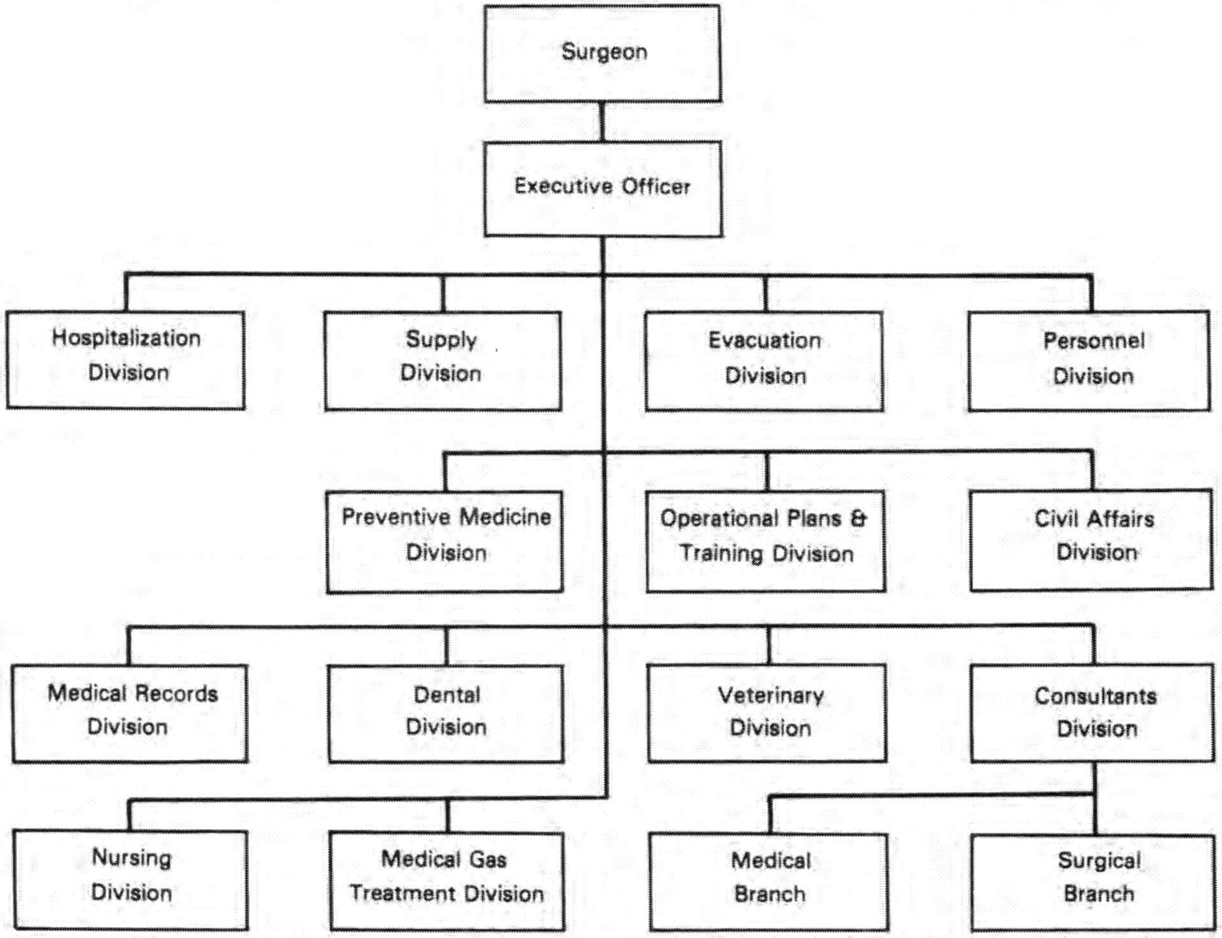

Source: Adapted by authors from Garand, Potter, and Vivette, "Medical Service in ETOUSA," ch. III, p. III–15, on file in CMH.

treacherous body of water, with limited shipping and port facilities.[14]

Support for the initial attack from the sea required the most complex arrangements and caused the planners the most controversy and soul-searching. The First Army tactical plan was straightforward. On D-Day the V Corps, with elements of the 1st and 29th Infantry Divisions, was to go ashore on the army's left on OMAHA beach, a stretch of Normandy coast backed by low bluffs northwest of Bayeaux. The VII Corps, with the 4th Infantry Division, was to land on the right on UTAH beach, near the base of the eastern side of the Cotentin Peninsula. The 82d and 101st Airborne Divisions, also under VII Corps, were to drop before the main attack, to secure crossings over the flooded areas immediately behind UTAH. Logistical support for the seaborne forces was to come from engineer special brigades—two, forming a provisional brigade group, for OMAHA and one for UTAH. These brigades were to begin landing soon after the first infantry elements. Assisted by shore party battalions of Rear Adm. Alan G. Kirk's Western Naval Task Force, which was responsible for transporting, landing, and supporting the American invasion troops, the special brigades would clear the beaches of wreckage, mines, and obstacles; open roads; and establish supply dumps. Their medical battalions would set up the first nondivisional medical facilities on the far shore.[15]

For medical support planners the number of casualties to be expected on and immediately after D-Day was the first crucial consideration. On this point COSSAC and SHAEF for a long time could not obtain agreement among the concerned staffs, although all expected losses to be very heavy. Different headquarters held to various estimates until February 1944, when General Kenner assembled the chief medical officers of the major invasion commands to reach a common figure "to establish our position for General Eisenhower." The conferees, after much debate, decided to assume for planning purposes that the assault force would suffer 12 percent wounded on D-Day and 6.5 percent on D+1 and D+2, with a declining proportion thereafter. Using this ratio, First Army surgeons had to think in terms of treating or evacuating over 7,200 wounded on D-Day and another 7,800 in the next forty-eight hours, of whom about 3 percent—at least 450—would be too severely injured to

[14] Unless otherwise noted, the following discussion is based on An. 6, Medical Plan (hereafter cited as An. 6—Medical), to First U.S. Army Operations Plan, Operation NEPTUNE (hereafter cited as FUSA Plan), 25 Feb 44; An. 8—Medical to ADSEC Plan, 30 Apr 44; and An. 9—Medical to FECOMZ Plan, 14 May 44. All in file HD 370 ETO. See also O/CS Continental SOP, 4 Apr 44, file 370.02. Additional sources are cited where appropriate.

[15] For the assault plan, see First U.S. Army Report of Operations, 20 Oct 43–1 Aug 44, bk. 1, p. 26; Harrison, *Cross-Channel*, pp. 174–97; and Ruppenthal, *Logistical Support*, 1:178, 269–70, 282–85, 324–44. Each engineer special brigade employed in NEPTUNE consisted of 1 medical and 3 engineer battalions, a DUKW battalion, and various small signal, military police, and quartermaster elements. The brigade group on OMAHA also included the 11th Port, to operate the MULBERRY artificial harbor. Special brigades could break down into battalion- or company-size composite beach groups to support regimental or battalion combat teams. The Western Naval Task Force, also designated by the U.S. Navy as Task Force 122, was the U.S. component of the Allied Naval Expeditionary Force, the overall naval command under SHAEF.

be transported any distance without definitive surgery. Even these estimates, the planners realized, were uncertain. Kenner noted: "If gas should be used, then these figures go by the board." [16]

On the basis of these estimates COSSAC, SHAEF, and army planners confronted the same problem of care and evacuation during the first days of the invasion that had preoccupied their ROUNDUP predecessors. COSSAC early reaffirmed the ROUNDUP decision to evacuate from the beaches to England all but the most lightly wounded and, conversely, those needing immediate surgery to keep them alive. COSSAC also reiterated the ROUNDUP staff's conclusion that most casualties must go out in returning landing craft. Unlike the earlier planners, those at COSSAC and SHAEF had available a vessel suited to their requirements: the LST (landing ship, tank), which had come into service since the end of ROUNDUP. This 330-foot oceangoing craft, designed to disembark tanks and other heavy vehicles directly onto a beach, also could embark large numbers of casualties in a comparatively short time through its bow doors and ramp, which could accommodate ambulances, litter-carrying jeeps, and a newly introduced amphibian truck, the DUKW. The latter vehicle also could swim out to and board an LST offshore. Within the ship the cavernous tank deck, extending the width and most of the length of the LST, could hold up to 300 litters, either fastened to bulkhead racks or lashed to the deck surface. When not transferred from vehicles directly onto the tank deck, casualties could be hoisted on board in small craft or on individual stretchers. The ship's upper decks and crew's quarters could hold 300 additional walking wounded. Any LST could be fitted for evacuation, and could accommodate a small emergency surgical facility, without reducing its ability to perform its main task of landing combat vehicles.

On 16 July 1943, at a conference attended by General Hawley and General Hood, the British Army medical chief, COSSAC adopted the LST as its principal evacuation craft. Reinforcing this decision, General Marshall directed in October that all cross-Channel movement of American wounded "will be handled in properly equipped combat LST[s]." [17] The U.S. Navy, which had charge of providing LSTs for the invasion, agreed to modify for casualty carrying 83 of the 98 ships allocated to the American forces and 70 of the 113 assigned to the British. After he became SHAEF's chief medical officer, General Kenner endorsed these arrangements. He directed medical planners to assume that only 75 litter and 75

[16] Quotations from MFR, Medical Section, SHAEF, sub: Meeting Held 26 Feb 44 in Gen Kenner's Office re Casualty Estimates for Operation OVERLORD, in Medical Division, COSSAC/SHAEF, War Diary, February 1944. See also VII Corps NEPTUNE Assault Plan and Medical Plan (hereafter cited as VII Corps Medical Plan), which gives corps-level casualty estimates using the SHAEF formula, encl. 1 to Surg, VII Corps, Annual Rpt, 1944; Dowling, Normandy Rpt, 11 Jan 45, p. 9. The OMAHA and UTAH assault forces included about 60,000 men, with an assault-loaded follow-up of 26,500 for OMAHA and further preloaded buildup of 43,500 for both beaches. See Ruppenthal, *Logistical Support*, 1:298.

[17] Msg, Marshall to Gen Devers, 30 Oct 43, in Medical Division, COSSAC/SHAEF, War Diary, February 1944.

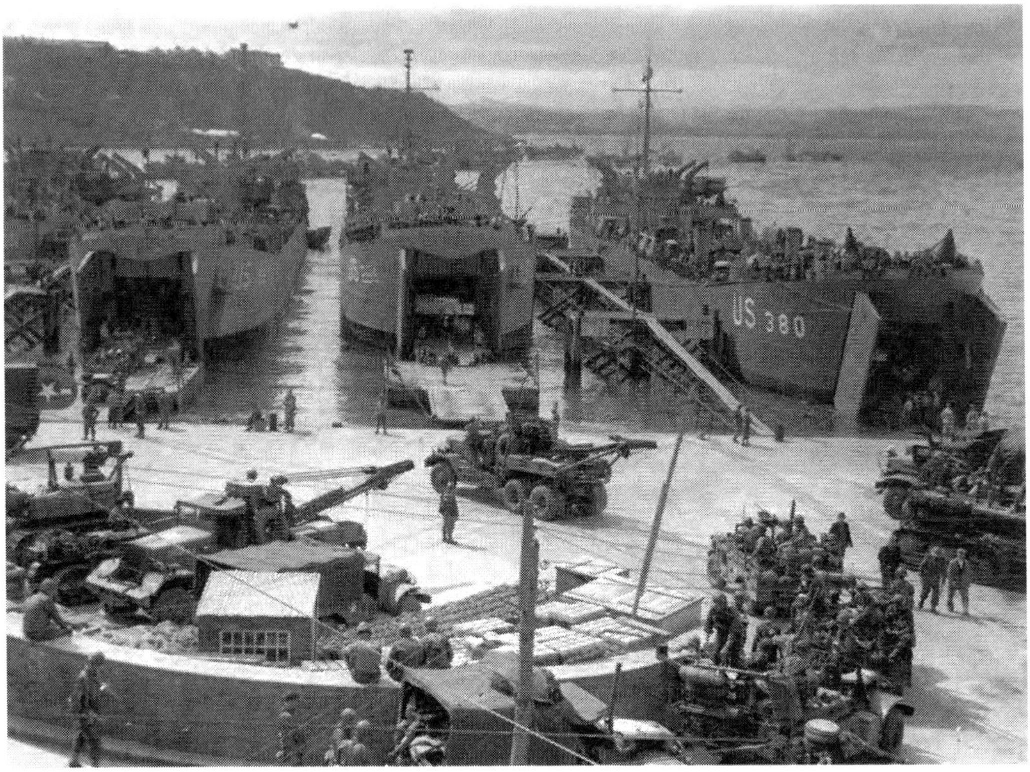

LSTs READYING FOR THE INVASION

walking patients would be moved on each voyage of an LST, to allow for the fact that few ships would be able to stay near the beach long enough to load to full capacity. If practicable, of course, the vessels were to take on more than this minimum.

To provide emergency surgery for casualties taken on board directly from clearing stations during the first days of the attack, the Western Naval Task Force surgeon, Capt. George B. Dowling, MC, planned to put two medical officers and twenty hospital corpsmen on each of his task force's LSTs. Because few of these Navy medical officers were experienced surgeons, General Hawley agreed to reinforce each LST medical complement with an Army surgical team of one officer and two enlisted technicians. To place still more emergency surgery capacity near the beaches, Kenner assigned 5 hospital carriers each to the British and American forces. These ships were to carry additional medical personnel and supplies to France and then embark patients requiring extensive early surgery.[18]

[18] Hawley Planning Directive No. 11, 21 Jul 43, box 2, Hawley Papers, MHI; Extract from Record of Meeting of Principal Staff Officers Held on 16 Jul 43, 20 Jul 43, in Medical Division, COSSAC/SHAEF, War Diary, February 1944; COSSAC Admin Instruction No. 8, 22 Dec 43, in ibid., De-

Continued

COSSAC and SHAEF based their evacuation plans on the LST reluctantly and in the face of much doubt about the feasibility of the whole system for removing wounded from the beaches. The doubters included General Hood. After inspecting an LST at Portsmouth, Hood called the vessel a "cold, dirty trap" for injured men. He carried unavailing protests against its use all the way to Churchill's War Cabinet. Colonel Cutler considered LSTs "rotten ships for care of wounded American boys," an opinion shared by many of his colleagues. The objectors had reason for concern. When emptied of their vehicular cargoes, LSTs rolled deeply in all but the calmest seas, creating, to say the least, an unstable platform for surgery. With any kind of sea running, DUKWs could not swim out to an LST and negotiate its ramp. Most important, as combatant vessels carrying troops and weapons outward bound, LSTs could not be protected with the Red Cross and were legitimate attack targets. If one foundered for any reason, the litter patients on board inevitably would go down with it. Kenner and Hawley shared their colleagues' uneasiness about the LST, Kenner calling use of the vessels "an improvised method of removing casualties forced upon the Medical Service by operational necessity." Nevertheless, they had to override all objections to employment of the LST, for it was the only available means of large-scale cross-Channel evacuation. They took comfort from the fact that LSTs had performed well in evacuation in the Pacific and could only hope that weather severe enough to prevent the loading of wounded on LSTs also would prevent the entire invasion.[19]

Until D-Day Allied medical planners considered their evacuation system a fragile structure, dependent for success on many uncontrollable variables. Kenner, in particular, feared that a "back-log" of unevacuated, untreated wounded would accumulate on the beaches, with demoralizing impact on the combat troops. He warned:

> The whole medical situation during the first few days hinges on two unknown factors, namely weather and the number of casualties. If both are in our favor then evacuation will be satisfactory. If weather is good and casualties heavy or if weather is bad and casualties light, the medical situation while becoming serious will probably remain under control. But if the weather is bad and the casualties heavy then it will be impossible to meet the situation either by local treatment or by

cember 1943; Memo, Kenner to ACofS, G-4, SHAEF, 25 Apr 44, sub: Casualty Lift of Converted LSTs, in ibid., April 1944. See also diary entries and correspondence for September and November 1943 and March 1944. On LST technical details, see Davis Interv, 19 Jun 45, pp. 2-3, box 222, RG 112, NARA; Crew, *AMS, Campaigns: North-West Europe,* 4:49-52; and Dowling, Normandy Rpt, 11 Jan 45, pp. 4-5, E-8, E-9, E-13. On LST surgeons, see Larkey "Hist," ch. 8, pp. 30-31, and correspondence in file HD 705 ETO (Medical Care on LSTs, 1944).

[19] Hood words as quoted in MFR, Col Cutler, 28 Feb 44, sub: Visit and Inspection of an LST at Portsmouth . . . , 21 Feb 44, file HD 705 ETO (Medical Care on LSTs 1944). Cutler quotation from Carter, ed., *Surgical Consultants,* 2:184. Kenner quotation from his memorandum of 6 Mar 44, in Medical Division, COSSAC/SHAEF, War Diary, March 1944; see also other entries and documents for this month. Crew, *AMS, Campaigns: North-West Europe,* 4:52-55, recounts Hood's appeal to the War Cabinet. See also Hartford Interv, 7-8 Oct 80, tape 1, side 1, CMH, and Davis Interv, 19 Jun 45, box 222, RG 112, NARA.

evacuation and a serious medical breakdown must inevitably occur.[20]

Colonel Rogers and his staff built their First Army medical support plans around the basic COSSAC-SHAEF evacuation decisions and attempted to provide against a breakdown of seaward evacuation. To this end Colonel Rogers arranged to reinforce each assault division medical battalion with an additional collecting company, to be landed as soon as possible after D-Day, and to attach six teams from the army's auxiliary surgical group to the clearing company of each engineer special brigade medical battalion. So augmented, these units—the only hospitals on shore during the first twenty-four hours or so of combat—would be able to care for a substantial number of severely wounded. On D-Day company aidmen and battalion medical sections were to go in with the first infantry waves, followed in close sequence by Navy shore party medical sections (one officer and eight hospital corpsmen per army battalion), division collecting companies, the engineer special brigade medical battalions, and the division clearing companies. This interlacing of division and special brigade elements, based on Mediterranean practice, would permit the division medical service to move inland at once and begin regular operations, leaving the shore party and special brigade medical units, in static beach positions, to collect wounded who fell in the first attack, to evacuate division medical installations, to set up emergency surgical hospitals, and to load all movable casualties on LSTs and other landing craft (*Diagram 1*). The beach medical elements also were to evacuate and support the airborne divisions, as soon as the seaborne forces made contact with them. Until then the airborne medical companies, landing by parachute or glider with attached surgical teams soon after the infantry touched down, would collect and treat all paratrooper wounded.[21]

After the assault and the securing of the beachhead, American reinforcements were to pour in, over OMAHA and UTAH beaches and later through Cherbourg and other captured ports, bringing U.S. strength on the Continent to over 1 million by D+90. The First Army and 1st Army Group before D-Day established a consolidated movement schedule for this buildup, detailing the size and shipping requirements of each unit, its date and place of embarkation, and its destination and assignment on the far shore. They divided each day's sealift among ground, air, and service forces so as to maintain a balanced flow of combat and support elements.

Medical units were interspersed throughout the schedule, on the basis of priorities developed by the First Army, ADSEC, and FECOMZ surgeons and worked into the troop list after tortuous negotiations with all the other forces vying for space (*see Table 3*). The First Army's nondivisional medical units were to go in

[20] Ltr, Kenner to Lt Gen Sir Humphrey Gale, 29 Feb 44, in Medical Division, COSSAC/SHAEF, War Diary, February 1944.

[21] VII Corps Medical Plan, encl. 1 to Surg, VII Corps, Annual Rpt, 1944; Surg, 1st Infantry Division, Annual Rpt, 1944, p. 8; Dowling, Normandy Rpt, 11 Jan 45, p. 8; Surg, 82d Airborne Division, Annual Rpt, 1944, an. 1; Surg, 101st Airborne Division, Annual Rpt, 1944, pp. 1–2; Editorial Advisory Board, 1962, pp. 70–71, 100–101, 112.

DIAGRAM 1—INFANTRY DIVISION LANDING PHASE EVACUATION PLAN

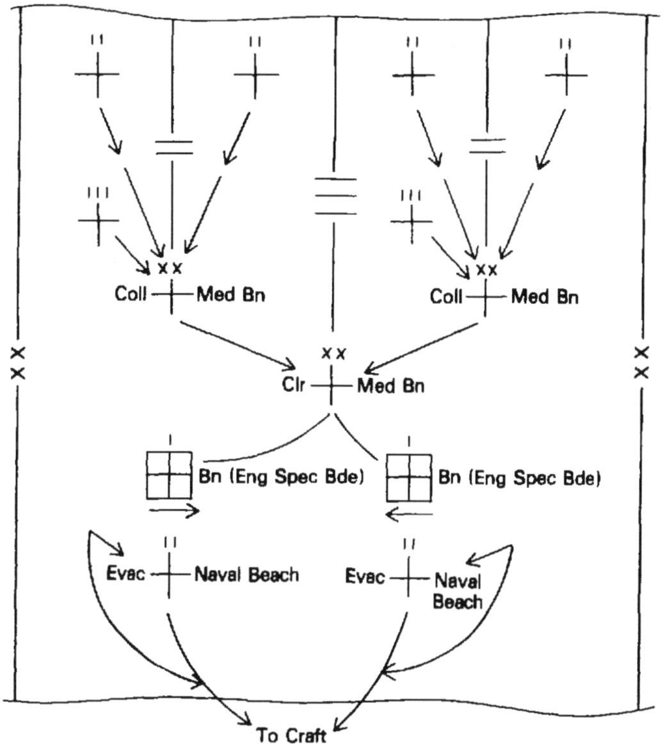

Source: Surg, 1st Infantry Division, Annual Rpt, 1944, p. 8a.

first, between D-Day and D+15, with field hospitals, auxiliary surgical teams, and the corps medical battalions leading. Evacuation hospitals were to follow, beginning on D+5, along with army medical battalions (separate) and groups, a supply depot company, a convalescent hospital, a laboratory unit, and a gas treatment battalion. A few ADSEC units were to be interspersed with those of the First Army, but most would arrive after D+12. The first scheduled to come were additional ambulance companies and evacuation and field hospitals, intended to function as station hospitals and holding units. On or about D+15 the first general hospital in France, the 298th, was to disembark and go into operation in Cherbourg. By D+90 both the Advance Section and Forward Echelon expected to have twenty-five general hospitals on the Continent, at preassigned locations in Normandy and Brittany, besides a full complement of supply depots and other COMZ medical units.[22]

Medical supplies in large quantities were to start arriving on the beaches as soon as the troops did. All First Army combat and support units land-

[22] In addition to the basic plans previously cited, see Surg, VII Corps, Annual Rpt, 1944, pp. 3-4 and 6-7. Memo, Surg, FECOMZ, to G-4, FECOMZ, 6 Apr 44, file HD 370 (HQ ADSEC Plans and Corresp, 1944); Larkey "Hist," ch. 8, app. 4.

TABLE 3—PLANNED LANDING OF MEDICAL UNITS, 6–14 JUNE 1944

UTAH Beach [a]	June	OMAHA Beach	June
6 auxiliary surgical teams	6	12 auxiliary surgical teams	6
1st Medical Depot Company, advance platoon	7	1st Medical Depot Company, advance platoon	6
42d Field Hospital	7	13th Field Hospital	6
45th Field Hospital	9	51st Field Hospital	8
3 auxiliary surgical teams	9	449th Collecting Company	11
463d Collecting Company	10	450th Collecting Company	11
564th Ambulance Company	11	577th Ambulance Company	11
464th Collecting Company	11	5th Evacuation Hospital	11
91st Evacuation Hospital	11	24th Evacuation Hospital	11
565th Ambulance Company	12	451st Collecting Company	12
493d Collecting Company	12	452d Collecting Company	12
128th Evacuation Hospital	14	575th Ambulance Company	12
566th Ambulance Company	14	41st Evacuation Hospital	12
501st Collecting Company	14		

[a] Small portion of troop buildup schedule, exclusive of brigade and corps units.
Source: First U.S. Army Report of Operations, 20 Oct 43–1 Aug 44, bk. II, an. 2, pp. 60–61.

ing on D-Day and the following 3 days were to carry reserves of rapidly consumable items, in the hands and on the backs of soldiers and loaded into vehicles. Each infantry, artillery, chemical warfare, engineer, and ranger battalion; each divisional collecting and clearing company; and each engineer special brigade medical battalion was to receive a special allowance of dressings, small implements, drugs, morphine, and dried plasma packed in waterproof containers portable by a single man. Each organization also would bring ashore extra litters, field medical chests, splints, and blankets. In the Advance Section mobile hospitals were to embark with reserves of expendable supplies sufficient for 10 days of operations; other medical units were to carry 3-day reserves.

Medical maintenance supplies were to be shipped automatically from the United Kingdom during the first 90 days of continental operations. Before D-Day the First Army, Advance Section, and Forward Echelon submitted requisitions to the chief surgeon's Supply Division for their periods of primary logistical responsibility, with allowances calculated to replace lost and consumed materiel and to establish 14- or 21-day reserves (depending on the echelon and the class of supplies) in army and COMZ depots by D+90. The supplies so requested were to be packed before the assault and loaded on ships on a daily schedule as the buildup proceeded.

From D-Day until about D+40 most maintenance supplies would consist of special division assault surgical and medical units, designed by the First Army and assembled by the Supply Division. Each of these units included dressings, drugs, and equipment for treating 500 casualties and was divided into 100-pound waterproof packages for easy, safe movement and storage. To ensure arrival of enough supplies on the beaches while the casualty rate was highest, the Supply Division based its scheduled shipments of these units on estimated numbers of wounded, rather than on total troop strength, as was the practice with regular medical maintenance units (which were not adapted to the assault situation in any case). As the buildup continued, standard 10,000-men-for-30-days maintenance units were to supplant the special ones. When enough depot companies reached France, the armies and the Communications Zone were to establish regular distribution procedures, with division medical supply officers drawing on army depots that those of the Advance Section would replenish. Whole blood, biologicals, and penicillin were to reach the front through special channels, delivered by the theater blood service.[23]

Hospitalization and evacuation in France were to evolve as the manpower and supply buildups progressed, with the aim throughout being to retain as many patients as possible on the Continent. From D-Day until about D+18 the First Army was to send back to England all sick and wounded except nontransportables (defined as men with severe abdominal, chest, and head injuries and compound fractures) and casualties who could be treated and returned to duty from division facilities. As First Army hospitals went into operation, the forces in France, at the army commander's direction, were to shift to a 7-day evacuation policy. Once COMZ fixed hospitals became available, the Advance Section was to evacuate to them from the armies casualties returnable to duty within 15 days, to be extended progressively to 30 days as still more hospitals arrived. Soldiers needing longer hospitalization, or eligible for return to the United States under the 180-day theater policy, were to go directly from army installations to hospitals in England.

Following the principles established by COSSAC, the NEPTUNE plans called for evacuation of wounded over the beaches during and after the assault, and for their transportation to Britain in LSTs and, after the first day or so, in hospital carriers. When the Allies captured and reopened Cherbourg, the Americans were to use that port, in addition to the beaches, for evacuation to the United Kingdom. U.S. hospital ships, eleven of which were expected to reach the European Theater between 29 May and 12 August, also would load wounded at Cherbourg for direct evacuation to the United States. Air evacuation to Britain, from both the field armies and the Communications Zone, was to begin as soon as the ground forces secured airstrips usable by the C–47s of the IX Troop Carrier Command. For overland movement of patients, the NEPTUNE plans provided for improvisation of hospital trains from captured rolling stock, but the armies and COMZ were to rely primarily on ambulances and, in emergencies, on trucks and jeeps, until about D+56. At that time hospital trains constructed in England were expected to begin

[23] First U.S. Army Report of Operations, 20 Oct 43–1 Aug 44, bk. VII, pp. 74–75; Supply Division, OofCSurg, HQ, ETOUSA, Annual Rpt, 1944, sec. IV, pp. 5–6, and sec. VI, pp. 5 and 7–8; Planning Branch, Operations Division, OofCSurg, HQ, ETOUSA, Annual Rpt, 1944, pp. 8–9; Interv, OSG with Col B. C. T. Fenton, MC, 7 Jun 45, box 222, RG 112, NARA.

rolling off ships at ports and beaches.[24]

The NEPTUNE planners concerned themselves with keeping the troops on the Continent healthy, as well as with treating them when sick and injured. Army and COMZ preventive medicine plans, based on information collected and collated by the chief surgeon's Medical Intelligence Branch, assessed the state of public health in occupied France and listed the likely major disease threats on the Continent. Troop commanders in France, the plans warned, could expect to find an ill-nourished, dirty civilian population whose hospitals and public health agencies were operating inefficiently because the occupying Germans had stripped them of much equipment and personnel. French water purification and sewage disposal facilities, never the best, could be assumed to have broken down under administrative neglect and combat damage.

Compared to what the Army faced in the Mediterranean, the Southwest Pacific, and other non-European tropical theaters, disease in northwestern Europe posed hardly any threat to the conduct of operations. Epidemic louse-borne typhus, which the planners considered likely to be introduced from eastern Europe by German troops and slave laborers, loomed as the disease of most potential danger. Commanders and surgeons also would have to guard against typhoid, but such familiar diseases of troops in the field as dysentery, diarrhea, influenza, venereal diseases, and infectious hepatitis, as well as a variety of skin ailments and vermin infestations, were likely to constitute the campaign's principal medical problems. Even though American troops had already been immunized against typhus, the field armies and the Communications Zone planned to issue insecticide powder to their troops and prepared for mass inspection and delousing of soldiers, civilians, and prisoners of war. NEPTUNE plans for combating other diseases depended on the standard immunizations, personal hygiene, mass sanitation, water treatment, sewage disposal, and pest eradication procedures, as well as on special supervision of soldier eating habits to prevent vitamin deficiencies among men subsisting for long periods on C- and K-rations.[25]

Preventive medicine planners expected venereal diseases, the incidence of which reportedly had increased threefold in France since 1941, to constitute "one of the most difficult control problems to be encountered." First Army and COMZ plans, backed up by a theater circular drafted by Colonel Gordon's Preventive Medicine Division in cooperation with the senior medical consultants

[24] Memo, Kenner to ACofS, G-4, SHAEF, 13 Apr 44; see also Mins, Conference of Gen Kenner with Brig Gen Grow, 11 Apr 44. Both in Medical Division, COSSAC/SHAEF, War Diary, April 1944. For a definition of nontransportables, see Ltr, Col E. C. Cutler to Lt Col Crisler, 16 Apr 44, box 3, Hawley Papers, MHI. See also Memo, Col F. H. Mowrey to Movements Division, Office of CofTrans, ETO, 29 May 44, EvacCorresp, 1942-45, file HD 024 ETO.

[25] For medical intelligence, see Medical Intelligence Branch, Operations Division, OofCSurg, HQ, ETOUSA, Annual Rpt, 1944, pp. 2-3, and Ltr, Hawley to TSG, 29 May 44, file HD 024 ETO O/CS (Hawley-SGO Corresp). See also Cir Ltr No. 53, OofCSurg, HQ, ETOUSA, 8 Apr 44, sub: Improvement of Nutrition of Combat Troops, in Larkey "Hist," ch. 8, app. 17.

and command venereal disease control officers, prescribed essentially the same precautions tested and proven in the United Kingdom: troop education, provision of healthful recreation, widespread issue of condoms and V-Packettes (even embarking assault troops were to be offered them), establishment of prophylactic stations, and—as far as language and local law and custom permitted—tracing of contacts. Repression of prostitution received special emphasis. In contrast to the unorganized, barely tolerated character of the business in Great Britain, continental prostitution was an accepted, legally regulated and sanctioned social institution, featuring numerous brothels. War Department policy, confirmed by practical experience in North Africa, Sicily, and Italy, ruled out any official Army attempt to license and regulate such establishments. Hence, ETO preventive medicine officers and medical consultants inserted in NEPTUNE plans and the theater circular a strongly worded policy statement:

> The practice of prostitution is contrary to the best principle[s] of public health and harmful to the health, morale and efficiency of troops. No member of this command will, directly or indirectly, condone prostitution, aid in or condone the establishment or maintenance of brothels, bordellos or similar establishments, or in any way supervise prostitutes in the practice of their profession or examine them for purpose of licensure or certification. Every member of this command will use all available measures to repress prostitution in areas in which troops of the command are quartered or through which they may pass.[26]

The NEPTUNE medical planners sought to anticipate and outline a solution for every foreseeable actual or potential problem. To keep seasickness from taking the fight out of the assault troops before they went ashore, the First Army prepared to issue newly developed antimotion sickness capsules—ten of them to be taken on a fixed schedule—to each embarking soldier, even though tests of the remedy in amphibious exercises had produced at best inconclusive results. Medical precautions against the threat of German gas attacks included intensive training for all troops in first aid for chemical warfare casualties and the issue of eye ointments and impregnated protective clothing. The various medical plans set policies and procedures for treating civilian sick and injured in Army hospitals (to be done only when necessary to save life), caring for and processing Allied casualties in the American evacuation chain, treating and evacuating wounded prisoners of war, and disposing of captured medical supplies. In detail and comprehensiveness the medical plans matched those for other aspects of NEPTUNE. They also shared in the essential rigidity of the overall plan, based as it was on the assumption that Allied forces would push the Germans back at a fairly steady pace. A radical slowdown or a radical acceleration of Allied progress would require complicated, difficult adjust-

[26] First quotation from An. 6—Medical to FUSA Plan, 25 Feb 44, file HD 370 ETO. Second quotation from Cir No. 49, HQ, ETO, 2 May 44, in Larkey "Hist," ch. 8, app. 19. See also Preventive Medicine Division, OofCSurg, HQ, ETOUSA, Annual Rpt, 1944, pp. 44–45; Middleton Interv, 1968–69, vol. 1, pp. 236–38, NLM. For North African and Italian experience, see Wiltse, *Mediterranean*, pp. 215, 257–58, 354.

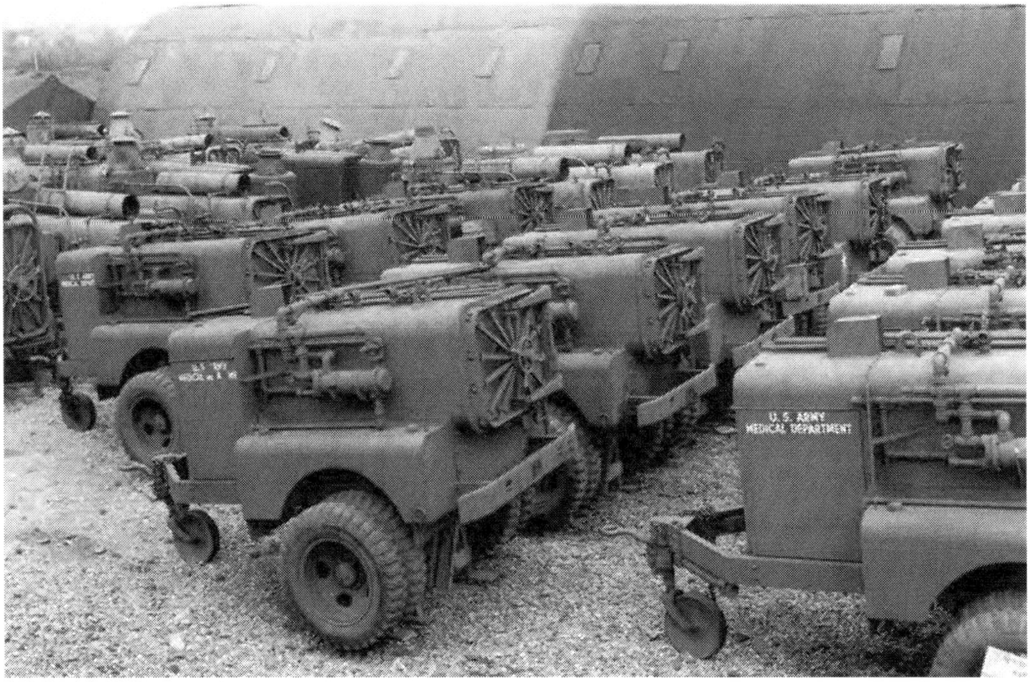

GAS DECONTAMINATION EQUIPMENT, *stockpiled at Thatcham supply depot as a precaution against a German gas attack*

ments throughout the elaborate medical support system.[27]

Technical Aspects

Even before the OVERLORD and NEPTUNE plans took definite shape, General Hawley and his staff began searching for solutions to a variety of technical problems connected with the invasion. The chief surgeon and his assistants paid special attention to three problems: providing whole blood to forward medical units, drafting guidelines for combat zone surgical practice, and devising a system for sheltering fixed hospitals on the Continent.

The Blood Program

U.S. Army surgeons in the European Theater learned from British experience in the Western Desert, and from early American operations in North Africa and Sicily, that whole blood—while highly perishable and difficult to store and transport—was indispensable for controlling shock in severely wounded soldiers. Blood, administered as far forward as possible in the evacuation chain, saved lives

[27] For the motion sickness preventive, see Medical Consultation Service sec., Professional Services Division, OofCSurg, HQ, ETOUSA, Annual Rpt, 1944, p. 15 and apps. J, K, and L; and Planning Branch, Operations Division, OofCSurg, HQ, ETOUSA, Annual Rpt, 1944, encl. 6. For antigas precautions, see Gas Casualty Division, OofCSurg, HQ, ETOUSA, Annual Rpt, 1944, and Memo, Col. C. B. Spruit to G-2/G-3, FECOMZ, 23 Mar 44, file HD 370 (HQ ADSEC Plans and Corresp, 1944).

that plasma alone could not. In response to this growing weight of evidence General Hawley in July 1943 decided to establish an ETO whole blood service, modeled on the highly successful British Army Transfusion Service.

The American blood bank took shape during late 1943 and early 1944, planned and supervised by an ad hoc committee headed by Colonel Mason, then chief of the Operations Division, and including Colonels Cutler and Middleton, the commander of the 1st Medical General Laboratory, and the chief of the Supply Division. No T/O blood bank unit existed, so General Hawley improvised one. He reorganized the 250-bed 152d Station Hospital into a base depot, located at the 1st Medical General Laboratory at Salisbury, and mobile advance depots—two for the Communications Zone and two for the armies. The base depot was to collect type O blood (the only kind used) from volunteer SOS donors, process it, and prepare it for daily shipment to France, where the advance depots, using truck-mounted refrigerators, would distribute it as far forward as the field hospital platoons attached to division clearing stations. Equipment for the units came from the United States, under a special project for continental operations (PROCO), and from the British, who furnished indispensable refrigerators, as well as bottles, tubing, and needles for bleeding and transfusion. By mid-April 1944 the blood bank, under the overall command of the 1st Medical General Laboratory and with Maj. Robert C. Hardin, MC, in immediate charge as executive officer, had secured most of its equipment and finished organizing and training the 11 officers and 143 enlisted men of its base, COMZ, and army depots. General Hawley meanwhile secured from the theater top priority for shipments of blood to France and from the Ninth Air Force a guarantee of daily space on aircraft.[28]

As the invasion approached, the ETO blood service faced a prospective supply shortage. Since whole blood could be stored for a maximum of fourteen days, the theater required a reliable flow of new blood about equal to the expected usage rate in the field, a rate which Colonel Mason's committee, applying the British planning ratio of 1 pint of blood for each 8–10 wounded, estimated as averaging about 200 pints per day during the first three months of combat. This amount was safely within the ETO blood bank's 600-pints-per-day collection and processing capacity. Even as the bank prepared for operations, however, the medical service, on the basis of reports from the Fifth Army in Italy, increased its estimate of requirements to 1 pint for every 2.2 casualties.

---

[28] For development of the concepts of shock and transfusion, see Douglas B. Kendrick, *Blood Program in World War II*, Medical Department, United States Army in World War II (Washington, D.C.: Office of the Surgeon General, Department of the Army, 1964), pp. ix, 15–17, 30–60, 459, 469–500, 508–12. For development of the ETO blood bank, see file 742 ETO General File (Blood Program). See also Professional Services Division, OofCSurg, HQ, ETOUSA, Annual Rpt, 1943, p. 8; James B. Mason, "Planning for the ETO Blood Bank," *The Military Surgeon* 102 (June 1948): 460–68; O/CS Continental SOP, 4 Apr 44, pp. 29–32, file HD 370.02. PROCO was an Army Service Forces system for tailoring equipment for particular tasks not covered by ordinary unit allowances or T/E. See Ruppenthal, *Logistical Support*, 1:260–61.

On this basis the blood bank, working at full capacity, would not be able to keep up with daily demands, and it became apparent that, even if collection and processing could be increased, the supply of raw material in the theater could not. When General Lee issued the planned call for volunteer donors early in 1944, response from the Services of Supply was disappointing. By mid-April the base sections, in spite of exhortations from Lee and Hawley, had enrolled only 35,000 of 80,000 potential type O donors. As early as May 1943 Colonel Cutler and Major Hardin had suggested flying in blood from the United States, but Surgeon General Kirk, until well after D-Day, vetoed this proposal. His staff underestimated the need for whole blood in field surgery and doubted the feasibility of transporting the perishable substance across the ocean. From the available donors the ETO blood bank, by starting collection well in advance and storing blood up to the maximum safe limit, could meet immediate invasion requirements. But, as the campaign expanded and the limited SOS donor pool diminished with the movement of service troops to France, the blood supply at some point would fall short of need unless the theater could find an additional source. On D-Day, such a source still was not in sight.[29]

The Surgical Program

The effort of General Hawley and his consultants to define uniform surgical practice for each step in the evacuation process had more satisfactory and definite results. During 1942 Colonel Cutler and the surgical consultants began rewriting War Department Technical Manual 8–210, *Guides to Therapy for Medical Officers,* to simplify it and make it more useful to surgeons in the field. Finished late in 1943, the resulting ETO *Manual of Therapy,* published as a pocket-sized booklet, reached medical officers before D-Day. Of the manual's three sections, two dealt with surgery in clearing stations and evacuation and fixed hospitals. Written in short, simple sentences, these sections concentrated on specific treatment of particular types of injury at each point in the evacuation chain and omitted lengthy expositions of theory. Generally, the manual emphasized the need to avoid definitive surgery in the forward areas, unless absolutely necessary to save life. The third section of the manual covered basic medical emergencies, from poisoning to neuropsychiatric disabilities. This manual, supplemented on 15 May 1944 by an ETO circular on "Principles of Surgical Management in the Care of Battle Casualties," which reiterated many of the same policies, constituted a concise practical guide for surgeons fresh from civilian practice and usually inexperienced at

[29] See file 742 ETO General File (Blood Program); Professional Services Division, OofCSurg, HQ, ETOUSA, Annual Rpt, 1944, pp. 5–6. Hawley Interv, 1962, pp. 43–44, CMH, recalls the disbelief with which the ETO surgeons greeted initial reports on blood use in Italy. For the policies of the Office of the Surgeon General, see Kendrick, *Blood Program,* pp. 476–84, 524–26, 530; Editorial Advisory Board, 1962, pp. 108–09; and Memo, Lt Col B. N. Carter to Gen Hillman, 28 Oct 43, sub: ETMD, ETO, and Ltr, Carter to Col E. C. Cutler, 4 Nov 43, both in file HD 024 ETO O/CS (Hawley-SGO Corresp).

treating severe injuries in primitive facilities under pressure of time.[30]

The Expeditionary Hospital

General Hawley's staff early took up the problem of housing general and station hospitals on the Continent, where they had to assume that the battle would leave behind few readily usable buildings. In late 1943, after almost a year of work, the Hospitalization Division and the ETO Office of the Chief of Engineers completed draft plans for an expeditionary tented-hutted hospital. Designed to house a 1,000-bed general or 750-bed station hospital, this standardized installation was to consist initially of tents on concrete bases, on a site improved with paved roads and with water, sewer, and power lines. Each tent was to have space beside it for a parallel hut, which the Engineers were to erect during hospital operations as circumstances permitted. Passing through several stages of development, from completely tented to completely hutted, an expeditionary hospital was supposed to be able to accommodate its full capacity of patients at each stage, even as construction and the transfer of facilities from under canvas to under roofs went on.

In October 1943, to test the newly completed plan, the Services of Supply sent the 12th Evacuation Hospital to Carmarthen, Wales, to erect and operate an expeditionary 750-bed station hospital serving troops in that area. The unit, and an Engineer company, arrived on the site, deliberately selected for unsuitability, early in November. In spite of rain, snow, obstructing hedgerows, and poorly drained marshy ground, the hospital unit and its supporting engineers had the plant in tented operation before the end of the year. The hospital was well into the hutted stage in March 1944, when the 12th turned it over to a station hospital unit. In March the Hospitalization Division issued a manual with construction specifications for the expeditionary hospital, incorporating lessons learned at Carmarthen. The system proved its worth even before the invasion, as the Services of Supply used it to set up several temporary plants needed to increase fixed bed capacity or receive casualties from France.[31]

Readying Medical Supply

As invasion planning neared completion, General Hawley viewed with increasing alarm one key element of his establishment: medical supply. Throughout the renewed BOLERO

[30] ETO, *Manual of Therapy*, 5 May 44, file Manual of Therapy, ETO, box 405, RG 112, NARA. For comparison, see War Department Technical Manual 8–210, *Guides to Therapy for Medical Officers*, 20 Mar 42. For the 15 May 44 circular, see Canter, ed., *Surgical Consultants*, 2:168–73 and app. B, p. 963. See also Hawley Interv, 1962, pp. 57–61, CMH; Ltrs, Col E. C. Cutler to Lt Col N. B. Carter, 5 Oct and 15 Nov 43, and Carter to Cutler, 30 Sep and 26 Oct 43, in file HD 024 ETO O/CS (Hawley-SGO Corresp).

[31] Hospitalization Division, OofCSurg, HQ, ETOUSA, Annual Rpts, 1943, pp. 3–5, and 1944, pp. 5–6; 12th Evacuation Hospital Annual Rpt, 1944, pp. 1–4; Spruit Diary, 7 Jul 43. See also Memo, Hospitalization Division to CSurg, ETO, 22 Jan 43; Memos, Hospitalization Division to DepCSurg (Cheltenham), 24 and 30 Jun 43; and Memo, Col J. R. Darnall to DepCSurg (Cheltenham), 8 Jul 43. All in HospDivGenCorresp, 1943, file HD 312 ETO.

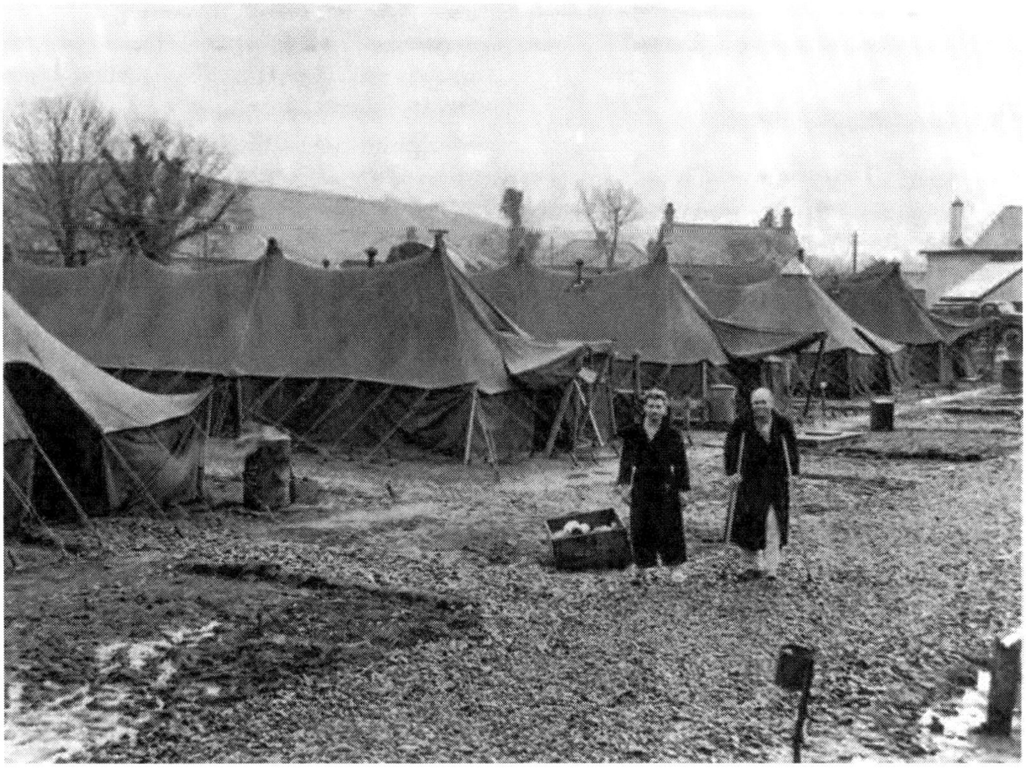

EXPEDITIONARY HOSPITAL AT CARMARTHEN

buildup persistent shortages and administrative deficiencies had made it difficult for the supply service even to support the troops in Britain. The Supply Division of the chief surgeon's office lacked qualified manpower and leadership to meet its expanding responsibilities, and the flow of materiel from American and British sources encountered diversions and dams at many points. By early 1944 both General Hawley and Surgeon General Kirk had been forced to realize that, unless drastically reorganized and reinforced, the medical supply service would fail in its effort to support the coming offensive.

The Supply Division during 1942 had been the weakest element in ETO medical administration; it improved only marginally in 1943. In March Col. Walter L. Perry, MC, arrived to take over the division, replacing the third in a series of unsatisfactory chiefs. General Hawley welcomed Perry, whom the surgeon general had picked for the position and who was experienced in depot operations, and gave him a free hand in reorganizing the supply system. Perry, however, like his predecessors, found the job too much for him. Most of his difficulties stemmed from a lack of trained men. Although his Cheltenham staff doubled during the year, from 8 to 16 officers and from 13 to 47 enlisted men, the size of the task grew even more rapidly, and few of the additional personnel possessed the specialized training needed to manage what was, in effect, a home base rather than a field supply service. Perry also lacked direct access to General Hawley after the latter moved to London in May. Instead, the supply chief had to communicate through Colonel Spruit, the deputy chief surgeon at Cheltenham, a circumstance which reduced Perry's ability to call attention to his requirements. Repeated Supply Division requests for more staff, for example, never went beyond Spruit's office.[32]

Manpower deficiencies plagued the theater's medical supply depots (*see Map 5*). Between the beginning of 1943 and early 1944 the number of medical branch depots and medical sections of Quartermaster general depots increased from five to sixteen. Eight of these depots issued supplies to units and hospitals in their geographical areas; the others held reserve stocks or performed specialized functions, such as outfitting tactical units, receiving British supplies, and repairing medical equipment. Of the 90 officers and 1,200 enlisted men who staffed these installations, about half were members of six field depot companies, units which arrived or were activated in the theater during the last half of 1943; the rest were on temporary assignment from replacement centers. Neither the depot companies, which were organized for mobile field operations, nor the attached casuals had received any training in the operation of large permanent depots. They learned their jobs by doing them. All were on temporary assignment—the depot companies awaiting orders for field service and the casuals subject to transfer on short notice. Without a sense of permanency and, in the case of the attached men, with no promotion prospects, these troops suffered from low morale and had little incentive to excel at their often hard, demanding work.[33]

Depot operations were inefficient at best and chaotic at worst. An officer who joined the medical section of Depot G–35 at Bristol early in 1944 reported: "There was no depot organization—it seemed as [if] everyone was doing what he chose to do. Responsibilities were not defined." Each depot commander improvised his own system for filling requisitions and his

[32] "Med Svc Hist, 1942–43," pp. 55–58, file HD 314.7–2 ETO; Supply Division, OofCSurg, HQ ETOUSA, Annual Rpt, 1944, sec. 1, p. 1. High hopes for Colonel Perry are expressed in Ltrs, Col F. C. Tyng, MC, to Hawley, 21 Jan 43, and Hawley to Tyng, 3 Mar 43, file HD 024 ETO O/CS (Hawley-SGO Corresp). See also Col T. S. Voorhees, "Resume of Trip to Survey Medical Supplies in ETO" (hereafter cited as "Resume"), 12 Apr 44, in Survey of the Medical Supply Situation in the ETO (hereafter cited as ETO Supply Survey), January–March 1944, file HD 333 ETO.

[33] At this time no standard T/O existed for the type of large, permanent depot established in the ETO. The field depot companies did not fit most depots and often had to be broken up between two or more installations. See "Med Svc Hist, 1942–43," pp. 55–56, file HD 314.7–2 ETO; Memo, Col T. S. Voorhees, H. C. Hangen, Col B. C. T. Fenton, and Lt Col L. H. Beers to TSG, 16 Feb 44, sub: Progress Report (hereafter cited as Progress Report, 16 Feb 44), and Voorhees, Fenton, Beers, and Hangen, Outline of Presentation to General Hawley of Supply Division Recommendations (hereafter cited as Outline Presentation), 7 Feb 44, both in ETO Supply Survey, January–March 1944, file HD 333 ETO; Interv, ETO with Lt Col Robert R. Kelley, MC (hereafter cited as Kelley Interv), 27 Jan 45, box 221, RG 112, NARA.

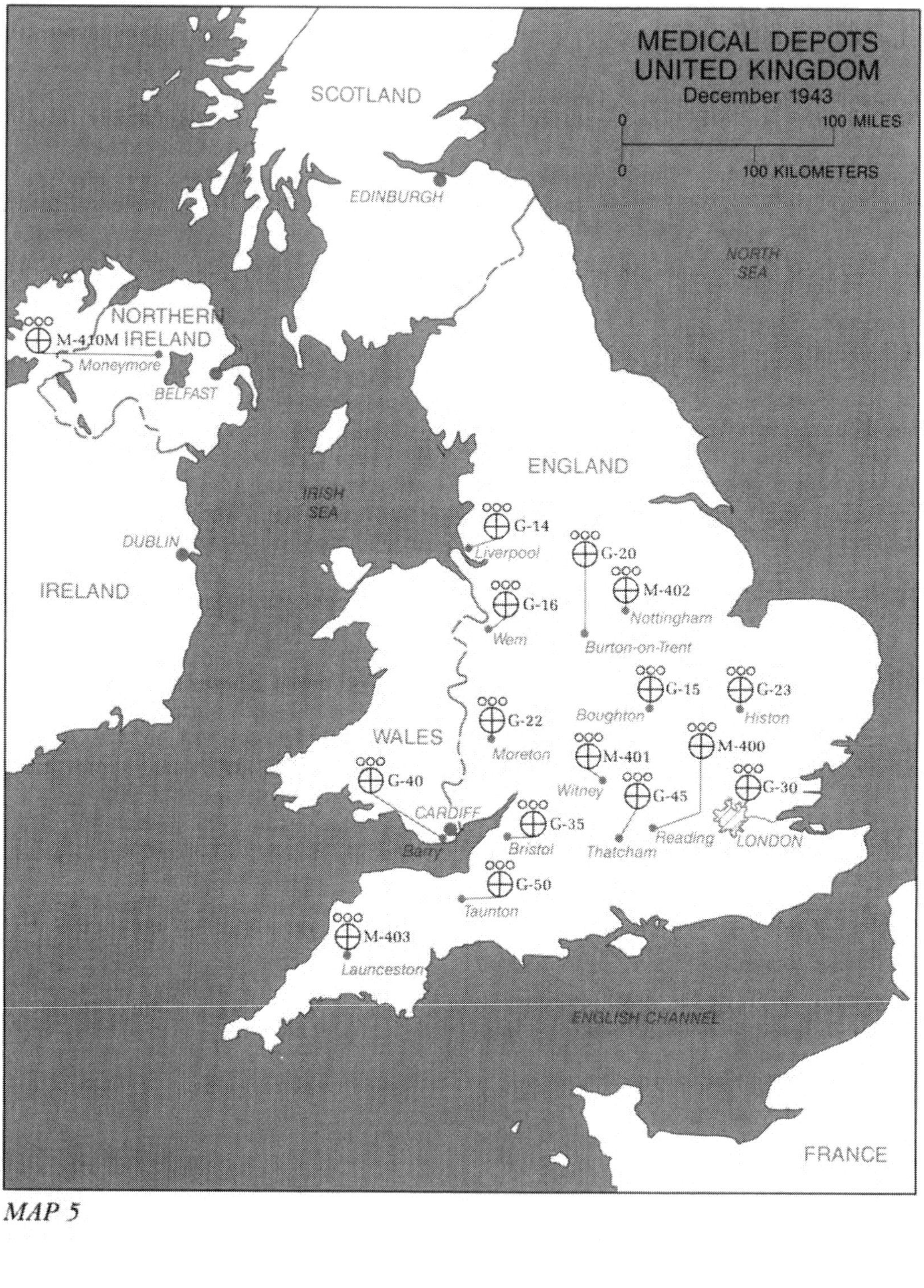
MEDICAL DEPOTS
UNITED KINGDOM
December 1943
0
100 MILES
0
100 KILOMETERS
SCOTLAND
EDINBURGH
NORTH SEA
NORTHERN IRELAND
M-410M
Moneymore
BELFAST
ENGLAND
IRISH SEA
DUBLIN
IRELAND
G-14
Liverpool
G-20
M-402
Nottingham
G-16
Wem
Burton-on-Trent
G-15
G-23
Boughton
Histon
G-22
WALES
Moreton
M-401
M-400
G-40
Witney
G-45
G-30
CARDIFF
G-35
Reading
LONDON
Barry
Bristol
Thatcham
G-50
Taunton
M-403
Launceston
ENGLISH CHANNEL
FRANCE

MAP 5

own stock control procedure. In most depots, record-keeping fell behind issues, leaving both local commanders and the Supply Division unaware of developing shortages until the shelves were empty. The Supply Division required periodic reports from the depots of stores on hand; but the depots' poor record-keeping rendered this information suspect, and the Cheltenham office lacked the staff and tabulating equipment to prepare up-to-date theater-wide reports on stock levels and distribution. With incomplete and outdated information, the Supply Division could not shift materiel between depots to even out local shortages and surpluses. The more enterprising depot commanders developed their own contacts for this purpose. Medical units and hospitals, in spite of instructions to the contrary, went from one depot to another until they secured not only the items they needed but also reserves considerably over authorized allowances. These field improvisations enabled the medical service to get along from day to day, but the resulting lack of accurate information disrupted theater-wide supply planning and hindered General Hawley in dealing with his sources of medical supply in Britain and the United States.[34]

During 1943, as American war production reached full momentum and the shipping shortage eased, the European Theater drew an increasing proportion of medical items, as well as other types of supply, from the United States. Small at the beginning of the year, the flow of materiel grew with the accelerating BOLERO buildup, but it by no means went smoothly. General Hawley complained throughout the year about delayed or only partly filled requisitions, while the surgeon general's office and the Port of New York insisted that they were meeting all ETO requirements. The stock control deficiencies in Hawley's depots contributed much to these disagreements, both by preventing timely dispatch of requisitions to the United States and by making it difficult to ascertain exactly what supplies actually had arrived.[35]

Shipment of preassembled and packed table-of-equipment (T/E) outfits for hospitals and field medical units continued to be trouble-plagued, in spite of War Department and ETO efforts to improve the system and in spite of the abandonment by the New York Port of Embarkation of the practice of earmarking particular outfits for individual organizations. Delivery of assemblies, instead of keeping pace with unit arrivals in Britain, fell behind. ETO depots then had to deplete their stocks to outfit disembarking units,

[34] As quoted in Wiltse, ed., *Medical Supply*, p. 274. See also Progress Report, 16 Feb 44, in ETO Supply Survey, January–March 1944, file HD 333 ETO; Kelley Interv, 27 Jan 45, box 221, RG 112, NARA; Memo, Hawley to DepCSurg (Cheltenham), 22 Sep 43, file HD 024 ETO O/CS (Spruit Policy Notebook). In latter file Cir Ltr No. 54 (Supply No. 6), OofCSurg, HQ, ETOUSA, 9 Apr 43, sub: Supply Policies and Procedures, ETO, outlines the prescribed—but often not followed—procedures. Ruppenthal, *Logistical Support*, 1:152–59, describes the organization, procedures, and problems of U.S. depots in Great Britain. The medical service had many difficulties in common with the other supply services.

[35] "Med Svc Hist, 1942–43," pp. 58–59, file HD 314.7-2 ETO. For typical complaints, see Ltrs, Hawley to TSG, 7 Dec 43; Hawley to Col S. B. Hays, MC, 7 Feb 44; and Hawley to Rankin, 16 Feb 44. All in file HD 024 ETO O/CS (Hawley-SGO Corresp).

with no assurance of early replenishment. Furthermore, most medical unit assemblies—especially those for hospitals—reached British depots short 15-30 percent of their components, in spite of strenuous efforts by the New York port to have them carefully marked and loaded on one ship. After much mutual recrimination between Hawley and the surgeon general's office, an investigation early in 1944 disclosed that most assemblies were entering English ports intact but that the Supply Division had made no special arrangements for keeping them together as they were unloaded. As a result, portions of hospitals and unit outfits turned up in different depots. These depots, uninstructed in handling this materiel, simply added it to their general stock without informing the Supply Division.[36]

Although shipments from the United States increased, the medical service during 1943 procured more than half of its supplies, by tonnage, from Great Britain. British materiel, in fact, comprised 49 percent of all the goods received by the medical service between mid-1942 and mid-1944. These supplies included most hospital furniture and housekeeping equipment, as well as quantities of over 900 other items, among them surgical instruments and many drugs.

British procurement had been invaluable in meeting TORCH requirements and in tiding the medical service over its period of low priorities and limited support from the United States, but it possessed many unsatisfactory aspects. The British insisted that the Americans place very large long-term orders far in advance of deliveries, a procedure that made it all but impossible to adjust procurement to changing requirements. At the same time British deliveries on these contracts were irregular in both timing and quantity. Few quality controls existed. In the emergency of 1942 General Hawley had disregarded American specifications in accepting British supplies. He used whatever his consultants, after examining samples, declared would serve the purpose. These items underwent no inspection as they came off the production lines; shipments reaching American units frequently were poorly packed, substandard in quality, or in unusable condition. Even when British materiel arrived in good condition, U.S. Army medical people were unaccustomed to its differences from their own and considered many items inferior to their American equivalents. Seemingly small differences in design and markings took getting used to, and at least one cost lives. British-supplied carbon dioxide, used in anesthesia, came in tanks painted green, the color used in the United States to denote oxygen. The resulting mixups caused at least eight deaths on operating tables before the Professional Services Division issued

[36] Memo, Col T. S. Voorhees to TSG, 17 Mar 44, sub: Report as to Splitting Up of Hospital Assemblies in Shipment From the U.S. to the ETO, in ETO Supply Survey, January-March 1944, file HD 333 ETO; "Med Svc Hist, 1942-43," p. 58, file HD 314.7-2 ETO; Supply Division, OofCSurg, HQ ETOUSA, Annual Rpt, 1944, sec. IV, pp. 1-4, sec. V, p. 1, and sec. VI, p. 2; Ltr, Tyng to Hawley, 21 Jan 43, and other 1943 letters, file HD 024 ETO O/CS (Hawley-SGO Corresp). Ruppenthal, *Logistical Support*, 1:132-46, describes the complex problems of shipping and marking ETO-bound supplies of all kinds.

warnings and arranged for relabeling of tanks.[37]

In August 1943 General Hawley began trying to reduce his dependency on the British. Aware of deficiencies in quality and slow deliveries, he also had discovered that his allies, while furnishing inferior goods to the European Theater, simultaneously were obtaining large quantities of standard American medical supplies and equipment from the United States under Lend-Lease. At Hawley's urging, Surgeon General Kirk authorized the theater chief surgeon to cancel contracts with the British for items duplicating lend-lease shipments and to requisition them directly from the New York Port of Embarkation. The War Department, at the same time, instructed the medical and other supply services to stop buying from the British a long list of items now overstocked in the United States. In spite of orders from Hawley, however, the Supply Division and its London procurement office, through poor coordination, made no real attempt to reduce local purchases. Instead, the procurement office placed large orders for British goods to be delivered in the first half of 1944.[38]

During the last few months of 1943, as more and more troops poured into the British Isles and invasion preparations got under way, the Supply Division obviously began to buckle under its steadily increasing work load. Disembarking units and newly opened hospitals waited for weeks for their basic equipment. The Air Force, to Hawley's embarrassment in his fight against an autonomous air medical service, continued to complain of shortages of field chests and other vital articles; the flight surgeons continued to resort, successfully, to their own channels to remedy these deficiencies. Early in 1944 the fixed hospitals in the Southern Base Section, where most American troops were concentrated, had only 75 percent of their authorized equipment. In response to complaints from all quarters, Hawley pressed the Supply Division for information but received only incomplete, inconsistent, or inaccurate replies. At the same time the tone of his correspondence with the surgeon general's office grew increasingly testy, as each side blamed the other for shortages and delays. On 7 December Hawley told General Kirk: "I have had a Hell of a lot of trouble with supply and am still having

[37] Memo, Col T. S. Voorhees to TSG, 14 Mar 44, sub: British Procurement, in ETO Supply Survey, January–March 1944, file HD 333 ETO; Ltr, Hawley to TSG, 14 Oct 43, file HD 024 ETO O/CS (Hawley-SGO Corresp). For statistics on British procurement, see Wiltse, ed., *Medical Supply*, p. 270, and Ruppenthal, *Logistical Support*, 1:256–57. See also Carter, ed., *Surgical Consultants*, 2:36–37. For the tank problem, see Senior Consultant in Anesthesiology sec., Professional Services Division, OofCSurg, HQ, ETOUSA, Annual Rpt, 1943; Mins, 18th Meeting of Base Section Surgeons, 27 Mar 44, p. 10, file HD 337; Editorial Advisory Board, 1962, p. 48; and Col T. S. Voorhees, "A Lawyer Among Army Doctors" (Fort Detrick, Md.: Historical Unit, U.S. Army Medical Department, n.d.), pp. 92–94.

[38] Ltrs, Hawley to TSG, 10 Aug and 17 Sep 43; Memo, Edward Reynolds to TSG, 24 Aug 43, sub: Letter From Gen Hawley . . . ; Ltr, TSG to Hawley, 24 Aug 43; Memo, Reynolds to TSG, 18 Nov 43, sub: Data for Reply to General Hawley's Letter. . . . All in file HD 024 ETO O/CS (Hawley-SGO Corresp). See also Voorhees, "Resume," 12 Apr 44, pp. 4–5, and Memo, Col T. S. Voorhees to CSurg, ETO, 18 Mar 44, sub: Report as to British Procurement, both in ETO Supply Survey, January–March 1944, file HD 333 ETO.

trouble. . . . Frankly, I am worried about my medical supply when I think of the approach of active operations." [39]

Hawley had reason to worry. His Supply Division barely was meeting the routine requirements of the forces stationed in the United Kingdom. With much delay and inefficiency it was equipping newly landed units and recently completed hospitals, the pressures of the latter task being eased by British construction delays. Additional missions to be accomplished in early 1944 promised to swamp the floundering division. Within about five months ETO medical depots would have to assemble and place on site equipment for all the hospitals still to be opened before D-Day. This entailed building thirty outfits for 1,000-bed general hospitals and twenty for 750-bed station hospitals, but the most efficient depot in late 1943 took three months to put together 60 percent of one 1,000-bed assembly. As if this were not enough, the depots would have to outfit still more incoming units, complete the equipment of organizations taking part in the assault, and pack dozens of waterproof maintenance units to supply the invasion force in its first weeks on shore. With the existing organization, personnel, and methods, these jobs could not be done in time.[40]

Fortunately for General Hawley, assistance was on the way. Late in 1943 Surgeon General Kirk, responding to the chief surgeon's repeated cries for help in supply, and at the suggestion of Colonel Gorby—then in Washington preparing to join Hawley's staff—decided to send a group of experts from his office to survey the ETO supply service and recommend comprehensive remedies. In doing so Kirk acted outside the established chain of command, which made the theater chief surgeon responsible only to the theater commander. The surgeon general's delegation would possess little authority beyond the moral force of its collective expertise. To lead the group, Kirk appointed the chief of his Control Division, Col. Tracy S. Voorhees, JAGD, a lawyer who had become well versed in medical organization and supply. Voorhees picked the other team members: Lt. Col. Bryan C. T. Fenton, MC; Lt. Col. Leonard H. Beers, MAC; and Mr. Herman C. Hangen, a civilian consultant to the surgeon general. All these men possessed extensive knowledge of medical supply distribution and depot operations; all earlier had helped reorganize the supply system in the United States.[41]

[39] Quotation from Ltr, Hawley to TSG, 7 Dec 43, file HD 024 ETO O/CS (Hawley-SGO Corresp). In same file, see other letters for late 1943 and early 1944. See also Hawley Interv, 1962, p. 36, CMH; Hawley Operational Directive No. 40, 13 Sep 43, box 2, Hawley Papers, MHI; file HD 024 ETO O/CS (Spruit Policy Notebook); "Med Svc Hist, 1942-43," p. 58, file 314.7-2 ETO; Supply Division, OofCSurg, HQ, ETOUSA, Annual Rpt, 1944, sec. IV, pp. 1-2, and sec. VI, p. 3; Mins, 15th Meeting of Base Section Surgeons, 14 Feb 44, p. 7, file HD 337.

[40] Outline Presentation, 7 Feb 44, in ETO Supply Survey, January-March 1944, file HD 333 ETO; Supply Division, OofCSurg, HQ, ETOUSA, Annual Rpt, 1944, sec. V, pp. 1-2; Voorhees, "Lawyer Among Army Doctors," pp. 85-86.

[41] Fenton was Chief, Issue Branch, and Beers, Chief, Stock Control Branch, in the Supply Division, Office of the Surgeon General. Hangen, an executive of J. C. Penney and Company, was a specialist in warehouse operations. Voorhees, a New York lawyer and friend of Under Secretary of War Robert

Continued

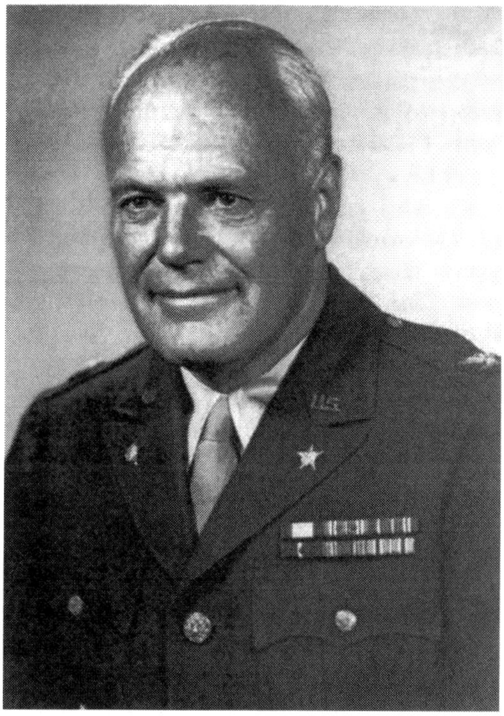

COL. TRACY S. VOORHEES

Voorhees and his party left Washington by plane on 24 January 1944, all but Beers (who was to join the European Theater to direct stock control), under orders for sixty days of temporary duty. Once in the theater, and with the full cooperation and assistance of Hawley and his staff, they visited the Supply Division at Cheltenham, inspected depots, and talked with U.S. Army medical officers of the Services of Supply and the air and ground forces. Very rapidly they learned the dimensions of the medical supply crisis. "Within 10 days," Voorhees recalled, "our team unanimously reached the conclusion that only a complete reorganization, undertaken immediately, would make it possible to furnish needed hospitals and medical supplies for the invasion." Breaking off any further gathering of evidence, they returned to London to report to Hawley.[42]

On 7 February the Voorhees team met with the chief surgeon to discuss not only the findings but also a plan for improvement. Voorhees and his colleagues disavowed any intention to "fix fault or blame," and they acknowledged Hawley's "entire executive authority and responsibility" and his complete freedom to accept or reject their proposals. However, "to the extent that the program involves bringing key people from the U.S., stripping The Surgeon General's Office and Depots of top-notch personnel in this field, we would not feel justified in recommending this unless the plan as a substantial whole is found acceptable by you." The group then told Hawley:

P. Patterson, initially headed the Legal Division, Office of the Surgeon General, and became involved in supply through his work on contracts. He became the confidential agent and troubleshooter of the surgeon general. The Control Division, which he headed, oversaw the operations of other divisions of Kirk's office. See Armfield, *Organization and Administration*, pp. 85–90 and 203–04, and Wiltse, ed., *Medical Supply*, pp. 18–21 and 280. See also Voorhees, "Resume," 12 Apr 44, in ETO Supply Survey, January–March 1944, file HD 333 ETO; Voorhees, "Lawyer Among Army Doctors," pp. 83–84; Gorby Interv, 1962, pp. 2–3, CMH; Editorial Advisory Board, 1962, p. 32.

[42] Quotation from Voorhees, "Lawyer Among Army Doctors," p. 84. See also Voorhees, "Resume," 12 Apr 44, pp. 1–2, in ETO Supply Survey, January–March 1944, file HD 333 ETO; correspondence for January–February 1944, file HD 024 ETO O/CS (Hawley-SGO Corresp); Hawley Planning Directive No. 24, 8 Jan 44, box 2, Hawley Papers, MHI; Memo, Hawley to Chief, Planning Division, 8 Jan 44, file HD 024 ETO O/CS (Spruit Policy Notebook); Supply Division, OofCSurg, HQ, ETOUSA, Annual Rpt, 1944, sec. I, p. 1.

> We believe that your own statements . . . as to the basic inadequacies of your supply service and the grave concern which you expressed as to it, are fully justified by the facts. . . . Unless sweeping reforms are immediately instituted, the Supply Division will fail to perform its mission of furnishing on an even reasonably adequate basis the hospital equipment, field equipment and supplies asked for.[43]

The committee laid before Hawley a three-part program, patterned, they pointed out, on the measures that had solved similar medical supply problems in the United States fifteen months earlier. First, to lighten the depots' impossible work load, they proposed that 37,000 hospital beds—almost all the general and station hospital assemblies needed before D-Day—and all the required medical maintenance units for the invasion be put together in the United States, where the surgeon general's depots now had ample stocks and manpower. The ETO depots then could concentrate on equipping tactical units and on the regular receipt, storage, and issue of supplies. Second, to establish effective stock controls, Voorhees' group proposed a streamlined but more comprehensive system of reports, the development of an SOP for depot operation, reduction of the number of issuing depots, and the creation of key depots to hold reserves of scarce items. Third, the delegation addressed quantitative and qualitative manpower deficiencies, confirming Hawley's long-standing belief that here lay the source of most of his other supply difficulties. They recommended doubling the Supply Division staff, to thirty-two officers and ninety-two enlisted men, and reorganization of the division into four functional branches: Administration and Finance, Stock Control, Depot Technical Control, and Issue. Voorhees and his colleagues urged relief of Colonel Perry "without reflection upon him," and Perry's replacement with Col. Silas B. Hays, MC, who was then head of the Distribution and Requirements Division in the surgeon general's office. They presented the names of other qualified officers whom General Kirk was willing to send from the United States to the European Theater if Hawley requested them. The Voorhees group also recommended that the existing on-the-job-trained depot complements be retained and organized in permanent units, both to improve efficiency and to permit morale-enhancing promotions.[44]

The chief surgeon without hesitation accepted all of the group's recommendations. To implement them—following still another Voorhees proposal—he assumed direct supervision of the Supply Division, superseding his Cheltenham deputy. On 10 February, in a transatlantic teletype conference, the surgeon general's office agreed to all the main points, including assembly in the United States of hospitals and maintenance units and the assignment of Hays and the other requested officers. Hangen, Beers, and Fenton moved to Cheltenham, where they effectively took over the Supply Division, with the full cooperation of Colonel Perry, who stayed on as nominal chief until Hays arrived

[43] Outline Presentation, 7 Feb 44, in ETO Supply Survey, January–March 1944, file HD 333 ETO.

[44] Ibid.

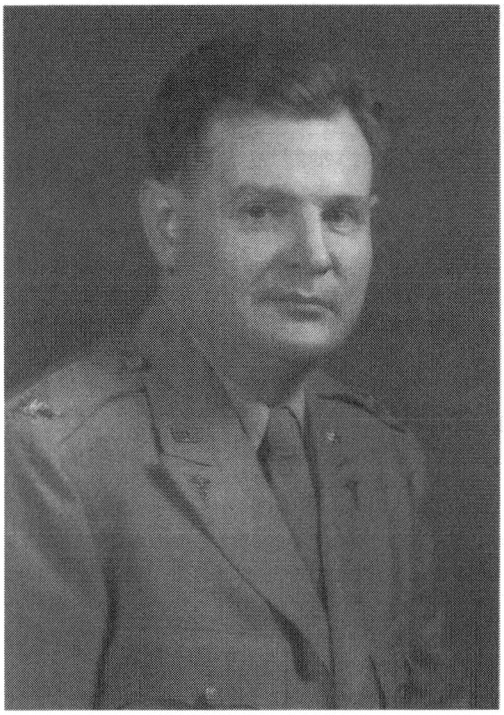

COL. SILAS P. HAYS

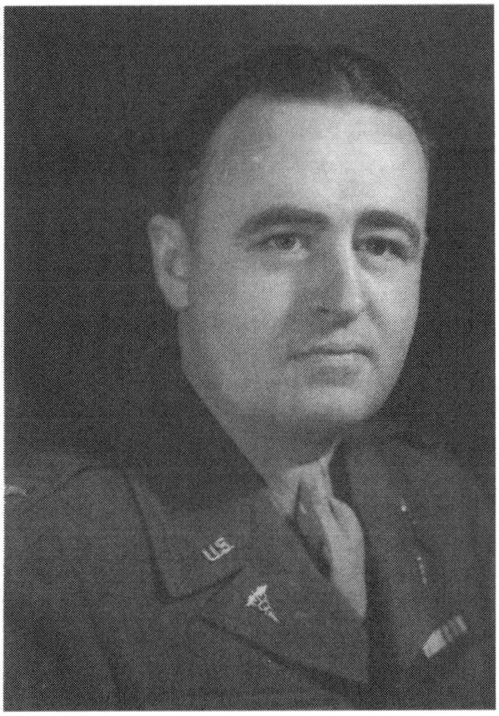

COL. BYRON C. T. FENTON
(Rank as of 15 August 1944)

in March. Colonel Voorhees remained in London, to work on permanent depot organization and begin a study of ways to reduce British procurement. The entire team spent February and March in sustained hard work, their efforts closely observed by General Kenner. The SHAEF chief medical officer received copies of Voorhees' reports and conferred on the supply situation with Hawley, Voorhees, and Colonel Fenton; but, as with hospital construction, he confined himself to supporting the chief surgeon's program.[45]

Voorhees' men rapidly reorganized the Supply Division, establishing the four new branches. By mid-March thirteen of the officers promised by the surgeon general had arrived and gone to work. The division staff expanded to thirty officers, eighty-four enlisted men, and thirteen British civilians, and for the first time in the history of the theater the reinforcements were thoroughly qualified for their jobs. After earnest and repeated pleas from Hawley, General Kirk al-

[45] Voorhees, "Resume," 12 Apr 44, pp. 2–5; OofCSurg, HQ, ETOUSA, Report of Teleprinter Conference . . . With Representatives of TSG, 10 Feb 44; Memo, Hawley to DepCSurg (Cheltenham), 11 Feb 44; Ltr, Voorhees to Edward Reynolds, 7 Mar 44. All in ETO Supply Survey, January–March 1944, file HD 333 ETO. See also Voorhees, "Lawyer Among Army Doctors," pp. 87–90; Ltr, TSG to Hawley, 12 Feb 44, file HD 024 ETO O/CS (Hawley-SGO Corresp). For Kenner's activities, see Medical Division, COSSAC/SHAEF, War Diary, February–April 1944.

TABLE 4—KEY DEPOT SYSTEM, UNITED KINGDOM, 1944

Depot	Location	Supplies
Medical Section, G-20	Burton-on-Trent	All items except for spare parts, lamps, batteries, teeth, blank forms, and veterinary supplies
Medical Section, G-30	London	Veterinary supplies and blank forms
M-400	Reading	Spare parts, batteries, and lamps
Medical Section, G-35	Bristol	Drugs, biologicals, surgical dressings, and instruments
Medical Section G-50	Taunton	Laboratory supplies and dental, X-ray, hospital, and field equipment
Medical Section, G-45	Thatcham	TO/E assemblies

Source: Wiltse, ed., *Medical Supply,* p. 285.

lowed the chief surgeon to retain Fenton as deputy Supply Division chief. Hawley held onto Fenton partly as a possible replacement for Hays, who suffered a severe gastric attack early in May; but, to the chief surgeon's immense relief, his supply chief recovered and was able to resume duty before D-Day.[46]

Depot reorganization went forward (*Table 4*). On 2 February Colonel Voorhees and the chief surgeon prevailed upon the ETO G-1 to halt all transfers of soldiers then working in medical supply depots. This action temporarily stabilized the depot force. After much negotiation between Hawley, Voorhees, and the theater G-1 and G-4, the ETO headquarters activated in Great Britain or called for from the United States eight additional field medical depot companies and assigned all depot personnel to them. While these field companies rarely matched in size and composition the requirements of any particular depot, and hence usually had to be divided among several installations, their establishment did end the transiency of depot personnel. They also provided an organization in which deserving soldiers could receive promotions.[47]

Hangen and Beers revamped depot operations and stock record-keeping. To better control supply issues, they reduced the number of depots distrib-

[46] Ltrs, Hawley to TSG, 20 Apr and 6 May 44; Ltr, TSG to Hawley, 26 Apr 44; Ltrs, Col E. Reynolds to Hawley, 16 May and 8 Jun 44; Ltr, Hawley to Reynolds, 15 Jun 44. All in file HD 024 ETO O/CS (Hawley-SGO Corresp). See also Supply Division, OofCSurg, HQ, ETOUSA, Annual Rpt, 1944, sec. I, p. 1, ex. III; Kelley Interv, 27 Jan 45, box 221, RG 112, NARA; Fenton Interv, 7 Jun 45, box 222, RG 112, NARA; Memo, Voorhees to Hawley, 25 Mar 44, sub: Review of Situation as to Medical Supply, in ETO Supply Survey, January-March 1944, file HD 333 ETO.

[47] The chief surgeon tried unsuccessfully to persuade the theater to authorize permanent non-T/O organizations adapted to the various depots, but the theater insisted on standard T/O units, leaving the field companies the only alternative. Each such company included 8 officers and 167 men. Of the fourteen such companies in the ETO by D-Day, eight were used in fixed depots; the rest were assigned to field armies or the SOS for mobile operations. See Supply Division, OofCSurg, HQ, ETOUSA, Annual Rpt, 1944, sec. II, pp. 1-2; Voorhees, "Resume," 12 Apr 44, and Ltr, Voorhees to TSG, 21 Feb 44, in ETO Supply Survey, January-March 1944, file HD 333 ETO; Kelley Interv, 27 Jan 45, box 221, RG 112, NARA.

uting to units from eight to five. They designated five key depots, each of which held the bulk of theater stocks of certain scarce items and filled requisitions for them passed on from issuing depots. A sixth key depot assembled and issued all tactical unit equipment. Other nonissuing depots performed maintenance and repair, received materiel from the ports, and stored reserve stocks. Hangen and Beers published a depot operations manual, establishing uniform issuing and inventory procedures that the Supply Division's Depot Technical Control Branch saw were carried out. They also set stock levels for each issuing depot, based on the number of troops it served, and redistributed on-hand materiel among installations to give each its proper allowance. To collect theater-wide supply information, Hangen and Beers replaced the three existing separate depot stock reports with a single comprehensive biweekly one. From this, the Supply Division, employing electric tabulating machines, compiled statistics on total supplies on hand and required. At the same time Hangen and Beers set a theater stock level of 75 days' supply of each item and provided for automatic reorder when quantities fell below that point plus an additional margin to allow for time taken in ordering and shipment. To bring all stocks to the 75-day level, the Supply Division placed large emergency requisitions on the New York port; it also sent initial orders for over 800 items in the surgeon general's catalog hitherto not used in the theater to reduce shipping requirements. With vessels and supplies now available, the European Theater thus expanded its supply table. By mid-May the ETO depots were well stocked, and the Supply Division knew what and how much was in them.[48]

While his associates reorganized the depots, Colonel Voorhees surveyed the record of British medical supply. Reviewing the orders placed late the previous year for 1944 delivery, he and his assistants discovered that, of over 800 items involved, all but several varieties of dental burs either were in oversupply in the United States or were being shipped from America under Lend-Lease for British use. After much negotiation with the Ministry of Supply and the War Department, Hawley and Voorhees canceled most supply requests with the British except those for dental burs and a few nonstandard articles; they also retained arrangements for small local emergency purchases. The British either stopped production of the no longer wanted items or diverted them to their own forces. To assure more effective control of any additional buying within the theater, the chief surgeon, at Voorhees' suggestion, placed the London procurement office within the Supply Division's new Stock Control

[48] Supply Division, OofCSurg, HQ, ETOUSA, Annual Rpt, 1944, sec. II, pp 2–4, and sec. VI, pp. 6–7; Ltr, Voorhees to Reynolds, 7 Mar 44, in ETO Supply Survey, January–March 1944, file HD 333 ETO; Memo, Medical Division, SHAEF, to ACofS, G–4, SHAEF, 7 Apr 44, in Medical Division, COSSAC/SHAEF, War Diary, April 1944; Kelley Interv, 27 Jan 45, box 221, RG 112, NARA; Memo, OofCSurg, HQ, ETOUSA, to Maj Gen LeRoy Lutes, 1 May 44, file HD 024 ETO CS (Hawley Chron); Wiltse, ed., *Medical Supply*, pp. 285–87. These additional medical supply shipments were only a small part of the massive last-minute flow of OVERLORD and BOLERO cargo into Britain. See Ruppenthal, *Logistical Support*, I:234–40 and 258–60.

Branch, ending procurement's semi-independent status.[49]

On both sides of the Atlantic, the Army Medical Department and the ETO medical service prepared to assemble and move equipment for hospitals containing a total of 35,000 beds. "This was roughly the equivalent," Voorhees pointed out, "of shipping about 12 complete New York City Bellevue Hospitals, except the buildings." By mid-March the surgeon general's office and the New York Port of Embarkation had worked out packing and loading schedules to ensure arrival of the required assemblies before the end of May. Combined with hospital assemblies requisitioned earlier, the materiel sent in response to Voorhees' special request would provide the European Theater with a large reserve of complete hospitals and components. In the United Kingdom the Supply Division, cooperating with port commanders, base section surgeons, and the Transportation Corps, established procedures for moving hospital assemblies directly from wharf to site, bypassing the depots and reducing the chance of units being broken up in transit. Under this system, between 30 March and 25 May, assemblies for twenty-nine 1,000-bed general hospitals and eight 750-bed station hospitals, as well as additional equipment for thousands of expansion beds, went from ships' holds to plants all over Britain with minimal loss or delay.[50]

Colonel Voorhees and Hangen returned to the United States early in April, to report personally to Surgeon General Kirk and to supervise the dispatch of hospitals and maintenance units. They left behind a medical supply service well on the way to complete transformation—a transformation accomplished in a few months by effective leadership, sufficient manpower, first-class priority for ETO requirements, and high-level command attention. By mid-May the depots possessed full, balanced stocks. The First Army, which would make the assault, had all its medical equipment in hand. The depots were packing for over-the-beach disembarkation maintenance units to sustain the first two weeks of combat. Additional medical maintenance units at sea or in depots contained supplies for the period D+14 to D+90. Most of the operating fixed hospitals in

[49] The War Department initially hesitated to stop ordering from the British because of warnings from the Allies that, without firm American orders, they would shut down production, thereby foreclosing later purchases which might become necessary. Hawley and Voorhees, however, persuaded the Army Service Forces that the sufficiency of shipping and supplies and the inadequacies of British procurement more than justified a complete cutoff. See Voorhees, "Resume," 12 Apr 44, pp. 4–5; Memo, Voorhees to TSG, 14 Mar 44, sub: British Procurement; Memo, Lt Col L. H. Beers, MAC, to Voorhees, 18 Mar 44, sub: British Procurement; Memo, Voorhees to Hawley, 25 Mar 44, sub: Review of Situation as to Medical Supply. All in ETO Supply Survey, January–March 1944, file HD 333 ETO.

[50] Before Voorhees made his request, the Office of the Surgeon General had plans to pack and ship twenty-four general hospitals for eventual use in France; it diverted these to Britain and then sent Voorhees' full request as well. Quotation from Voorhees, "Lawyer Among Army Doctors," p. 89. See also Memo, Voorhees to CSurg, ETO, Col Liston, Col Hays, and Maj Marshall, 16 Mar 44, sub: Status of Requirements for Hospital Assemblies, Dates of Expected Arrival, and Proposed Steps To Assure Timely Deliveries, in ETO Supply Survey, January–March 1944, file HD 333 ETO; Supply Division, OofCSurg, HQ, ETOUSA, Annual Rpt, 1944, sec. V, pp. 1–2, and sec. VI, pp. 2–3; Mins, 16th Meeting of Base Section Surgeons, 28 Feb 44, p. 3, file HD 337; Wiltse, ed., *Medical Supply*, pp. 297–98.

Britain had received their full equipment and held at least sixty days of reserve supplies. Even the Air Force now relied for medical supply more upon SOS channels than upon its own. Three days before the invasion, a still-cautious Hawley declared: "We have just barely squeaked through on our supply. . . . I shall not, however, breathe really easily about it for another month." He had no further cause for worry. ETO medical supply, as reorganized by the Voorhees mission, was ready for war.[51]

Mounting the Attack

Preparations for mounting NEPTUNE—equipping, organizing, and embarking the assault troops and reinforcements so as to ensure their arrival on the far shore in the right order with the right materiel—merged with the final stages of invasion planning. For its part in this process the medical service selected, assigned, and completed the training of army and COMZ units, equipped them, and packed their supplies. It furnished treatment and evacuation to troops assembling for embarkation, and it prepared to receive and care for wounded from the opening battle in Normandy.

During the final months before D-Day the surgeons of the First and Third Armies, Advance Section, and Forward Echelon, in consultation with General Hawley, developed medical troop lists for their respective commands. The ETO headquarters then assigned the requested units from the huge pool accumulating in the United Kingdom. The First Army's preinvasion allocation included one 750-bed and ten 400-bed evacuation hospitals, five field hospitals, a convalescent hospital, headquarters of three medical groups and eight medical battalions (separate), a medical gas treatment battalion, an auxiliary surgical group, a medical laboratory, a medical depot company, and eleven collecting, six clearing, and seven ambulance companies (separate). These units underwent personnel augmentations and rearrangements. To provide ready replacements for invasion casualties, medical elements of the engineer special brigades and of the assault and early buildup divisions received extra officers and men above T/O strength. Army mobile hospitals transferred doctors to balance their professional staffs. First Army field and evacuation hospitals had the painful task of replacing 95 veteran nurses who were considered too old or physically unfit for active campaigning.[52]

The Advance Section and Forward Echelon also received their full allotments of units before D-Day. ADSEC included over 1,800 medical officers, 2,300 nurses, and 16,000 enlisted men when the campaign began.

[51] Quotation from Ltr, Hawley to TSG, 3 Jun 44, file HD 024 ETO O/CS (Hawley-SGO Corresp). See also Memo, Col T. S. Voorhees and H. C. Hangen to TSG, 5 Apr 44, sub: Final Report as to Survey of Medical Supplies in E.T.O., in ETO Supply Survey, January–March 1944, file HD 333 ETO; Memo, OofCSurg, HQ, ETOUSA, to Lutes, 1 May 44, file HD 024 ETO CS (Hawley Chron). The medical supply situation more or less paralleled that in other technical services and the theater as a whole. See Ruppenthal, *Logistical Support*, 1:261–66.

[52] First U.S. Army Report of Operations, 20 Oct 43–1 Aug 44, bk. VII, p. 61. For personnel arrangements, see Surg, Third U.S. Army, Annual Rpt, 1944, pp. 16, 102, 105, and Nursing Division, OofCSurg, HQ, ETOUSA, Annual Rpt, 1944, p. 9.

Unlike those attached to the armies, most units assigned to the Communications Zone were operating fixed installations in Great Britain or had marshaling and casualty reception duties that would continue until embarkation; hence, they remained under base section control, except on matters directly connected with preparing for continental operations—a dual command chain that forced unit staffs to thread their way among duplicate, occasionally conflicting, directives and reporting requirements. Especially in selecting the twenty-five ADSEC and FECOMZ general hospitals, General Hawley recommended SOS units for early shipment to France on the basis of superior performance in Britain. He angrily deleted from the list one general hospital that he found "inexcusably dirty and disorderly" on a pre-D-Day visit.[53]

Medical units designated for early movement to France added instruction and exercises in amphibious warfare and field operations to their already crowded training schedules. The First Army, at Colonel Roger's recommendation, attached medical battalion elements to combat units early in the attack preparations so that the medical troops and the battalions they were to support could go together through the entire invasion training sequence, including the amphibious landing exercise at the army's assault training center on the Devon coast. COMZ organizations usually trained at their stations, supervised and inspected by their assigned headquarters. They also sent key people to special courses. Commanders of the twenty-five ADSEC and FECOMZ general hospitals, for instance, attended a five-day school on erecting the expeditionary tented-hutted plant. First Army and COMZ medical elements participated together in the final division and corps invasion rehearsals covering the entire process of marshaling, embarkation, and assault—TIGER, held late in April for VII Corps; and FABIUS, in early May, for V Corps and the initial buildup force. During TIGER U.S. Army medical units had real casualties to handle, the result of German torpedo boat attacks in the Channel that sank two LSTs and severely damaged a third, with the loss of some 700 American lives. At Portland-Weymouth, in an unplanned but effective test of the system for receiving wounded from France, the 33d Medical Battalion, its attached ambulance and sanitary companies, and the 50th Field Hospital efficiently met the emergency under "particularly trying and difficult conditions." [54]

[53] ADSEC Hist, p. 8; Surg, ADSEC, COMZ, Annual Rpt, 1944, pp. 3 and 38–39; Larkey "Hist," ch. 8, pp. 23–25; file HD 370 (HQ ADSEC Plans and Corresp, 1944). For the hospital deletion, see Ltr (source of quotation), Hawley to Col A. A. Albright, MC, 19 May 44 (marked "not sent"), file HD 024 ETO CS (Hawley Chron), and Hawley Interv, 1962, p. 58, CMH.

[54] For a general account of invasion training and exercises, see Ruppenthal, *Logistical Support*, 1:191 and 334–54, and Harrison, *Cross-Channel*, pp. 162–64 and 269–70. See also remarks of Maj Gen J. L. Snyder, MC, in Editorial Advisory Board, 1962, pp. 69–70. For examples of training, see Surg, VII Corps, Annual Rpt, 1944, pp. 4–5; Surg, 1st Infantry Division, Annual Rpt, 1944, p. 2; 53d Medical Battalion Annual Rpt, 1944, p. 2; and Force U Operations Order 2–44, an. NAN, 18 Apr 44, file HD 370 (Evaluation, Annex JIG); Surg, ADSEC, COMZ, Annual Rpt, 144, pp. 13–15, 31, 48; Hospitalization Division, OofCSurg, HQ, ETOUSA, Annual Rpt, 1944, p. 5. Description of the medical response to the torpedo boat incident, from which the quotation

Continued

Equipment and supply of the assault and early buildup units required cooperation between the First Army and the chief surgeon's Supply Division. On the basis of a First Army study of assault requirements, the Supply Division issued supplemental equipment, above T/E allowances, to army medical units of all types. In spite of duplicated and misdirected shipments, the result of frequent unit movements during marshaling, most First Army organizations had received their extra allotments, as well as nearly 100 percent of their authorized equipment, before they embarked, a tribute to the effectiveness of the newly reorganized depots. Amphibious packing received careful attention from all echelons. The Supply Division distributed standard watertight shipping boxes to First Army field and evacuation hospitals and sent an officer to advise units on how best to protect their materiel against the hazards of sea, weather, and battle. Army units prepared thousands of hand-portable assault supply containers, each a waterproof cylinder 21 inches long and 9.5 inches in diameter, originally used to ship 60-mm. mortar shells. Each case, with a carrying strap attached and painted with a Red Cross in a white circle, weighed about 14 pounds when filled with first aid dressings, sulfa crystals, dried plasma, and other small items. Each container would float, serving the medical soldier hauling it as a life preserver that he could take inland with him as he advanced or could drop on the beach for later retrieval. Eight such cases constituted a single unit of these supplies, and every battalion or company received an allowance of units. The 4th Infantry Division landed with 285 of these cases, containing over 3,500 pounds of supplies.[55]

Following theater policy, the Supply Division loaded all scheduled maintenance supplies for the first sixty days on standard wooden skids, each a sled-like device weighing about 1,700 pounds with cargo, designed to be dragged across beaches and stored in open-air depots. By 8 May medical depots had finished loading these supplies for D-Day through D+15. Piled onto 955 skids, this materiel included ninety-two surgical and twenty-two medical division assault units and twenty regular maintenance units, as well as other freight. General Hawley, meanwhile, secured from the Ninth Air Force a guarantee to airlift daily across the Channel 4,000 pounds of blood, penicillin, and other perishable items, which Depot G-45 at Thatcham was to pack for emplaning at a nearby Army airfield. Late in May the theater blood bank began collecting and processing; its detachments made their first deliveries, over 1,100 pints, to LSTs and hospital carriers. The latter vessels, fitting out at English, Scottish, and Welsh ports, took on blood and biologicals, both

---

is taken, is in OofSurg, United Kingdom Base, Historical Resume of the Planning for and Staging of Operation OVERLORD and the Preceding Exercises (hereafter cited as Surg, UKB, OVERLORD Resume), n.d., pp. 1–8, file HD 370.

[55] First U.S. Army Operations Report, 20 Oct 43–1 Aug 44, bk. VII, pp. 73–74 and 114–16; Supply Division, OofCSurg, HQ, ETOUSA, Annual Rpt, 1944, secs. II, IV, and VI; Kelley Interv, 27 Jan 45, box 221, RG 112, NARA; Surg, United Kingdom Base, Annual Rpt, 1944, p. 35; Mins, 18th Meeting of Base Section Surgeons, 27 Mar 44, pp. 2–3, file HD 337. Surg, VII Corps, Annual Rpt, 1944, pp. 6–8, contains a detailed description of the hand-carried container.

for their own use and to supply the beachheads.[56]

To embark the 130,000 troops and 17,000 vehicles of the assault and initial buildup forces, the U.S. Army used a system worked out by the British early in the ROUNDUP planning. Under it each organization, in prearranged sequence, went from its permanent station through a concentration area to a dockside marshaling camp. In the course of this movement the unit dropped off men and materiel not needed for the attack, waterproofed its vehicles, and picked up assault equipment. Finally, in a marshaling camp sealed off by barbed wire and security patrols, the unit received its mission briefing and organized into ship and landing craft loads. The First Army directed these troop movements and the embarkation, while the Services of Supply built and manned the concentration and marshaling camps and provided messing, medical, and other administrative support for the combat units passing through them. The SOS headquarters, in turn, delegated most mounting tasks to the Southern Base Section, which embarked the OMAHA and UTAH seaborne attack forces and the glider elements of the airborne divisions, and to the Western Base Section, which loaded the first buildup divisions and the airborne paratroopers. Medical support for the mounting, accordingly, rested principally with Col. Robert E. Thomas, MC, the Southern Base Section surgeon, and Col. Mack M. Green, MC, the Western Base Section surgeon.[57]

Medical support provisions for the embarkation were limited and straightforward. In the marshaling camps the base sections established medical supply points to make emergency preembarkation issues and over 150 camp dispensaries, each staffed with 1 officer and 4 enlisted men, to serve units that had dropped off or packed up their own medical detachments. Most of the officers and men for these dispensaries, and for 24 mess teams that helped feed the transient soldiers, came on temporary assignment from station and general hospitals throughout Great Britain. From the same sources the Dental Division of the chief surgeon's office assigned a dentist and an assistant to the marshaling camps for each 3,000 troops, to do last-minute fillings, extractions, and prosthesis repairs. Taken as they were from fixed hospitals, many of these temporary camp doctors had little experience and only brief predeployment training in field medicine and sanitation.[58]

---

[56] Supply Division, OofCSurg, HQ, ETOUSA, Annual Rpt, 1944, secs. II and VI; Surg, ADSEC, COMZ, Annual Rpt, 1944, p. 25; HQ, SOS, ETOUSA, Mounting Plan, an. 8, Medical Corps (hereafter cited as SOS Mounting Plan), 20 Mar 44, in Larkey "Hist," ch. 8, app. 3; Evacuation Branch, Operations Division, OofCSurg, HQ, ETOUSA, Daily Diary, 19 May 44, file HD 024 ETO; Kendrick, *Blood Program*, p. 512; Kelley Interv, 27 Jan 45, box 221, RG 112, NARA.

[57] For the mounting system, see Ruppenthal, *Logistical Support*, 1:218 and 357–62, and Southern Base Section History, August 1943–August 1944, pp. 6–7. See also Surg, UKB, OVERLORD Resume, pp. 1–4, file HD 370; SOS Mounting Plan, 20 Mar 44, in Larkey "Hist," ch. 8, app. 3; Planning Branch, Operations Division, OofCSurg, HQ, ETOUSA, Annual Rpt, 1944, p. 6.

[58] Each mess team included 1 officer, 4 cooks, and 11 men. The latter medical troops were only a few of the 4,500 new cooks hastily assembled for the camps. See Ruppenthal, *Logistical Support*, 1:361. See also Larkey "Hist," ch. 8, pp. 28–31; SOS Mounting Plan, 20 Mar 44, in ibid., app. 3; Surg, UKB, OVERLORD Resume, pp. 11–12, file HD 370; Surg, West-

Continued

The abilities of the camp surgeons, fortunately, were not sorely taxed. Marshaling and embarkation began early in May, after General Eisenhower set D-Day for 5 June, and went forward with no major enemy harassment and, from a medical standpoint, few problems. As planned, the embarking troops enjoyed hot meals of fresh, tasty food. They donned uniforms treated to resist gas and picked up seasickness preventives, insecticide powder, and water purification tablets. They heard a final one-hour preventive medicine lecture that emphasized proper eating habits, personal cleanliness in the field, and precautions against venereal disease. In many marshaling camps, sanitation left much to be desired—the result of inevitable carelessness among transient soldiers and of mistakes by the hastily assembled, sketchily trained camp and mess hall staffs. Base section preventive medicine officers, aided much of the time by Colonel Gordon and members of his division, quickly corrected these deficiencies, although lapses in mess hall cleanliness caused a few battalion-wide outbreaks of diarrhea. Filing a gap in the planning, Gordon's officers devised a system for feeding hot meals to troops held for hours on the docks by embarkation delays. One anticipated problem did not develop. The base section surgeons, expecting a rash of preinvasion emotional disorders, assigned psychiatrists to the marshaling camps. Few cases appeared, and the psychiatrists spent their time giving impromptu short courses in battlefield neuropsychiatry to unit medics.[59]

As the Army embarked, the medical service completed its preparations for receiving invasion casualties (*see Diagram 2*). The chief surgeon's office and Southern Base Section, working closely with the British Southern Command, drafted plans for this operation, which was a complicated task in itself. Under the final plan, published in mid-March, evacuation LSTs and hospital carriers were to unload American wounded at three Channel coast ports: Brixham, Portland-Weymouth, and Southampton. The arriving patients were to undergo two stages of triage and emergency treatment. Holding units at the docks and hards (concrete ramps at which LSTs could load and unload through their bow doors) were to give surgical treatment to men tagged by LST doctors as requiring immediate attention before further transportation. The rest of the patients were to go by ambulance directly from the ships to transit hospitals, designated station and general hospitals 15–30 miles inland. These hospitals again were to separate out wounded who were unable to travel further and prepare the transportables for rail movement to general hospitals for definitive

ern Base Section, Rpt, 1 Jan–31 Aug 44, pp. 5–6; Mins, 13th and 15th Meetings of Base Section Surgeons, 17 Jan and 14 Feb 44, file HD 337; Surg, United Kingdom Base, Annual Rpt, 1944, p. 22; Dental Division, OofCSurg, HQ, ETOUSA, Annual Rpt, 1944, pp. 4–5.

[59] For the course of the embarkation, see Harrison, *Cross-Channel*, pp. 188–90 and 269–74; Ruppenthal, *Logistical Support*, 1:363–73; and Southern Base Section History, August 1943–August 1944, pp. 42–52. See also Surg, UKB, OVERLORD Resume, pp. 14–15, file HD 370; Surg, Infantry Division, Annual Rpt, 1944, pp. 2 and 5; ADSEC Hist, p. 8; Surg, United Kingdom Base, Annual Rpt, 1944, pp. 79–81; Surg, Western Base Section, Rpt, 1 Jan–31 Aug 44, pp. 5–6; Gordon "Hist," vol. 2, pt. 4, pp. 38–39, CMH. For the preventive medicine briefing, see Larkey "Hist," ch. 8, app. 15.

DIAGRAM 2—CASUALTY RECEPTION SYSTEM IN GREAT BRITAIN, JUNE 1944

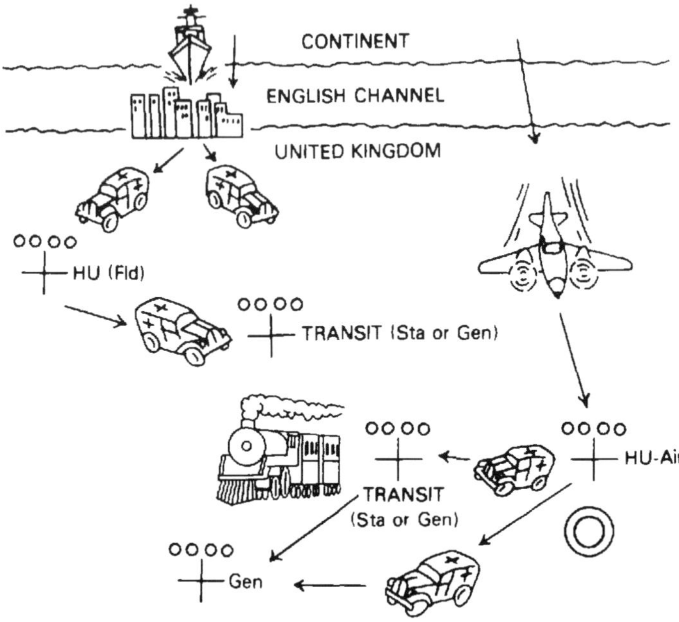

Source: Evacuation Branch, Operations Division, OofCsurg, HQ, ETOUSA, Annual Rpt, 1944, encl. 3.

treatment. Port evacuation officers, under the base section surgeons, were to direct patient movements as far as the transit hospitals; transfers beyond that point would be controlled by the chief surgeon's office. During the first days of combat, when the beachhead was shallowest, this system not only would enable holding units and transit hospitals to assume many functions of division clearing stations and army evacuation hospitals but also would keep wounded flowing from the coast to the large hospital centers in the north and west of England.[60]

The medical service tested this evacuation plan in two exercises: CRACKSHOT, in February 1944, for movement of wounded into and out of transit hospitals; and CADUCEUS, in April for unloading evacuation LSTs. Then the casualty reception forces deployed. At each of the three major receiving ports, and at many minor ones, the base sections established field hospitals under canvas or in requisitioned buildings to serve as holding units, often with platoons placed only a short litter carry from hards and wharves (*Map 6*). Separate medi-

[60] SOS Mounting Plan, 20 Mar 44, in Larkey "Hist," ch. 8, app. 3; Carter, ed., *Surgical Consultants*, 2:173–75. See also MFR, 5 Jan 44, sub: Decisions Made by Gen Hawley at Informal Conference With Cols Hartford and Peyton; Memo, Lt Col F. H. Mowrey, MC, n.d. sub: Evacuation and Medical Service at Hards; Memo, Col J. H. McNinch, MC, to OofCSurg, HQ, ETOUSA, 15 Feb 44; Memo, Chief, Passenger Branch, Office of CofTrans, ETO, to ACofTrans, Movements, 2 Mar 44, sub: Evacuation of Sick and Wounded From the Continent. . . . All in EvacCorresp, 1942–44, file HD 024 ETO.

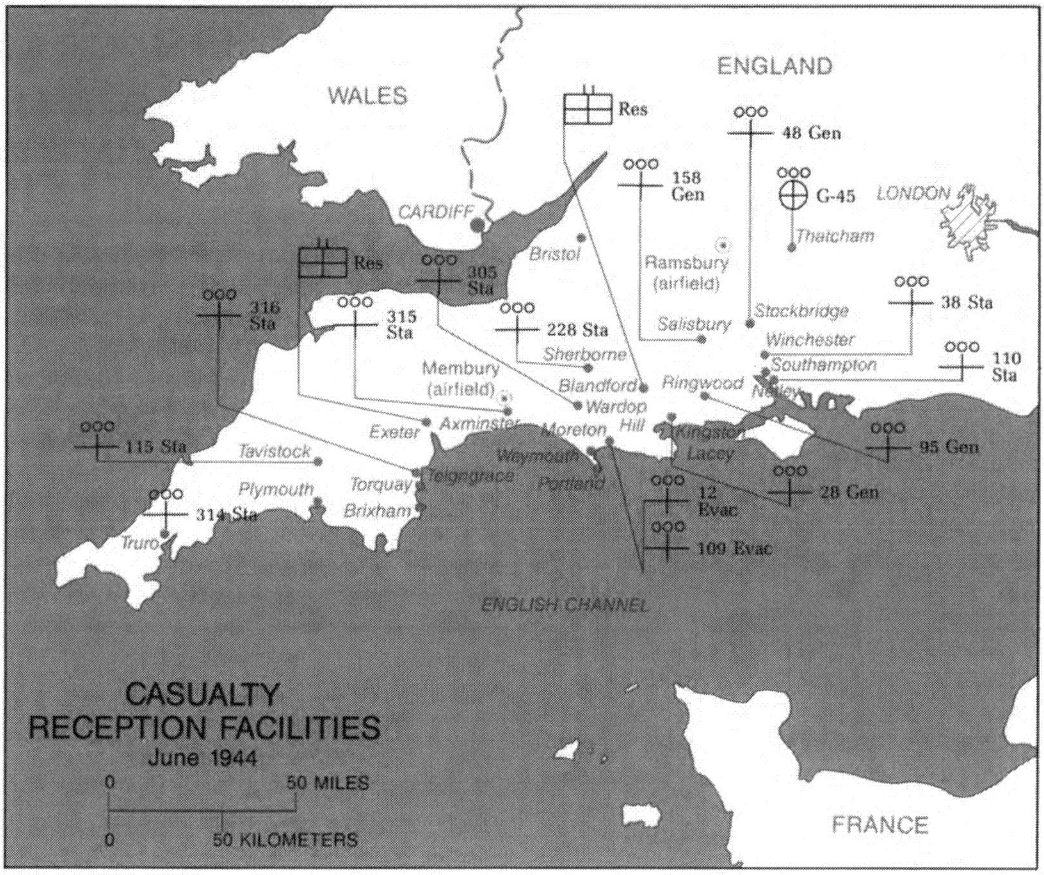

MAP 6

cal battalions at Brixham and Portland and a gas treatment battalion at Southampton, each with sanitary, ambulance, and collecting companies attached, prepared to unload ships and transport patients between holding units and transit hospitals. Each battalion commander acted as evacuation officer for his port. Two more medical battalions, at Blandford and Exeter, held collecting, clearing, and ambulance companies in reserve for commitment at General Hawley's direction. At Ramsbury and Membury airfields, the nearshore terminals for cross-Channel air evacuation, still other field hospital platoon holding units and ambulance detachments awaited patients. Forty-nine units (nine field hospitals; one gas treatment and four medical battalions; and five sanitary, seventeen ambulance, four collecting, and two clearing companies), all temporarily detached from the Communications Zone and the field armies, made ready to receive wounded from Normandy.[61]

---

[61] Surg, UKB, OVERLORD Resume, pp. 4–5, 8–13, 18, file HD 370; Larkey "Hist," ch. 8, pp. 31–

Continued

To assist in casualty reception, treatment, and evacuation, the medical service improvised a variety of teams and special units. General Hawley drew almost 500 doctors and a comparable number of enlisted technicians from Third Army, the air forces, and station and general hospitals, to staff marshaling camp dispensaries, to form LST surgical teams, and to assist the 1st Auxiliary Surgical Group in reinforcing the staffs of holding units and transit hospitals. Hawley and the base section surgeons tried to distribute the burden of these details evenly, but some fixed hospitals suffered significant temporary losses. In the Eastern Base Section, for instance, the 303d Station Hospital, which treated Eighth Air Force battle casualties, had to give up 2 officers and 8 men for dispensaries, 2 mess sergeants and 31 enlisted people for marshaling camp details, and 1 officer for a district inspection team. To provide professional staffs for three of the British-crewed hospital carriers, the Evacuation Branch, lacking T/O units for this purpose, placed a hospital train unit and a medical hospital ship platoon on each vessel. The Western Base Section, needing a holding unit for two Welsh ports, improvised one by augmenting an engineer regiment's medical detachment with doctors from dispensaries in the marshaling camps.[62]

The chief surgeon backed up his receiving units with reserves of transportation and supplies. General Hawley established a pool of 350 extra ambulances—American ¾-ton vehicles not yet issued to units and surplus British Austins. He distributed these, and 18 bus ambulances, to the Southern and Western Base Sections to reinforce ambulance companies and transit hospitals. The Evacuation Branch, unable to obtain any more home ambulance trains than the 5 then in service, persuaded the Ministry of Transport to adapt 10 overseas trains to run on British lines, ensuring enough rolling stock to keep the transit hospitals cleared. The Supply Division set up temporary advance depots at Plymouth, Torquay, Winterborne Steepleton, and Lockerley in the Southern Base Section. Besides holding reserves needed by the hospitals, these dumps, and others on the docks and hards, stored Navy supplies to replenish evacuation LSTs. They also contained exchange units

32, 55–56, and ch. 13, p. 7; Evacuation Branch, Operations Division, OofCSurg, HQ, ETOUSA, Annual Rpt, 1944, pp. 2–4; Surg, United Kingdom Base, Annual Rpt, 1944, pp. 20–21, 24, 44–46. For unit procurement, see Planning Branch, Operations Division, OofCSurg, HQ, ETOUSA, Annual Rpt, 1944, p. 8; SOS Mounting Plan, 20 Mar 44, in Larkey "Hist," ch. 8, app. 3; and file HD 370 (HQ ADSEC Plans and Corresp, 1944). On unit activities, see 33d Medical Battalion Annual Rpt, 1944, pp. 5–8; 93d Medical Gas Treatment Battalion Unit History, 1943–44, pp. 3–6; and 12th and 50th Field Hospitals Annual Rpts, 1944.

[62] Larkey "Hist," ch. 8, pp. 28–31; Personnel Division, OofCSurg, HQ, ETOUSA, Annual Rpt, 1944, pp. 10–11; Mins, 14th, 18th, and 19th Meetings of Base Section Surgeons, respectively 31 Jan, 27 Mar, and 10 Apr 44, file HD 337; Surg, Western Base Section, Rpt, 1 Jan–31 Aug 44, p. 6. On LST teams, see Dowling, Normany Rpt, 11 Jan 45, pp. 6–8, and file HD 705 ETO (Medical Care on LSTs, 1944). On drafts from hospitals, see Ltrs, Hawley to Col R. E. Thomas, MC, 27 Apr 44, and Hawley to Col M. M. Green, MC, 5 May 44, file HD 024 ETO CS (Hawley Chron); see also 5th General Hospital Annual Rpt, 1944, p. 5, and 12th Evacuation Hospital Annual Rpt, 1944, p. 8. On hospital carriers, see Evacuation Branch, Operations Division, OofCSurg, HQ, ETOUSA, Daily Diary, 16–30 May 44, file HD 024 ETO.

of stretchers, blankets, and splints, designed and assembled jointly by the Supply Division and the Western Naval Task Force to prevent the planned near-total evacuation policy from stripping the beachhead of these vital items. LSTs were to deliver 300 of these units—containing in all 30,000 litters, 96,000 blankets, and quantities of splints and plasma—to Normandy on their first and subsequent voyages. Permanent Southern Base Section medical depots accumulated still more supplies of all classes, among them most of the theater's available oxygen cylinders, stockpiled for possible use in treating gas casualties.[63]

Fixed hospitals made preparations of their own. The eight station and four general hospitals assigned to transit duty cleared out patients, streamlined admission and evacuation procedures, and trained extra ambulance drivers and litterbearers. To provide more transit beds at Portland-Weymouth, where most wounded were expected to arrive, the 12th and 109th Evacuation Hospitals, detached from the Third Army, established a temporary expeditionary tented plant. General hospitals, prodded by Hawley and his consultants, sped up the return of convalescents to duty and increased the number of eligible patients evacuated to the United States. By 1 June the Southern Base Section had available for invasion wounded over 10,000 beds in transit hospitals and 18,000 more in regular station and general hospitals.[64]

By 3 June the assault forces had embarked. After a 24-hour delay caused by storms over the Channel and Normandy, the 5,000-ship invasion fleet set course for France, for a landing scheduled for first light on the sixth. For many medical troops in southern England not yet embarking or preparing to do so, the first notice that the long-awaited invasion was under way came on the night of 5 June, in the form of a sky filled with the navigation lights and engine sound of hundreds of planes heading for the airborne drop zone behind Utah beach. For General Hawley, two years of planning and preparation had reached their goal and climax. "We are all set for the kick-off," he wrote after a final tour of his holding units and transit hospitals, "and I, personally, feel as nervous as players usually feel just prior to the whistle." The chief surgeon and his SHAEF superi-

[63] On reserve ambulances and trains, see file HD ETO 451.8 (Amb), 1942–44; Evacuation Branch, Operations Division, OofCSurg, HQ, ETOUSA, Daily Diary, 19, 22, and 27 May 44, file HD 024 ETO. On supplies, see Surg, UKB, OVERLORD Resume, p. 12, file HD 370; Supply Division, OofCSurg, HQ, ETOUSA, Annual Rpt, 1944, sec. VI; Fenton Interv, 7 Jun 45, box 222, RG 112, NARA; Surg, United Kingdom Base, Annual Rpt. 1944, pp. 34–35. On exchange units, see First U.S. Army Report of Operations, 20 Oct 43–1 Aug 44, bk. VII, p. 75; Directive, HQ, ETOUSA, to CG, FUSAG, and Cdr, US Fleet, TF 122, 19 May 44, sub: Initial Evacuation of Casualties From Far to Near Shore . . . , in Larkey "Hist," ch. 8, app. 5.

[64] For number of beds, see Memo, Maj D. J. Twohig, MC, to CSurg, 1 Jun 44, sub: Status of Evaucation, EvacCorresp, 1944–45, file HD 370.05 ETO. See also Surg, UKB, OVERLORD Resume, pp. 13–14, file HD 370; Larkey "Hist," ch. 8, pp. 49–50; Surg, United Kingdom Base, Annual Rpt, 1944, p. 16; Hospitalization Division, OofCSurg, HQ, ETOUSA, Annual Rpt, 1944, p. 21; 12th Evacuation Hospital Annual Rpt, 1944, pp. 6–8. For bed clearing, see EvacCorresp, 1942–44, file HD 024 ETO; file HD 024 ETO CS (Hawley Chron) for April–June 1944; and Hawley Interv, 1962, p. 58, CMH.

or, General Kenner, expressed guarded confidence in the sufficiency of their preparations. Kenner declared: "The British and U.S. medical services are organized and prepared to adequately support Operation OVERLORD." Confirmation of the truth of Hawley's and Kenner's estimates no longer rested in their hands. It depended on the performance of thousands of aidmen, doctors, technicians, and nurses on the ships and in the aircraft heading for Normandy.[65]

[65] First and second quotations from Ltr, Hawley to TSG, 3 Jun 44, file HD 024 ETO O/CS (Hawley-SGO Corresp). Third quotation from Memo, Kenner to CofS, via ACofS, G-4, and CAdminOff, 20 May 44, sub: Report of Inspection of Medical Facilities, SBS, 9-13 May 44, in Medical Division, COSSAC/SHAEF, War Diary, May 1944.

CHAPTER VII

Introduction to Battle

On 6 June 1944 U.S. and British forces went ashore along a 40-mile stretch of the Normandy coast. Following the NEPTUNE plan, 13,000 parachute and glider troops of the 82d and 101st Airborne Divisions, who landed just after midnight in the Cotentin countryside behind UTAH beach, opened the American part of the attack. Widely scattered and badly disorganized in the drop due to navigation errors, high winds, and enemy antiaircraft fire, each division managed to assemble enough men and equipment to accomplish at least part of its D-Day mission. In confused vicious fighting against initially uncoordinated but increasingly stubborn and aggressive German opponents, the airborne troops by the end of D-Day had opened the way inland for the seaborne forces across the flooded areas behind UTAH beach, and they were well on the way to securing the lodgement's western and southern flanks.

The amphibious assault task forces, Force U for UTAH and Force O for OMAHA, dropped anchor in their assembly areas 12 miles off the coast at about 0230. H-hour for the first landings was 0630, when low tide would uncover for demolition the German obstacles that studded both UTAH and OMAHA between high and low water lines. As the troops transferred from transports to landing craft, a gusty northwest wind kicked up a choppy sea, tossing about the smaller craft and quickly overcoming antiseasickness efforts. At about 0530 the Germans, hitherto passive, opened artillery fire; fifteen minutes later the final Allied naval bombardment began, as the assault waves headed for the beaches. About on schedule, the first bow ramps went down.

At UTAH Maj. Gen. J. Lawton Collins' VII Corps, the 4th Infantry Division leading, went ashore almost unopposed. Quickly overcoming beach defenders, who were few in numbers and were distracted by the airborne attack behind them, the infantry pushed inland over causeways crossing the inundated areas. Elements of the 1st Engineer Special Brigade, supporting this assault, cleared away mines and obstacles; opened vehicle routes across the beach; readied the causeways for heavy traffic; and set up supply dumps, harassed only by a few snipers and by sporadic German shelling. By the end of the day 23,000 of the 32,000 troops of the initial UTAH assault force were ashore. The

4th Division had established contact with the 101st but, as yet, not with the 82d.

At OMAHA the V Corps, under Maj. Gen. Leonard T. Gerow, had the day's hardest, costliest fight. The corps landed with two regiments abreast, both under operational control of the 1st Infantry Division: the 116th Infantry of the 29th Infantry Division on the right, and the 1st Division's own 16th Infantry on the left. Two engineer units supported the infantry, the 6th Engineer Special Brigade going in with the 116th and the 5th Engineer Special Brigade with the 16th. The first assault waves ran into a strong, well-entrenched German infantry division not previously spotted by Allied reconnaissance, its defense little affected by preliminary air strikes and naval bombardments. Losses among troops and landing craft were heavy, and the attackers were pinned down along the high water mark for much of the day. Gradually, aided by naval gunfire and reinforced by later landing waves, they overcame the defenders and worked their way inland. By nightfall about 34,000 troops of the 55,000-man assault force were ashore. The corps, however, had fallen far short of its D-Day objective. Its advance position constituted more a series of islands than a continuous line. German snipers and strongpoints remained unsubdued at many points on the beach, most of which still was under enemy artillery fire.

The ordeal on OMAHA notwithstanding, the Allies on D-Day had broken the Nazi coastal defenses. During the next few days troops and supplies flowed in over increasingly secure and well-organized beaches. Inland from OMAHA the 1st and 29th Divisions, reinforced by the 2d Infantry Division, expanded their lodgement to the south, southwest, and west, against weakening resistance. The 4th Division at UTAH made firm contact with the airborne divisions and attacked northward. At the same time the 82d pushed westward in the Cotentin, while the 101st drove south to link up the two beachheads, an objective it achieved on 11 June (D+5).[1]

The human cost of securing the lodgement was substantial, but much less than expected. On D-Day the hard-hit V Corps suffered about 2,400 dead, wounded, and missing; the 4th Division, by contrast, reported only 200 casualties; and the two airborne divisions together lost about 2,400 men. Of these 5,000 casualties, perhaps 3,000 were wounded—a total well under the anticipated 12 percent of the assault force. This number was within the treatment and evacuation capabilities of the medical forces ashore on D-Day, even though those forces endured their share of the losses and vicissitudes of battle.[2]

---

[1] This summary of the tactical situation is based on Harrison, *Cross-Channel*, chs. VIII and IX; Ruppenthal, *Logistical Support*, 1:10; First U.S. Army Report of Operations, 20 Oct 43–1 Aug 44, bk. I, pp. 40–46; Rpt, Provisional Engineer Special Brigade Group (hereafter cited as ProvESBGp), 30 Sep 44, sub: Operation NEPTUNE, 26 Feb–26 Jun 44, pp. 75–103.

[2] D-Day casualties are summarized in Charles B. MacDonald, *The Mighty Endeavor: American Armed Forces in the European Theater in World War II* (New York: Oxford University Press, 1969), p. 279. V Corps casualties are broken down into dead, wounded, and missing in Rpt, V Corps, sub: Operations in the ETO, 6 January 1942 to 9 May 1945, p. 64. For airborne losses, see Harrison, *Cross-Channel*, pp. 28 n and 300.

The Assault

The burden of treating and evacuating First Army casualties on D-Day and during the days immediately thereafter fell largely on the medical elements of the airborne and infantry divisions and the engineer special brigades, and on the teams of the 3d Auxiliary Surgical Group. These forces worked under control of the assault corps surgeons: Col. Charles E. Brenn, MC, of V Corps on OMAHA and Col. Paul Hayes, MC, of VII Corps on UTAH.[3] Hayes' area of responsibility included the airborne divisions, as well as the seaborne forces. Until the beachheads joined, these officers performed most of the tasks of an army surgeon, rather than the more limited duties usually done at corps level.

Regimental and battalion surgeons and aidmen of the two airborne divisions were the first Army Medical Department soldiers to set foot in Normandy. In each division they dropped by parachute or rode in on gliders with their organizations—nine officers and sixty enlisted men with each parachute regiment and seven officers and sixty-four men with each regiment of glider infantry. Anticipating heavy drop losses and days of isolation behind enemy lines, unit medics landed with all the extra supplies and equipment they could collect—either carried on their persons, parachuted down in special containers, or packed in glider-borne vehicles. The 101st Division, for example, went into Normandy with 250 litters and 2,500 blankets above its regular allowance, 25 instead of the regulation 7 aerial delivery containers per regiment, and 2,000 units of plasma. The 101st's field artillery battalion brought along 2 complete sets of aid station equipment. Each paratrooper carried 2 British-made individual dressings and a copper sulphate sponge for use on phosphorus burns.[4]

Much of this equipment—and many of the people carrying it—were lost, as paratroopers and gliders plunged into the hedgerow-lined fields and marshy river bottoms of the Cotentin and as men in the early morning darkness began the tense, deadly hide-and-seek game of finding comrades, assembling units, and getting on with their missions. Airborne medical personnel were as badly scattered in the drops as everyone else. In the 82d Division 50 percent of the medical officers were unaccounted for during the first seventy-two hours of combat; in one of the 101st's battalions, which landed in swamps, only two members of a sixteen-man medical detachment initially rallied with the unit. For some medics the war ended quickly as they ran into Germans and were captured or—rarely, if clearly identified—shot. The 101st during June lost 20 percent of its medical personnel, most of them in the first days. Equipment losses were equally heavy. The 101st recovered only 30 percent of its air-dropped supply containers, and its surgeon later concluded that it was a mistake to drop so much materiel in the early

[3] Col. Hayes was replaced as VII Corps surgeon on 4 July 1944 by Lt. Col. Robert H. Barr.

[4] Surg, 82d Airborne Division, Annual Rpt, 1944, an. I, p. 1; Surg, 101st Airborne Division, Annual Rpt, 1944, pp. 1–2; Interv, OSG with Capt Ernest Gruenberg (hereafter cited as Gruenberg Interv), 13 Jun 45, box 222, RG 112, NARA.

hours, when the surgeons did not yet need it and darkness made it almost impossible to find.

During the first hours on the ground, medical officers and aidmen collected what supplies they could locate. They made contact with other paratroopers, gave first aid to men injured in the jump or in glider crashes and in the first firefights, and worked their way toward battalion assembly areas. Especially in the 82d Division, elements of which landed farthest inland, small groups of paratroopers were cut off from their units for days. Injured and wounded soldiers with these groups received at best improvised care, even if their chance-met companions included medical officers and aidmen. Some groups, forced to maneuver to avoid Germans or driven from their positions by counterattacks, had to leave their wounded behind to be captured, frequently along with medical personnel who voluntarily stayed with their patients. At isolated positions, wounded men died for lack of plasma. Other cut-off groups were more fortunate. Medical officers with them managed to salvage equipment for adequate first aid and in at least one case secured milk and food for the wounded from French farmers.

Medical officers and men who reached their battalion assembly areas set up rough-and-ready aid stations, usually near their unit command posts. At these stations improvisation was the common practice, as surgeons scavenged for supplies and commandeered farm wagons and captured enemy vehicles to collect wounded from widespread company positions. In the 1st Battalion, 502d Parachute Infantry, a 101st Division unit, the battalion commander, Lt. Col. Patrick J. Cassidy, and his surgeon, Capt. Frank Choy, MC, secured a small cart and a horse to pull it and drafted a dental technician to drive it. "All day long," according to a battalion report, "this boy drove up and down the roads, exposing himself to sniper fire, working like a Trojan, to bring in the wounded and the parachutists who had been hurt on the jump; his energy saved countless lives." During much of the day Colonel Cassidy, who had to send his surgeon to treat an untransportable casualty at an outlying position, acted as his own medical officer. Cassidy, and the medical sergeant who remained with him, decided which badly wounded men should receive their limited supply of plasma, and the battalion commander personally helped retrieve medical supply bundles from the surrounding fields. Because his drop zone was just inland from UTAH, Cassidy was able to evacuate many of his casualties to the beach late in the afternoon, after making contact with the 4th Division.[5]

Although a few units, such as Cassidy's, sent casualties directly to the beach, most airborne wounded went from battalion aid stations, and often from where they fell, to the clearing stations set up by their division medical companies. These companies, each of which included an attached team from the 3d Auxiliary Surgical Group, deployed in Normandy on D-

[5]This account of unit medical support is based on Surg, 82d Airborne Division, Annual Rpt, 1944, an. I, pp. 1–2; Surg, 101st Airborne Division, Annual Rpt, 1944, pp. 2–6; Gruenberg Interv, 13 Jun 45, box 222, RG 112, NARA, and in RG 407, NARA, 82d Airborne Division Combat Intervs, box 24057, and 101st Airborne Division Combat Intervs (source of quotation), box 24072.

Day in several echelons. An advance element of each company, with the division surgeon and the auxiliary surgical team, went in by glider around dawn with enough hand-carried and air-dropped instruments and equipment for a small emergency surgical station. The rest of the personnel, with the company vehicles and the balance of the clearing station outfit, arrived during the late afternoon by glider and, in the case of the 101st Division, partly by sea.

An advance element of the 101st's 326th Airborne Medical Company parachuted in with the infantry at 0100. As many of the four officers and forty-five men of this detachment as could reach their rendezvous improvised a small hospital in a French farmhouse near Hiesville, the division command post site about 5 miles from UTAH beach. The group performed first aid and emergency surgery here until well into D+1 (7 June), when it joined the rest of the company. About two hours behind this advance group two gliders arrived carrying the 326th Company commander, Maj. William E. Barfield, MC, and seven officers and twenty-one men, including the auxiliary surgical team, with four jeeps and trailers. Although both gliders crash-landed, painfully injuring every member of the surgical team, the men retrieved most of their gear and maneuvered around German positions toward the Chateau Colombierre, just north of Hiesville, selected on the basis of preinvasion aerial reconnaissance as the site for the division clearing station. They arrived at about 0700, just as paratroopers were driving German defenders out of the buildings.

By early afternoon the members of the original party, reinforced by other medical officers and men who straggled in, had a rudimentary surgical hospital and clearing station in operation. Surgeons worked at three tables, as the chateau courtyard filled with casualties brought in on improvised litters, horses, and captured trucks. Living on D-bars and Benzedrine, the surgeons treated about 300 patients during the day. In the evening another glider lift of the company and the seaborne element, which had landed on UTAH, reached the chateau. But even with this reinforcement, which included Lt. Col. David Gold, MC, the 101st Division surgeon, the number of wounded arriving all but overwhelmed the staff. The surgical team leader, Maj. Albert J. Crandall, MC, recalled: "We had to maintain a careful priority system, operating on those who were most in need of surgery and giving the others emergency treatment." In surgery, "first we did the heads and chest and next the abdomens and extremities." [6]

An advance group of the 82d Division's 307th Airborne Medical Company, with the division surgeon, Col. Wolcott L. Etienne, MC, and a surgical team, also went in by glider before dawn. Shrapnel from German antiaircraft fire wounded Colonel Etienne before he even touched ground; the same fire caused the gliders to overshoot their planned landing zone at Blosville near Ste.-Mere-Eglise, a

[6] Surg, 101st Airborne Division, Annual Rpt, 1944, pp. 2–3; 3d Auxiliary Surgical Group Annual Rpt, 1944, pp. 17–19; Capt W. P. McKee Recorded Rpt, pp. 2–4. Quotation from Interv, OSG with Maj A. J. Crandall (hereafter cited as Crandall Interv), 8 Jun 45, box 222, RG 112, NARA.

major division objective, and crash land at Hiesville. Medics were scattered in the landing and lost much equipment. Some of them, including the surgical team leader, Maj. James J. Whitsitt, MC, found their way to Chateau Colombierre, where they assisted 326th Company doctors for the rest of the day. The bulk of the 307th Company arrived in gliders near Ste.-Mere-Eglise in the late afternoon and also ran into hard luck. Many gliders plunged into flooded areas, and the landing zone came under shelling that killed the company commander. In spite of these setbacks, the company pulled itself together and had its clearing station in operation at Blosville by morning of the seventh.[7]

During the first few days after D-Day the airborne division medical service lost its improvised, irregular character and gradually came to resemble that of a conventional infantry division. Both the 82d and the 101st Divisions remained fully committed to hard offensive combat, and the flow of wounded through their aid stations and clearing companies was steady and substantial. On 8 June alone the 326th Company treated and evacuated over 400 casualties. On the ninth the 326th was bombed out of its chateau, fortunately just after evacuating most of its patients. The company, however, lost 5 officers and 9 enlisted men wounded and 8 enlisted men killed, as well as much of its equipment. Obtaining new equipment and personnel replacements from VII Corps, the company resumed work the next day at a new site near Hiesville. On D-Day the 326th Company evacuated a few wounded to the 261st Medical Battalion of the 1st Engineer Special Brigade at UTAH beach and then kept up a steady seaward flow of patients, mostly carried in Quartermaster Corps trucks *(Map 7)*. Ambulances of the VII Corps medical battalion began evacuating the company on the ninth. The 82d Division's clearing station had accumulated 300 patients before starting evacuation to the beach on the seventh, using borrowed trucks and ambulances, many of them from the 4th Division's 4th Medical Battalion. The clearing company of the latter unit received, treated, and evacuated many airborne soldiers during its first days on shore; at times half the wounded passing through the infantry division clearing station were parachute and glider troops.[8]

On UTAH beach, the landing of medical units and the establishment of the initial chain of evacuation went about as smoothly as an operation could go under combat conditions. Company aidmen and battalion medical sections of the 4th Division landed first, followed closely by the nine officers and seventy-two hospital corpsmen of the 2d Naval Beach Battalion. Collecting companies of the 4th Medical Battalion came in with the regiments they supported, bringing most

[7]VII Corps Medical Plan, pp. 14–15, encl. 1 to Surg, VII Corps, Annual Rpt, 1944; Surg, 82d Airborne Division, Annual Rpt, 1944, pp. 3–4 and an. I, p. 1; 3d Auxiliary Surgical Group Annual Rpt, 1944, pp. 16–17; 307th Airborne Medical Company Annual Rpt, 1944.

[8]First U.S. Army Report of Operations, 20 Oct 43–1 Aug 44, bk. VII, pp. 65–66; VII Corps Medical Plan, p. 15, encl. 1 to Surg, VII Corps, Annual Rpt, 1944; Surg, 82d Airborne Division, Annual Rpt, 1944, an. I; Surg, 101st Airborne Division, Annual Rpt, 1944, p. 2; Medical Service, 101st Airborne Division, After-Action Rpt, 6–25 Jun 44; Crandall Interv, 8 Jun 45, box 222, RG 112, NARA.

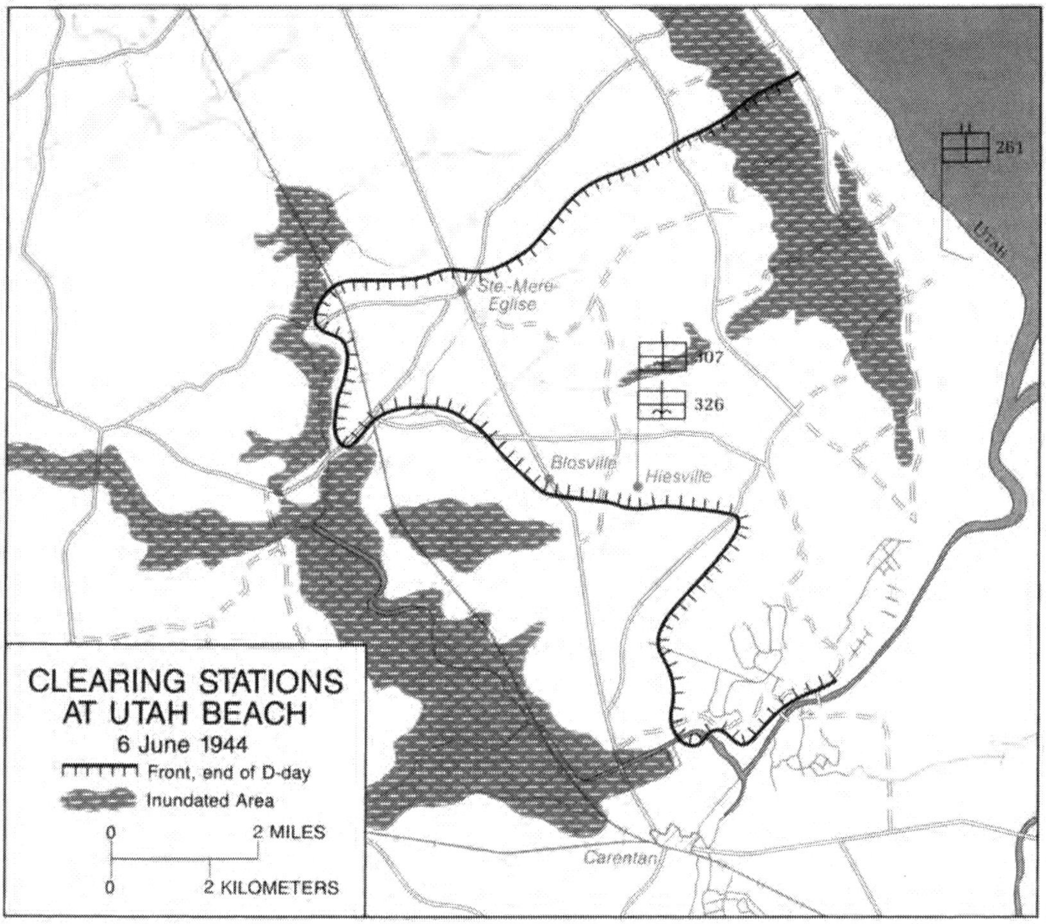

MAP 7

of their thirty ambulances. In spite of day-long sporadic artillery fire, which killed a medical officer and several enlisted men on the beach, wounded the regimental surgeon of the 12th Infantry, and peppered the 4th Medical Battalion's ambulances with shrapnel, the division medical elements rapidly moved inland. The Navy corpsmen organized two beach aid stations, collected the few casualties of the assault, and loaded on DUKWs and landing craft for movement to LSTs offshore. At about 1000 the first engineer special brigade unit, Company C, 261st Medical Battalion, arrived on the beach, followed two hours later by Company A. These two "collecto-clearing" companies, formed by combining the litter and ambulance elements of a collecting company with a platoon from the battalion's clearing company, set up stations at a crossroads just behind the flooded area. Their attached surgical teams began performing operations at around 1800, carrying out their mission of providing emergency surgery for nontransportable patients. These clearing stations evacuated few wounded to the beach during the first hours, as casualties from the airborne divisions and the 4th Medical Battalion did not start flowing back in significant numbers until the following day. Between 2100 and 2130 the VII Corps surgeon, Colonel Hayes, and the 4th Division surgeon, Lt. Col. Robert H. Barr, MC, landed with members of their staff sections.

During the next three days VII Corps medical support expanded, as did the corps and its beachead. The 4th Division's clearing company, scheduled to land late on D-Day but held back in favor of additional combat units, came ashore on 7 June and went into operation at Hebert, a crossroads village just beyond the inundated area. Later the company followed the 4th northward. By the ninth two more infantry divisions—the 9th and 90th—had disembarked, each with its full medical complement. Clearing stations of these divisions opened in the general vicinity of Ste.-Mere-Eglise. The rest of the 261st Medical Battalion, meanwhile, landed on the seventh. The battalion established a medical supply depot. Its surgical teams worked around the clock to handle an increasing flow of casualties, as the divisions attacking northward and westward from UTAH met strong German opposition. Between 8 and 12 June the VII Corps' 50th Medical Battalion disembarked. The battalion's clearing company, besides supporting corps troops, its normal role, took part of the burden of general medical and surgical care from the 261st's companies, and its collecting and ambulance companies evacuated division clearing stations to the 261st and helped move patients from that unit to the Navy beach stations. On the ninth the *Lady Connaught*, first of what was to be a regular series of hospital carriers, anchored off UTAH. She discharged supplies and six additional surgical teams for the 261st Medical Battalion, allowing relief to the battalion's original teams that had worked for 36 hours with little rest. The carrier took on board 400 wounded for the return voyage to England. As the first army field and evacuation hospitals opened on 10 and 11 June, the VII Corps medical service was well into the transition from an amphibious to a conventional land organization and system of support.[9]

On OMAHA the story was different. This beach, about 5 miles from end to end, consisted of a tidal flat bordered at the high water mark by an embankment of loose stones, called shingle, backed on the eastern portion by sand dunes and on the western by a wooden seawall 4–5 feet high. At varying distances from the shingle, usually 200–300 yards, rose low bluffs, too steep to be negotiated by vehicles except through five draws that the Germans had mined and blocked with obstacles. The defenders, entrenched on and in front of the bluffs in pillboxes and machine-gun nests, met the first assault waves with

[9] First U.S. Army Report of Operations, 20 Oct 43–1 Aug 44, bk. VII, pp. 65–67 and 96; Surg, First U.S. Army, Annual Rpt, 1944, p. 33; VII Corps Medical Plan, pp. 13–17, encl. 1 to Surg, VII Corps, Annual Rpt, 1944; Dowling, Normandy Rpt, 11 Jan 45, pp. 17–18; 3d Auxiliary Surgical Group Annual Rpt, 1944, pp. 13 and 20; 4th Medical Battalion Report of Operations, 6–30 Jun 44, box 6727, RG 407, NARA; 50th Medical Battalion Annual Rpt, 1944, pp. 2–3.

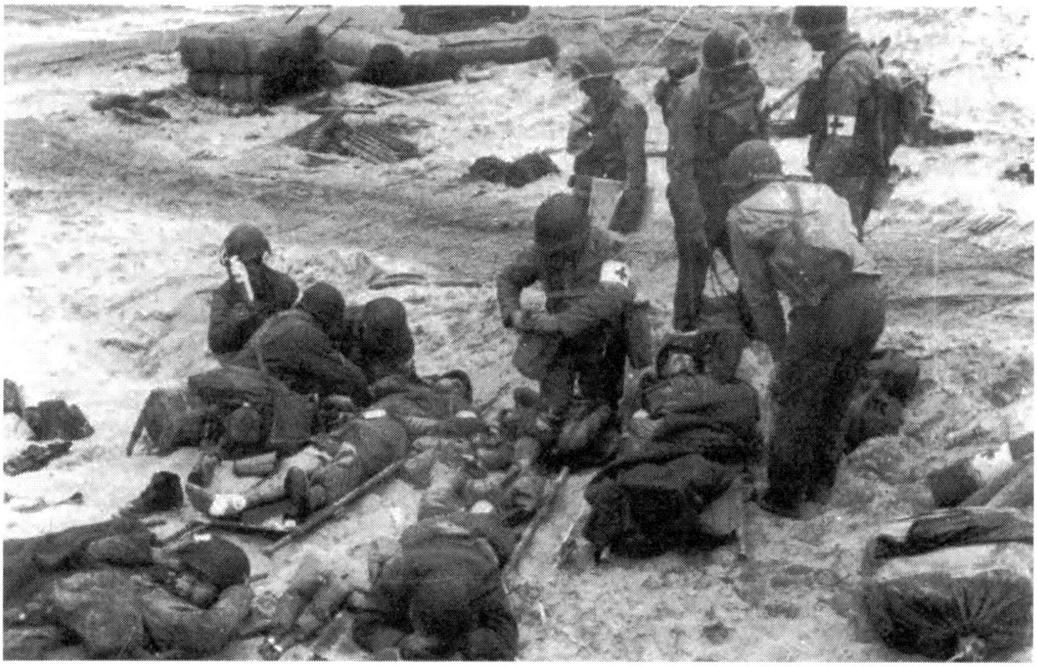

MEDICS ADMINISTERING FIRST AID TO INVASION CASUALTIES ON UTAH *(top)* AND OMAHA *(bottom)*

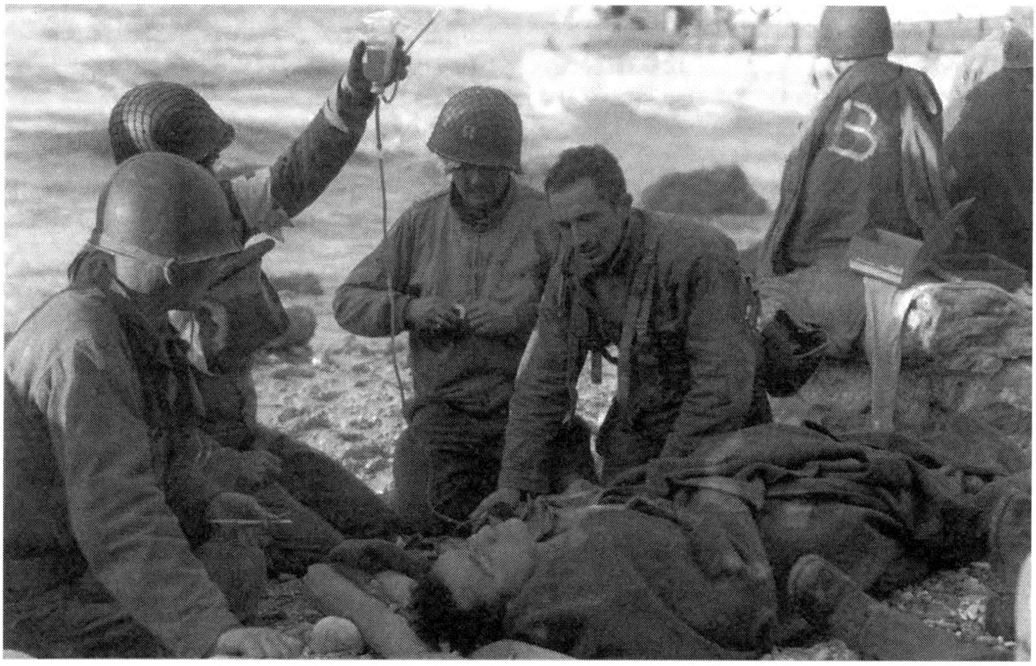

heavy fire. As the landing craft nosed into shore, German machine-gun nests cut down many Americans before they even left the bow ramps and others as they struggled across the tidal flat. Artillery shells sank, set on fire, or blew up one landing craft after another. Wading and crawling across the sand, pushed by the now rising tide, dragging their wounded, and losing or abandoning weapons, radios, and equipment, the assault troops sought cover from the searching fire behind the seawall and shingle pile. The American units took their heaviest losses of the day in this movement up to the high water line; one 16th Infantry company suffered most of its 105 D-Day casualties here. Exhausted from seasickness and the struggle ashore, the survivors tried to clear sand-clogged weapons, to rescue and tend wounded, to demolish beach obstacles, and to cut the barbed wire the Germans had laid along the shingle pile.

Troops and vehicles of the first and subsequent landing waves remained bunched along the high water line for much of the day. Around 0800 small intrepid groups began pushing across the beach to the foot of the bluffs and then working their way up the hills. One by one, they eliminated German strongpoints, aided after about 1030 by point-blank naval gunfire. Landing of reinforcements, temporarily halted when high tide covered the beach obstacles, resumed when landing craft commanders discovered that they could ram through safely. During the afternoon the trickle of men across the beach and over the bluff became a flood. The arrival of two additional infantry regiments gave still more momentum to the inland drive. As darkness fell, the infantry had partially secured the objective towns of Vierville on the western end of the beach, St.-Laurent in the center, and Colleville on the east. The engineers, using what equipment they could salvage, cleared mines, bulldozed openings for vehicles through the shingle opposite several of the beach exit draws, and began developing roads through the draws themselves.[10]

The near-catastrophe of D-Day morning and the resulting delay of the advance inland telescoped the elaborately sequenced arrival of medical units. Organizations landed off schedule and on the wrong beach sectors, often losing much of their equipment. Regardless of type or intended function, each unit and detachment, as it plunged into the welter between the low tide line and the bluffs, dissolved into scattered groups of men, working desperately under fire to drag wounded to places of relative safety, to give first aid, and to salvage supplies.

The battalion and regimental medical sections and attached divisional collecting companies of the 16th and 116th Regimental Combat Teams, closely followed by the officers and hospital corpsmen of the 6th and 7th Naval Beach Battalions, came ashore early in the morning, just after the first assault companies had been shot to pieces. The medical soldiers took their share of casualties. The 2d Battalion, 116th Infantry, lost five aidmen, killed leaving their landing craft, and its surgeon, wounded on

[10] This account is based on 1st Infantry Division Combat Intervs, box 24011, and 29th Infantry Division Combat Intervs, box 24034, RG 407, NARA.

the beach by shrapnel. Other medics quickly fell as they tried to drag casualties out of the rising water. As German artillery blasted the landing craft, medical supplies went up in flames or disappeared under the waves; the 116th Infantry lost its entire regimental supply of plasma in two LCIs (landing craft, infantry) sunk off the beach.[11]

Maj. Charles E. Tegtmeyer, MC, regimental surgeon of the 16th Infantry, who landed at about 0815, described what faced those medical troops who survived the wade and crawl through the obstacles to the shingle pile:

> The shelf on which I rested was about ten yards in width sloping upward from the water's edge to a height of from two to ten feet at an angle of roughly 35 degrees. Face downward, as far as eyes could see in either direction were the huddled bodies of men living, wounded and dead, as tightly packed together as a layer of cigars in a box. Some were frantically but ineffectually attempting to dig into the shale shelf, a few were raising themselves above the parapet-like edge and firing toward the concrete protected enemy and those on the cliff above but the majority merely huddled together face downward. Artillery . . . and mortar shells exploded on the beach and in the water . . . and threw fragments in all directions. Uncomfortably close, overhead, machine gun and rifle bullets grazed the top of the ledge . . . and plunged into the water behind us with innumerable sharp hisses or whined away in to the distance as they richocheted off the stones of the beach. At the water's edge floating face downward with arched backs were innumerable human forms eddying to and fro with each incoming wave, the water above them a muddy pink in color. Floating equipment of all types like flotsam and jetsam rolled in the surf mingled with the bodies. . . . Everywhere, the frantic cry, 'Medics, hey, Medics,' could be heard above the horrible din.[12]

Among the company aidmen on OMAHA, heroism was the only standard procedure. Under the punishing fire, often themselves wounded, these soldiers worked up and down the shingle pile, bandaging, splinting, giving morphine and plasma if they had any. Many ventured repeatedly back into the water to pull in the disabled and drowning or to retrieve medical supplies. Others went into minefields to carry out injured men. A 29th Division staff officer with 116th Infantry recalled: "First-aid men of all units were the most active members of the group that huddled against the seawall. With the limited . . . facilities available to them, they did not hesitate to treat the most severe casualties. Gaping head and belly wounds were bandaged with the same rapid efficiency that was dealt to the more minor wounds." As the infantry filtered in to the base of the bluff, the medics took additional risks to drag wounded to the shelter of the hill. Paradoxically, most evacuation on OMAHA in these first hours was forward, toward the enemy.[13]

---

[11] For overviews of D-Day medical operations on OMAHA, see First U.S. Army Report of Operations, 20 Oct 43–1 Aug 44, bk. VII, pp. 62–63; Surg, V Corps, Annual Rpt, 1944, pp. 2–3; Surg, 1st Infantry Division, Annual Rpt, 1944, p. 9. For medical losses in the initial assault, see 1st Infantry Division Combat Intervs, box 24011, and 29th Infantry Division Combat Intervs, box 24034, RG 407, NARA.

[12] Col Charles E. Tegtmeyer, MC, "Personal Military Diary" (hereafter cited as Tegtmeyer "Diary"), pt. 1, ch. 20, pp. 1–5.

[13] Quotation from Lt. Jack Shea, D-Day Narrative, in 29th Infantry Division Combat Intervs, box 24034. See also other company narratives in this collection and in the 1st Infantry Division Combat Intervs, box 24011. All in RG 407, NARA.

The work of Major Tegtmeyer and his 16th Infantry medical section typified the character of regimental medical support on OMAHA.[14] Landing with the regimental commander, Col. George A. Taylor, and his staff on Easy Red sector, the left center of the beach, Tegtmeyer and his aidmen followed the command group back and forth along the shingle pile as Taylor tried to organize an advance toward the bluffs. The medical soldiers, now wading, now stumbling over prone men, bandaged and splinted wounded as they came upon them, then left them in the shelter of the embankment with instructions to call for help and evacuation to incoming landing craft. "I examined scores as I went," Tegtmeyer declared, "telling the men who to dress and who not to bother with."

At around 1040 the medical section followed the rifle companies off the beach and set up an aid station near the regimental command post, dug into the seaward slope of the bluff, which sheltered them from direct enemy fire. The group used what supplies they had carried ashore, plus two litters and some other materiel they picked up on the beach. Troops from the first waves were still thick on the shore below Tegtmeyer's position, and landing craft kept bringing in more under shelling that steadily added to the number of dead and wounded littering the sand. Tegtmeyer sent aidmen down to the beach and along the bluff to collect casualties and by nightfall had over eighty wounded at his station. Running low on blankets and plasma, he secured more from a passing battalion of the newly landed 26th Infantry, the commander of which he knew. Even with these supplies, men came in that emergency care could not save, such as the infantryman with one leg traumatically amputated and multiple compound fractures of the other. "He was conscious and cheerful," Tegtmeyer reports, "but his only hope was rapid evacuation, and at this time evacuation did not exist. An hour later he was dead."

Around 2200 an auxiliary surgical team, which had become separated from its engineer special brigade, reached Tegtmeyer's position, but the surgeons lacked equipment and did little but dig foxholes for shelter against the continuing artillery bombardment. More useful were the twelve litterbearers of Company A, 1st Medical Battalion, the 16th Infantry's attached collecting company, who appeared with their commander, Captain Ralston, shortly after the surgical team. This company was scheduled to land with the regiment in the morning, but enemy guns had set their landing craft on fire during two unsuccessful attempts to beach. Ralston and his men had worked heroically, rescuing soldiers and sailors from burning holds and compartments and treating the injured who encumbered the decks. After the craft limped seaward to a transport and unloaded its casualties, Ralston rallied his tired, shocked company; got them onto another craft; and disembarked them on OMAHA at about 1700. Then

[14] This account is based on Tegtmeyer "Diary," pt. 1, ch. 20, pp. 5–15, from which the quotations come; Rpt, Maj Charles E. Tegtmeyer, sub: Activities of Medical Detachment, 16th Infantry, and Company A, 1st Medical Battalion, After-Action Rpt, both in 1st Infantry Division Combat Intervs, box 24011, RG 407, NARA.

he and part of his command found their way to Tegtmeyer.

With the help of Ralston's litterbearers Tegtmeyer began moving his patients down to the beach, the ambulatory cases walking and the rest laboriously carried on litters. All but about ten of the most severely injured arrived at the beach station the Navy now had in operation before renewed shelling halted the evacuation. Because no more landing craft were coming in, the wounded on the beach stayed there all night, tended by Navy corpsmen. Tegtmeyer's group and the remaining patients spent a cold, damp night in foxholes, during which time four more of the injured died.

During the early afternoon the engineer special brigade medical battalions began landing. Both special brigades—the 6th, responsible for organizing the western half of OMAHA behind the 116th Infantry; and the 5th, in charge of the eastern half behind the 16th Infantry—were formed into battalion beach groups for the assault, with a group attached to each regimental combat team. Each beach group included one or more companies from the brigade medical battalion. The 6th Brigade's 60th Medical Battalion was organized conventionally in one clearing and three collecting companies; its 500th Collecting Company and a platoon of the 634th Clearing Company came ashore with the battalion beach group supporting the 116th Infantry. The 5th Brigade's 61st Medical Battalion, like its UTAH beach counterpart, had formed three provisional collecto-clearing companies. Of these, the 391st Collecto-Clearing Company landed first, behind the 16th Infantry. Each clearing and collecto-clearing company had attached teams of the 3d Auxiliary Surgical Group. Besides the clearing station and operating room equipment packed into their trucks, each company went in heavily laden with hand-carried supplies. Men of the 61st's 393d Collecto-Clearing Company, for example, landed with mortar shell casing containers and waterproofed dufflebags filled with dressings, bandages, tourniquets, sulfa powder, and plasma. Every litterbearer took along an extra litter with a life belt attached, to float the litter ashore if he lost hold of it.[15]

During D-Day these medical battalions were only partially able to perform their evacuation tasks, and they could not undertake emergency surgery at all. For the most part, their officers and men simply joined in the general effort at casualty collection, first aid, and supply salvage. Such was the fate of the small advance party of the 60th Medical Battalion, which landed at 0855 on Easy Green sector below St.-Laurent, to reconnoiter a previously selected clearing station site. German troops still controlled the site, and the officer and enlisted men of the advance party worked all day with regimental and Navy medics along the beach. Between 1400 and 1500 the bulk of the 500th Collecting Company and part of the 634th Clearing Company came ashore on

[15] For the assault, the 5th Brigade had operational control of all 6th Brigade elements, even as the 1st Division controlled the first 29th Division elements on shore. When the brigade group headquarters landed, which occurred late on D-Day, 6th Brigade units reverted to control of their parent brigade. See Rpt, ProvESBGp, 30 Sep 44, sub: Operation NEPTUNE, pp. 36–38 and 327–28; 61st Medical Battalion Annual Rpt, 1944, pp. 1–6; 393d Collecto-Clearing Company Annual Rpt, 1944, p. 8.

Easy Green. The units lost men and equipment on the way in. Casualties included Lt. Col. Bernard E. Bullock, MC, the battalion commander, who landed with the 500th Company, only to be mortally wounded within minutes. Men of these two companies spread out along most of the western half of OMAHA, setting up casualty collecting points and helping Navy beach detachments load evacuation craft. Late in the day the 634th Company platoon, which had managed to land a truckload of ward and operating room equipment, moved off the beach through exit D–3 and set up an aid station part way up the draw toward St.-Laurent.[16]

Due to a breakdown of the landing sequence, the first men of the 61st Medical Battalion to wade ashore on Easy Red sector at about 1345 were members of the headquarters detachment. They landed with typewriters, files, and office supplies on a beach still strewn with dead and wounded. Putting this materiel aside (they later managed to save the battalion records), the headquarters men scavenged for medical equipment and went to work on the casualties around them. Around 1400 the 391st Collecto-Clearing Company, which should have landed before the headquarters element, came in on Easy Red and set up a dressing station in a captured pillbox; this unit also had to rely on hand-carried and scavenged equipment, as its heavy gear remained on board ship. A couple of hours later the 393d Collecto-Clearing Company disembarked with the 18th Infantry, far to the right of the 391st and almost in the 6th Brigade sector. This company set up a collecting station in an antitank ditch under the bluff northeast of St.-Laurent. These companies, and the 61st Battalion headquarters, suffered five enlisted men killed and five officers and twenty men wounded on D-Day.[17]

Forward emergency surgery never got started on OMAHA during the first twenty-four hours. Of twelve teams attached to the 60th and 61st Medical Battalions, eight succeeded in reaching shore between 1130 and 1730, after various harrowing adventures on board misdirected, damaged, and sunk landing craft. Invariably, they arrived on the beach without operating equipment. Even if they reached their assigned collecto-clearing and clearing companies, they could do little but pitch in with everyone else in basic first aid, evacuation, and salvage. The Provisional Engineer Special Brigade Group commander commented that, although the auxiliary surgeons "did heroic work on D-Day and D+1, their skill probably was not put to its greatest use."[18]

Throughout the day the naval beach medical sections, aided during the afternoon by the engineer special brigade companies, tried to keep wounded moving off the beach onto landing craft. Enemy fire, the inability of craft to approach some sectors of the beach, and the reluctance of some

[16] Rpt, ProvESBGp, 30 Sep 44, sub: Operation NEPTUNE, pp. 328–29; 60th Medical Battalion Annual Rpt, 1944, pp. 5–6, 8–9, 15.

[17] Rpt, ProvESBGp, 30 Sep 44, sub: Operation NEPTUNE, pp. 329–31; 61st Medical Battalion Annual Rpt, 1944, pp. 4–5, 10–11, app. 3.

[18] Rpt, ProvESBGp, 30 Sep 44, sub: Operation NEPTUNE, p. 334; 3d Auxiliary Surgical Group Annual Rpt, 1944, pp. 13–14 and 22–29; Tegtmeyer "Diary," pt. 1, ch. 20, p. 11.

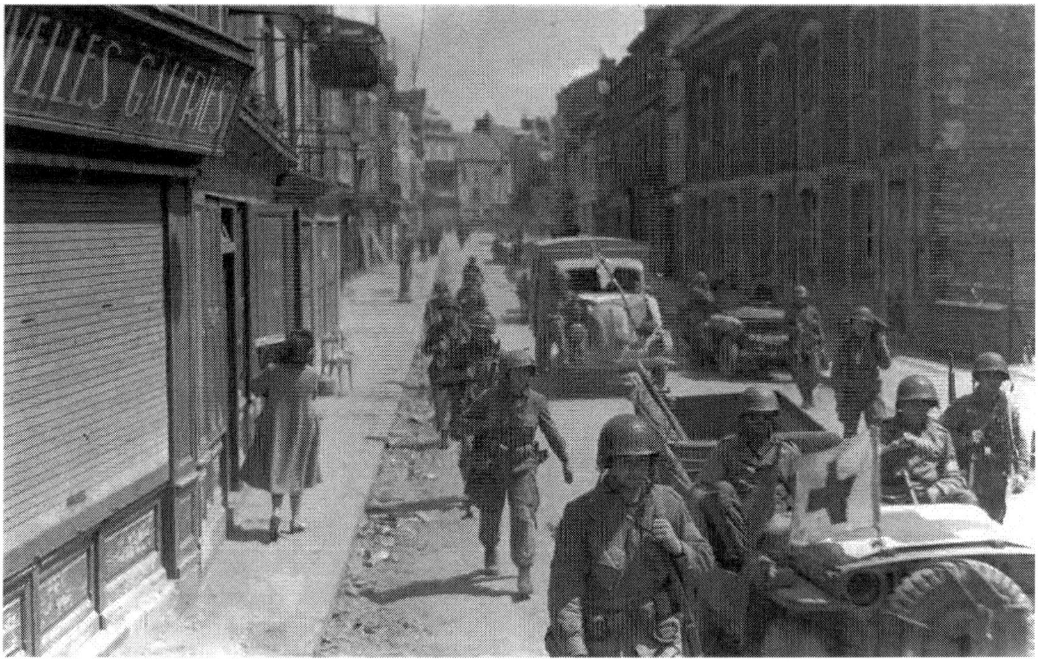

MEN AND EQUIPMENT IN SUPPORT OF THE NORMANDY BUILDUP. *Troops, with medical evacuation vehicles, enter Carentan, and ambulances disembark across a beach.*

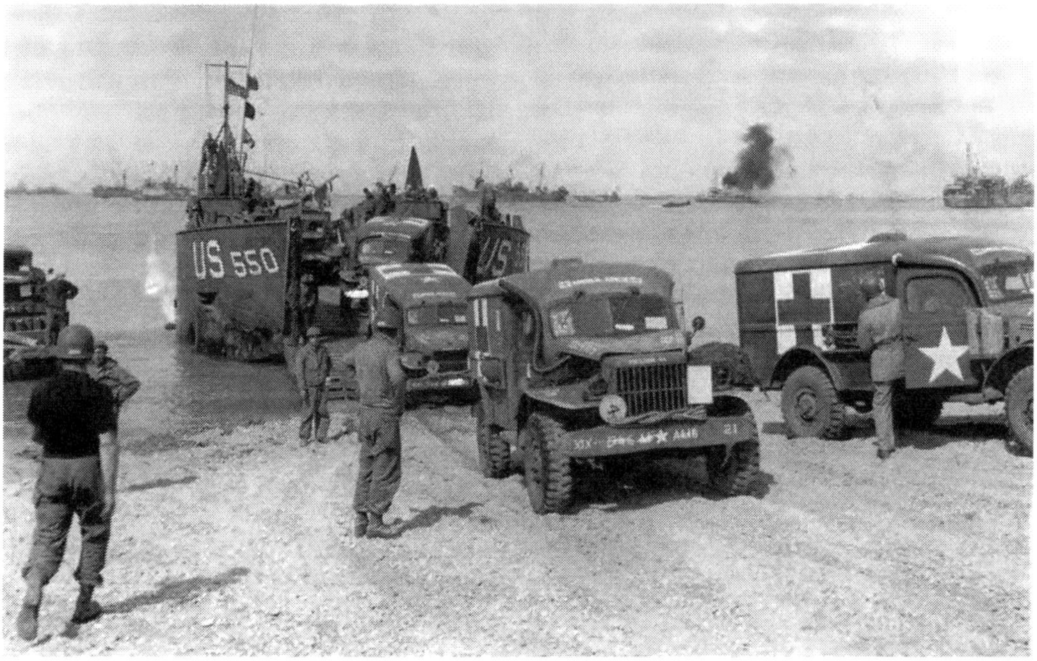

crews to stay exposed near shore long enough to load, limited seaward evacuation and in many places prevented it entirely. By the end of the day medics had cleared about 830 casualties off the beach. Hundreds more remained, huddled under blankets at collecting points or still lying where they fell. Long after sunset, carrying parties and a few ambulances continued to seek and pick up wounded.[19]

During D+1 (7 June) the organizations that had landed on D-Day gradually assembled or finished bringing ashore their men and equipment and began performing more or less their intended functions *(Map 8)*. Regimental and battalion aid stations and collecting companies of the 1st and 29th Divisions evacuated their accumulated casualties to the beach and headed inland with their units. Early in the morning the 1st Medical Battalion's clearing company, which had landed late on D-Day, opened its station on the bluffs northeast of St.-Laurent. Reinforced with two auxiliary surgical teams sent up by the 61st Medical Battalion, this station was one of the first facilities on OMAHA able to operate on nontransportable cases. The 29th Division, on the other hand, had to rely for clearing for several days on the 60th Medical Battalion, as the clearing company of the division's 104th Medical Battalion was slow to disembark its equipment and could not begin work until 12 June. Most of the 60th Medical Battalion came ashore on the seventh. Its collecting companies helped Navy elements remove dead and evacuate casualties from the western half of OMAHA. In the afternoon the 634th Clearing Company opened a station just northwest of St.-Laurent, where its attached surgical teams began operating at about 2000 under generator-powered lights. The 61st Battalion's two companies on the eastern half of OMAHA, still unable to bring most of their equipment ashore, continued to function as aid and collecting stations.

Colonel Brenn, the V Corps surgeon, had landed on D-Day with part of his section, losing most of his personal equipment and office records in the process. On the seventh he toured his units on foot, finding most of them short of men and materiel but doing their best with what they had. Evacuation to the beach and seaward, Brenn reported, was proceeding "in dribbles," but with "no stagnation." Part of the 1st Medical Depot Company arrived with supplies, which it and the special brigade units began organizing into rudimentary dumps. At 1900 the hospital carrier *Naushon,* anchored off the beach, unloaded a stock of whole blood for the clearing stations and took wounded on board. The vessel remained overnight, its surgeons operating on emergency cases, and sailed for England on the eighth.[20]

---

[19] First U.S. Army Report of Operations, 20 Oct 43–1 Aug 44, bk. VII, pp. 62–63, estimates the number evacuated. See also Dowling, Normandy Rpt, 11 Jan 45, p. 16, and Rpt, ProvESBGp, 30 Sep 44, sub: Operation NEPTUNE, pp. 88 and 331. For firsthand views, see Maj Gen C. H. Gerhardt, "Battle Lessons and Conclusions"; and Lt. Jack Shea, Narrative, both in 29th Infantry Division Combat Intervs, box 24034, RG 407, NARA.

[20] Quotation from Surg, V Corps, Annual Rpt, 1944, pp. 2–3. See First U.S. Army Report of Operations, 20 Oct 43–1 Aug 44, bk. VII, p. 63; Surg, 1st Infantry Division, Annual Rpt, 1944, p. 9; Rpt,

Continued

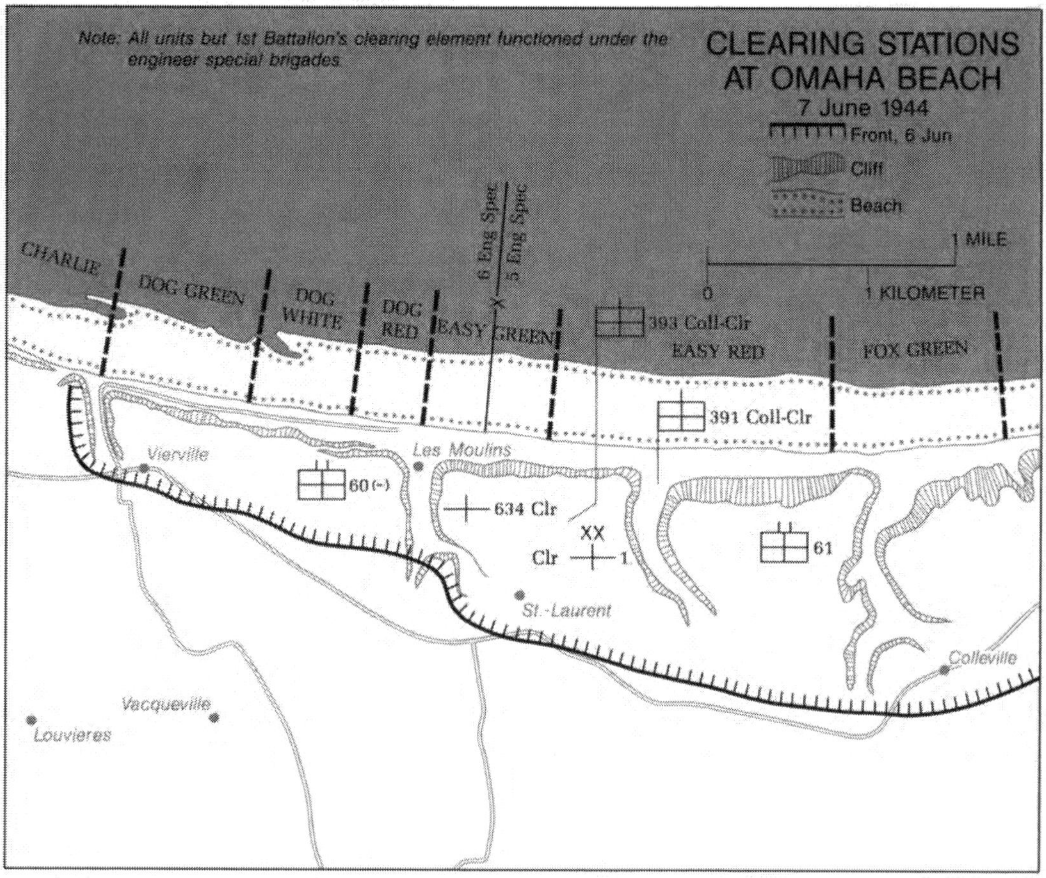

MAP 8

During the period 8–11 June, as the advance gathered momentum, the V Corps medical service fully assumed its planned shape, and its operations displayed increasing regularity. Division clearing stations moved inland. The ambulance platoons of the engineer special brigades and of the V Corps, 53d Medical Battalion, which disembarked between the seventh and the ninth, transported wounded over the increasing distance separating the divisions and beach clearing stations. On the eleventh, as the evacuation network expanded, Colonel Brenn and the medical section moved with the corps command post from St.-Laurent to La Poterie, about 5 miles deeper in the Norman countryside. Back at the beach the 60th and 61st Medical Battalions, no longer under enemy harassment except for ineffectual night air raids, brought their remaining men and equipment ashore and developed into full-fledged clear-

ProvESBGp, 30 Sep 44, sub: Operation NEPTUNE, p. 333; Tegtmeyer "Diary," pt. 2, ch. 1, pp. 1–6; 60th Medical Battalion Annual Rpt, 1944, pp. 6–9, 12, 15–16; 104th Medical Battalion After-Action Rpt, June 1944; 1st Medical Battalion After-Action Rpt, May–June 1944, box 5966, RG 407, NARA.

ing and emergency surgical facilities. The 60th Battalion clearing station stayed near St.-Laurent, and the three 61st Battalion companies one by one moved up from the beach onto the bluffs east of that town. These movements, and a consolidation of naval shore medical activities, established a single line of seaward evacuation across roughly the center of OMAHA beach. By 11 June over 3,160 patients had passed through this chain of evacuation.[21]

The NEPTUNE medical planners concentrated on two objectives in their arrangements for supporting the initial assault: the provision of emergency surgery on the far shore during the first hours of combat, and the early and complete seaward evacuation of the wounded. Measured by these objectives, medical results on D-Day were mixed. The First Army's decision to place as much consumable medical materiel—splints, litters, blankets, plasma, morphine, and other such items—as possible on shore with the first troops in a wide variety of packaging and means of transportation proved to be a lifesaver, in the most literal sense of the term. Even medics who reached dry land with little more than the clothes they stood up in seem to have been able to pick up on the beach or, in the airborne, scattered in the fields, enough supplies to do their jobs. Further, the ability of Medical Department officers and men to take individual initiative and improvise in carrying out their missions amid great danger and confusion testified to the effectiveness of the months of preattack training and indoctrination, both military and medical.

On the other hand, especially on heavily contested OMAHA, evacuation and forward surgery arrangements came near collapse. The tactical situation restricted early loading of wounded on landing craft and prevented the auxiliary surgical teams from doing any more than could have been done by battalion medical officers and company aidmen. The commanders of the engineer special brigade group and the 61st Medical Battalion later criticized the rigidly scheduled landing of surgical teams and clearing companies, arguing that it had resulted in the unproductive exposure to danger of valuable specialists and equipment. Instead, they suggested, the clearing companies and attached teams should have been held on vessels offshore, to be called in when beach conditions permitted orderly disembarkation and the immediate performance of their intended functions. In the meantime a few companies and teams could have staffed shipboard surgical facilities for care of wounded brought out to them in landing craft.[22]

Whatever the merits of these suggestions, experience on OMAHA—where casualties, though heavy, still were fewer than planners had antici-

[21] First U.S. Army Report of Operations, 20 Oct 43-1 Aug 44, bk. VII, pp. 63-65 and 69; Dowling, Normandy Rpt, 11 Jan 45, p. 4; Surg, V Corps, Annual Rpt, 1944, pp. 3-7; 53d Medical Battalion Annual Rpt, 1944, pp. 4-5; Rpt, ProvESBGp, 30 Sep 44, sub: Operation NEPTUNE, pp. 333-34; 60th Medical Battalion Annual Rpt, 1944, pp. 6-7, 9-10, 12-14; 61st Medical Battalion Annual Rpt, 1944, p. 5; 104th Medical Battalion After-Action Rpt, June 1944.

[22] Rpt, ProvESBGp, 30 Sep 44, sub: Operation NEPTUNE, pp. 334 and 337-38; 61st Medical Battalion Annual Rpt, 1944, pp. 5-6.

pated, and where, after the coastal assault, the rapid collapse of German resistance allowed early organization of the beach—did much to substantiate the fears of General Kenner and other officers that untreated, unevacuated wounded would pile up on the far shore. In summary, the medical service on D-Day benefited from careful planning and meticulous preparation, but the success achieved also owed much to individual courage and competence, and to good fortune.

First Army Medical Buildup

Between the linkup of the beachheads on 10–11 June and the end of July, reinforcements enlarged the First Army to over 437,000 officers and men in eighteen divisions and four corps. So augmented, the army fought a hard, costly battle to take Cherbourg, to expand its continental lodgement, and to break out toward Brittany and the interior of France. In this same period the army medical service brought all of its elements into Normandy, completed its organization, and treated and evacuated a constant flow of casualties (*see Map 9*).

Tactically, the First Army shifted its strength and most of its offensive effort to its right wing while holding its ground on the left. Inland from OMAHA, the V Corps, reinforced after 13 June by the XIX, pushed forward about 20 miles and then stood fast. Meanwhile, in the Cotentin, the heavily reinforced VII Corps drove on Cherbourg, the Americans' most important early objective of the campaign. That major port fell on the twenty-sixth, after a stubborn German defense. With the harbor obstructed and the wharves damaged, full use of the port by the Allies was delayed for many weeks.

After the capture of Cherbourg, the First Army redeployed its Cotentin forces southward. On 3 July most of the army attacked into the swamp and hedgerow country at the base of the peninsula, with the objective of gaining roads and open ground for an armored breakout. This offensive led to bitter, apparently inconclusive fighting. The Germans, prevented by Allied air power and French partisans from massing for a major early counterattack on the beaches, nevertheless stiffened their line with a steady stream of infantry and armor. Taking advantage of very favorable defensive terrain and of rainy and cloudy weather, which limited Allied air support, the Germans fought to confine their more mobile foes within a narrow perimeter. When the so-called Battle of the Hedgerows ended on the nineteenth, with the American capture of the key road center of St.-Lo, it seemed as though the Nazis had succeeded. They had restricted the First Army to a maximum advance of 7 miles, at the cost of about 40,000 casualties. In this offensive, and indeed in the entire campaign thus far, the Americans, and the British (who were stalled around Caen), fell far short of their planned objectives. Their continental lodgement at the end of July included only a fraction of the territory that NEPTUNE planners had expected to hold by that time. The Germans, however, also lost heavily in the Cotentin and the hedgerows; their defensive crust had worn very thin and was ready to crack, if the Allies

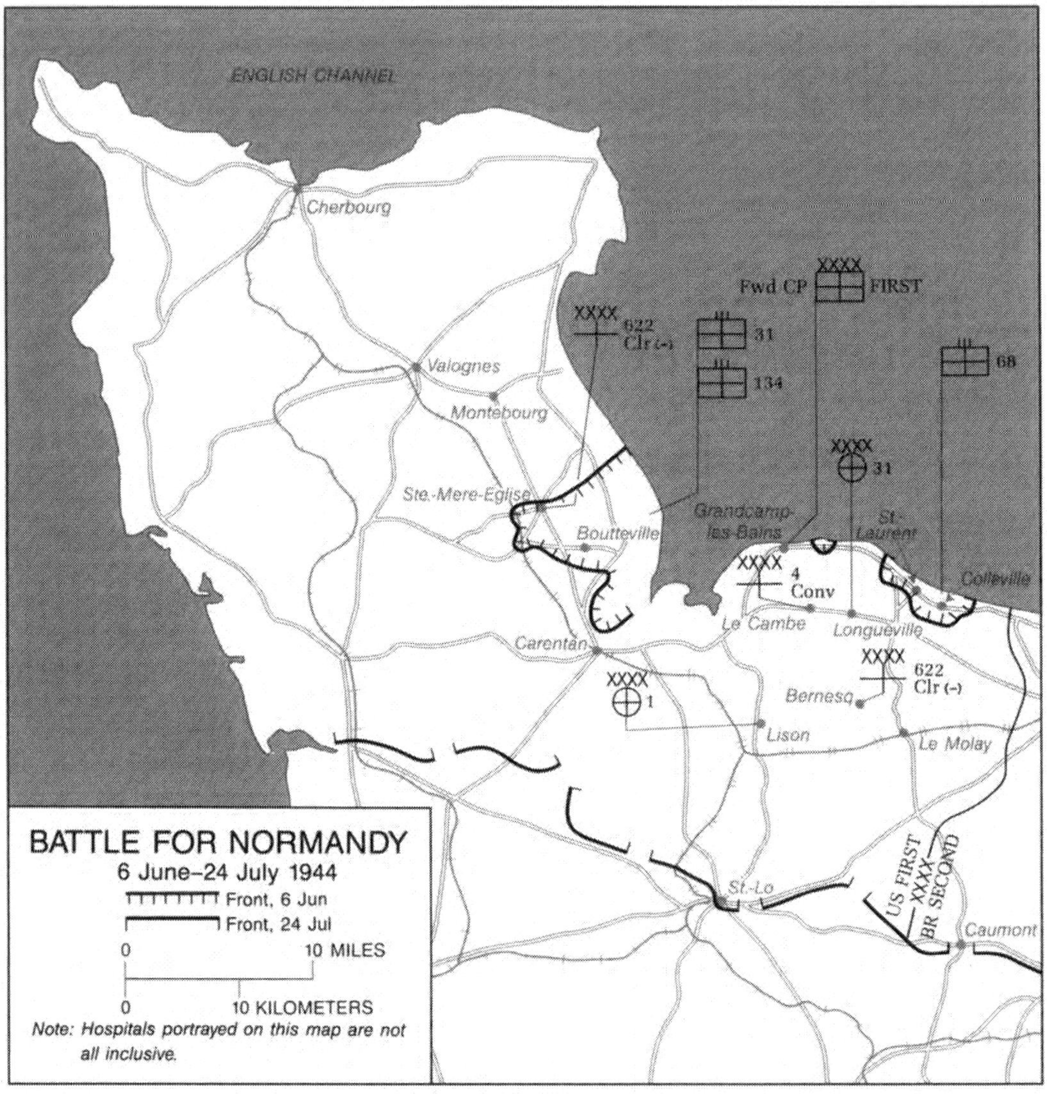

MAP 9

could pierce it with a hard enough blow.[23]

As the Normandy battle expanded, medical reinforcements flowed in across OMAHA and UTAH beaches. The first medical units not attached to corps, divisions, or engineer special brigades to arrive, First Army Medical Detachments A and B, disembarked respectively at OMAHA and UTAH on 8 and 9 June, having crossed the Chan-

[23] This account of tactical developments is drawn from Harrison, *Cross-Channel*, chs. IX–X, and Martin Blumenson, *Breakout and Pursuit*, United States Army in World War II (Washington, D.C.: Office of the Chief of Military History, Department of the Army, 1961), chs. I–IX.

nel on hospital carriers. Each detachment included station and litter platoons of two separate collecting companies, six teams of the 4th Auxiliary Surgical Group, a platoon of a supply depot company, headquarters personnel of a medical group, and liaison officers from various medical and nonmedical commands. The collecting elements and surgical teams, and many of the other medical officers, temporarily replaced assault casualties in the divisions or reinforced the special brigade clearing stations. The group staff and liaison officers made plans for landing and setting up hospitals and other facilities and arranged for engineers to clear selected sites and prepare them for occupation. On the ninth the army surgeon, Colonel Rogers, and an advance party of his staff landed on OMAHA and established themselves at the First Army forward command post near Grandcamp-les-Bains. Rogers at once began a round of inspections and conferences with his corps surgeons, but temporarily left those officers in charge of all medical activities.[24]

The first field hospitals came ashore on 7 and 8 June, the 13th and 51st at OMAHA and the 42d and 45th at UTAH, bringing with them the first Army nurses to enter the beachhead. After collecting their equipment, scattered in landing on the congested and as yet only partially organized beaches, these units went into operation near the coast on the tenth and eleventh. The engineer special brigade clearing stations subsequently transferred their auxiliary surgical teams to them. So reinforced, the field hospitals took over performance of most emergency surgery. During their first days on shore they functioned as evacuation hospitals, receiving and treating all types of patients.

Even as the field hospitals were opening, the first evacuation hospital in Normandy, the 128th, disembarked at UTAH beach on 10 June and set up the next day near Boutteville, about 6 miles from the coast. Other evacuation hospitals followed at both beaches until, at the end of June, the First Army had fourteen 400-bed units in operation. The evacuation hospitals behind V and XIX Corps were concentrated around Le Cambe, just east of Carentan, and at Le Molay, well forward toward the advance V Corps positions around Caumont. Those supporting VII and VIII Corps moved more frequently during the first weeks of fighting, advancing northward up the highways toward Cherbourg and westward across the Cotentin. As the evacuation hospitals arrived, the field hospitals assumed their intended role, attaching separate platoons to division clearing stations to care for nontransportable wounded.[25]

[24] Surg, First U.S. Army, Annual Rpt, 1944, pp. 30 and 33; First U.S. Army Rpt of Operations, 20 Oct 43–1 Aug 44, bk. VII, pp. 64 and 70–71; Surg, V Corps, Annual Rpt, 1944, p. 4; 68th Medical Group Annual Rpt, 1944, pp. 4–5.

[25] Surg, First U.S. Army, Annual Rpt, 1944, pp. 105–06; First U.S. Army Report of Operations, 20 Oct 43–1 Aug 44, bk. VII, pp. 67–69, 96–97, 104; Surg, V Corps, Annual Rpt, 1944, pp. 4–8; VII Corps Medical Plan, pp. 16–22, encl. 1 to Surg, VII Corps, Annual Rpt, 1944; 60th Medical Battalion Annual Rpt, 1944, pp. 10–11; 13th, 45th, and 51st Field Hospitals Annual Rpts, 1944; 5th, 24th, 41st, 91st, and 128th Evacuation Hospitals Annual Rpts, 1944.

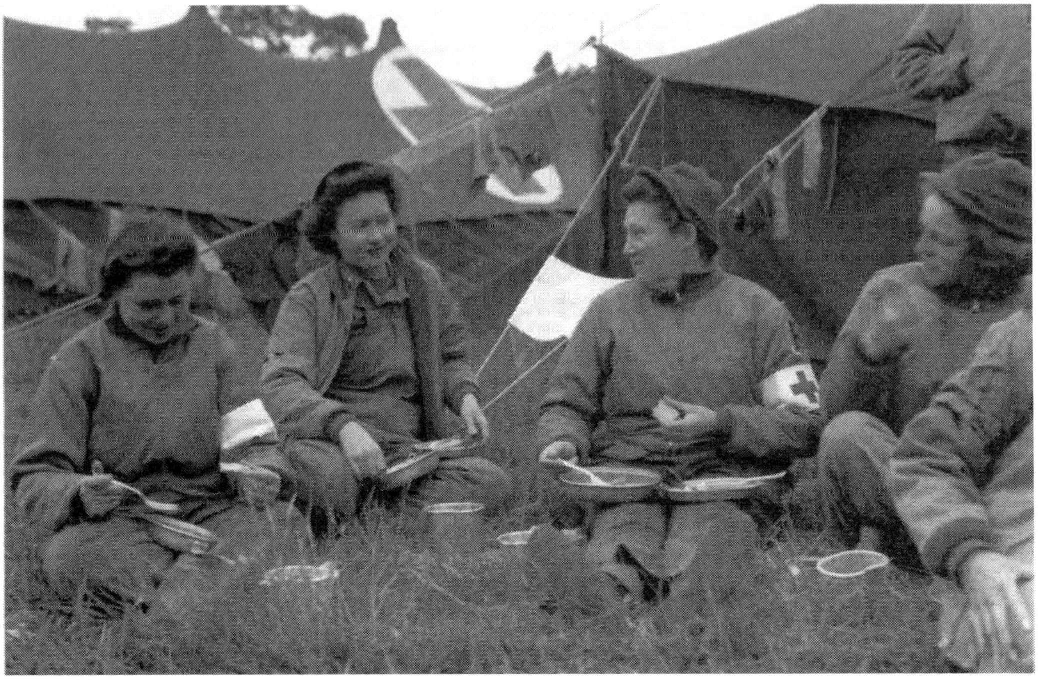

NURSES OF THE 13TH FIELD HOSPITAL, *first to land in Normandy to tend the wounded, take time out for a meal*

Still more hospitals entered Normandy during late June and the July weeks of hedgerow fighting. The First Army convalescent hospital, the 4th, disembarked in two detachments, beginning on 24 June, and opened at Le Cambe. As the army expanded beyond its planned strength of three corps, the theater reinforced it with one field and eleven evacuation hospitals, temporarily transferred from the Third Army and intended to revert to that army when it finally went into operation. All of these units deployed between 26 June and 1 August.[26]

As hospitals came ashore on and after D-Day, so did elements of the First Army's three medical groups—the 31st, 68th, and 134th. Rogers organized the 31st and 68th primarily for evacuation, assigning to them three medical battalion headquarters each and all of his separate collecting and ambulance companies, and the 134th primarily for a variety of tasks, assigning to it two battalion headquarters and all of his clearing companies. Between 10 and 23 June the 31st and 68th Medical Groups and their attached units disembarked respectively at UTAH and OMAHA. Each group deployed to control and conduct evacuation for a wing of the army, the 68th supporting the V and XIX Corps and the 31st the VII and

[26] 4th Convalescent Hospital Annual Rpt, 1944, p. 1; First U.S. Army Report of Operations, 20 Oct 43–1 Aug 44, bk. VII, p. 72.

VIII. During the same period the 134th Medical Group landed on UTAH. Its 622d Clearing Company, specially trained for this mission, on the seventeenth opened holding and treatment units for neuropsychiatric casualties at Bernescq in the OMAHA sector and at Ste.-Mere-Eglise in the Cotentin. Other clearing companies reinforced field and evacuation hospitals and division clearing stations, and one set up an air evacuation holding unit at Ste.-Mere-Eglise.[27]

The army medical supply system also developed, following the general pattern of temporary beach dumps during the first week on shore and then establishment of more permanent, thoroughly organized depots inland. On D-Day and in the days immediately thereafter, elements of the 1st Medical Depot Company, reinforced with portions of the 31st and 32d Medical Depot Companies, temporarily attached respectively from the Advance Section and the Third Army, landed at OMAHA and UTAH. They issued supplies from improvised beach dumps near the engineer special brigade clearing stations and then set up depots in open fields a short distance inland, at St.-Laurent, Colleville, and later Le Molay behind OMAHA and at Le Grand Chemin behind UTAH. Initially, the companies stocked their dumps with salvage from the invasion flotsam on the beaches. The first scheduled medical maintenance units arrived on OMAHA on 7 and 8 June, but were lost when the tide came in and engulfed them before they could be dragged to the beach. On UTAH, as the result of early difficulties in discharging cargo, no significant amount of medical supplies came ashore until the twelfth. Supply deliveries soon increased in volume and regularity, however, as the engineers by the end of the second week in France brought cargo flow over both beaches up to over 95 percent of its planned tonnage rate. Even the storm of 19–22 June, which wrecked or beached numerous landing craft and destroyed the artificial harbor at OMAHA, only temporarily disrupted the accelerating influx. To receive, store, and issue the medical supplies arriving in such volume, the ADSEC 31st Depot Company on the thirtieth opened a new rear facility at Longueville to replace those at St.-Laurent and Colleville, while a section of the 1st Depot Company on 17 July set up an advance dump at Lison Junction, convenient to the units battling for St.-Lo.[28]

Well before all these units were in place, Colonel Rogers established centralized control of First Army hospitalization, evacuation, and medical supply. Between 12 and 19 June, after the headquarters and sufficient companies of his medical groups had landed for immediate operations, Rogers relieved the V and VII Corps surgeons of responsibility for all med-

[27] VII Corps Medical Plan, p. 22, encl. 1 to Surg, VII Corps, Annual Rpt, 1944; 31st, 68th, and 134th Medical Groups Annual Rpts, 1944.

[28] For a general view of the supply situation, see Ruppenthal, *Logistical Support*, 1:391–422, 439, 464–74; Harrison *Cross-Channel*, pp. 422–23; Supply Division, OofCSurg, HQ, ETOUSA, Annual Rpt, sec. II, pp. 7–8; Surg, First U.S. Army, Annual Rpt, 1944, p. 14; First U.S. Army Report of Operations, 20 Oct 43–1 Aug 44, bk. VII, p. 76; Surg, V Corps, Annual Rpt, 1944, pp. 4 and 8; VII Corps Medical Plan, pp. 18–19, encl. 1 to Surg, VII Corps, Annual Rpt, 1944; 1st and 32d Medical Depot Companies Annual Rpts, 1944; Wiltse, ed., *Medical Supply*, pp. 307–13.

ical support to the rear of the divisions. Evacuation, field, and convalescent hospitals and supply depots now reported directly to the army surgeon. His office, through the 31st and 68th Medical Groups, directed the flow of patients from division clearing stations to the beaches. On the twenty-first, deviating slightly from the NEPTUNE plan, Rogers put into effect a ten-day evacuation policy, allowing retention in France of many sick and lightly wounded men hitherto sent back across the Channel.[29]

During the first two months of the campaign, the buildup of the First Army medical service went essentially according to the NEPTUNE plan. By the end of the period over 35,000 army medical people were on shore. For them, and for the organization to which they belonged, these early summer weeks of activity—the first combat experience for the majority of personnel and units—provided a test of doctrine and training, taught practical lessons, brought forth field improvisations, and revealed certain anticipated and unanticipated problems.

Cherbourg and the Hedgerows

During the fighting for Cherbourg and St.-Lo, First Army medical units admitted 95,172 Army personnel; they returned 22,639 of these patients to duty, evacuated 60,317 to the United Kingdom, and lost 2,027 to death. Sick men, including neuropsychiatric patients, accounted for almost 27 percent of these admissions, soldiers with nonbattle injuries for 8 percent, and combat wounded for the rest. Of the 60,279 battle casualties, the majority received their injuries from shell and bomb fragments, most often in the arms and legs—a pattern of causative agents and anatomical locations similar to that in other theaters—and over one-third suffered multiple wounds (*Chart 8*).[30]

Throughout the drive to Cherbourg and the struggle among the hedgerows, about 90 percent of all battle casualties occurred in the infantry rifle companies. For the company aidmen and battalion and regimental surgeons who first cared for these injured, as for the riflemen they accompanied, the Normandy hedgerows became the dominant fact of life, and too often of death. These earthen banks, overgrown with trees and brush, crisscrossed most of the countryside outside the marshes, transforming roads into sunken lanes ideal for ambush and breaking up the landscape into easily defended terrain compartments that had to be cleared one at a time by teams of tanks and riflemen. Each 100- or 200-yard-long rectangle of plowed ground, pasture, or orchard had its price in American dead and wounded. In five days of fighting during the July offensive one 4th Division regiment, the 22d Infantry, suffered 729 casualties, including

[29] First U.S. Army Report of Operations, 20 Oct 43–1 Aug 44, bk. VII, pp. 70–71 and 87–91; VII Corps Medical Plan, pp. 18–19, 22–23, 25, encl. 1 to Surg, VII Corps, Annual Rpt, 1944; Surg, V Corps, Annual Rpt, 1944; 31st Medical Group Annual Rpt, 1944, p. 8.

[30] In addition to U.S. soldiers, the army hospitals admitted 337 U.S. Navy men, 486 Allied personnel, 6,207 enemy POWs, and 812 civilians. For statistics, see: First U.S. Army Report of Operations, 20 Oct 43–1 Aug 44, bk. VII, apps. 11, 17, 26, and 29; VII Corps Medical Plan, p. 29, encl. 1 to Surg, VII Corps, Annual Rpt, 1944; Medical Bulletins, 2d Infantry Division, June and July 1944, box 388, RG 112, NARA.

Chart 8—Causes and Locations of Wounds, Battle of Normandy, June–July 1944

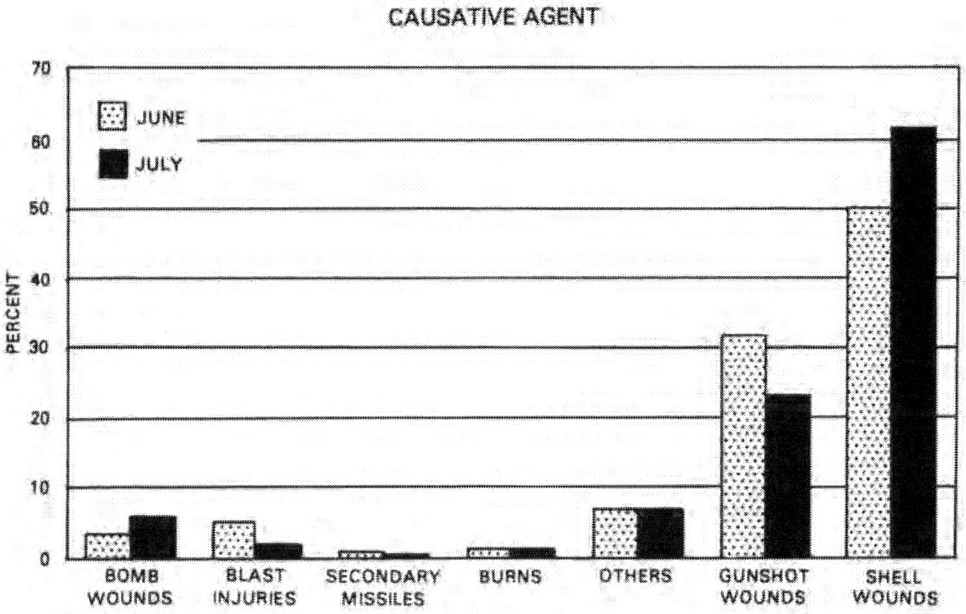

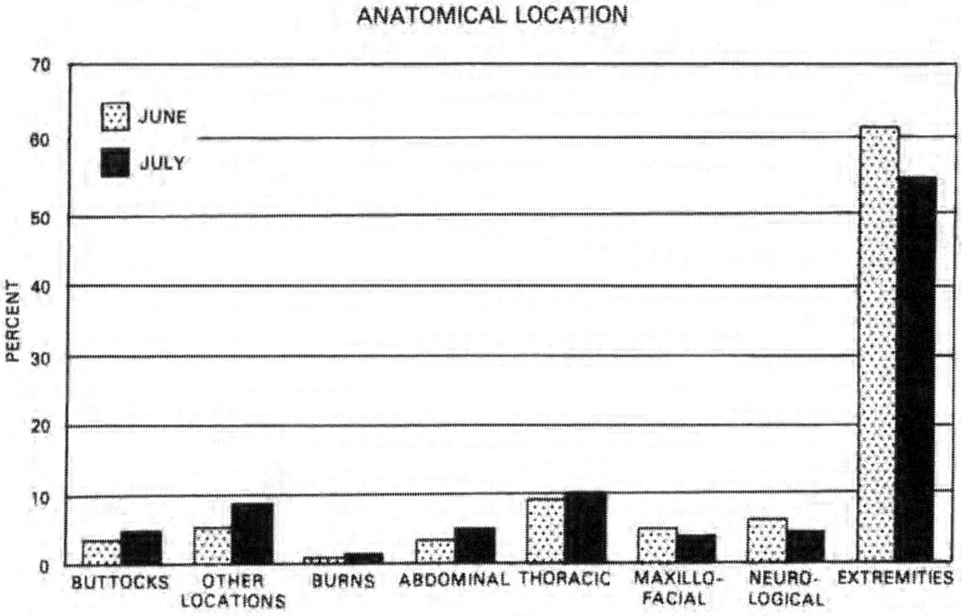

a battalion commander, a battalion executive officer, and five rifle company commanders. In one rifle company, stated a division report, there were "only five noncoms left who had been with the company more than two weeks. Four of these according to the first sergeant were battle exhaustion cases and would not have been tolerated as noncoms if there had been anyone else available." [31]

In this environment company aidmen who survived for any length of time acquired many skills and learned many lessons very quickly. They mastered the art of going over hedgerows low and fast. Instead of jumping up and running under fire at the first cries of "Medics," they learned to wait for a lull and then crawl to their objectives. Once an aidman reached a group of wounded, he had to make an instant decision as to who were beyond any help, who could help themselves, and who would benefit most from medical intervention. "We soon figured out," a 30th Infantry Division medic recalled,

> that our most useful . . . aids were compresses and morphine. We usually used the individual soldier's sulfa powder and compress. Tourniquets were very rarely used to control bleeding, since most wounds were puncture[s] . . . and bled very little or were amputations or hits caused by hot and high velocity shell or mortar fragments which seared the wound shut.

Aidmen discarded much equipment, found to be unnecessary, and discovered unplanned use for other items. The carriers for thrown-away gas masks conveniently held extra compresses. A patch cut from the tail of a raincoat, applied with the compress to a sucking chest wound, helped keep respiration from drawing in dust and dirt. Bandage scissors also could cut through clothing, and carrying an extra pair proved to be worthwhile.[32]

With an extensive, if tortuous, road network behind the front, and with most medical service jeeps equipped with litter brackets, division surgeons early discovered that almost all evacuation to the rear of the battalion aid stations could be done by motor vehicles. This was fortunate, because some divisions, to avoid medical personnel casualties from artillery and mortar fire, placed their battalion aid stations as far as 1.5 miles behind their forward elements and their collecting stations, correspondingly, as much as 5 miles farther to the rear. Collecting company litter platoons, in a departure from doctrine, worked almost entirely forward of the battalion aid stations, functioning in effect as part of the unit medical detachments and often under operational control of the battalion surgeons. Even with the collecting company squads available for relief and reinforcement, litterbearers were in chronically short supply in the infantry regiments. Casualties and exhaustion, both physical and emotional, further thinned their ranks. An

[31] Quotation from "Operation 4th Division between Carentan and Perriers, 6–15 July 1944," in 4th Infantry Division Combat Intervs, box 24020, RG 407, NARA. For general descriptions of hedgerow terrain and combat, see Harrison, *Cross-Channel*, p. 284, and Blumenson, *Breakout and Pursuit*, pp. 12–13 and 40–45.

[32] Quotation from Bradley, *Aid Man*, p. 51. See also ibid., pp. 48–70; Tegtmeyer "Dairy," bk. II, pp. 15–16.

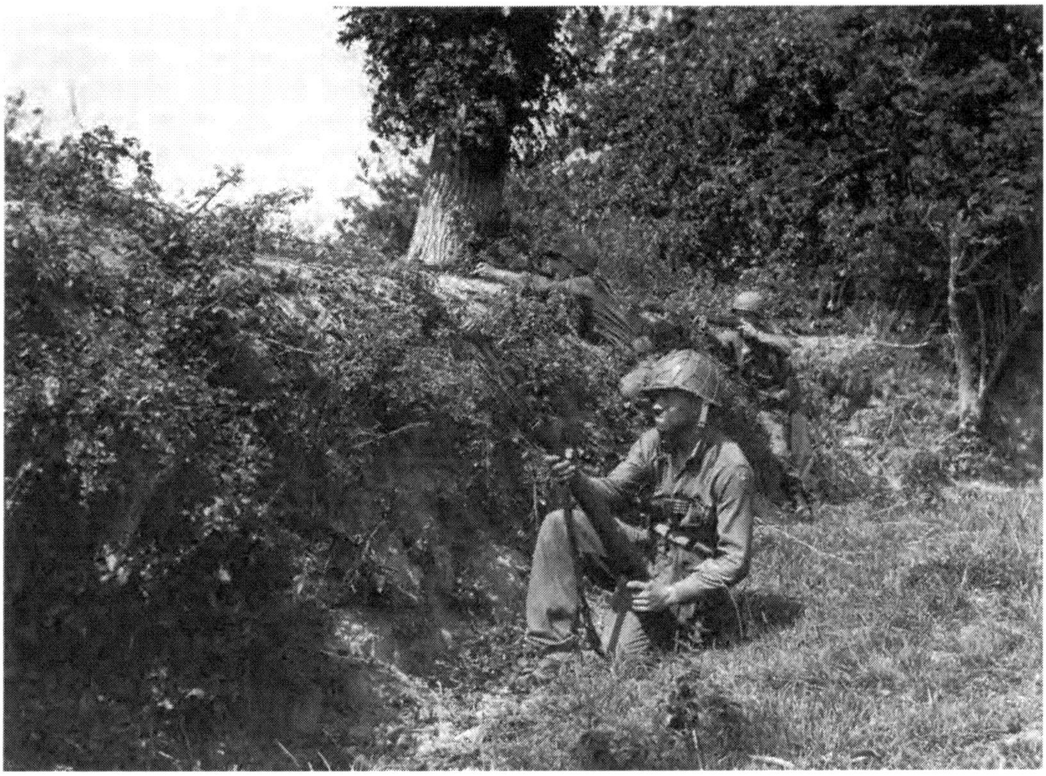

INFANTRYMEN IN ACTION IN THE HEDGEROWS

aidman recalled: "I have picked up a litter with a wounded man on it and had my fingers uncurl from the handles, even though I was exerting all my willpower to keep my hands closed." For extra litterbearers during heavy, sustained combat, divisions regularly had to draw upon collecting companies of the corps medical battalions and army medical groups, or they temporarily drafted infantrymen for the additional duty—an especially unsatisfactory solution when the rifle companies were themselves understrength from battle losses.[33]

The hedgerow fighting imposed special strains on the first-echelon medical service of the armored divisions, principally the 2d and 3d. These divisions, instead of operating in concentrated mobile combat com-

[33] Quotation from Bradley, *Aid Man*, p. 59. See Surg, First U.S. Army, Annual Rpt, 1944, p. 79; Surg, VIII Corps, Annual Rpt, 1944, p. 5; Surg, XIX Corps, Annual Rpt, 1944, encl. 14 and an. E, p. 1; Memo, CO, 104th Medical Battalion, to Surg, Ninth Army, 12 Jun 45, sub: Division Medical Service, box 355, RG 112, NARA; Medical Bulletins, 2d Infantry Division, June and July 1944, box 388, RG 112, NARA; Rpt, Surg, 9th Infantry Division, 1944, sub: Medical Activities—Marigny Sector, box 388, RG 112, NARA; 4th Medical Battalion Report of Operations, 6–30 Jun 44, box 6727, RG 407, NARA; Interv, Medical History Branch, CMH, with Ambassador Elliot Richardson (hereafter cited as Richardson Interv), 8 Nov 79, tape 1, sides 1 and 2, CMH; Surg, Ninth U.S. Army, Daily Journal, 9 Jul 44, in William E. Shambora Papers, MHI; 53d Medical Battalion Annual Rpt, 1944, pp. 6–7.

mands, had to split up their tank and armored infantry battalions into platoons to help the infantry clear ground, hedgerow by hedgerow. The divisions then had to attach aidmen and litterbearers to each separate platoon, in violation of their doctrine, under which tank battalions, especially, kept all their enlisted medical personnel at their aid stations. Because tank and mechanized infantry battalions included only half as many enlisted medical people as standard infantry battalions, the armored divisions had to strip their medical battalions to build up their unit detachments. After the initial weeks of hedgerow combat, the 3d Armored Division surgeon, Col. James L. Salmon, MC, requested an additional eighty-four medical enlisted men for his division so that tank and mechanized infantry battalions could maintain what was, in effect, a conventional infantry system of evacuation. In the absence of such permanent reinforcements the XIX Corps surgeon temporarily attached men from his corps medical battalion to the armored units.[34]

Collecting and clearing station operations conformed closely to doctrine. Collecting stations, usually located near the command posts of the regiments they supported, changed bandages on incoming wounded, adjusted splints, administered plasma, and combated shock while preparing patients for further evacuation. Clearing stations, 4–6 miles behind the collecting companies, performed triage, maintained wards for care of shock and of minor sickness and injuries, and transferred men needing immediate emergency surgery to adjacent field hospital platoons. Moving frequently to keep up with their divisions, clearing companies handled a large volume of casualties. The 4th Division clearing station, for example, received, treated, and evacuated over 6,100 patients—an average of about 245 per day—during its first twenty-five days in operation. During the battle for St.-Lo in July, the 83d Infantry Division clearing station processed 1,600 wounded in three days. To relieve the exhausted staff of this company, the VII Corps surgeon reinforced it temporarily with elements of the corps medical battalion and with an entire clearing company borrowed from the 134th Medical Group. As it had in other theaters, the combination of clearing station and field hospital platoon worked smoothly, freeing the clearing company of nontransportable patients and saving the lives of severely injured men. General Kenner reported after a mid-July inspection tour: "Many men, wounded within the hour, were receiving emergency major surgical treatment in these installations. The forward disposition of these elements is responsible in large measure for the . . . low mortality rate amongst our casualties." [35]

[34] Surg, XIX Corps, Annual Rpt, 1994, encls. 15–16.

[35] Quotation from Memo, Kenner, 13 Jul 44, sub: Report of Inspection of Medical Service in Liberated Areas, in Medical Division, COSSAC/SHAEF, War Diary, July 1944. For 4th Medical Battalion statistics, see 4th Medical Battalion Report of Operations, 6–30 Jun 44, box 6727, RG 407, NARA. On the 83d Division, see VII Corps Medical Plan, pp. 33 and 35, encl. 1 to Surg, VII Corps, Annual Rpt, 1944, and 134th Medical Group Annual Rpt, 1944, p. 8. For other examples of collecting and clearing station activities, see Medical Bulletin, 2d Infantry

Continued

Division medical elements, especially the infantry regimental detachments and the collecting company litter platoons, suffered substantial casualties. Colonel Hayes, the VII Corps surgeon, reported as early as 14 June: "All divisions in the line have lost from one to eight medical officers and from five to forty enlisted men." Between 10 and 24 July, in the already understrength regimental detachments of the 9th Division, 1 medical officer and 20 enlisted men were killed, 4 officers and 155 men wounded, and 2 officers and 19 men captured. The 83d Division, in the July offensive, had two entire battalion aid stations overrun and taken prisoner during a local German counterattack.[36]

Random artillery and mortar fire accounted for most medical troop casualties, as well as for frequent damage to medical service vehicles and installations. However, the killing and wounding of aidmen, litterbearers, and aid station personnel by aimed rifle fire, usually from snipers, raised the question whether the enemy, as general policy, was respecting the Geneva Convention rights of unarmed Red Cross-marked medical personnel. After two months of combat and careful analysis of many incidents, most corps, division, and lower-echelon surgeons and medical unit commanders concluded that, except for isolated cases, the Germans were following the rules. The commander of the 4th Medical Battalion, which had had men killed and wounded and ambulances damaged by artillery and machine-gun fire, summed up the prevailing opinion: "It is the consensus . . . that little of this damage was deliberate and that for the most part the enemy respects the Rules of Land Warfare. . . ." According to German prisoners, sniper incidents often resulted from difficulty in seeing Red Cross arm brassards on men moving along the hedgerows; medics in some divisions noted that a high proportion of their small-arms casualties were shot from the unbrassarded right side. Aidmen and litterbearers accordingly began wearing brassards on both arms and painted nonregulation red crosses in white squares on their helmets. The XIX Corps surgeon late in July officially authorized these and other measures to make Geneva Convention markings on men and vehicles more conspicuous.[37]

Division, June 1944, box 388, RG 112, NARA; Rpt, Surg, 9th Infantry Division, 1944, sub: Medical Activities—Marigny Sector, box 388, RG 112, NARA; 1st Medical Battalion After-Action Rpts, May, June, and July 1944, box 5966, RG 407, NARA; Richardson Interv, tape 2, side 1, CMH.

[36] VII Corps Medical Plan, p. 20, encl. 1 to Surg, VII Corps, Annual Rpt, 1944; Rpt, Surg, 9th Infantry Division, 1944, sub: Medical Activities—Marigny Sector, box 388, RG 112, NARA; Surg, 83d Infantry Division, Annual Rpt, 1944, p. 3.

[37] Quotation from 4th Medical Battalion Report of Operations, 6–30 Jun 44, box 6727, RG 407, NARA. For other expressions of this view, see Memo, Kenner to CofS, SHAEF, 20 Jun 44, sub: Report of Inspection ETO, and Memo, Kenner, 13 Jul 44, sub: Report of Inspection of Medical Service in Liberated Areas, both in Medical Division, COSSAC/SHAEF, War Diary, June and July 1944; and Medical Bulletin, 2d Infantry Division, box 388, RG 112, NARA. Less favorable views of the Germans are in VII Corps Medical Plan, p. 20, encl. 1 to Surg, VII Corps, Annual Rpt, 1944; Tegtmeyer "Diary," bk. II, p. 15; Richardson Interv, tape 1, side 2, CMH; and Bradley, *Aid Man*, p. 49. On Red Cross markings, see Surg, XIX Corps, Annual Rpt, 1944; Surg, 29th Infantry Division, Annual Rpt, 1944, p. 13; Surg, 35th Infantry Division, Annual Rpt, 1944, pp. 4–5; and Rpt, Lt Col C. L. Milburn, Jr., 28 Jun 44, sub: Report of Medical Officer Observer in France, 19–26 Jun 1944, in Shambora Papers, MHI.

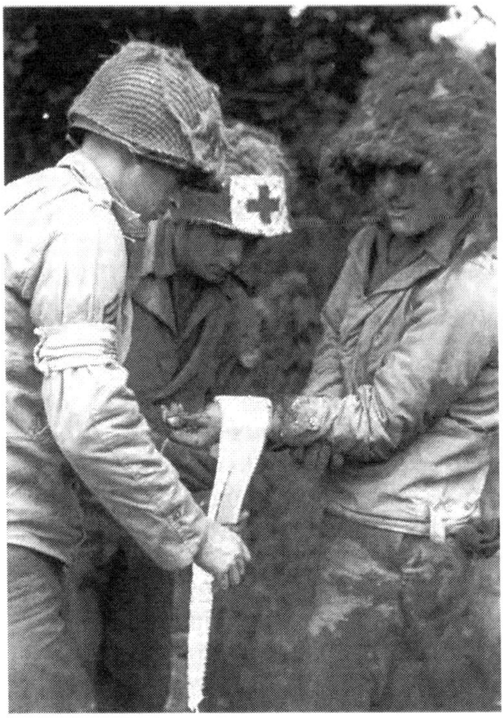

MEDICS WITH IMPROVISED RED CROSS INSIGNIA *on their arms and helmets*

Gestures of a chivalry supposedly dead in mechanized total war occasionally graced the Normandy battlefield. Soldiers of both sides, either as the result of formal temporary truces or more often by tacit mutual consent, at times ceased fire to allow aidmen to reach casualties. A 30th Division aidman remembered "deliberately exposing myself to enemy view and waiving at machine-gun crews in order to get them to lift fire so I could remove wounded. . . . The fire was often lifted." On D-Day a trooper in the 82d Division saw German and American medics rush toward some wounded lying near a tank that had just been knocked out. "There was no firing by either side upon these aid men as they went to work." Early in July the First Army returned sixteen German nurses captured in Cherbourg to their own forces under a flag of truce. The commander of a German parachute regiment in the hedgerows sent back 83d Division medics his troops had captured. Such incidents were exceptional in the bitter fighting, but they did indicate that, in dealing with wounded and those who treated and evacuated them, both sides were following as best they could the conventions of civilized warfare.[38]

To the rear of the divisions the 31st and 68th Medical Groups managed the flow of casualties to evacuation hospitals and then to convalescent facilities and beach holding units. The groups deployed their attached ambulance companies as well as the ambulance platoons of their collecting companies at division clearing stations, at field hospitals, and at other installations. They placed liaison officers at clearing stations and hospitals and set up ambulance control points on the roads. Based on evacuation hospital reports, relayed through Colonel Rogers' office twice daily and containing current statistics on empty beds, on patients awaiting surgery, and on patients ready for transportation, the groups routed am-

[38] First quotation from Bradley, *Aid Man*, p. 62. Second quotation from Statement by Lt. Joseph Kormylo, in 82d Airborne Division Combat Intervs, box 24057, RG 407, NARA. See also Blumenson, *Breakout and Pursuit*, pp. 83–84 and 137; Surg, First U.S. Army, Annual Rpt, 1944, pp. 117–18; First U.S. Army Report of Operations, 20 Oct 43–1 Aug 44, bk. VII, p. 105; 68th Medical Group, Report of Evacuation of Enemy Casualties From Vicinity Cherbourg, 19 Jul 44, in 68th Medical Group Annual Rpt, 1944.

bulance convoys from the divisions to hospitals in their sectors and from the hospitals to UTAH and OMAHA beaches. Each group transported as many as 2,500 patients a day, keeping its ambulances rolling steadily in the constant bumper-to-bumper traffic of the congested beachhead. Occasionally, they massed forces to meet sudden emergencies. Between 28 June and 1 July, for instance, the 68th Group, which normally worked in the OMAHA area, sent men, trucks, and ambulances to Cherbourg to evacuate to UTAH beach over 1,300 wounded German prisoners. During July, as the intensity of combat and the number of divisions in Normandy increased, Colonel Rogers reinforced the medical groups with additional ambulance and collecting companies temporarily detached from the Third Army and with ambulance companies taken from the corps medical battalions.[39]

At OMAHA and UTAH the engineer special brigade medical battalions, rearmost evacuation elements of the First Army, received patients from the medical groups and prepared them for cross-Channel movement, by ship and, for an increasing proportion, by airplane. The NEPTUNE plans called for the beginning of mass air evacuation from France around D+14 (20 June), but the engineer special brigades managed to complete a temporary airstrip near St.-Laurent on the eighth. A IX Troop Carrier Command C–47 lifted out the first 13 patients, including 7 wounded POWs, two days later. With passable flying weather much of the time and plenty of returning cargo planes, the 60th and 61st Medical Battalions on some days flew out as many as 600 patients, while the number leaving OMAHA daily by ship dwindled to less than 20. On UTAH beach, by contrast, sea evacuation continued to predominate. A company of the 134th Medical Group opened an air evacuation holding unit at Ste.-Mere-Eglise on the eighteenth, but it closed after eleven days of limited operation because transport flights there interfered with combat air activities. Not until 20 July did the medical service secure more or less regular evacuation use of an airfield in the Cotentin. Air evacuation at once proved its worth. With the flight itself taking no longer than ninety minutes, General Kenner reported, "men wounded in the morning are often on the operating table of a general hospital in the UK within 10 hours." With such rapid evacuation available, surgeons could send to Britain many severely wounded men hitherto classified nontransportable, reducing the surgical burden on hard-pressed field and evacuation hospitals.[40]

[39] First U.S. Army Report of Operations, 20 Oct 43–1 Aug 44, bk. VII, p. 71; 31st and 68th Medical Groups Annual Rpts, 1944; Surg, V Corps, Annual Rpt, 1944, p. 9; Surg, VII Corps, Annual Rpt, 1944, p. 10; Surg, XIX Corps, Annual Rpt, p. 5.

[40] Quotation from Memo, Kenner to CofS, SHAEF, 20 Jun 44, sub: Report of Inspection ETO, in Medical Division, COSSAC/SHAEF, War Diary, July 1944. In same file, see Memo, Kenner to CAdminOff, 26 Jul 44, sub: Evacuation of Casualties by Air. See also Professional Services Division, OofCSurg, HQ, ETOUSA, Annual Rpt, 1944, Chief Consultant in Surgery sec., pp. 12–13; First U.S. Army Report of Operations, 20 Oct 43–1 Aug 44, bk. VII, pp. 69–70; John W. Pace, "Air Evacuation in the European Theater of Operations," *Air Surgeon's Bulletin* 2 (October 1945): 324; Dowling, Normandy Rpt, 11 Jan 45, p. 17; Rpt, ProvESBGp, 30 Sep 44, sub: Operation NEPTUNE, pp. 115, 335, 339; VII Corps Medical Plan, pp. 21–22, encl. 1 to Surg, VII Corps, Annual Rpt, 1944; 134th Medical Group Annual Rpt, 1944, p. 8.

On OMAHA the engineer special brigade units reorganized to take maximum advantage of both air and sea transportation. The Provisional Engineer Special Brigade Group, between 18 and 22 June, consolidated most of the 60th and 61st Medical Battalions into an evacuation center under the command of the group surgeon, Lt. Col. George D. Newton, MC. The 61st Battalion, of which the 393d Collecto-Clearing Company had acted as a holding unit for the St.-Laurent strip since air evacuation began, deployed its other companies with the 393d to form a 750-bed tented holding facility for litter patients. A platoon of the 60th Battalion's 634th Clearing Company maintained temporary accommodations for 250 walking wounded, and the 499th Collecting Company sorted incoming patients and furnished litterbearers and ambulances. Working with attached Air Force liaison personnel and in direct telephone contact with the airstrip and the naval beach station, the center's evacuation control officer, borrowed from the 11th Port, dispatched patients as LSTs, hospital carriers, and aircraft became available. The center normally gave stretcher cases priority for cross-Channel flights and sent the walking wounded by ship. As Captain Dowling, the Western Naval Task Force surgeon, later reported, "This system was easily regulated and maintained, and greatly facilitated speed and ease in handling casualties. . . ." [41]

While the medical battalions on OMAHA beach concentrated on air evacuation, the 261st Medical Battalion on UTAH handled most of the seaward movement of casualties out of Normandy. Acting almost entirely as a holding unit after the field and evacuation hospitals opened, the battalion funneled patients to the 2d Naval Beach Battalion, which embarked them on LSTs and hospital carriers. The naval unit stationed a radio-equipped liaison team at each 261st Battalion clearing company to keep the Army units promptly informed of ship arrivals. Evacuation across UTAH beach proceeded at a steady rate, averaging about 570 men per week throughout June and July. [42]

Most wounded men who passed through the army evacuation chain underwent surgery in field or evacuation hospitals. Field hospital platoons, located close to division clearing stations, received the most urgent nontransportable cases, primarily, General Hawley observed, "perforating wounds of the belly and sucking wounds of the chest." Each platoon had auxiliary surgical teams attached as operating staff, and between them the three platoons of a field hospital, if all were active, could perform about thirty major and usually complex procedures a day. Death rates in these installations ranged from 11 to 14 percent of surgical admissions, about three times the rate for evacuation hospitals, which reflected the desperate nature of the cases the field units received. As the commander of the

[41] Dowling, Normandy Rpt, 11 Jan 45, p. 17; Rpt, ProvESBGp, 30 Sep 44, sub: Operation NEPTUNE, pp. 335–36; 60th Medical Battalion Annual Rpt, 1944, pp. 11–13; 61st Medical Battalion Annual Rpt, 1944, pp. 6–7 and 10; 393d Collecto-Clearing Company Annual Rpt, 1944, pp. 11–12.

[42] First U.S. Army Report of Operations, 20 Oct 43–1 Aug 44, bk. VII, pp. 69–70; Dowling, Normandy Rpt, 11 Jan 45, pp. 17–18 and app. N; 261st Medical Battalion Annual Rpt, 1944, p. 3.

51st Field Hospital put it, "Exsanguination, eviscerations, cardio-respiratory difficulties, and deep shock" were the normal fare of his doctors. For the attached teams, who had complete authority over the surgical service, field hospital work, while hard and demanding, offered a high level of professional challenge and satisfaction. With perhaps some exaggeration, a 3d Auxiliary Surgical Group report referred to this duty as "the surgeon's paradise." The first weeks of operation revealed only a few deficiencies in platoon organization and equipment: a shortage of litter-bearers; a need for extra officers and nurses to stay behind with patients when the unit moved; and requirements for larger generators and additional suction, anesthesia, and oxygen apparatus.[43]

While the field hosptials proved more than equal to their task, the 400-bed army evacuation hospitals found themselves consistently overburdened. Processing all patients who were transportable and needed more than the most elementary treatment, these hospitals worked in rotation, some receiving casualties while others, cleared of patients, rested or moved forward behind the divisions. During the first weeks evacuation hospitals lived from crisis to crisis. "When a hospital moved in and set up," the 41st Evacuation Hospital commander complained, "there would always be a big influx of patients, which continued until every bed was filled and this hospital bogged down. Then the hospital would be closed and left to work itself out of the mess." [44]

With the arrival of more evacuation hospitals the flow of patients evened out, but in more units a chronic surgical backlog persisted. The majority of the casualties reaching these hospitals were injured men who needed surgery—for example, 894 patients out of 1,302 admitted by the 5th Evacuation Hospital during its first two weeks in Normandy and all but 360 out of 3,200 treated at the 128th Evacuation Hospital in a similar space of time. The T/O surgical staff of this type installation, working twelve-hour shifts and reinforced by as many auxiliary surgical teams as the hospital's 40 nurses and 217 enlisted men could support, could perform about 100 major operations every twenty-four hours; the patient influx during heavy combat occurred at about double that rate. Inevitably, the less urgent cases had to wait their turn on the operating tables, often developing infections in undebrided wounds or suffering other complications. To help its hospitals overcome this backlog, the First Army deployed surgical teams and mobile truck-mounted surgical and X-ray units of the 3d Auxiliary Surgical Group and, when these proved insufficient, added provisional teams from COMZ hospitals landed but not yet

---

[43] First quotation from Ltr, Hawley to TSG, 26 Jun 44, file HD 024 ETO O/CS (Hawley-SGO Corresp). Second quotation from 51st Field Hospital Annual Rpt, 1944, pp. 24–25; see also pp. 8–11. Third quotation from 3d Auxiliary Surgical Group Annual Rpt, 1944, p. 33; see also pp. 3–4, 32, 34–35, 44–46. See First U.S. Army Report of Operations, 20 Oct 43–1 Aug 44, bk. VII, pp. 72–73 and 96–97; Rpt, Milburn, 28 Jun 44, sub: Report of Medical Officer Observer in France, 19–26 June 1944, Shambora Papers, MHI.

[44] Quotation from 41st Evacuation Hospital Annual Rpt, 1944, p. 60. See also First U.S. Army Report of Operations, 20 Oct 43–1 Aug 44, bk. VII, p. 72.

functioning. The medical groups assigned a collecting company to each evacuation hospital, to provide reliefs for ward officers, additional litter-bearers, and ambulances to help in moving out patients. Clearing companies, from the 134th Medical Group or the corps medical battalions, set up near evacuation hospitals to relieve them of the sick and minor surgical patients. For unskilled labor, the hospitals obtained German prisoners from the First Army provost marshal.

The First Army tried to manage evacuation so as to reduce the surgical log jam. The 31st and 68th Medical Groups directed ambulances from clearing stations to the evacuation hospitals on the basis of surgical backlog, rather than proximity or number of empty beds. As a final expedient, on 28 June, Colonel Rogers, at the urging of General Hawley and Colonel Cutler, authorized hospital commanders to send transportable minor surgery patients directly to the beach holding units for air evacuation, whenever, in their judgment, that course of action would bring the patient earlier treatment. Under this policy, evacuation hospitals could relieve themselves of between 15 and 25 percent of their surgical patients; but, even with this assistance, it was clear that this type of unit needed constant augmentation to carry out its mission.[45]

Clinically, surgery during the first two months of combat produced few surprises. Surgeons were impressed by the frequency and severity of the multiple wounds from artillery fire. On his July inspection trip General Kenner saw patients "with a penetrating wound of the skull, sucking wound of the chest, partial evisceration and a compound fracture. This means that one surgical team, on that one individual, must perform four major operations." The rate of use of whole blood about matched the highest pre-D-Day projections, running about one pint for each pint of plasma. According to Colonel Rogers, the *Manual of Therapy* "met all expectations" as a practical guide to forward surgery. Rogers' staff, working closely with the theater consultants, issued a steady stream of directives to clarify certain points in the *Manual* and to correct surgeons' minor deviations from it. Early debridement and liberal use of penicillin and sulfa drugs kept the incidence of serious wound infection low, in spite of surgical backlog, and in spite of the fact that many casualties occurred on pastures and farmland contaminated with animal and human feces. Of the wounded men treated in First Army installations and then evacuated across the Channel less than 1 percent died after reaching England, a result which Kenner attributed to "the echeloning of skilled surgical care throughout the evacuation chain." Colonel Cutler, after a visit to

[45]First U.S. Army Report of Operations, 20 Oct 43–1 Aug 44, bk. VII, pp. 73, 81–82, 98–99; First U.S. Army Command Journal, 27 Jun 44; Mins, First U.S. Army Surgeons Conference, 25 Jun 44, in First U.S. Army Log, D-Day through D+56; Medical News No. 10, First U.S. Army, 28 Jun 44; 3d Auxiliary Surgical Group Annual Rpt, 1944, pp. 32–35 and 44–46; 31st Medical Group Annual Rpt, 1944, pp. 10–11 and 13; Surg, XIX Corps, Annual Rpt, 1944, p. 5 and an. B; Carter, ed., *Surgical Consultants,* 2:220–22 and 227. For examples of the problem and its solutions in various units, see 24th, 32d, 41st, 91st, and 128th Evacuation Hospitals Annual Rpts, 1944.

army hospitals in late June, concluded:

It is my overall opinion that the level of professional care is very high, certainly better than in the last war. . . . The low incidence of serious infection was striking and must be related to the bacteriostatic agents . . . now employed in military surgery. The incidence of amputations seemed happily low, the incidence of gas gangrene also much lower than was expected or was present in the European War, 1914–1918.[46]

The First Army suffered little from disease during its early battles. Minor outbreaks of diarrhea occurred; the cool, rainy weather resulted in respiratory ailments; and prolonged diet of C- and K-rations led to cases of vitamin deficiency. Recurrent malaria continued to flare up in divisions that had served in the Mediterranean, with an Army-wide total of 175–250 hospital admissions each week during June and July. The affected units put their men back on prophylactic doses of Atabrine, and the army evacuated men with complicated malaria to the United Kingdom while retaining those with simple cases in evacuation hospitals. Late in July, to save evacuation hospital space for the wounded, the army concentrated its malaria and other communicable disease patients at the 16th Field Hospital, a newly arrived Third Army unit. With women largely absent from the beachhead towns, the army's venereal disease rate remained low, 8.5 cases per 1,000 men in June and 4.2 per 1,000 in July. Only 398 new infections appeared in the period, all traceable to preinvasion contacts in England.[47]

Neuropsychiatric casualties, increasing in incidence as the fighting intensified, taxed First Army medical facilities. During the July battles most infantry divisions sent one man to the rear with combat exhaustion for each three or four wounded. Before the invasion Colonel Rogers and his staff, seeking to profit by the experience of other theaters, made preparations to treat as many neuropsychiatric patients as possible near the front and return them promptly to duty. Accordingly, once operations began, battalion and regimental surgeons held the mildest cases—those likely to recover after twenty-four hours or so of sedation, rest, and food—at their unit aid stations. Men more severely disturbed went to clearing stations where division psychiatrists supervised up to seventy-two hours of treatment. Setting up and equipping these facilities taxed the ingenuity of the officers in charge. The equipment authorized a division psychiatrist included only "a sphygmomanometer, a set of five . . . tuning forks, a percus-

[46]Kenner quotations from Memo, Kenner, 13 Jul 44, sub: Report of Inspection of Medical Service in Liberated Areas, and Memo, Kenner to CofS, SHAEF, 20 Jun 44, sub: Report of Inspection ETO, 20 Jun 44, both in Medical Division, COSSAC/SHAEF, War Diary, June–July 1944. Rogers quotation from First U.S. Army Report of Operations, 20 Oct 43–1 Aug 44, bk. VII, pp. 100–101. Cutler quotations from Carter, ed., *Surgical Consultants*, 2:220–21 (see 2:217–18). See also Ltr, Hawley to TSG, 26 Jun 44, file HD 024 ETO O/CS (Hawley-SGO Corresp); VII Corps Medical Plan, p. 30, encl. 1 to Surg, VII Corps, Annual Rpt, 1944. For environmental conditions, see Company D, 4th Medical Battalion, Monthly Sanitary Rpts, June and July 1944, box 6730, RG 407, NARA.

[47]First U.S. Army Report of Operations, 20 Oct 43–1 Aug 44, bk. VII, pp. 88–93; VII Corps Medical Plan, pp. 29, 32, 43, encl. 1 to Surg, VII Corps, Annual Rpt, 1944; Rpt, Milburn, 28 Jun 44, sub: Report of Medical Officer Observer in France, 19–26 June 1944, Shambora Papers, MHI. For orders on Atabrine, see, for example, 1st Medical Battalion Journal, 19 Jul 44, box 5967, RG 407, NARA.

sion hammer, and an ophthalmoscope," and he had to pick up enlisted staff, tentage, cots, blankets, and a medical chest by the time-honored Army method of scrounging. Division clearing stations evacuated soldiers who required more lengthy treatment and reconditioning but were still deemed salvageable to one of the two First Army exhaustion centers, opened at Bernescq and Ste.-Mere-Eglise on 19 June by the 622d Clearing Company and staffed with psychiatrists from the evacuation hospitals. Here, patients underwent extended sedation, received counseling and limited individual and group therapy, and took part in calisthenics and military drill, followed by final examination and either return to duty or evacuation across the Channel.[48]

The psychiatric toll of the hedgerows forced expansion of both divisional and army facilities. Each of the army exhaustion centers doubled in size, from 500 to 1,000 beds, and the staffs worked sixteen- and eighteen-hour days. The army assigned a second clearing company, the 618th, to take over the Bernescq center, allowing the 622d to concentrate at Ste.-Mere-Eglise. Still overcrowded, even with this reinforcement, the army facilities in mid-July began turning all but the worst-off patients back to their divisions. In response, some infantry divisions, notably the 29th and 35th, enlarged their clearing station psychiatric facilities into full-fledged 250-bed exhaustion centers, which kept men for up to seven days of treatment comparable to that in the army units. Between them, the division clearing stations and army exhaustion centers returned to combat duty about 62 percent of the 11,150 neuropsychiatric patients they admitted; they released another 13 percent to noncombat service and evacuated the balance to Great Britain.[49]

The medical supply system, which had been the subject of so much theater concern until the eve of the invasion, proved efficient and responsive in Normandy. Between them, the First Army and Hawley's Supply Division managed to include enough materiel in the assault forces to sustain the medical service in its first days on the beach. As the buildup went on, the arrival of prescheduled shipments and maintenance units, besides meeting day-to-day needs, allowed the First Army to accumulate seven-day reserves of most items by the end of June. Using theater systems for express air and sea shipment of urgently needed materiel, the army depots obtained additional oxygen, X-ray, and transfusion equipment for field and evacuation hospitals. They put together outfits for improvised non-T/E installations, such as the exhaustion centers, and they remedied omissions and inadequacies in the medical maintenance units. The medical service encountered such perennial problems

[48]Quotation from Memo, Maj D. L. Weintrob, 20 Oct 44, sub: Meeting the Problem of Combat Exhaustion, in 29th Infantry Division Combat Intervs, box 24035, RG 407, NARA; in same file, see Weintrob Interv, 2 Oct 44. See also First U.S. Army Report of Operations, 20 Oct 43–1 Aug 44, bk. VII, pp. 82–85 and 106; Surg, First U.S. Army, Annual Rpt, 1944, pp. 130–34; Surg, XIX Corps, Annual Rpt, 1944, encl. 16; 134th Medical Group Annual Rpt, 1944, p. 8; 618th and 622d Clearing Companies Annual Rpts, 1944.

[49]For an extended clinical and administrative review of neuropsychiatry in the ETO, see Chapter XI of this volume.

as equipment lost and damaged in landing or separated from the owning units; unexpectedly high breakdown rates for key equipment, such as autoclaves; and an unreplaced cross-Channel drainage from Normandy of pajamas, litters, and tracheal tubes with evacuated casualties. These difficulties however, remained at the nuisance rather than the crisis level. Medical maintenance units imposed extra labor on the depots in that most of the items they included were scattered among a number of containers, requiring supply people to open as many as thirty boxes of miscellaneous goods to fill a single requisition. In the shallow beachhead, with a nearly static front, divisions and other units had little difficulty drawing medical stores from army depots. Nevertheless, Colonel Rogers expressed concern late in July that the size of the reinforced army was straining the distribution capacity of his depots and that they would be unable to sustain the force if it broke through and began a rapid advance.[50]

Whole blood and penicillin reached the army in ample supply through a separate logistics channel. Refrigerated trucks of the 152d Station Hospital, the ETO blood bank unit, went ashore fully loaded on OMAHA beach on 7 June and on UTAH two days later; hospital carriers and LSTs landed some 3,000 additional pints of blood early in the invasion. On the twelfth, Detachment A of the blood bank disembarked and set up at the St.-Laurent airstrip to receive regular flights of blood from England, 250 pints a day until 24 June, when the theater increased the shipment to 500 pints. Refrigerated trucks of the unit, as planned, carried blood forward to hospitals and clearing stations. The same trucks also distributed penicillin, flown in on the transports that brought in blood. The First Army suffered from a penicillin shortage in mid-June, the result of temporary exhaustion of stocks in the United Kingdom, and had to restrict use of the antibiotic to only the most urgent cases. But by the end of that month the chief surgeon's Supply Division, with its depots in Britain replenished from the United States, had resumed air deliveries to Normandy at a rate of 500 million units per day. These shipments continued throughout the Battle of the Hedgerows.[51]

The first two months of battle tested the European Theater version of a field army medical service and in the main proved it sound. Except for the understaffed 400-bed evacuation hospitals, army medical units functioned as the NEPTUNE planners hoped and expected. Colonel Rogers, in his assessment of this period of operations, praised the field hospital platoon–clearing station combination, and he also expressed satisfaction

[50] First U.S. Army Report of Operations, 20 Oct 43–1 Aug 44, bk. VII, pp. 70, 77–79, 148–53; Rpt, Milburn, 28 Jun 44, sub: Report of Medical Officer Observer in France, 19–26 June 1944, Shambora Papers, MHI; Surg, XIX Corps, Annual Rpt, 1944, encl. 14; Surg, 1st Infantry Division, Annual Rpt, 1944, p. 10.

[51] First U.S. Army Report of Operations, 20 Oct 43–1 Aug 44, bk. VII, pp. 77 and 100; Chief Consultant in Surgery sec., Professional Services Division, OofCSurg, HQ, ETOUSA, Annual Rpt, 1944, p. 11; Kendrick, *Blood Program*, pp. 484–86 and 553–54; Wiltse, ed., *Medical Supply*, p. 302; HQ, ETOUSA, Blood Bank (152d Station Hospital) Annual Rpt, 1944, pp. 3–4; Rpt, Milburn, 28 Jun 44, sub: Report of Medical Officer Observer in France, 19–26 June 1944, Shambora Papers, MHI.

with the flexibility and adaptability of his medical groups. Nevertheless, unresolved questions existed as the First Army paused after the capture of St.-Lo and prepared for new attacks. Thus far, the army medical service had supported a static or slow-moving force; how well prepared was it to perform if the army broke out of the beachhead into truly mobile warfare? Further, if the army did start moving rapidly away from the beaches, its medical service would need a continental Communications Zone to fill in behind it and relieve it of its rearmost hospitalization, evacuation, and supply tasks. However, as the campaign approached D+50, a point well beyond the date the NEPTUNE planners had set for drawing the army rear boundary, no such boundary yet existed. The Advance Section barely had shouldered its way ashore and was in only limited operation. The slow advance of the front in June and July had disrupted COMZ plans for movement across the Channel, even as the base sections in England received and cared for the First Army's wounded as well as supported its operations.[52]

[52] First U.S. Army Report of Operations, 20 Oct 43–1 Aug 44, bk. VII, pp. 108–09; Rpt, Milburn, 28 Jun 44, sub: Report of Medical Officer Observer in France, 19–26 June 1944, Shambora Papers, MHI; Memo, Kenner to ACofS, G–4, SHAEF, 21 Jul 44, sub: Present Status of Fixed US Hospital Beds, UK and Continent, in Medical Division, COSSAC/SHAEF, War Diary, July 1944, which reflects the concern at the delay in organizing the Normandy COMZ.

CHAPTER VIII

COMZ Reaches the Continent

When the Battle of the Hedgerows ended late in July 1944, the British and American armies controlled a little over 1,500 square miles of the Cotentin Peninsula and the Normandy countryside, about one-tenth of the area the NEPTUNE planners had expected them to occupy by that time. This delay in the tactical advance upset most aspects of the development and operations of the Communications Zone.[1]

To begin with, SHAEF, on General Bradley's recommendation, postponed the scheduled cross-Channel movement of many COMZ units in order to speed up shipment of the infantry and armor needed to reinforce the stubbornly resisted attack. When COMZ troops reached the crowded beachhead of Normandy, they intermingled with First Army and Air Force support elements, which had been unable to move forward. The Communications Zone had to negotiate with the other commands for space for its units and often for alternate sites to replace planned locations still in German hands. With Cherbourg captured ten days behind schedule and not opened even for limited traffic until 17 July, COMZ supply activities, as well as the disembarkation of additional men and equipment, were sharply restricted. Slow expansion of the lodgement telescoped and partially nullified the elaborate program for transferring logistical responsibilities at phased intervals from the First Army to the Advance Section and then to the Forward Echelon. ADSEC headquarters moved to Normandy in increments during June and established itself at Catz, a village near Carentan on the road joining the OMAHA and UTAH beachheads. ADSEC staff sections worked closely and harmoniously with their First Army counterparts. However, the army, with its own support elements still closely intermingled with the arriving ADSEC units, refused to draw its rear boundary, as had been planned, around the end of June. Instead, it retained direct authority over the entire American portion of the lodgement area, gradually delegating particular logistical functions to the Advance Section. On the twentieth the First Army drew a forward boundary for ADSEC, giving the section, which remained a subordinate com-

[1] From this point on in the narrative, the term *Communications Zone* will be used in place of *Services of Supply*, in accord with the formal redesignation of the command. See GO No. 60, HQ, ETOUSA, 7 Jun 44.

mand under the army, a narrow strip of territory along OMAHA beach, later enlarged to include UTAH beach and the upper Cotentin around Cherbourg. SHAEF, increasingly impatient at the army's delay in relinquishing logistical responsibilities, on 14 July nominally detached ADSEC from the First Army and placed it under General Lee, the COMZ commander, but under provisions that, for practical purposes, left the section under field army control.

The Advance Section at least performed its intended functions, although under different command arrangements than initially contemplated. Forward Echelon, organized to direct all continental COMZ activities from roughly D+41 (17 July) to D+90, never really went into operation at all. A FECOMZ advance party occupied a chateau in Valognes, at the hub of the Cotentin road network, on 18 June, and the headquarters formally opened a month later. However, it had nothing to command, because the Advance Section remained under the First Army. General Lee, in mid-July, decided to move the main COMZ headquarters to France ahead of schedule and to take direct charge of the developing rear area. FECOMZ, as a result, spent its brief time in operation preparing facilities at Valognes for its parent headquarters.[2]

As the Communications Zone struggled to adapt to the changing circumstances of the campaign, its medical service concentrated on two principal tasks. In the United Kingdom the medical service put into execution preinvasion plans for receiving and caring for battle casualties from the Continent. In France it revised and then tried to implement plans for evacuating patients from the field forces, setting up supply depots, and establishing general hospitals.

Cross-Channel Evacuation

During the invasion COMZ responsibility for battle casualties began at the water's edge in Normandy, where Navy shore parties loaded the wounded onto LSTs and other vessels for the voyage back to England. Under the NEPTUNE plans the Army and Navy shared the task of cross-Channel evacuation, and medical relations between the two services were close and cordial throughout the operation. General Hawley characterized his naval counterpart, Captain Dowling of the Western Naval Task Force, as "a man whose middle name is cooperation." Dowling, on his part, praised the Army Medical Department for "one of the finest examples of unstinted cooperation I have ever experienced."[3]

The Army and Navy medical services worked together to make the LST, upon which the NEPTUNE planners based their arrangements for early casualty clearance from the beaches, into an effective carrier of sick and wounded. The Western Naval Task Force, which anticipated transporting 5,000 patients per day

[2] Ruppenthal, *Logistical Support*, 1:430, 433-37, 449-58; ADSEC Hist, pp. 26-28 and 40; Memo, Brig Gen R. G. Moses to Gen Bradley, 9 Oct 44, sub: Responsibility for COMZ, Raymond G. Moses Papers, MHI.

[3] First quotation from Ltr, Hawley to TSG, n.d. [1944]. Second quotation from Ltr, Capt G. B. Dowling to Hawley, 12 Jul 44. Both in file HD 024 ETO O/CS (Hawley-SGO Corresp).

across the Channel during the first ten days of the campaign, structurally converted 54 of its 103 LSTs to accommodate casualties. The task force installed tiers of removable bulkhead litter brackets and a platform, lights, and plumbing for a surgical station on the tank deck of each vessel. So equipped, an LST could hold 144 stretcher patients suspended from the bulkheads and 150 more lashed to the deck surface. Another 150 walking wounded could ride in the troop compartments, making a maximum capacity several times the conservative average load of 75 litter and 75 ambulatory patients used in planning. Converted LSTs, and the 49 that were not converted but were able to take on casualties if necessary, all received allowances of dressings, morphine, sulfa, splints, whole blood, plasma, and penicillin. These supplies came partly from Army and partly from Navy stocks, and Southern Base Section medical facilities at the ports and hards issued and replenished them. On its first outbound voyage each LST carried an exchange unit of blankets, litters, splints, surgical dressings, and plasma, to be deposited on the beach to replace materiel taken off with the wounded. Each vessel embarked another such package on subsequent trips until 300 exchange units, containing in all 30,000 litters and 96,000 blankets, had been landed in France.[4]

Hawley and Dowling anticipated, as did the NEPTUNE planners, that during the first days of the assault many wounded would reach the LSTs having received only minimal first aid and requiring emergency surgery to keep them alive. The Western Naval Task Force, accordingly, reinforced the medical complement of each LST, both converted and unconverted, with 2 additional medical officers and 20 hospital corpsmen. These Navy doctors, although given a short course in amphibious warfare medical support at the Navy's training center in Cornwall, were not experienced surgeons. To ensure adequate shipboard emergency care, Hawley, at Dowling's request, placed 1 Army medical officer and 2 enlisted surgical technicians on each LST. Colonel Cutler, the theater chief surgical consultant, handpicked the 100-odd officers, mostly captains and majors, from the Third Army, the Communications Zone, and the air forces on the basis of their surgical training and qualifications. In mid-May, before joining their ships, the officers and their supporting technicians assembled at three station hospitals for orientation to their mission and for a refresher course, taught by the ETO senior consultants, in shock, anesthesia, transfusion, and surgical management of trauma.

Hawley and Dowling, concerned lest the LST doctors attempt too much surgery, issued a directive carefully defining the shipboard officers' task. In general, they declared, "treatment on board LSTs should be similar to that of a Division Clearing Sta-

[4] Dowling, Normandy Rpt, 11 Jan 45, p. 19, app. A, pp. 6–7, app. M, p. 3, app. N, pp. 3–4; Essential Technical Medical Data Rpt, HQ, ETOUSA, June 1944, encl. 2; Supply Division, OofCSurg, HQ, ETOUSA, Annual Rpt, 1944, sec. VI, p. 6; Directive, HQ, ETOUSA, to CG, FUSAG, and Cdr, US Fleet, TF 122, 19 May 44, sub: Initial Evacuation of Casualties From Far to Near Shore . . . , in Larkey "Hist," ch. 8, app. 5; First U.S. Army Report of Operations, 20 Oct 43–1 Aug 44, bk. VII, p. 75.

tion." It should consist principally of control of bleeding, shock, and pain; blood and plasma transfusions; immobilization of fractures; and maintenance of airway, if necessary by tracheotomy. The surgeons were to perform extensive debridements and major operations only as "a life saving measure," decided upon after "careful consideration in favor of conservatism." During the voyage the surgeons were to sort and tag their patients as transportable, that is, able to travel a distance overland before undergoing definitive treatment, and nontransportable, that is, needing attention as soon as they reached the dock. The chief surgeon felt apprehensive about placing relatively junior officers in positions of such physical risk (the combat LSTs had no Geneva Convention protection) and clinical discretion. He recalled: "This was a damn dangerous thing, putting young surgeons on those LSTs and I felt very, very concerned about that."[5]

The activities of 1st Lt. Frank Davis, Jr., MC, typified the work of these Army surgeons on Navy vessels during the first days of the invasion. Davis, an orthopedist and general surgeon, arrived in England in March 1944 with the 68th General Hospital. On 10 May, soon after the 68th occupied its plant at Whitchurch, the hospital received orders to send two surgeons to the 316th Station Hospital at Teingrace, Devonshire, for unspecified detached service. In the absence of an available senior in rank, Davis received the assignment. With two accompanying surgical technicians from the 68th—actually, he recalled, they were "both PFCs and neither had ever scrubbed on a major operation before"—Davis reported to the 316th. After the training course he and his technicians traveled to Plymouth, where they boarded LST No. 496 on 26 May. Davis brought with him an Army surgical kit, and the Navy furnished him a supplementary one. Because No. 496 had been casualty converted, the vessel had operating room floodlights installed over a space far aft on her tank deck, but Davis and his two Navy colleagues had to improvise a sterilizer from a galley steam table and put together their own operating table. The ship received a supply of blood, plasma, and penicillin, delivered to the dock by ambulance, just before it sailed with the invasion convoys.[6]

LST No. 496 arrived off OMAHA beach on D-Day and during the afternoon, much behind schedule, began discharging troops and vehicles of the 29th Infantry Division and its 115 Infantry. Even before the tank deck was emptied, DUKWs and LCVPs (landing craft, vehicle/personnel), tossing in the choppy sea, came alongside the anchored LST with wounded. Navy crewmen hoisted the casualties on their litters to the top deck, then laboriously maneuvered the stretchers down ladders and through passageways to the cavernous vehicle deck and Davis' surgical station. Patient loading speeded up after the vessel

[5] First, second, and third quotations from correspondence in file HD 705 ETO (Medical Care on LSTs, 1944). Fourth quotation from Hawley Interv, 1962, pp. 41–44, CMH. See also Dowling, Normandy Rpt, 11 Jan 45, pp. 6–8, app. E, pp. 8–9, app. N, p. 2; Mins, 14th and 18th Meetings of Base Section Surgeons, 31 Jan and 27 Mar 44, file HD 337.

[6] Interv, OSG with 1st Lt Frank Davis, Jr., 24 Nov 44, box 220, RG 112, NARA.

finished discharging her troops and cargo, with wounded coming directly in through the bow doors. LST No. 496 spent three days and nights off OMAHA. She took on for evacuation over 100 wounded, and her medics treated and sent back to the beach another 96 men with minor injuries who had been embarked by mistake. Davis' small surgical unit used up their whole blood, plasma, and penicillin; performed numerous debridements, as well as an appendectomy; and splinted fractures. The Army surgical technicians, Davis declared, were "all right" after some initial instruction; the Navy surgeons acted as anesthetists; and a chief pharmacist's mate also assisted. The LST left French waters on 9 June and a day later anchored off Weymouth to disembark her load of wounded, 30 of whom Davis had tagged as nontransportable. Only 1 death occurred during the voyage: a crewman accidently killed by a falling elevator.[7]

During the first eleven days of the campaign, LSTs transported about 80 percent of the wounded evacuated from Normandy. Of the LSTs used in the operation 95 carried casualties on one or more return voyages. While patient loads occasionally exceeded 300, the average number carried per trip was about 78, and few ships brought back more than 200 at a time. LSTs proved easy to load by a variety of means. Afloat, they hoisted wounded over their sides on stretchers from smaller craft, or transferred them through their bow doors. Once the vessels began beaching and "drying out" between tides, ambulances, jeeps, and DUKWs simply drove on board directly from clearing stations. Especially during the period immediately after D-Day, LST medical officers complained that shore evacuation units overloaded some ships with patients, while others, beached or anchored nearby, waited for hours, even days, and then sailed for the United Kingdom empty. Soon after D-Day the Navy beach battalion on OMAHA began designating a single LST per tide to receive casualties, thus permitting quick turnaround for the others.[8]

On board the LSTs, as Lieutenant Davis' experience indicated, the mixed Army-Navy medical staffs, for the most part, worked as effective teams. Army doctors on a couple of vessels complained of conflicts of authority with their Navy counterparts, but most of the Navy men, as one Army doctor put it, "made the integration of medical effort between the two forces a workable and delightful experience." Navy line officers and crewmen assisted in loading and unloading the wounded and occasionally helped with treatment. On at least one vessel, even ground troops waiting to disembark helped bring casualties on board. The ship medical complements proved adequate in size, except when the number of litter patients exceeded 200 or so. In such in-

---

[7] Ibid. LST No. 496 made only one evacuation trip. Outbound on her second voyage she hit a mine in the Channel and sank. Davis survived the sinking, but with a severe back injury that forced his evacuation to the United States.

[8] Dowling, Normandy Rpt, 11 Jan 45, pp. 16, 25, app. N, pp. 8–10; 261st Medical Battalion Annual Rpt, 1944, p. 3; 4th Infantry Division Supplementary Notes—Landing, p. 5, in 4th Infantry Division Combat Intervs, box 24020, RG 407, NARA; correspondence in file HD 705 ETO (Medical Care on LSTs, 1944) and file Evacuation on LSTs, June 1944.

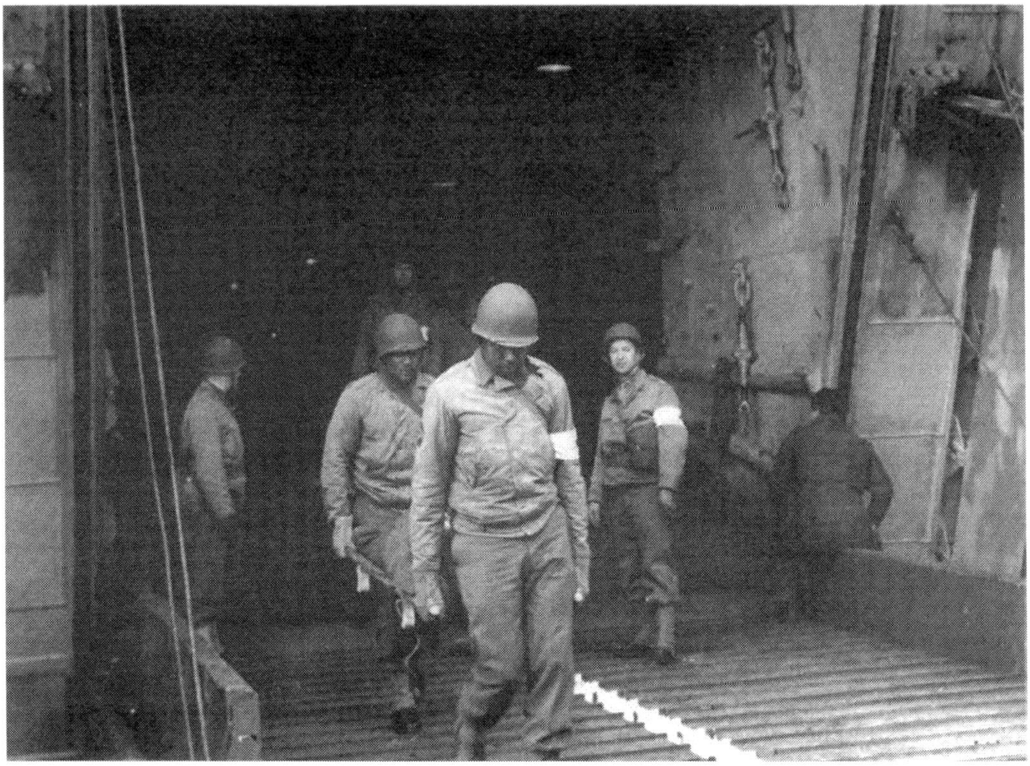

REMOVING A CASUALTY FROM AN LST

stances officers and corpsmen were too busy checking dressings, adjusting splints, and administering medicine and transfusions to perform much surgery. LST surgeons, generally following preinvasion directives, avoided major operations and concentrated mainly on debridement, immobilizing fractures, and occasional amputations. In rare cases they successfully operated on severe chest and abdominal injuries. Most of the wounded survived the cross-Channel voyage in good condition. General Hawley, who boarded one of the first returning LSTs as soon as it entered harbor, recalled: "I went down on the tank deck . . . and looked at all those wounded . . . . They were in beautiful shape. The morale was up. Their dressings were clean. . . ."[9]

While LSTs continued to transport patients throughout the first two months of fighting, the opening of field and evacuation hospitals in France quickly eliminated the need for emergency surgery on board the ships. In late June, therefore, General

[9] First quotation from correspondence in file Evacuation on LSTs, June 1944. See also Essential Technical Medical Data Rpt, HQ, ETOUSA, June 1944, p. 4. Second quotation from Hawley Interv, 1962, p. 54, CMH. On the condition of the wounded, see Memo, Lt Col R. M. Zollinger to Col Kimbrough, 10 Jun 44, sub: Observations on Receipt of Casualties, file HD 705 ETO (Medical Care on LSTs, 1944).

TABLE 5—PERSONNEL AND PATIENT CAPACITY OF HOSPITAL CARRIERS [a]

Hospital Carriers	Personnel			Patient Capacity		
	Officers	Nurses	Enlisted Men	Litter	Ambulatory	Total
Dinard	5	5	49	62	146	208
Naushon	5	5	49	124	176	300
Lady Connaught	5	5	49	95	246	341
Prague	5	6	49	194	228	422
Total	20	21	136	475	796	1,271

[a] On loan to U.S. Navy from Great Britain.

Source: Encl 2, Report of Evacuation Operations, 10 Jul 44, p. 2, of Essential Technical Medical Data Rpt, HQ, ETOUSA, July 1944.

Hawley withdrew his Army surgeons and technicians from the vessels and sent them back to their units. By the time he did so, it was clear to senior consultants and shipboard surgeons alike that preinvasion forebodings about the use of the LST had been exaggerated. The tank landing ship, although cold, damp and vulnerable to attack, had demonstrated its effectiveness for moving casualties.[10]

Except for 560 men taken out on assault transports, those sea-evacuated casualties who did not travel on LSTs crossed the Channel on hospital carriers (*Table 5*). Four of these white-painted, Red Cross–marked converted ferries and coastal steamers supported the American Army: the *Dinard, Naushon, Lady Connaught,* and *Prague.* With British crews and, in three, U.S. Army medical complements, these vessels operated under the British Ministry of Transportation, which dispatched them at the request of the First Army, transmitted through the Western Naval Task Force and SHAEF. Beginning soon after D-Day, the carriers shuttled between Southampton and Normandy, on a schedule that placed one off each invasion beach every day. For their size (patient capacities ranged from 62 litter and 146 ambulatory on the smallest, the *Dinard,* to 194 stretcher and 228 ambulatory on the largest, the *Prague*) they moved a substantial number of casualties. The *Prague* alone, in her first eleven trips, transported 3,280 patients.

Hospital carriers, which had Geneva Convention protective markings, were safer from attack than LSTs. Heated inside and equipped with bunk beds, they were more comfortable for patients than the landing vessels and, with fully outfitted operating rooms, could provide more complete medical and surgical care. Nevertheless, the carriers had major deficiencies beyond their limited patient capacity. Outside a regular port where they could tie up to wharves, they were difficult to load. The carriers, unlike the LSTs, could not take casualties on board directly from DUKWs and other landing craft, forc-

[10] Correspondence in file Evacuation on LSTs, June 1944; Ltr, Hawley to TSG, 26 Jun 44, file HD 024 ETO O/CS (Hawley-SGO Corresp); Dowling, Normandy Rpt, 11 Jan 45, pp. 23–26.

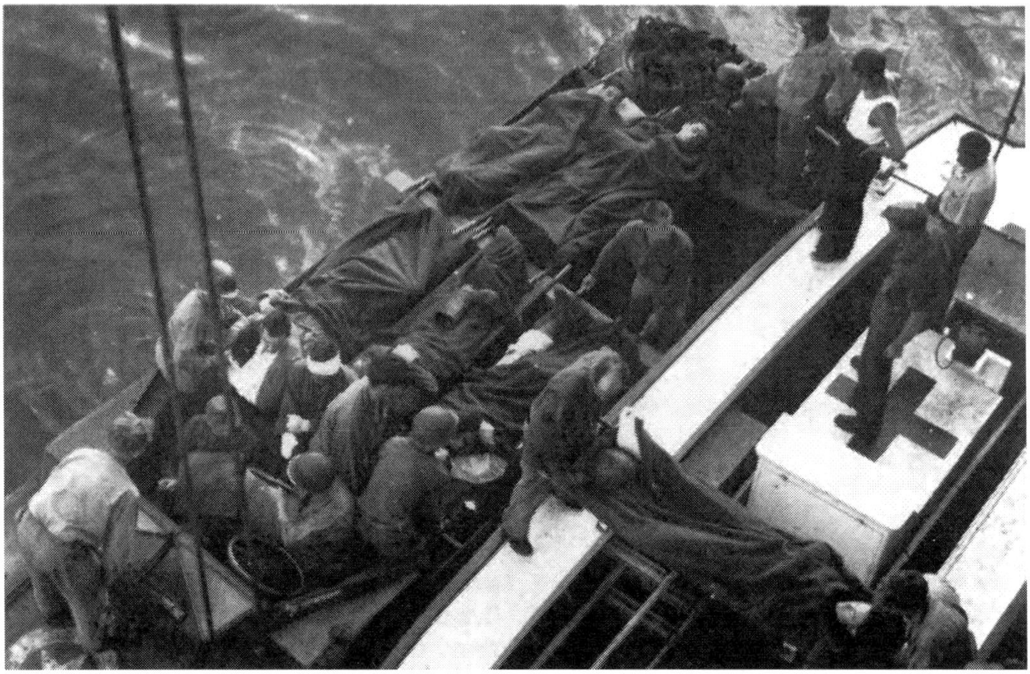

TRANSFERRING CASUALTIES FROM A DUKW TO A WATER AMBULANCE *for embarkation on the hospital carrier Prague*

ing awkward, hazardous offshore transfers from craft to the carriers' own small water ambulances. Once on a carrier, litter cases had to be manhandled from the top deck down ladders and passages and then transferred from stretchers to double-decked bunks. The Army medical staffs of these ships, drawn from hospital train units and hospital ship platoons, lacked experience in working on carriers. They quarreled with the British ships' crews and made errors in loading and care of patients. On the first voyage of the *Lady Connaught* the medical staff reduced the vessel to "complete chaos" by overcrowding her with litter patients and trying to do too much surgery. The complex Anglo-American chain of command governing carrier movements made availability of these vessels always uncertain. Army and Navy evacuation officers perferred the more easily loaded LST and, as casualty flow diminished late in June, stopped employing the carriers. General Hawley, however, directed resumption of their use, if only to transport ambulatory patients. Hawley believed that the carriers would be of value once Cherbourg opened and wanted to forestall a British attempt to reclaim them. The chief surgeon also had public relations in mind. He declared:

The arguments that LSTs are easier to load and that airplanes are more convenient, are no good. Neither LSTs nor planes are protected by the Geneva Convention; and, if we lose a single casualty by enemy action when we are not using

TABLE 6—CASUALTY RECEPTION AT PORTS, JUNE 1944

Date	At Portland	At Southampton
D	19	
D+1	543	
D+2	17	280
D+3	1,466	138
D+4	2,269	1,439
D+5	971	419
D+6	1,052	486
D+7	1,102	194
D+8	854	280
D+9	329	279
D+10	1,144	204
D+11	1	579
D+12	464	309
D+13	562	258
D+14	800	1
D+15	291	324
D+16	3	
D+17	1	
D+18	301	227
D+19	240	1
D+20	185	86
D+21	7	263
D+22	213	298

Source: Dowling, Normandy Rpt, 11 Jan 45, app. N, p. 6.

protected transport to its fullest capacity, we are laying ourselves wide open to terrific criticism. . . . I want protected hospital carriers used to their fullest capacity.[11]

After D-Day the seaborne movement of wounded back across the Channel began slowly. A few casualties, mostly soldiers and sailors hurt on board ships and landing craft, reached England during the first forty-eight hours. On 9 June (D+3) returning convoys of LSTs made port, carrying casualties from the initial assaults. Thereafter daily patient arrivals numbered in the hundreds and, on some days, in the thousands *(Table 6)*. Most Americans evacuated from Normandy landed at Southampton and Portland-Weymouth, although the medical service also had made major reception preparations at Brixham and more limited provisions at other Channel ports. Between 6

[11] First quotation from Evacuation Branch, Operations Division, OofCSurg, HQ, ETOUSA, Daily Diary, 11 Jun 44, file HD 024 ETO. See also 9–10 Jun 44 and 1, 4, and 31 Jul 44. Second quotation from Ltr, Hawley to Col C. H. Beasley, 4 Jul 44, file HD 024 ETO CS (Hawley Chron). See also Ltr, Hawley to TSG, 26 Jun 44, file HD 024 ETO O/CS (Hawley-SGO Corresp); Dowling, Normandy Rpt, 11 Jan 45, pp. 19, 26, app. N. pp. 5 and 10; Surg, United Kingdom Base, Annual Rpt, 1944, p. 27; Professional Services Division, OofCSurg, HQ, ETOUSA, Annual Rpt, 1944, Chief Consultant in Surgery sec., p. 12; Essential Technical Medical Data Rpt, HQ, ETOUSA, June 1944; Memo, Col J. K. Davis to CMedOff, SHAEF, 7 Aug 44, sub: Visit to Medical Facilities, Southampton, in Medical Division, COSSAC/SHAEF, War Diary, August 1944; Memo, Col F. H. Mowrey to Hawley, 27 Jul 44, sub: Report on Trip to Continent, file 370.05.

and 22 June Portland-Weymouth disembarked over 12,800 wounded and Southampton, used jointly with the British, more than 6,000.[12]

As casualties arrived, the medical service put into execution its preinvasion plans for disembarking wounded and processing them in port holding units and transit and general hospitals. Through the transit hospital stage the Southern Base Section surgeon, Colonel Thomas, directed evacuation, under close supervision during the first days from General Hawley. Hawley and Colonel Cutler, using the 1st Medical General Laboratory at Salisbury as a field command post, roved continually among ports and medical units. They observed disembarkation, triage, and treatment; made sure that units were following prescribed procedures; and issued orders or made suggestions for solving unanticipated problems. Further ensuring direct control of operations by the chief surgeon's staff, Cutler stationed a senior surgical consultant at each main LST port, to aid in separating transportable from nontransportable cases and to keep holding units from succumbing to the common hospital tendency to retain patients for too long. Other surgical consultants performed a similar function, as well as assisting in professional care, in transit hospitals.[13]

Before D-Day the Southern Base Section deployed the 33d Medical Battalion, with one collecting, six ambulance, and two sanitary companies attached, at Portland-Weymouth. At Southampton the base section stationed the 93d Medical Gas Treatment Battalion with elements of its own organic companies, as well as one sanitary and two ambulance companies. The battalion commanders, Lt. Col. Frederick J. Knoblauch, MC, of the 33d and Col. Joseph W. Palmer, MC, of the 93d, as port evacuation officers, had immediate charge of removal of patients from LSTs and their distribution to holding units and transit hospitals.

As landing ships pulled in to the wharves and hards, medical officers from the receiving battalions boarded them to recheck the triage done on the voyage by the LST surgeons and to make sure that nontransportables bound for the port holding units were positioned on the deck for first removal. Teams of sanitary company men then carried the stretcher patients and helped the walking wounded to lines of ambulances parked near the ships. The black sanitary company soldiers, many of whom had arrived in the theater trained only for malaria control, distinguished themselves at this unloading task, for gentleness in handling the severely injured and for speed in emptying LSTs. The 724th Medical Sanitary Company, under the 33d Medical Battalion, could take off as many as 175 stretcher cases in less than thirty minutes. Ambulances shuttled constantly between docks and

---

[12] Dowling, Normandy Rpt, 11 Jan 45, pp. 18–20 and app. N, p. 6; Surg, United Kingdom Base, Annual Rpt, 1944, pp. 25–26; Evacuation Branch, Operations Division, OofCSurg, HQ, ETOUSA, Annual Rpt, 1944, p. 3, and, in file HD 024 ETO, ibid., Daily Diary, 7–10 Jun 44.

[13] Ltr, Hawley to TSG, 26 Jun 44, file HD 024 ETO O/CS (Hawley-SGO Corresp); Carter, ed., *Surgical Consultants,* 2:204–24; Professional Services Division, OofCSurg, HQ, ETOUSA, Annual Rpt, 1944, Chief Consultant in Surgery sec., pp. 7–9; Hawley Interv, 1962, pp. 62–63, CMH; correspondence for June–July 1944 in file HD 024 ETO CS (Hawley Chron).

hospitals, following routes previously mapped out and tested. At Portland-Weymouth Colonel Knoblauch combined the vehicles and crews of his ambulance companies into a single transportation pool, from which he dispatched convoys as required. Ambulances of one of Knoblauch's units, the 590th Medical Ambulance Company, carried 7,000 passengers and drove over 150,000 miles before the company was relieved in mid-July to prepare for shipment to France. When convoys came in, ambulance and sanitary troops alike worked around the clock, at times handling an average of 1 casualty per minute throughout an entire day. On duty at the docks for up to sixteen hours without a break, men snatched what sleep they could and ate hurried meals from mobile kitchen trucks.[14]

At Portland-Weymouth local improvisation overcame a disembarkation crisis. Between 10 and 13 June three convoys, including sixty-seven LSTs with almost 2,000 wounded on board, reached these ports at the same time. The wharves and hards could accommodate only five LSTs at once. While the ships could be cleared of casualties in minutes, they then had to remain docked or beached until reloaded with troops and freight vitally needed in France, a process which took up to six hours. In the meantime other LSTs, with men on board urgently requiring medical care, remained tossing at anchor outside the breakwater. After ineffectual experiments with small landing and harbor craft, the port medical officers, at Colonel Cutler's urging, arranged with the Navy for LCTs (landing craft, tank) to go out to the waiting LSTs and link bow ramps with them. Sanitary company troops on board the LCTs transferred patients to the smaller craft, which could unload at hards not usable by LSTs. By this expedient, which also kept ambulances from interfering with cargo movement at the LST hards, the Army and

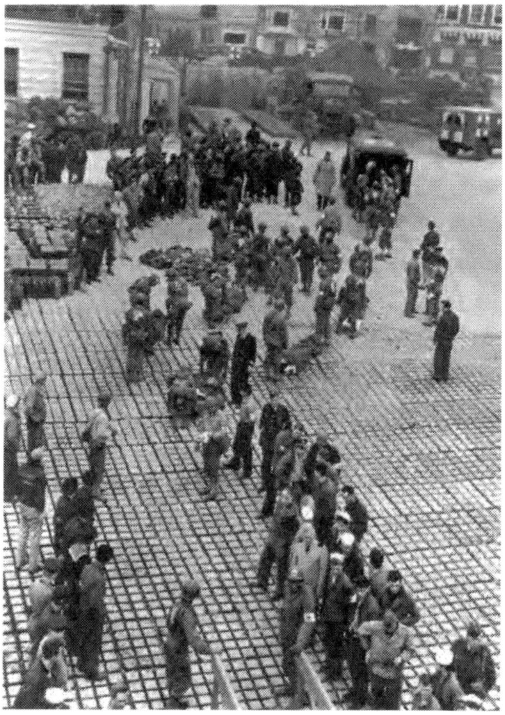

CASUALTY RECEPTION IN BRITAIN

[14] Evacuation Branch, Operations Division, OofCSurg, HQ, ETOUSA, Annual Rpt, 1944, pp. 3-4; Larkey "Hist," ch. 13, pp. 8-10; Surg, United Kingdom Base, Annual Rpt, 1944, p. 28; Ltr, Hawley to TSG, 26 Jun 44, file HD 024 ETO O/CS (Hawley-SGO Corresp); 33d Medical Battalion Annual Rpt, 1944, pp. 8-9 and 11-12; 93d Medical Gas Treatment Battalion Annual Rpt, 1944, p. 4; 724th Sanitary Company Hists, 1 Apr-30 Jun 44, 1 Jul-30 Sep 44, and 1st Semiannual Rpt, 1945; 740th Sanitary Company Annual Rpt, 1944, pp. 4-5; 570th, 590th, and 598th Ambulance Companies Annual Rpts, 1944.

Navy landed about 1,100 wounded in a little over three hours.[15]

Minor inefficiencies plagued casualty disembarkation. The port medical units never could obtain reliable advance notice when LSTs were returning with casualties. Triage officers disagreed on which patients were transportable and which were not, in spite of the advice of the consultants. Evacuation officers had a tendency to overload the nearest transit hospitals while leaving those farther inland with few patients. Yet, even with these difficulties, the disembarkation of patients and their dispatch to hospitals in the main went smoothly, thanks to thorough planning and preparation, sufficient manpower and equipment, and close high-level supervision. In at least one respect the U.S. receiving system proved superior to its generally similar British counterpart. The British relied almost entirely on hospital trains to take wounded from wharves to transit hospitals, a practice that often kept men in need of treatment and rest waiting for hours on the waterfront until a train was filled. The Americans, on the other hand, by using ambulances for the first stage of land evacuation could start the wounded on their way as soon as they came off the ships.[16]

Patients tagged nontransportable by LST surgeons or dockside triage officers went at once to holding units of the 12th and 50th Field Hospitals at Portland-Weymouth and of the 28th and 46th Field Hospitals at Southampton. Directly under base section command, these units placed detachments only blocks from wharves and hards to receive the most urgent cases. At Southampton, for example, a platoon of the 28th occupied a bombed-out brewery on the waterfront. The platoon used the intact cellar for wards, operating room, and X-ray department and placed supply, staff quarters, and other facilities in tents in the rubble above. The main bodies of the field hospitals, established under canvas on the city outskirts, received most of the nontransportables and were organized for short-notice mass admissions and evacuations. At the 50th ambulances

> pulled up in front of the admitting tents where wooden horses were placed for the litters. Here the admitting officer quickly checked the emergency medical tag and on the basis of the diagnosis thereon sent the patient to the appropriate ward [while] making out a new record. The number of beds available in any tented ward was indicated on a board with a circular tab for each bed. As the patient was allocated to a ward one of these tabs was pinned to his records and this was returned to its place when the patient was further evacuated. In this way the bed

[15] The LCT could carry several medium tanks and was the Allies' principal small vehicle landing craft, in contrast to the LST, an oceangoing ship capable of beaching. See Dowling, Normandy Rpt, 11 Jan 45, app. N, p. 6; Carter, ed., *Surgical Consultants*, 2:209 and 213–14; Surg, United Kingdom Base, Annual Rpt, pp. 27–28; Larkey "Hist," ch. 13, p. 9.

[16] Memo, Kenner, sub: Report of Inspection—Reception of Casualties of Southampton, 7–8 Jun 44, and Memo, Kenner to CofS, SHAEF, 20 Jun 44, sub: Report of Inspection ETO During . . . Period 7–17 Jun 44, both in Medical Division, COSSAC/SHAEF, War Diary, June 1944; Memo, Lt Col M. E. Glock to Chief, Operations Division, OofCSurg, HQ, ETOUSA, 6 Jul 44, sub: Report on Medical Operations, SBS, EvacCorresp, 1942–44, file HD 024 ETO; Evacuation Branch, Operations Division, OofCSurg, HQ, ETOUSA, Daily Diary, 11, 14, 18 Jun 44 and 16, 23 Jul 44, file HD 024 ETO. On the British evacuation system, see Crew, *AMS, Campaigns: North-West Europe*, 4:61–69. The U.S. comparison is in Evacuation Branch, Operations Division, OofCSurg, HQ, ETOUSA, Annual Rpt, 1944, p. 5.

status was instantly known. The whole procedure of admission took only one or two minutes and the litter bearers then carried the patient out through the side door of the admission tent. The patients in shock were taken to the shock wards for transfusion. . . . The patients requiring immediate surgery were taken to the surgical wards and prepared for operation. . . .[17]

These units, reinforced with auxiliary surgical and shock teams and often with gas treatment elements, performed much the same function as did their continental counterparts attached to division clearing stations. Generally, they kept patients no longer than twenty-four hours before sending them by ambulance to the larger transit hospitals. Field hospitals did most of their emergency surgery during the first couple of weeks of the invasion, before First Army hospitals were in position to retain nontransportables on the far shore. As the campaign went on, their work dwindled to dealing with emergencies and complications developing on the voyage and to caring for occasional severe cases that slipped through the sorting process farther forward. The field hospitals also were supposed to handle injured from enemy air attacks on the embarkation ports or on vessels left off shore, but the number of these was negligible. Even during the first weeks after D-Day, lighter than expected casualties left many holding units with little to do. The 46th Field Hospital at Southampton and the 50th at Portland-Weymouth, which received most of the nontransportables, kept constantly busy. By contrast, the platoon of the 28th in the Southampton brewery admitted only 81 patients before it closed on 4 July. The 7th Field Hospital at Brixham, where casualties had been expected to land but did not, "ran a hotel for . . . casual troops . . . engaged in various duties on the hards" and treated occasional road accident victims.[18]

Most of the ambulances leaving the docks headed directly for the station and general hospitals that General Hawley, before D-Day, had designated to serve as transit hospitals. If the field hospitals at the ports resembled in mission those at division clearing stations, the transit units, located within 30 miles of the coast, acted much like army evacuation hospitals. Indeed, two of them actually were evacuation hospitals—the 12th and 109th, established side by side near Portland-Weymouth to provide additional transit beds.

The fixed hospitals assigned to transit duty had to adjust their procedures and routines for rapid reception, short-term treatment, and disposition of patients. During the final hours before D-Day they cleared out their wards often hastily and informally because the process, for security reasons, could start only at the last minute. A surgeon at the 228th Station Hospital recalled: "We succeed-

[17] Quotation from Larkey "Hist," ch. 13, pp. 10–11; as theater medical historian, Larkey was an eyewitness of these operations. See also 50th Field Hospital Annual Rpt, 1944, pp. 1–8; 28th Field Hospital Hist, 1944, pp. 27–28, box 412, RG 112, NARA.

[18] Professional Services Division, OofCSurg, HO, ETOUSA, Annual Rpt, 1944, Chief Consultant in Surgery sec., p. 13; 7th, 12th, 46th, and 50th Field Hospitals Annual Rpts, 1944; 28th Field Hospital Hist, 1944, box 412, RG 112, NARA. An eyewitness description of holding unit reception is in Larkey "Hist," ch. 13, pp. 10–11.

ed in emptying the hospital simply by throwing some of the patients on trains, loading some on convoys [of ambulances], and summarily giving discharges to many others." Some convalescents, realizing that the invasion was imminent, helped by departing without leave to rejoin their units. "We knew they were going, but we didn't try to stop them." [19] Transit hospitals revamped their methods for admitting patients and initiating their clinical records, some decentralizing the entire process to a number of wards. Staffs reorganized to keep all departments and services open around the clock. Shifts for doctors, nurses, and enlisted men averaged twelve hours a day. One unit, the 315th Station Hospital, divided its personnel into three sixteen-hour shifts, two of which were always on duty. Station hospitals, especially, received reinforcements of surgical teams, nurses, and enlisted men. The 110th Station Hospital at Southampton had 80 officers and 150 nurses from eleven different units attached at various times, as well as a sanitary company platoon for litterbearers and a military police detachment to guard wounded POWs.

Transit hospitals were supposed to examine incoming patients, retain those needing immediate definitive care or requiring rest before further travel, and prepare the remainder for early rail movement to regular general hospitals. In practice, they adopted flexible evacuation policies. The 228th Station Hospital, for example, "operated under a very informal holding policy. . . . When a patient could be moved, he was moved. Sometimes that meant 24 hours, sometimes five days." Individual units processed large number of casualties within a short time. One of the most active, the 834-bed 110th Station Hospital, only 6 miles from the Southampton waterfront, handled 7,000 patients during June and July, admitting and evacuating as many as 1,700 in one week. Another heavily used unit, the 48th General Hospital at Stockbridge, processed about 3,000 casualties in eight days. The load, however, was unequally distributed, depending on a hospital's location and the decisions of port evacuation officers. The 314th Station Hospital at Truro, well away from the main receiving ports, admitted only two groups of wounded during a month of transit operations.[20]

Early in the campaign, transit hospital staffs were uncertain how much surgery they were expected to do. Their preinvasion directives from General Hawley indicated that they were not to engage in surgery on patients capable of continued travel; some hospitals, adhering rigidly to these instructions, held this category of cases on their wards for lengthy periods, awaiting accumulation of a trainload of evacuees. Appropriate when casualties were coming in rapidly, this policy at other times resulted in idle surgical teams and in the denial of early definitive treatment to

[19] Interv, OSG with Maj Harry R. Grau, 18 Jul 45, box 223, RG 112, NARA.

[20] Quotations from ibid. See also 110th Station Hospital, 28th and 48th General Hospitals, and 12th Evacuation Hospital Annual Rpts, 1944; 28th General Hospital Supplementary Hist, 15 Apr–15 Jul 44; 38th Station Hospital Hist, 1 Jan–31 Dec 44; 314th Station Hospital Annual Hist, 1944; 305th and 315th Station Hospitals Supplementary Hists, 1 Apr–30 Jun 44.

men who could have benefited from it. Within a week of D-Day Colonel Cutler directed transit hospitals to do as much definitive surgery as the availability of staff and their admission rates permitted, which often turned out to be a great deal. Surgeons of the 48th General Hospital found that they could operate on almost all the wounded soldiers they received and hold them as nontransportable for a day or so of recovery without clogging the flow of patients through their unit. On the other hand, surgeons at the busy 110th Station Hospital confined themselves largely to "supportive and revisional surgery in the interests, mainly, of continued transportability," such as debridements, fragment extractions, hemorrhage control, and splint and cast reconstruction. As did the holding units, the transit hospitals encountered their heaviest surgical burden during the weeks immediately after D-Day, often working on men who "for all practical purposes, were admitted from the field." The increasing proportion of incoming wounded who had undergone surgery on the far shore generally reached the transit hospitals in good condition, except for occasional patients with inadequate debridements and improperly applied casts and for a few prematurely transported chest injury cases. The transit hospitals' own mortality rates were low, averaging about 0.2 percent of the patients received.[21]

Beyond the transit hospitals the Evacuation Branch of General Hawley's office, headed by Col. Fred H. Mowrey, MC, controlled the routing of patients to the general hospitals, where they would stay until they recovered or were evacuated from the theater. For this stage of evacuation the branch employed fifteen British-built and -operated and U.S. Army-staffed hospital trains based in southwest England. Working with U.S. and British transportation authorities, Mowrey's staff dispatched these trains on the basis of Southern Base Section reports, received four times each day, giving the number and location of transit hospital patients ready to travel. The transit hospitals used their own ambulances and trucks, and vehicles borrowed from other units, to bring prescribed loads of patients to their assigned railheads. The Evacuation Branch usually kept its trains running on time, in spite of the complexity and occasional lack of responsiveness of the Anglo-American rail traffic control system, and in spite of frequent breakdowns of the ten overseas hospital trains, originally constructed to operate on the Continent and hastily modified to run on British tracks. The transit hospitals, on their side, quickly learned to synchronize ambulance movements with train schedules. Their drivers and litter-bearers developed proficiency in shifting wounded from ambulances to railroad cars, often filling a train to its 300-patient capacity in less than an hour. By the end of June the Evacu-

[21] Quotations from 110th Station Hospital Annual Rpt, 1944, pp. 1–3 and 7. See also Professional Services Division, OofCSurg, HQ, ETOUSA, Annual Rpt, 1944, Chief Consultant in Surgery sec., p. 11; Carter, ed., *Surgical Consultants*, 2:208–09; 48th General Hospital Annual Rpt, 1944, pp. 31–33; Memo, sub: Inspection by Gen Kenner—Transit Hospitals, SBS, 28–29 June 1944, and Memo, Col J. K. Davis, 10 Aug 44, sub: Visit to UK Transit Hospitals, both in Medical Division, COSSAC/SHAEF, War Diary, July–August 1944.

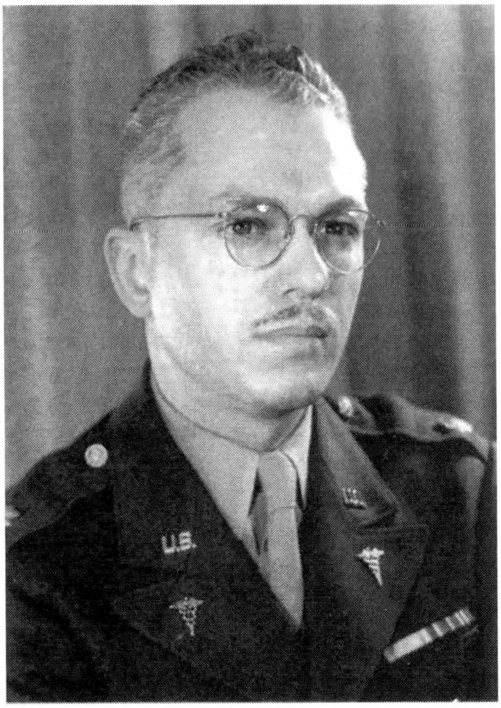

COL. FRED H. MOWREY

ation Branch had moved over 23,800 casualties in eighty-four trainloads, safely and in reasonable comfort.[22]

Throughout the evacuation chain property exchanges required constant attention from the chief surgeon's Supply Division. In theory, one-for-one exchanges of blankets, litters, sheets, pillows, pajamas, splints, and tracheal and abdominal tubes were to occur at each point along the route, for example, between hospital trains and transit hospitals. In practice, each element tried to build up its own reserves so that items steadily disappeared from the system. This process eventually left the far shore elements short, in spite of such expedients as the LST exchange units. The hospitals in Normandy then drew on the depots in the United Kingdom, which found their own stocks steadily diminishing. Colonel Hays, the Supply Division chief, partially solved this problem by imposing rigid ceilings (for example, an average of 3.2 blankets per bed) on fixed hospitals stocks of key items. He sent out liaison officers to make sure that hospitals regularly turned in excesses to the depots, which packed the return materiel and shipped it back to France. Leakage, nevertheless, continued. At the end of July Colonel Hays warned base section surgeons of the need for "constant vigilance" to ensure that exchange items "stayed in the stream and not in the eddies." [23]

Beginning on 10 June, trainloads of battle casualties reached the end of the evacuation chain: the European Theater general hospitals, especially those grouped under the 12th and 15th Hospital Centers at Great Mal-

[22] The British had three train types: Ministry of Health casualty evacuation trains intended for civilian air raid victims, military home ambulance trains, and military overseas ambulance trains. Of these, the British used all twenty-one of the first type and all but five of the second. These five went to the Americans, as did all ten overseas trains. See Crew, *AMS, Campaigns: North-West Europe*, 4:64–65; Dunn, *EMS*, 1:287–88; Evacuation Branch, Operations Division, OofCSurg, HQ, ETOUSA, Annual Rpt, pp. 4–5, and, in file HD 024 ETO, ibid., Daily Diary, June–July 1944; 28th, 48th, and 95th General Hospitals Annual Rpts, 1944; 110th and 315th Station Hospitals Annual Rpts, 1944; Memo, Lt Col M. E. Glock to Chief, Operations Division, OofCSurg, HQ, ETOUSA, 6 Jul 44, sub: Report on Medical Operations, SBS, EvacCorresp, 1942–44, file HD 024 ETO.

[23] Quotation from Mins, 26th Meeting of Base Section Surgeons, 31 Jul 44, p. 2, file HD 337. In same file, see also Mins, 24th and 25th Meetings of Base Section Surgeons, 19 Jun and 3 Jul 44. See Kelley Interv, 27 Jan 45, box 221, RG 112, NARA.

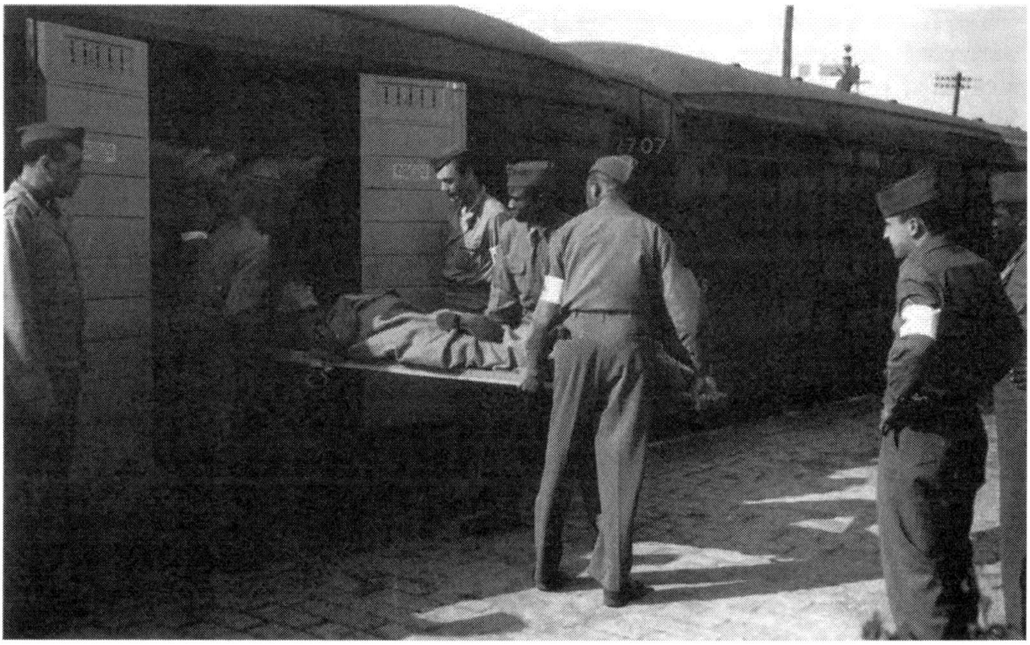

DETRAINING A CASUALTY IN BRITAIN FOR TRANSPORT TO A GENERAL HOSPITAL

vern and Cirencester. The centers now proved their value in organizing and directing the rapid transfer of wounded and sick soldiers from railroad cars to hutted wards. After early difficulties with late-arriving and unannounced trains and with confusion in unloading, the centers rapidly reduced mass admissions to routine. The 15th Hospital Center, for instance, designated one of its attached general hospitals to receive each trainload of patients and pooled ambulances and litterbearers from the others to empty the railcars. By such means the hospital center could have a wounded man in bed in a ward thirty-five minutes after the train carrying him pulled into the station. Hospital personnel, an observer noted, "consider this time as their actual 'battle participation' and all work long hours and hard on receipt of the casualties." Indicating the quality of work done at holding and transit units, most patients arrived at the general hospitals with fractures properly immobilized, wounds debrided and ready for secondary closure, and relatively little infection or gas gangrene. Patient deaths on the way to general hospitals, and after arrival there, were very few.[24]

---

[24] Quotation from Surg, Ninth U.S. Army, Daily Journal, 9 Jul 44, Shambora Papers, MHI. See also Professional Services Division, OofCSurg, HQ, ETOUSA, Annual Rpt, 1944, Chief Consultant in Surgery sec., pp. 9 and 13–14; Rpt, Kenner, 17 Jun 44, sub: Visit of CMO to 91st and 97th General Hospitals, Oxford, in Medical Division, COSSAC/SHAEF, War Diary, June 1944; Evacuation Branch, Operations Division, OofCSurg, HQ, ETOUSA, Daily Diary, 10 Jun 44, file HD 024 ETO; 12th Hospital Center Annual Rpt, 1944, pp. 31–32; 15th Hospital Center Hist, 1944, pp. 21–22.

The fixed hospital system in Britain continued to change and expand, even as it received and treated battle casualties. In the Western Base Section the number of beds increased from about 42,000 on D-Day to 50,000 at the end of July, as units finished their planned tented additions and other organizations occupied late-completed plants or took over recently vacated militia and conversion camps. Many plants experienced turnover in occupying units. The 99th General Hospital, for instance, which landed at Liverpool on 20 April and staged at Llandudno, opened a hutted hospital at Foxley, Hertfordshire, on 12 June. After treating battle casualties for about a month, the unit turned over its facility and patients to the 156th General Hospital and then returned to Llandudno to prepare for movement to France. Troop departures for the Continent left many station hospitals all but unemployed. To prevent waste of plants and highly qualified staffs, the Professional Services, Operations, and Hospitalization Divisions of Hawley's office, in consultation with the base sections, late in July designated eight of the professionally strongest station hospitals to function as general hospitals and made plans for using others to care for lightly wounded, sick, and convalescents.[25]

[25] Surg, Western Base Section, Rpt, 1 Jan–31 Aug 44, pp. 10–12; Larkey "Hist," ch. 8, p. 25; 99th General Hospital Annual Rpt, pp. 2–3. The reassigned station hospitals were the 49th, 115th, 121st, 136th, 208th, 231st, 303d, and 327th. See Evacuation Branch, Operations Division, OofCSurg, HQ, ETOUSA, Daily Diary, 4, 12 and 29 Jul 44, file HD 024 ETO; Mins, 25th Meeting of Base Section Surgeons, 3 Jul 44, pp. 12–13, file HD 337.

Air Evacuation Begins

A separate system of holding units and transit hospitals handled the growing number of wounded evacuated to Great Britain by air. All the NEPTUNE plans called for early, extensive use of returning cargo planes to carry casualties, but the actual scale and effectiveness of air evacuation remained uncertain as the campaign began. Throughout the planning General Grow, the USSTAF surgeon, made only the most conservative air evacuation commitments. He insisted that the field armies and the Communications Zone operate on the assumption that they would have to move all their wounded by sea, with provisions for use of aircraft if available. Experience quickly showed that Grow had been overly pessimistic.

Cross-Channel casualty flights began on 10 June, sooner than expected, and proved both efficient and beneficial for the patients. Air evacuation grew rapidly in volume so that by the end of July over 25,900 American wounded, more than one-third of the total number evacuated, had returned from France by plane (*Table* 7). As envisioned in the NEPTUNE plans, ground and air forces shared responsibility for air evacuation. The First Army's engineer special brigade medical battalions delivered patients to designated landing fields in Normandy. The IX Troop Carrier Command assigned an air evacuation officer to coordinate its efforts with those of the army and also furnished C–47 transports to care for the wounded in flight. In Britain the Communications Zone unloaded casualties from air-

TABLE 7—CROSS-CHANNEL EVACUATION, JUNE–JULY 1944

Month	Air	Water	Total
June	6,469	20,923	27,392
July	19,490	18,195	37,685
Total	25,959	39,118	65,077

Source: Evacuation Branch, Operations Division, OofCSurg, HQ, ETOUSA, Annual Rpt, 1944, encl. 10.

craft and dispatched them to hospitals.[26]

Most air-evacuated casualties landed at the Ramsbury and Membury airfields in the Southern Base Section, which the Ninth Air Force had designated for this purpose before D-Day. At each base a field hospital platoon (the 3d of the 6th at Ramsbury and the 2d of the 28th at Membury), reinforced by an auxiliary surgical team, acted as a holding unit. Set up in tents close to the runways, these hospitals retained nontransportables selected by plane-side triage officers for emergency surgery and resuscitation. Ambulances, from the field hospitals and an attached ambulance company, took evacuees able to travel to two station and two general hospitals within a 30-mile radius, which served as transit facilities. From then on, the evacuation pattern was the same as that for seaborne patients. The airstrip holding units, which could remove a C–47's cargo of 24 litter cases in no more than eight minutes, between them could process 1,000 wounded a day, although actual daily flow averaged about half that number. Patients generally showed no ill effects from their flight, except for a few with chest and abdominal injuries who were evacuated too early after surgery in France.[27]

As the logistical efficiency and medical advantages of air evacuation became apparent, the medical service and the Air Force opened additional receiving facilities at Merryfield, Rednall, and Tarrant Rushton airfields. Located close to general hospitals, these fields required no elaborate holding and transit arrangements. The medical service, accordingly, stationed only a small holding element at Merryfield and placed detachments of litterbearers and ambulances at the

[26] Link and Coleman *AAF Medical Support*, pp. 598–600; Surg, Ninth Air Force, Annual Rpt, 1944, pp. 16 and 21–22; Surg, IX Troop Carrier Command, Annual Rpt, 1944, p. 9. On the NEPTUNE plans, see An. 6—Medical, pp. 13–14, to FUSA Plan, 25 Feb 44; An. 8—Medical, p. 8, to ADSEC Plan, 30 Apr 44; and An. 9—Medical, pp. 13–14, to FECOMZ Plan, 14 May 44. All in file HD 370 ETO. See also O/CS Continental SOP, 4 Apr 44, pp. 12–13, file 370.02. On statistics, see Evacuation Branch, Operations Division, OofCSurg, HQ, ETOUSA, Annual Rpt, 1944, p. 13 and encl. 10; Memo, Kenner, 26 Jul 44, sub: Evacuation of Casualties by Air, in Medical Division, COSSAC/SHAEF, War Diary, July 1944.

[27] Surg, United Kingdom Base, Annual Rpt, 1944, p. 24; 6th Field Hospital Annual Rpt, 1944, pp. 3–4; 28th Field Hospital Hist, 1944, pp. 5–6 and 30, box 412, RG 112, NARA; Evacuation Branch, Operations Division, OofCSurg, HQ, ETOUSA, Daily Diary, June–July 1944, file HD 024 ETO; 98th General Hospital Annual Rpt, 1944, pp. 2 and 38–39; 598th Ambulance Company Annual Rpt, 1944, p. 3; correspondence in Medical Division, COSSAC/SHAEF, War Diary, June–August 1944; Ltr, Hawley to Col Thomas, 28 Jul 44, file HD 024 ETO CS (Hawley Chron).

other two fields. Meanwhile, the two original evacuation air bases, Ramsbury and Membury, continued in operation, with the 6th Field Hospital during July taking over the entire holding mission at both places. The number of nontransportable wounded arriving at these fields dwindled steadily, reducing the hospital to the tasks of triage and ambulance-loading, much to the discontent of the unit's professional staff. With all these bases available, the medical service by late July had the capacity to handle 6,000 air-evacuated casualties per day. General Kenner and Colonel Cutler hoped that air transportation on this scale would permit the service to abandon the LST as a means of carrying wounded, especially as the opening of continental ports facilitated use of the hospital carriers. Air evacuation, however, was subject to other limitations than the capacity of receiving fields in England, and Kenner's and Cutler's hopes were not to be realized.[28]

The expansion of air evacuation, combined with the lighter-than-expected invasion casualties and the opening of First Army hospitals, rendered superfluous much of the elaborate network of port holding units and transit hospitals. Accordingly, the Communications Zone during June redeployed two of the four field hospitals, the 12th and 28th, from Portland-Weymouth and Southampton and gradually detached ambulance and collecting companies from the 33d Medical and 93d Medical Gas Treatment Battalions. All the medical receiving units left the smaller Channel ports. In late June General Hawley's office returned all but five of the Southern Base Section transit hospitals to regular duty. Nevertheless, sea evacuation by LSTs was to continue. On 18 July the theater commander and the commander of the United States Naval Forces in Europe agreed that the Navy would furnish landing ships, in diminishing numbers, for transport of wounded through 1 October, by which date French ports should be open for hospital ships and carriers and the autumn storms would cause all logistical activity on the beaches to cease.[29]

During the first two months of the campaign over 65,000 casualties

[28] Surg, United Kingdom Base, Annual Rpt, 1944, pp. 24–25; Evacuation Branch, Operations Division, OofCSurg, HQ, ETOUSA, Daily Diary, June–July 1944, file HD 024 ETO; Surg, Western Base Section, Rpt, 1 Jan–31 Aug 44, pp. 9–10; 6th Field Hospital Annual Rpt, pp. 3–4 and 6; Memo, Kenner, 26 Jul 44, sub: Evacuation of Casualties by Air, in Medical Division, COSSAC/SHAEF, War Diary, July 1944; Memo, Cutler to Hawley, 30 Jun 44, in Professional Services Division, OofCSurg, HQ, ETOUSA, Annual Rpt, 1944, Chief Consultant in Surgery sec., p. 12.

[29] The remaining transit hospitals, all station hospitals, were: 38th (Winchester), 110th (Netley), 228th (Sherbourne Park), 305th (Wardon Hill), and 315th (Axminster), with a total of 5,093 beds. This list does not include the hospitals doing air evacuation transit duty, usually in addition to regular functions. See Essential Technical Medical Data Rpt, HQ, ETOUSA, June 1944, encl. 2; 33d Medical and 93d Medical Gas Treatment Battalions Annual Rpts, 1944; 7th and 12th Field Hospitals Annual Rpts, 1944; 28th Field Hospital Hist, 1944, box 412, RG 112, NARA; 48th General Hospital Annual Rpt, 1944, p. 5; Evacuation Branch, Operations Division, OofCSurg, HQ, ETOUSA, Daily Diary, 22 Jun 44, file HD 024 ETO; Memo, Col D. E. Liston to G–4, ETO, 10 Jun 44, EvacCorresp, 1942–44, file HD 024 ETO. See also in EvacCorresp, 1944–45, file HD 370.05 ETO, the following: Memo, Liston to Capt J. H. Chambers, MC, USN, 13 Jul 44, sub: LST Requirements for Evacuation of Patients; Ltr, Cdr, NAVFOREU, to CG, ETO, 18 Jul 44, sub: Intra-Theater Evacuation of Casualties; Ltr, Liston to G–4, ETO, 30 Jul 44.

passed across the Channel into the hospitals so laboriously constructed under the BOLERO program. Except for the fact that the casualty receiving system turned out to have been overbuilt for the number of patients it handled, this portion of COMZ medical support went essentially according to plan. The same could not be said for the effort to establish COMZ medical support in Normandy. On the Continent the medical service, like the other technical services, ran afoul of the slow progress of the attack. By late July the resulting delays in opening facilities, especially general hospitals, had compelled major revisions in the COMZ medical plan.[30]

ADSEC Medics in Normandy

Shortly before D-Day the ADSEC surgeon, Colonel Beasley, and his staff were alerted and began staging for movement to France. Officers of Beasley's section landed at OMAHA and UTAH beaches on 12 June, and Beasley himself came ashore on the sixteenth. Two days later Beasley and the advance elements of his office established themselves at Auville-sur-le-Vey near Carentan, close by the main ADSEC headquarters at Catz. During the next month the rest of the 100-man section, in prearranged increments, disembarked at UTAH; marched to concentration areas; and then rode in trucks to Auville. Housed in battle-damaged dwellings and in tents in an apple orchard, the medical section until late in July was only a few miles behind the front, shaken constantly by the blast of nearby American artillery and in danger from German shelling and air raids aimed at a nearby bridge.[31]

During their first month in Normandy, Beasley and his growing staff, in keeping with the subordinate status of ADSEC, worked under Colonel Rogers, the First Army surgeon. Beasley, who initially had little to do but keep up with army activities, attended Rogers' daily conferences. The heads of the various divisions of Beasley's office established close liaison with their First Army counterparts, and with the medical staffs of 21 Army Group and the Ninth Air Force. Gradually, they found employment in overseeing the disembarkation and positioning of ADSEC medical units, and they prepared to take over particular support functions as Rogers directed. The latter process began on 19 July, when Rogers transferred to Beasley responsibility for the receipt, storage, and issue of medical supplies arriving on the beaches and at Cherbourg.[32]

In the crucial matter of evacuation the ADSEC surgeon's role was still evolving when the Battle of the Hedgerows ended. In accordance with NEPTUNE plans the Advance Section was to assume command of the engineer special brigades around D+25 (1 July) and was to be directing most

[30] Evacuation Branch, Operations Division, OofCSurg, HQ, ETOUSA, Annual Rpt, 1944, encl. 10.

[31] Surg, ADSEC, COMZ, Annual Rpt, 1944, pp. 6–7 and 14–15; Joseph R. Darnall, "Scouting for Hospital Sites in Normandy," *The Military Surgeon* 101 (September 1947): 192–93 and 196.

[32] Surg, ADSEC, COMZ, Annual Rpt, 1944, pp. 7 and 26. See also in Charles H. Beasley Papers, MHI, the following: Surg, ADSEC, Daily Activities Rpts, June–July 1944; Supply Division, OofSurg, ADSEC, Weekly Activities Rpts, weeks ending 8 and 22 Jul 44.

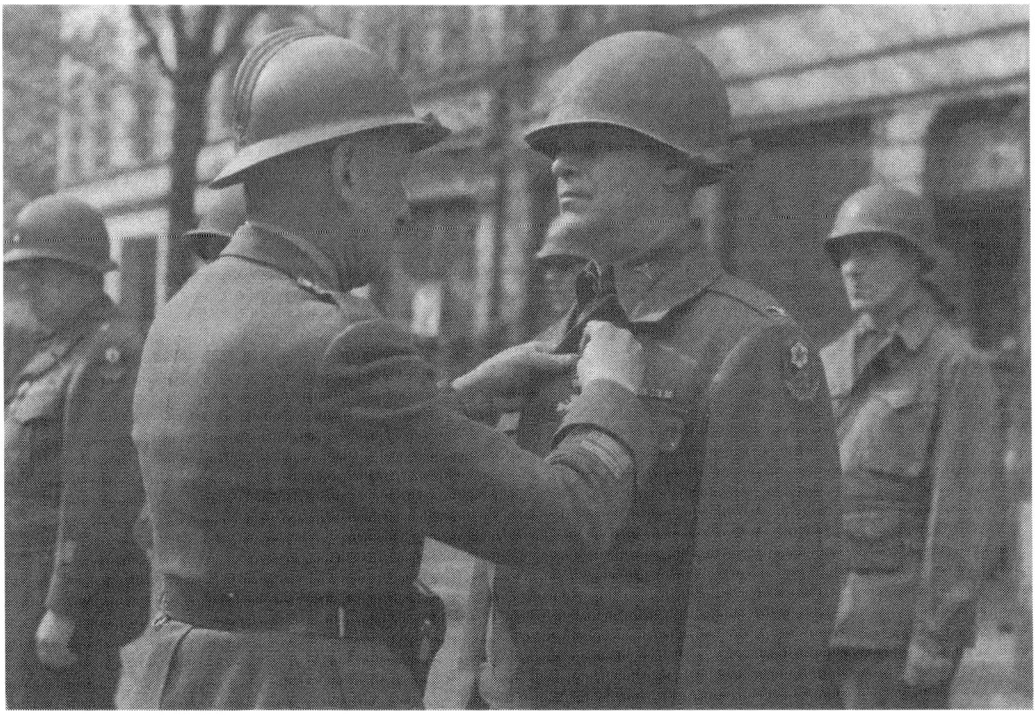

COL. CHARLES A. BEASLEY, *the ADSEC surgeon, receiving a decoration from the French in April 1945*

evacuation to the rear of the army hospitals by the forty-first day of the campaign. In practice, the transfer went more slowly and in a less orderly manner. Not until 8 July did Beasley's office begin receiving daily First Army reports on the number of patients being evacuated by air and sea. As the army finally drew an ADSEC forward boundary, Beasley assumed control of most evacuation in the northern Cotentin, for both army and COMZ units, and on the twenty-fourth the First Army turned over to the Advance Section command of its holding facility at OMAHA and of the evacuation center at UTAH. At the end of the month, however, no single headquarters coordinated the flow of patients out of Normandy. Evacuation officers of the Advance Section, First Army, and Ninth Air Force, as well as the engineer special brigade medical battalion commanders, all had a hand in the process. As a result, according to General Hawley's chief of evacuation,

> there is no clear delineation of responsibility, and evacuation just occurs . . . . In the Omaha sector casualties are evacuated from evacuation hospitals, field hospitals, and the 4th Convalescent Hospital to the 'holding unit' . . . whenever the respective hospital commanders feel like evacuating patients. In some instances, individual hospitals have put patients directly on planes without passing through the 'holding unit'. . . . In the Utah sector, ASCZ [ADSEC] has allotted ten . . . ambulances to each evacuation hos-

pital. These hospitals evacuate patients whenever they desire to either the 'holding unit' [set up by ADSEC] near the airstrip at Binniville [*sic*] or to the holding unit at Utah Beach. ASCZ attempts to designate which 'holding unit' will be used . . . . The problem is a difficult one and all appear to be cooperating, but there is no central control [to] coordinate all evacuation operations which is most essential.[33]

During the last days of June, as the First Army completed the conquest of Cherbourg and the northern Cotentin Peninsula, ADSEC medical units began landing and going into operation (*see Map 10*). Medical battalions and field and evacuation hospitals led the way, their mission to support the other ADSEC troops pouring into Normandy and to supplement army facilities as required. Most of these units arrived behind schedule, their sailings from England postponed to make way for combat forces. Many, their planned sites still German-occupied or in use by other organizations, waited in temporary bivouacs while the ADSEC G-4 went through the complicated process of negotiating with his First Army counterpart for new locations. Because the army allowed troops to stay only twenty-four hours in its beach assembly areas, Colonel Beasley used early-arriving field hospitals to run transit camps for his units at OMAHA and UTAH.[34]

One of the first ADSEC medical organizations to reach Normandy, the 12th Field Hospital, had no need to wait long in transit camp. This hospital, early relieved from duty as a holding unit at Portland-Weymouth, disembarked at OMAHA beach on 26 June and three days later went directly to its previously assigned location: the French Naval Hospital at Cherbourg, where the 12th was to care for patients while preparing the premises for later occupation by a general hospital. The men and women of the 12th rode to Cherbourg in vehicles of the 68th Medical Group, which was clearing wounded German prisoners from the port city. When they entered the Naval Hospital, they found filth and chaos. The building, a huge quadrangle dating from the 1860s with flanking modern pavilions, had housed one of the three large German medical installations overrun when Cherbourg fell. During the siege an inadequate German staff, augmented by two captured U.S. Army doctors, had tried to care for over 1,000 of their own wounded and about 150 American prisoners. Before the 12th moved in, the 68th Medical Group had evacuated all the freed Americans and the transportable Germans, but about 400 POW patients remained, many of them nontransportables shifted from the other two captured hospitals. The Naval Hospital

[33] Quotation from Memo, Col Mowrey to Hawley, 27 Jul 44, sub: Report on Trip to Continent, file 370.05. See also An. 8—Medical, pp. 4-5, to ADSEC Plan, 30 Apr 44, file 370 ETO; Evacuation Branch, Operations Division, OofCSurg, HQ ETOUSA, Annual Rpt, 1944, pp. 5-6; First U.S. Army Report of Operations, 20 Oct 43-1 Aug 44, bk. VII, p. 72; Surg, ADSEC, COMZ, Annual Rpt, 1944, pp. 8 and 16; and, in the Beasley Papers, MHI, Surg, ADSEC, Daily Activities Rpts, 3, 10, 13 and 17 Jul 44, and Evacuation Branch, OofSurg, ADSEC, Weekly Activities Rpts, weeks ending 23 Jun and 10 Jul 44.

[34] Surg, ADSEC, Daily Activities Rpts, 5-31 Jul 44, Beasley Papers, MHI; ADSEC Hist, pp. 28-30; Surg, ADSEC, COMZ, Annual Rpt, 1944, pp. 7-8 and 14. See also An. 8—Medical, p. 6 and encls. 1-2, to ADSEC Plan, 30 Apr 44, file 370 ETO, which gives original unit location and missions.

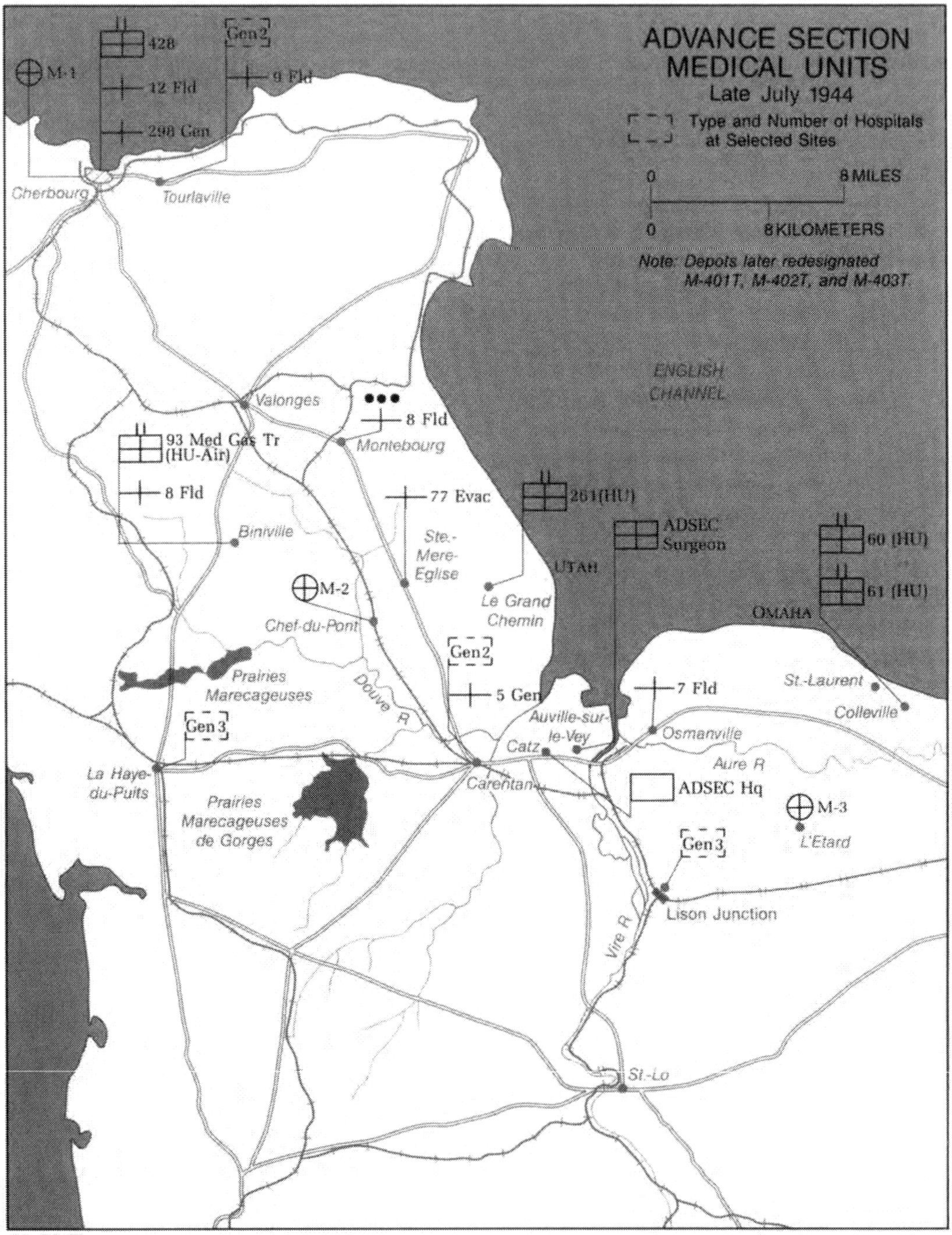
ADVANCE SECTION
MEDICAL UNITS
Late July 1944
Type and Number of Hospitals at Selected Sites
0
8 MILES
0
8 KILOMETERS
Note: Depots later redesignated M-401T, M-402T, and M-403T.
428
M-1
12 Fld
298 Gen
Gen 2
9 Fld
Cherbourg
Tourlaville
ENGLISH CHANNEL
Valonges
8 Fld
Montebourg
93 Med Gas Tr (HU-Air)
8 Fld
77 Evac
261(HU)
Biniville
Ste.-Mere-Eglise
ADSEC Surgeon
60 (HU)
UTAH
M-2
Le Grand Chemin
61 (HU)
OMAHA
Chef-du-Pont
Gen 2
Prairies Marecageuses
Douve R
5 Gen
7 Fld
St.-Laurent
Colleville
Gen 3
Auville-sur-le-Vey
Osmanville
Catz
Aure R
La Haye-du-Puits
Carentan
ADSEC Hq
M-3
Prairies Marecageuses de Gorges
Gen 3
L'Etard
Lison Junction
Vire R
St.-Lo

MAP 10

had had no running water for the last week of the siege; discipline had broken down; and French civilian doctors, who had used part of the building under the occupation, now were looting the supplies of their former conquerors. According to the 12th's commander,

> the sanitary facilities were virtually non-existent—bed pans and urinals were used again and again without being cleaned and . . . were at the bedside of the patients; no attempt has been made to provide for any form of laundry facilities and thus filth was evident on the bedding and on the patients themselves. The stench which emanated from these wards is one that can never be dismissed from the minds of those who worked therein. Perhaps the operating theater, an underground set-up, presented the most ghastly scene. Surgeons of the German staff had been operating for . . . 72 hours non-stop and with water unavailable, no attempt had been made to clean up the place. Debris from amputations lay in various receptacles about the operating . . . tables and blood and filth was evident throughout the rooms. On the grounds in back of the hospital, as well as in the morgue, still remained the unburied bodies of soldiers and civilians; and dumped on the ground near the mess hall, amputated extremities were in abundance, brought there from the operating room.[35]

Medics of the 12th Field Hospital fell to work, cleaning up and repairing wards, operating rooms, kitchen, and mess hall. They restored the water supply. They supervised captured German medical personnel, assembled from all three overrun hospitals, in caring for their wounded countrymen until the last POWs were evacuated early in July. Supplementing their equipment and medical supplies with confiscated German articles, the Americans opened 400 beds for their own patients on 30 June. The 12th functioned as a small general hospital, receiving sick and injured from the Cherbourg area, including many mine and booby-trap casualties from the port clearing operations. Under the First Army evacuation policy the hospital retained men returnable to duty within ten days; it sent other patients by ambulance to UTAH beach for transportation to England. In addition to its other tasks, the 12th housed and fed medical organizations awaiting deployment in the upper Cotentin.[36]

Other ADSEC medical units went into operation throughout the Cotentin and in the crowded space inland of OMAHA beach. Typically, these organizations moved to their assigned locations in their own vehicles, or in transport borrowed from other units, over roads marked "Mines Cleared to Hedges Only." Usually setting up in hedged fields, the medical people had to clear away battle debris—discarded equipment, glider wreckage, and occasionally bodies or parts of bodies—before they could erect their facilities. The more enterprising organizations found uses for some of the litter. Salvaged wood from glider frames, for example, went into floors and furniture for living quarters and work spaces.[37]

[35] Quotation from 12th Field Hospital Annual Rpt, 1944, p. 5. See also Surg, ADSEC, COMZ, Annual Rpt, 1944, p. 7; Darnall, "Hospital Sites in Normandy," p. 194. On clearing captured hospitals, see VII Corps Medical Plan, pp. 27–28, encl. 1 to Surg, VII Corps, Annual Rpt, 1944; 68th Medical Group Annual Rpt, 1944.

[36] 12th Field Hospital Annual Rpt, 1944, pp. 5–6.

[37] For typical descriptions of countryside, cleanup, and salvage, see 8th Field Hospital Annual Rpt, 1944, p. 5, and Allen, ed., *Medicine Under Canvas*, pp. 108–11.

The 428th Medical Battalion, with four attached ambulance companies, disembarked between 28 June and 8 July. With its headquarters at Cherbourg and its companies spread throughout the Cotentin, the battalion evacuated First Army and ADSEC units and hospitals. The 7th Field Hospital opened at Osmanville, in the OMAHA area, early in July; it treated patients from the Advance Section, received some battle casualties, and administered one of the medical transit camps. Another field hospital, the 8th, set up one of its platoons at Montebourg in the Cotentin to perform similar functions. On 12 July still another field hospital, the 9th, occupied a site at Tourlaville, on the outskirts of Cherbourg, but it could not go into operation until the thirtieth, when its equipment, lost in disembarkation, at last was delivered. The 77th Evacuation Hospital, a 750-bed unit, again after a frustrating wait for a misdirected equipment assembly, opened near Ste.-Mere-Eglise on the fifteenth. This unit admitted casualties from First Army evacuation hospitals so that the latter could clear their wards and move forward; it also received wounded directly from division clearing stations.[38]

Under an agreement with the First Army, made on 17 July, the Advance Section opened an air evacuation holding unit at Biniville, about 15 miles south of Cherbourg, to support the army's right wing. For this purpose Colonel Beasley employed the 93d Medical Gas Treatment Battalion, which had landed on the fifteenth, reinforced for emergency surgery by a platoon of the 8th Field Hospital. The units opened their installations on the twentieth, in a tented camp spread over several hedgerow-lined fields. Later augmented by the rest of the 8th, the Biniville holding unit could accommodate almost 900 patients. It received casualties from army hospitals, and at times from battalion aid stations; held them for treatment when required; and, when they were ready to travel, loaded them on aircraft at a nearby airstrip used exclusively for evacuation. The unit assembled planeloads and moved them out on short notice, to minimize waits by the C-47s on a runway still subject to *Luftwaffe* attacks. This ADSEC holding unit supplemented the OMAHA beach facility operated by the 60th and 61st Medical Battalions. The latter installation, which had moved on the sixteenth from its St.-Laurent site to an airfield 2 miles south of Colleville, came under ADSEC command on the twenty-fourth.[39]

[38] First U.S. Army Report of Operations, 20 Oct 43-1 Aug 44, bk. VII, p. 72; ADSEC Hist, p. 19; Surg, ADSEC, COMZ, Annual Rpt, 1944, pp. 14, 16, ex. J; 7th Field Hospital Annual Rpt, 1944, pp. 1-2; 8th Field Hospital Annual Rpt, 1944, pp. 3-7; 9th Field Hospital Annual Rpt, 1944, pp. 3-6; 77th Evacuation Hospital Annual Rpt, 1944, pp. 1-7; Allen, ed., *Medicine Under Canvas*, pp. 108-11; Darnall, "Hospital Sites in Normandy," p. 198. See also in Beasley Papers, MHI, the following: Surg, ADSEC, Daily Activities Rpts, 8 and 12 Jul 44; Evacuation Division, OofSurg, ADSEC, Weekly Activities Rpts, weeks ending 10 and 22 Jul 44; Hospitalization Division, OofSurg, ADSEC, Weekly Activities Rpt, week ending 9 Jul 44.

[39] Surg, ADSEC, Daily Activities Rpts, 16-17 and 20 Jul 44, and Evacuation Division, OofSurg, ADSEC, Weekly Activities Rpt, week ending 22 Jul 44, in Beasley Papers, MHI; 93d Medical Gas Treatment Battalion Annual Rpt, 1944, pp. 6-9; 8th Field Hospital Annual Rpt, 1944, pp. 6-7; Memo, Mowrey to Hawley, 27 Jul 44, sub: Report on Trip to Continent, file 370.05.

In connection with its assumption of responsibility for medical supply to the rear of First Army, the Advance Section during July reclaimed from the army command of its 30th and 31st Medical Depot Companies and brought in another, the 13th, to reinforce them. Colonel Beasley's Supply Division set up three new depots. On the tenth a platoon of the 30th Company established Depot M–1 (later redesignated M–401T) in a taken-over building in Cherbourg, to distribute medical supplies to units in the northern Cotentin and to receive and store materiel landed at the port once it opened. Ten days later, the 32d Medical Depot Company, a Third Army unit soon replaced by the 13th Company, organized Depot M–2 (M–402T) at Chef-du-Pont, to receive, store, and issue supplies brought in over UTAH beach. This depot drew its initial stock from the First Army dump at Le Grand Chemin, which then closed. To handle supplies coming in at OMAHA, the 31st Company set up Depot M–3 (M–403T) at L'Etard on the nineteenth. This depot also replaced the rearmost First Army dumps and took over their stocks. Both the Chef-du-Pont and L'Etard depots, part of larger ADSEC storage areas, consisted simply of open fields in which crated supplies were stacked, with a few ward tents sheltering loose items and administration offices.[40]

[40] Supply Division, OofCSurg, HQ, ETOUSA, Annual Rpt, 1944, sec. II, pp. 1–2 and 7–8; Surg, ADSEC, COMZ, Annual Rpt, 1944, pp. 25–26 and ex. K; Supply Division, OofSurg, ADSEC, Weekly Activities Rpts, weeks ending 15 and 22 Jul 44, and ADSEC Stock Control Team Progress Rpts, 25 Jul and 1 Aug 44, in Beasley Papers, MHI. Ruppenthal, *Logistical Support,* 1:431–33, covers overall development of ADSEC depots.

For the most part, the establishment of ADSEC supply facilities and field and evacuation hospitals in Normandy followed preinvasion NEPTUNE plans, with modifications due to delayed movement and the occasional need to find alternate locations. The same could not be said of the section's effort to set up 1,000-bed general hospitals on the Continent. Execution of this part of the medical program became snarled in confusion and delay, resulting largely from the First Army's failure to attain its planned tactical objectives.

Before D-Day the Advance Section and the Forward Echelon had made detailed plans for moving twenty-five general hospitals, selected by General Hawley on the basis of performance in Great Britain, into various French cities during the first ninety days of the campaign. Early in May, following a schedule contained in the plans, the first of these general hospitals began turning over their British plants, complete with furnishings and supplies, to units newly arrived from the United States. Relieved about a month before their sailing dates, the deploying hospitals went into temporary billets, usually in the Western Base Section. There, they conducted training and prepared vehicles and personal equipment for the cross-Channel voyage. For each hospital Hawley's Supply Division set up a complete equipment assembly—a block of materiel filling almost sixty small British freight cars—at one of its depots, where the unit medical supply officer checked it for completeness and oversaw its crating for shipment. While hospitals waited to be called forward for embarkation, they furnished surgical teams, nurses, and enlisted men for mounting and casualty reception assignments; and they provided custodial details for newly completed but not yet occupied hospital plants.[41]

The first two general hospitals to reach Normandy, the 5th and 298th, stood down from operations in Britain respectively on 7 and 10 May. Col. Maxwell G. Keeler's 5th General Hospital, the initial unit of its type to enter the European Theater back in 1942, staged at Tidworth until its embarkation on 3 July. Three days later the unit's 58 officers, 102 nurses, and 500 enlisted men, with their vehicles, came ashore at OMAHA beach; however, its hospital assembly, sent from England on a different vessel, did not. Keeler's supply officer searched beachhead dumps to no avail, only to discover eventually that the assembly, scheduled to be landed at still unusable Cherbourg, had been held on shipboard awaiting discharge at one of the beaches. Even if the equipment had been immediately available, the 5th would have had no place to set it up; the hospital's assigned location at St.-Lo still was German-held. Fortunately, the unit was prepared to operate in an expeditionary tented plant. On the tenth Colonel Keeler and Colonel Beasley decided to place it on a new site, a low-lying field near Carentan. The 5th spent the next twenty-one days bivouacked with the 7th Field Hospital at Osmanville, waiting for engineers to complete construction of its facility. In the meantime it detached surgical and shock teams to First Army evacuation hospitals and sent most of its remaining medical officers, all its nurses, and 100 enlisted men to help the 12th Field Hospital with cleaning and repairs at Cherbourg.[42]

The second general hospital to land in Normandy, the 298th, a University of Michigan-affiliated unit under Lt. Col. Walter G. Maddock, MC, was assigned to occupy the Cherbourg Naval Hospital that the 12th Field Hospital was rehabilitating. A victim of shipping schedule changes, the 298th spent two months shuttling between camps in Wales and England, ending up only a few miles from its former site at Frenchay Park, near Bristol. The unit personnel at last embarked at Plymouth on 15 July and waded ashore on UTAH beach the next day, again separated from their equipment assembly. They moved into billets in houses and barracks in Cherbourg on the seventeenth. The 298th at least had a plant to occupy. It prepared to relieve the 12th in the Naval Hospital and continued the smaller unit's work of cleaning and refurbishing, while engineers began the extensive alternations needed to fit the old plant for a 1,000-bed general hospital.[43]

---

[41] Troop Movements and Training Branch, Operations Division, OofCSurg, HQ, ETOUSA, Annual Rpt, 1944, pp. 13–14 and encl. 15; Surg, ADSEC, COMZ, Annual Rpt, 1944, p. 14; Technical Directive No. 1, OofCSurg, HQ, ETOUSA, 17 May 44, sub: Procedure for Equipping General Hospitals To Be Utilized in Continental Operations, in Supply Division, OofCSurg, HQ, ETOUSA, Annual Rpt, sec. V, ex. 1 (see also sec. II, p. 6).

[42] Darnall, "Hospital Sites in Normandy," pp. 191–92; 5th General Hospital Annual Rpt, 1944, pp. 4–7; Keeler Interv, 11 Jul 45, box 223, RG 112, NARA; Surg, ADSEC, Daily Activities Rpts, 9–11 Jul 44, Beasley Papers, MHI.

[43] 298th General Hospital Annual Rpt, 1944, pp. 1, 61–65, 72–74, 78, 233–34, 299–300.

Even as the 298th was settling down in Cherbourg, the Advance Section and the chief surgeon's office undertook a major revision of fixed hospital plans. Those plans had called for twelve of the continental general hospitals, including the two already landed, to be functioning in France by mid-July; but at that time the 5th and 298th still were not open. The ground forces had yet to capture the sites of the other ten hospitals. General Hawley now confronted a sudden fixed bed shortage. His plans for providing beds to care for the still expanding American force in the theater depended on the prompt establishment of hospitals in France, since completion of the pre-D-Day program would use up the supply of available United Kingdom locations. Twenty-five of Hawley's best general hospitals, those staging for movement, were out of action. At the same time, with no fixed COMZ beds in France, the field forces had to evacuate even their lightly wounded back across the Channel, threatening to overload the nearshore hospitals. Colonel Mowrey, the Evacuation Branch chief, warned Hawley on 21 July that the general hospitals had room for only about 6,900 more patients. "The patient census has increased 14,533 in the past two weeks," he reported, "or an average increase of 1,032 per day; hence, it is anticipated that general hospitals will be filled within approximately eight days." At SHAEF General Kenner, whose calculations of the impending bed shortage reached about the same conclusion as Mowrey's, pressed for speed in setting up fixed hospitals in Normandy. Even before receiving Kenner's and Mowrey's pessimistic forecasts, Hawley adopted the only feasible solution to the problem: He scrapped the originally planned sites and ordered Colonel Beasley immediately to set up as many general hospitals as possible wherever they would fit in the existing beachhead. "We simply must get beds operating over there," he told Beasley, "regardless of changes in locations." [44]

The chief surgeon and his staff intervened directly to get the revised hospitalization program moving. Between 15 and 19 July Hawley's Hospitalization Division chief, Colonel Darnall, conferred at Auville with Beasley and his staff. In these discussions Darnall emphasized the need for rapid action, and in company with ADSEC and First Army officers he did preliminary reconnaissance throughout the beachhead for general hospital sites. Hawley himself visited the Advance Section on the seventeenth, escorting Secretary of War Henry L. Stimson, Surgeon General Kirk, and General Lee. Shortly thereafter, the chief surgeon by letter exhorted Beasley, whom he considered overly influenced by geographical phase lines, to move rapidly and flexibly. On 22 July Colonel Mowrey flew over to coordinate plans with the

[44] First quotation from Ltr, Mowrey to DepCSurg, HQ, ETOUSA, 21 Jul 44, sub: Evacuation Policy to ZI, EvacCorresp, 1944–45, file HD 370.05 ETO. Mowrey's calculations included only fixed beds for definitive long-term care, excluding transit and holding beds. Second quotation from Ltr, Hawley to Beasley, 19 Jul 44, file HD 024 ETO CS (Hawley Chron). See also Memo, Kenner to ACofS, G–4, SHAEF, 21 Jul 44, sub: Present Status of Fixed US Hospital Beds, UK and Continent, in Medical Division, COSSAC/SHAEF, War Diary, July 1944; Darnall, "Hospital Sites in Normandy," p. 191; Hospitalization Division, OofCSurg, HQ, ETOUSA, Annual Rpt, 1944, p. 8.

ADSEC and First Army medical and engineer authorities and again to press for swift action. Working under this high-level pressure, Beasley's staff, between the twenty-third and twenty-ninth, secured from the First Army ten sites for expeditionary-type tented general hospitals. In the OMAHA area the Advance Section obtained five locations: three at Lison Junction, on a rail line to Cherbourg; and two at Carentan, including the one previously selected for the 5th General Hospital. The remaining five sites were in the Cotentin: three at La Haye-du-Puits, at the base of the peninsula, and two at Tourlaville, just outside Cherbourg.[45]

The ADSEC surgeon, under peremptory direction from Hawley, expedited the opening of the two general hospitals already in Normandy, the 5th and 298th. Construction of the 5th's tented plant at Carentan had begun on 14 July, but neither that unit nor the 298th had received its equipment assembly. On the twenty-second Colonel Beasley's Supply Division finally released to these units two hospital assemblies that had arrived for other organizations not yet landed. This action resulted in the opening of the 298th on the twenty-ninth and that of the 5th two days later. Both units initially had less than half their beds in operation. The 298th began work amid the noise and debris of construction, as engineers struggled to renovate "a building for which they had no . . . plans, whose wiring and plumbing was a composite of 80 years' development, a continental hodgepodge that often defied analysis." Major alterations continued until shortly before the 298th left in October. In the meantime the staff, besides caring for patients in temporary facilities, kept busy with a host of minor repairs and tried to make do with barely adequate, always unreliable, water and power supplies. At Carentan the 5th also began operations while still under construction, receiving patients before it had either electric lights or running water. Its hastily chosen, poorly drained site was mosquito infested and turned into a quagmire with every rainstorm.[46]

Both general hospitals eventually expanded beyond their rated capacities, each attaining a size of about 1,500 beds. Under a First Army-ADSEC agreement on 1 August the 5th and 298th, besides acting as area station hospitals, admitted lightly wounded men returnable to duty within ten days. They thereby relieved army installations of these patients

[45] Darnall, "Hospital Sites in Normandy," pp. 191–201; Ltr, Hawley to Beasley, 19 Jul 44, and Memo, Hawley to G-4, ETO, 5 Aug 44, sub: Hospitalization and Evacuation—Cherbourg Peninsula, file HD 024 ETO CS (Hawley Chron); Memo, Mowrey to Hawley, 27 Jul 44, sub: Report on Trip to Continent, file 370.05; Surg, ADSEC, COMZ, Annual Rpt, 1944, pp. 8 and 21–22; Hospitalization Division, OofCSurg, HQ, ETOUSA, Annual Rpt, 1944, pp. 8–9; Surg, ADSEC, Daily Activities Rpts, 23 and 25 Jul 44, and Hospitalization Division, OofSurg, ADSEC, Weekly Activities Rpt, week ending 29 Jul 44, Beasley Papers, MHI.

[46] Quotation from 298th General Hospital Annual Rpt, pp. 78–81. See also 5th General Hospital Annual Rpt, 1944, pp. 7–8, 10–11, 13–15; Hospitalization Division, OofSurg, ADSEC, Weekly Activities Rpt, week ending 29 Jul 44, and Supply Division, OofSurg, ADSEC, Weekly Activities Rpt, week ending 30 Jul 44, Beasley Papers, MHI; Lt Col J. E. Dunphy and Maj. S. O. Hoerr, "A General Hospital in the Normandy Campaign," *The Bulletin of the U.S. Army Medical Department* 6 (November 1946): 594–602.

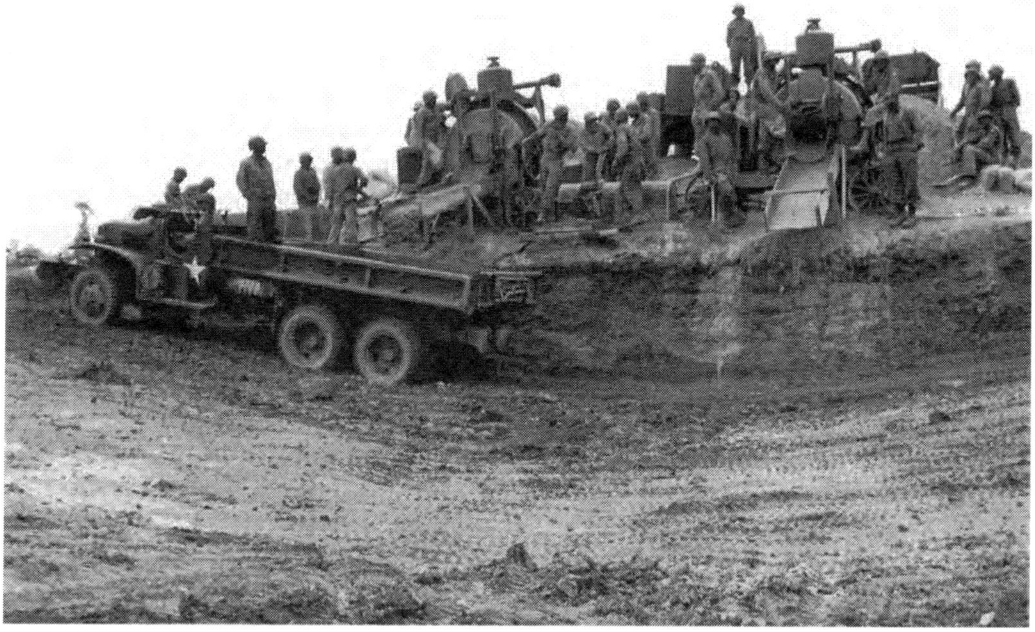

CONSTRUCTING THE 5TH GENERAL HOSPITAL TENTED PLANT AT CARENTAN.
Engineers prepare concrete for the ward platforms, and a completed ward tent with beds.

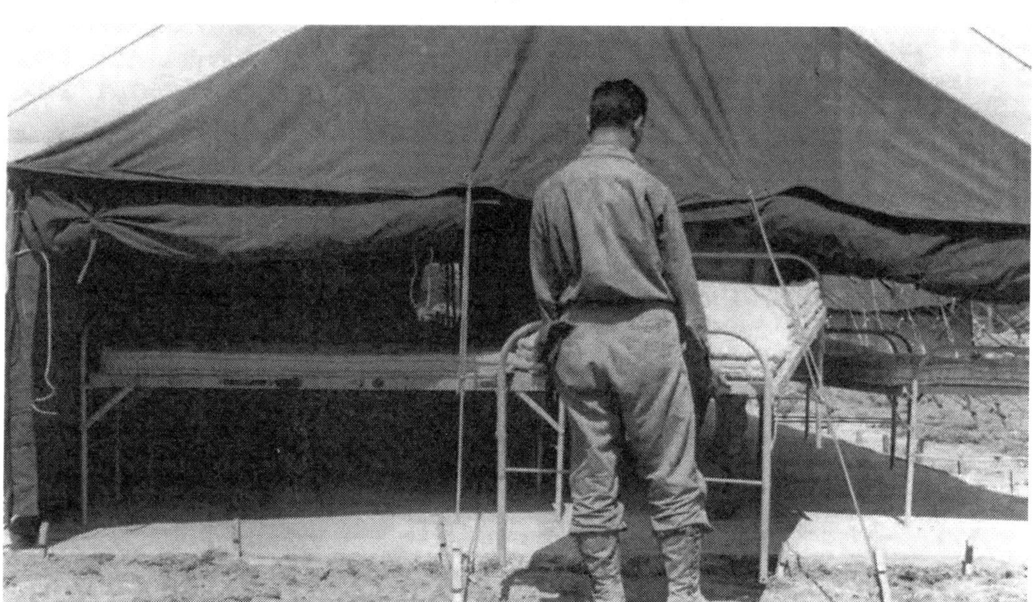

while ensuring their retention on the Continent, a manpower conserving measure strongly desired by General Bradley. The 5th, located close to the fighting line, also became a collecting point for combat exhaustion patients and for soldiers with suspected self-inflicted wounds, a circumstance that led General Kenner to complain that the unit's surgical capabilities were being wasted on the mission of a convalescent hospital. By contrast, the 298th had no lack of emergency surgical patients, mostly mine casualties from the Cherbourg port. For its short-term patients the 298th, without guidance on the point from higher headquarters, during the first weeks followed an informal evacuation procedure. The hospital used its own ambulances to return recovered men directly to their units, or, if the organization were nearby, simply discharged patients and let them find their own way back. Casualties requiring extended care went by ambulance to the Biniville holding unit for evacuation to England.[47]

Establishment of the other nine general hospitals, meanwhile, got under way. General Hawley worked with SHAEF and ETOUSA to hasten the dispatch of more 1,000-bed units to Normandy; and, as these organizations arrived, the Advance Section sent them to bivouac at their assigned operating sites. Most were in position by 5 August. While they awaited completion of their facilities and delivery of their equipment, these general hospitals furnished surgical teams to field force installations and enlisted details to aid the engineers preparing their plants.

ADSEC engineers began construction at the sites between 21 July and 2 August. At each installation the engineer officer in charge and the hospital commander cooperated in adapting standard plans, developed and tested in Britain before D-Day, to ground conditions and to unit preferences. Enlisted medics and engineers labored side by side, pouring concrete tent bases, grading roads and paths, and installing wiring and plumbing. They worked under handicaps. Engineers, few in numbers and in heavy demand, frequently were abruptly transferred to other jobs. Building supplies arrived irregularly, forcing periodic work stoppages at most plants. Short of American materials, the engineers substituted German and French cement and pipe, among other items. The cement often failed to set properly, requiring time-consuming tearing up and repouring of foundations. The mixture of ill-fitting pipe that made up water and sewage systems had to be welded at every joint. Engineers and enlisted medics overcame these obstacles, but slowly. By the third week of August the engineers had managed to finish one plant and had completed 65 to

[47] Surg, ADSEC, Daily Activities Rpt, 1 Aug 44, Beasley Papers, MHI; Memo, Hawley to G-4, ETO, 5 Aug 44, sub: Hospitalization and Evacuation—Cherbourg Peninsula, file HD 024 ETO CS (Hawley Chron); Rpt, Kenner, sub: Inspection of Medical Troops and Installations—12th AG, ADSEC, CZ, and 21 AG, 2-13 August 1944, in Medical Division, COSSAC/SHAEF, War Diary, August 1944; 5th General Hospital Annual Rpt, 1944, p. 8; 298th General Hospital Annual Rpt, 1944, pp. 101-03 and 107; Keeler Interv, 11 Jul 45, box 223, RG 112, NARA.

75 percent of the work on most of the others.[48]

Besides construction delays, missing unit assemblies plagued the hospital program. The transportation system simply could not deliver the personnel of a general hospital and their assigned equipment to the same place at the same time. Changes in unit movement dates, timely notice of which often failed to reach the sending depots, helped to desynchronize shipments. Even when a unit and its assembly left England together, they rarely traveled on the same vessel; frequently, the assembly would be split among several ships that discharged cargo on different beaches. The theater chief of transportation never permitted hospital detachments to accompany their assemblies; hence, equipment arrived on the beaches unescorted and disappeared into various dumps unless a unit representative was there to claim it immediately. Colonel Beasley and his supply officer, Maj. Thomas A. Carilia, MAC, repeatedly remonstrated with the ADSEC G–4 and the Transportation Corps about the assembly problem, but to little avail. Beasley finally resorted to sending one of his officers to visit the OMAHA and UTAH dumps on alternate days, for the sole purpose of finding and redirecting lost equipment. His staff continued the practice, begun with the 5th and 298th, of assigning whatever general hospital assembly was available to any unit otherwise ready to open. This expedient delivered equipment to hospitals that could use it, but it required much exchanging later between organizations that had packed personal property with their assemblies.[49]

The new general hospitals gradually went into operation, most of them initially at less than their rated 1,000 beds. Two Lison units, one at La Haye-du-Puits, and the second Carentan hospital opened on 15 August; another hospital at La Haye became active on the twenty-fourth. The remaining four units, however, did not open until September and October. Long before they did, it had become apparent that the continental Communications Zone would not meet its NEPTUNE goal of having 25,500 fixed hospital beds in operation by D+90.[50]

[48] Hospitalization Division, OofCSurg, HQ, ETOUSA, Annual Rpt, 1944, pp. 9-10; Surg, ADSEC, COMZ, Annual Rpt, 1944, pp. 22 and 63; Surg, ADSEC, Daily Activities Rpts, 11-12, 26 and 28 Jul 44, and Hospitalization Division, OofSurg, ADSEC, Weekly Activities Rpts, weeks ending 5 and 19 Aug 44, Beasley Papers, MHI; Keeler Interv, 11 Jul 45, box 223, RG 112, NARA; Memo, Mowrey to Hawley, 27 Jul 44, sub: Report on Trip to Continent, file 370.05; Memo, Maj S. Blumenthal to Lt Col Meador, 1 Aug 44, EvacCorresp, 1942–44, file HD 024 ETO.

[49] Supply Division, OofCSurg, HQ, ETOUSA, Annual Rpt, 1944, sec. V, pp. 2–3; Supply Division, OofSurg, ADSEC, Weekly Activities Rpts, weeks ending 15 and 22 Jul 44, and Hospitalization Division, OofSurg, ADSEC, Weekly Activities Rpt, week ending 19 Aug 44, Beasley Papers, MHI; Surg, ADSEC, COMZ, Annual Rpt, 1944, pp. 26–27; Ltr, Hawley to Beasley, 19 Jul 44, file HD 024 ETO CS (Hawley Chron). For the exchange problem, see 298th General Hospital Annual Rpt, 1944, pp. 233–34.

[50] Hospitalization Division, OofCSurg, HQ, ETOUSA, Annual Rpt, 1944, p. 9; Surg, ADSEC, Daily Activities Rpts, 14–15 Aug 44, and Hospitalization Division, OofSurg, ADSEC, Weekly Activities Rpts, weeks ending 5 and 19 Aug 44, Beasley Papers, MHI; Rpt, Kenner, sub: Inspection of Medical Troops and Installations—12th AG, ADSEC, CZ, and 21 AG, 2–13 August 1944, in Medical Division, COSSAC/SHAEF, War Diary, August 1944.

At the end of July the Advance Section medical service gradually was carving out its sphere of influence in the Normandy beachhead. Colonel Beasley and his staff were acquiring an increasing amount of control over supply, evacuation, and hospitalization. ADSEC depots and field and evacuation hospitals were in operation, beginning to relieve First Army units of part of the support task. Establishment of general hospitals, delayed by slow adaptation of preinvasion plans to the tactical situation, at last was under way. Ironically, even as the Advance Section thus adjusted to operations in a constricted lodgement, the battlefront broke wide open, initiating a period of mobile warfare that again would force radical change in COMZ medical plans and hasty improvisation in operations.

CHAPTER IX

Breakout and Pursuit

On 25 July 1944, after a week of rest and refitting following the capture of St.-Lo, the First Army launched a new offensive, Operation COBRA, planned by General Bradley as an effort to break completely through a narrow segment of what was looking discouragingly like a stabilized front. The VII Corps, heavily reinforced with infantry and armor and supported by all the artillery that the First Army could assemble, conducted the breakthrough attack. Ahead of the VII Corps, yet so close that misdirected bombs killed 111 American soldiers and wounded 490, were all the available Eighth Air Force heavy bombers and over 1,000 smaller tactical aircraft, which saturated the German front with high explosives and napalm, nearly obliterating the defending division. After a slow start on the twenty-fifth, caused in part by the bombing errors, the COBRA attack and its exploitation by massed American armor rapidly escalated from a breakthrough into a breakout.[1]

The German *Seventh Army,* weakened by the earlier attrition battles and with most of its reserves drawn away by British attacks at Caen, disintegrated before the fast-moving American tank-infantry combat teams and their supporting tactical air power. Coutances, the initial objective of the attack, fell on the twenty-eighth. The VIII Corps, attacking on the right of the VII, took Avranches, 30 miles farther south, on 1 August, positioning American troops to move either westward into Brittany or eastward toward Paris and the Seine. The German armies, now pressed all along the line by the First Army and by Montgomery's British and Canadian forces, had lost their western anchor. Hitler's effort to bottle up the Allies in the Cotentin had collapsed.

With their Normandy confinement at an end, the Americans implemented their NEPTUNE plans for activating a second field army and an army group. On 1 August General Bradley placed in operation General Patton's Third Army, the headquarters of which had moved into the Cotentin during July. Bradley gave the Third

---

[1] This section is based on Blumenson, *Breakout and Pursuit,* chs. X-XXII; Charles B. MacDonald, *The Siegfried Line Campaign,* United States Army in World War II (Washington, D.C.: Office of the Chief of Military History, Department of the Army, 1963), chs. I-VIII; and Hugh M. Cole, *The Lorraine Campaign,* United States Army in World War II (Washington, D.C.: Historical Division, Department of the Army, 1950), chs. I-VI.

Army control of the already committed VIII Corps and of the newly arrived XV and XX Corps. Most divisions and supporting elements of the new army had been in France for some time, attached to the First Army; they now reverted to their original command. Also on the first Bradley activated the 12th Army Group (actually the 1st Army Group headquarters, redesignated as part of the Allied effort to convince the Germans that another invasion still was coming in the Pas-de-Calais). Bradley took command of this army group, while Lt. Gen. Courtney Hodges replaced him at the First Army. General Montgomery remained in overall Allied ground command for another month, until SHAEF opened its continental headquarters on 1 September.

The reorganized Allied ground forces rapidly exploited the success of COBRA. Departing from the original plan so as to take advantage of German disintegration in the western Cotentin, the Third Army used only one of its corps, the VIII, to secure Brittany. This corps, which met only disorganized resistance, quickly overrun the entire peninsula, captured Nantes without a fight, and took St.-Malo after a stubbornly contested siege. By the end of August it had penned up the remaining major German forces in Lorient and Brest. However, the Brittany ports, considered essential as entry points for supplies and reinforcements, were either too badly damaged for early use or, as in the case of Brest, were occupied by garrisons determined to hold them as long as militarily possible.

To the eastward of Brittany, the Allies fanned out to seize their planned lodgement area between the Seine and the Loire and in the process destroyed much of the German army opposing them (*see Map 11*). On the American right, the Third Army rolled ahead almost unimpeded; its XV Corps took Le Mans on 8 August after driving 75 miles in three days. On the Third Army's left, the First Army pushed forward slowly against a still solid German line. The Germans now compounded their own difficulties. On the seventh they had attacked westward toward Avranches with most of their remaining armor, trying to cut the Third Army's line of communications at its narrowest point, but after five days of bitter fighting around Mortain the 30th Infantry Division and other First Army units blocked the German thrust. Eisenhower, Montgomery, and Bradley, meanwhile, set in motion a large-scale envelopment of the attackers, turning Third Army elements north from Le Mans while the British and Canadians pushed southward from Caen. The ensuing battle of the Falaise pocket between 16 and 20 August, eliminated the German army in Normandy as an effective fighting force, the First and Third Armies, quickly following up success, reached and bridged the Seine, respectively east and west of Paris, by the twenty-fifth. The French capital itself fell to the Allies on the twenty-ninth.

The OVERLORD and NEPTUNE planners had assumed that the Germans would form a strong defense line along the Seine and that the Allies would halt at that river for a month or so, to reorganize and bring forward supplies. However, the completeness of the German collapse compelled continuation of the pursuit. Accordingly, during the last days of August and the first two weeks of September the British and Americans swept forward over 200 miles. They overran or outflanked weak German rear guards, gathered in tens of thousands of prisoners, and liberated town after town to the tumultuous delight of the inhabitants, who pressed liquor, food, flowers, and kisses on the passing soldiery. On the Allied left, 21 Army Group cleared the Channel coast and captured Brussels and Antwerp before halting at the Belgian-Dutch border. To the right of the British and Canadians, Hodges' First Army followed the historic invasion route to the Ruhr along the northern edge of the Ardennes. First Army troops encircled another 25,000 Germans at Mons, then took Liege and by 11 September were fighting on the German frontier. Patton's Third Army, meanwhile, headed eastward through Orleans, Troyes, and Verdun toward Lorraine and the upper Rhine. Early in September, before halting for lack of gasoline, the Third Army's XII and XX Corps seized bridgeheads over the Meuse.

As the pursuit went on, the roster of Allied armies further expanded. On 15 August the U.S. Seventh and French First Armies landed on the French Riviera and advanced up the Rhone valley, making contact with the Third Army on 11 September and extending the Allied front to the Swiss border. The U.S. Ninth Army, activated on 5 September, relieved the Third Army of responsibility for the forces in Brittany and protected the Americans' southern flank along the Loire. This new army had as its principal element the VIII Corps, engaged since 25 August in a bunker-by-bunker assault on Brest. At a cost of about 9,800 American casualties, the VIII Corps forced the 30,000 defenders of Brest to surrender on 19 September. The Ninth Army then began preparations to move into the main line in Belgium.

By the time Brest fell, the pursuit had given way to a slow, laborious advance against stiffening resistance. The rush across France left the Allied supply depots far behind near the beaches so that army and COMZ motor transport barely sufficed to haul forward enough fuel and ammunition to keep the combat elements going, with nothing to spare to build up advance dumps. By mid-September daily replenishment of gasoline, ammunition, food, and other vital commodities had fallen below the minimum requirements for sustaining an offensive. At the same time the Germans began to recover from their August rout. Aided by rough terrain, by the partially built fortifications of the West Wall,[2] and by clouds and rain which diminished air support, hastily improvised battle groups first slowed and then halted the weakening British and American drives. Behind this screen the Nazi regime, in a display of ruthless efficiency, collected men and equipment to rebuild divisions around the cadres that had escaped from Normandy and to form new ones. By late September these

[2] According to MacDonald, *Siegfried Line*, p. 30, "this was the fortified belt extending along the western borders of Germany from the vicinity of Kleve on the Dutch frontier to Lorrach near Basle on the Swiss border." Americans referred to this man-made obstacle as the Siegfried Line. However, from a World War II standpoint, this was a misnomer, derived from the fact that there had been a similarly designated position in World War I.

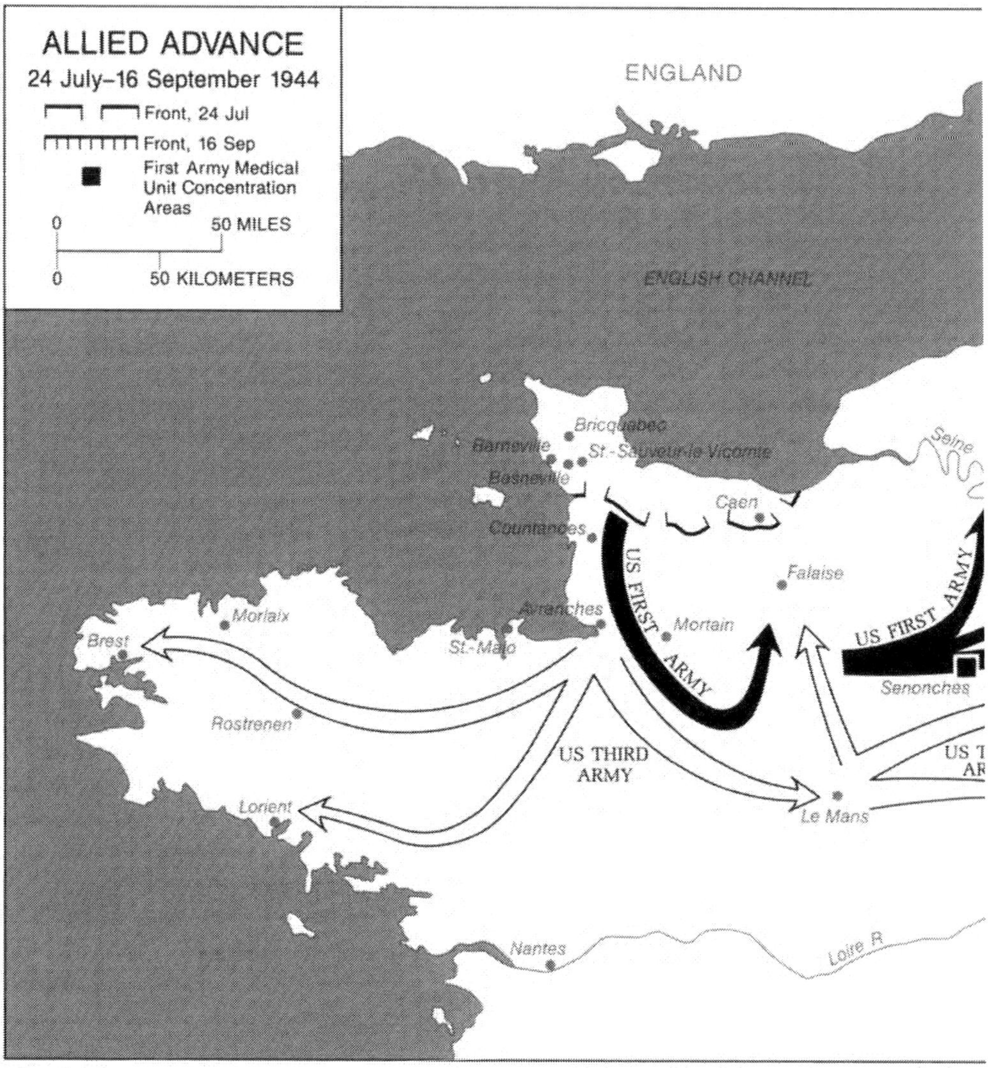
ALLIED ADVANCE
24 July–16 September 1944
Front, 24 Jul
Front, 16 Sep
First Army Medical Unit Concentration Areas
0 50 MILES
0 50 KILOMETERS
ENGLAND
ENGLISH CHANNEL
Bricquebec
Barneville
St.-Sauveur-le-Vicomte
Basneville
Coutances
Caen
Seine
Falaise
Avranches
Mortain
St.-Malo
Morlaix
Brest
Rostrenen
Lorient
Nantes
Loire R
Le Mans
Senonches
US FIRST ARMY
US FIRST ARMY
US THIRD ARMY

MAP 11

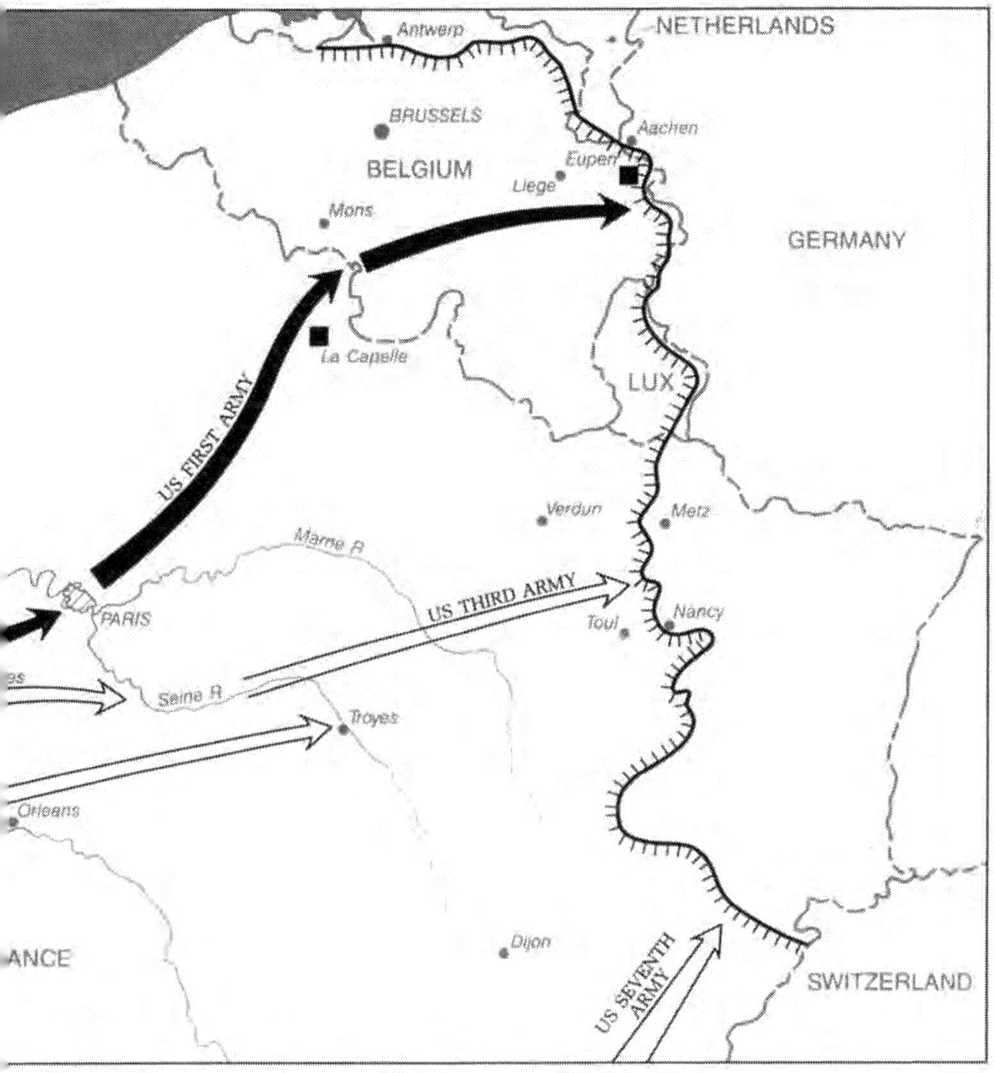
NETHERLANDS
Antwerp
BRUSSELS
BELGIUM
Aachen
Eupen
Liege
Mons
GERMANY
La Capelle
LUX
US FIRST ARMY
Verdun
Metz
Marne R
US THIRD ARMY
PARIS
Toul
Nancy
Seine R
Troyes
Orleans
Dijon
ANCE
SWITZERLAND
US SEVENTH ARMY

units were moving into and reinforcing the line.

Renewed First and Third Army offensives, accordingly, produced heavier casualties and disappointing results. Between 10 and 22 September the First Army penetrated the West Wall in the Ardennes and partially encircled Aachen, the first major German city to come under attack, but supply shortages and enemy reinforcements stalled the offensive short of a breakthrough. South of the Ardennes the Third Army forced its way across the Moselle against desperate resistance and fierce counterattacks. Patton's troops captured Nancy, but they failed to take the fortress of Metz and from 19–30 September had to fight off a major armored assault on their southern flank. Then the Third Army, too, had to halt for rest and replenishment.

On the British front, General Montgomery persuaded SHAEF to try a final audacious effort to maintain the momentum of the pursuit. On 17 September, in Operation MARKET-GARDEN, one British and two American airborne divisions dropped into Holland, to seize bridges over the rivers between the Belgian border and the lower Rhine and to open a corridor through which the British XXX Corps could drive to secure a bridgehead in Germany and flank the West Wall. The airborne assault achieved most of its objectives. However, the British 1st Airborne Division, which had landed farthest north, could not hold its Rhine bridgehead at Arnhem against armored counterattack, and the tanks and mechanized infantry of the XXX Corps could not get through the corridor before the paratroopers' perimeter collapsed. By the twenty-fifth, as the survivors of the shattered 1st withdrew to the south bank of the lower Rhine, it was clear that MARKET-GARDEN, too, had failed to break the solidifying German defense.

These final setbacks notwithstanding, the Battle of France was a substantial Allied victory. In four months of campaigning, the British and Americans killed, captured, or penned up in coastal fortresses about 500,000 German soldiers, at a cost to themselves of about 40,000 dead, 164,000 wounded, and 20,000 missing. The German debacle in Normandy permitted the Allied advance to surge far ahead of schedule. By 11 September (D+97) the Anglo-Americans already had reached a line that the OVERLORD planners had not expected them to attain until D+330 (2 May 1945). This sharp acceleration of Allied progress, while a tactical triumph, forced upon the theater medical service, as upon all the technical services, a period of often frantic adjustment and improvisation.

First Army Medical Support

Since D-Day the First Army medical service had supported a slow-moving advance with high casualty rates and short lines of evacuation. The army's larger medical units had changed position only a few at a time and at long intervals. In the breakout and pursuit the medical service had to adapt itself to just the opposite conditions: a rapidly moving front, low casualty rates, long lines of evacuation, and frequent repositioning of even the least mobile medical units. Colonel Rogers, the army surgeon, assembled his forces to support the breakthrough attack, reorganized them to keep up with the accelerating pursuit, and finally regrouped them behind another solid, slow-moving front.

Operation COBRA confronted the army medical service with a support problem hitherto not encountered in the campaign. In the First Army's previous broad frontal attacks, each division could receive medical support along a separate axis of communications. In COBRA, by contrast, medical units and supplies for seven divisions would have to go forward, and casualties come back, along a few roads through a corridor no more than 5 miles wide. If the attack went as planned, the distance to be covered in this corridor between front and rear medical installations steadily would increase, as would the flow of traffic through the constricted communications arteries.

The task of finding a solution to this problem fell primarily to the VII Corps surgeon, Colonel Barr. Under a plan developed by him, the First Army made preparations on the assumption that the assault divisions, once they broke through, would suffer relatively low casualties—a maximum of 300 severely wounded and the same number of lightly wounded per day for each division. To move these casualties up the corridor, the army attached 15 extra ambulances and 15 trucks (for ambulatory patients) to each assault division clearing station. It worked into its complex traffic control plan provision for rearward movement of as many as 1,300 ambulances a day and also planned for holding patients up to twenty-four hours in clearing stations and field hospital platoons if traffic congestion temporarily blocked evacuation. The evacuation vehicles, besides carrying casualties back, were to haul medical supplies forward to the divisions from an advance dump set up close to the breakthrough point.

As the hedgerow fields of the VII Corps sector filled with infantry, armor, and artillery massing for the attack, the army reequipped the assault division medical elements and brought them up to strength with replacements. It assembled numerous evacuation hospitals in rear of the corps, ready either to receive casualties or to follow the pursuit. Colonel Barr at the same time established communications and coordinated plans with the commanders of the 31st and 68th Medical Groups, which were to evacuate respectively the left and right wings of the VII Corps. He visited each division surgeon to explain the corps medical plan and to ensure that all preparations were complete. In the divisions the regimental surgeons, briefed at the last moment, hurriedly made their own plans and preparations, usually in informal coordination with the commanders of their supporting collecting companies.[3]

In the light of these elaborate preliminaries, the execution of COBRA, from the standpoint of the theater medical service, was anticlimactic. The preparatory bombing killed, injured, or stunned dozens of infantrymen in a few battalions, and the breakthrough area presented an ap-

[3] VII Corps Medical Plan, pp. 36–43 and 52, encl. 1 to Surg, VII Corps, Annual Rpt, 1944; 68th Medical Group Annual Rpt, 1944, p. 7. Tegtmeyer "Diary," bk. II, pp. 34 and 38–40, illustrates regimental preparations.

palling spectacle of craters, shattered trees, flattened villages, smashed vehicles, and dismembered, disemboweled German corpses. Nevertheless, from the beginning, the VII Corps suffered far fewer casualties than the planners had estimated it would. During the first two days of COBRA the clearing stations of the three lead infantry divisions, the 4th, 9th, and 30th, handled respectively 171, 362, and 480 patients. In the 1st Infantry Division, part of the exploitation force, aidmen and battalion surgeons occasionally had difficulty evacuating wounded from units temporarily surrounded in the increasingly fluid combat, but the division clearing station received so few patients that its attached field hospital platoon seldom even had to set up. While casualties were light for individual divisions, the cumulative flow of wounded through the breakthrough corridor quickly filled the foremost evacuation hospitals and forced the medical groups to divert ambulances to installations farther to the rear. As the penetration deepened, the road distance between open evacuation hospitals and division clearing stations expanded to as much as 60 miles. The medical groups had to commit an ever-growing larger number of ambulances to move the same or a diminishing number of patients. By 30 July the 57th Medical Battalion, which supported the left half of the VII Corps, was using 95 ambulances to evacuate a single fast-moving armored division.[4]

On 4 August, as breakthrough became breakout, Colonel Barr in his diary summed up the developing medical problem of the next stage of the campaign:

> Everything seems to be going well except that the ambulance hauls are becoming longer as the front progresses and hospital installations are left to the rear. The transportation of sick and wounded . . . is becoming a problem. We are daily more concerned at the possibility that the system might bog down owing to the inherent difficulties of supporting a rapid and sustained advance.[5]

After the capture of Avranches the First Army, now composed of three corps, attacked continuously, protecting the flank of the Third Army as it broke out to the west, south, and east. For better control of evacuation as the distance between clearing stations and hospitals increased and as medical units became dispersed over a wider area, Colonel Rogers on 2 August redefined the missions of his 31st and 68th Medical Groups. In the campaign thus far, each group had managed all stages of evacuation, from clearing stations to the beaches, for about half the army. Under the new arrangement the 68th Medical Group evacuated division and corps clearing stations and field hospitals across the entire army front; the 31st conducted all patient movement to the rear of the evacuation hospitals, as well as reinforcing them with elements from its collecting companies. The army's third medical group, the 134th, continued to control all the

[4] VII Corps Medical Plan, pp. 44–52, encl. 1 to Surg, VII Corps, Annual Rpt, 1944; 31st Medical Group Annual Rpt, 1944, p. 14; 68th Medical Group Annual Rpt, 1944, p. 7; Surg, 1st Infantry Division, Annual Rpt, 1944, pp. 12–14; Bradley, *Aid Man*, pp. 65–66; Tegtmeyer "Diary," bk. II, pp. 43–48; 57th Medical Battalion Annual Rpt, 1944, pp. 11–13.

[5] VII Corps Medical Plan, p. 56, encl. 1 to Surg, VII Corps, Annual Rpt, 1944.

separate clearing companies, including the two treating neuropsychiatric casualties.[6]

Preparing for the pursuit across the Seine, Colonel Rogers regrouped his medical units, which the Falaise encirclement left spread out in an arc from the beaches to the outskirts of Paris. Between 25 and 31 August Rogers collected most of his hospitals, depot companies, and groups around Senonches, 50 miles southeast of the French capital, on the line of evacuation from the advancing infantry and armor to the beaches. Such concentration of the evacuation hospitals and other less mobile units was to be the First Army's practice for the rest of the campaign; it facilitated communications and control, made handling of casualties more efficient, and simplified forward movement. Most of the units at Senonches, not immediately needed to treat the few sick and wounded of the early pursuit, went into bivouac for a welcome rest. They gave their people time off from duty—in many organizations the first since early June—and also repaired and replaced equipment.[7]

The concentration at Senonches included the First Army's five field hospitals, which Colonel Rogers detached from the division clearing stations and assigned a new mission. It had become obvious to Rogers and his staff early in the advance that the 400-bed evacuation hospitals could not move rapidly enough to stay within a practicable ambulance haul of the clearing stations. On the other hand, with casualty rates falling, fewer but more mobile forward-area beds would be needed. To provide these beds, Rogers pressed his field hospitals into service as evacuation rather than emergency surgery units and attached them to the 68th Medical Group. (Hitherto, Rogers' own office had directed deployment of these units.) On 27 August Rogers instructed the group to assign a complete field hospital to each of the three corps while keeping two in reserve. The units supporting corps were to receive all types of casualties. While performing surgery on nontransportable and emergency cases, they were to avoid definitive treatment of other patients and promptly send them rearward—those deemed returnable to duty within ten days to army evacuation, convalescent, or specialized hospitals, and the rest directly to the Communications Zone.[8]

With the field hospitals attached, the 68th Medical Group, under Col. Francis P. Kintz, MC, included 2,400 officers and men and 90 nurses and was, Kintz claimed, "the largest medical group in the history of the . . .

[6] Ibid., p. 59; 31st Medical Group Annual Rpt, pp 14–16; 68th Medical Group Annual Rpt, 1944, pp. 7–11; 134th Medical Group Rpt, 1944, pp. 7–9.

[7] Surg, First U.S. Army, Annual Rpt, 1944, pp. 44 and 59; VII Corps Medical Plan, p. 68, encl. 1 to Surg, VII Corps, Annual Rpt, 1944; 31st Medical Group Annual Rpt, 1944, p. 16; 68th Medical Group Annual Rpt, 1944, pp. 8–9. For samples of unit activity, see 5th Evacuation Hospital Annual Rpt, 1944, pp. 11–12, and 41st Evacuation Hospital Annual Rpt, 1944, p. 10.

[8] Surg, First U.S. Army, Annual Rpt, 1944, pp. 42, 44, 64–65; Memo, Col J. L. Snyder to CO, 68th Medical Group, 18 Aug 44, sub: Employment of Field Hospitals, and Memo, Snyder to COs of Army Hospitals, 68th Medical Group, and Army Medical Units, 27 Aug 44, sub: Utilization of Field Hospitals, both in 68th Medical Group Annual Rpt, 1944. Division and corps surgeons initially protested the loss of their attached field hospital platoons. See Surg, V Corps, Annual Rpt, 1944, p. 16, and VII Corps Medical Plan, p. 61, encl. 1 to Surg, VII Corps, Annual Rpt, 1944.

Medical Department." The group oversaw most medical support operations north of the Seine as the pursuit accelerated. It maintained contact with the fast-moving combat forces; it coordinated hospitalization, evacuation, and medical supply; and it reconnoitered hospital and depot sites for the heavier units struggling up from the rear.[9]

The group's field hospitals, operating under control of the 177th Medical Battalion, leapfrogged platoons forward across northern France and into Belgium, using trucks borrowed from other medical and nonmedical units. Ordinarily, only one of a hospital's three platoons (often called "hospitalization units") set up at a time, reinforced by the personnel of a second. The third platoon held itself ready for the next advance. When an active platoon closed, it turned over its remaining nontransportable patients to a clearing platoon from the 134th Medical Group. Each field hospital, augmented with half a dozen auxiliary surgical teams, could keep six operating tables, and in emergencies nine, working around the clock. A collecting company traveled with each hospital to provide clerks, litter-bearers, and general labor for mass triage, treatment, feeding, and evacuation of transportable wounded and sick. Employed in this fashion until 19 September, the field hospitals maintained treatment and evacuation facilities within 20 miles of the forward clearing stations. They efficiently handled the light casualties of the pursuit, some 300–600 a day for the entire army.[10]

As the forces north of the Seine rolled forward almost 200 miles in fifteen days, First Army medical units other than those of the 68th Medical Group fell steadily farther behind. The speed of the pursuit outran army medical planning. Early in September Colonel Rogers began shifting evacuation hospitals northward from Senonches to a new concentration point at La Capelle on the Franco-Belgian border. However, by the time the first units, delayed in movement by shortages of trucks and gasoline and by heavy traffic, reached La Capelle, the area already was too far behind the line for convenient use and the medics had to pack up and move again to another site further on. At the end of the first week of September army medical units were strung out along the entire path of the pursuit. A few evacuation hospitals—too few for the peace of mind of corps surgeons anticipating heavier casualties from the intensified German resistance—were in the process of opening in Belgium. The least movable installations, such as the 4th Convalescent Hosptial, still were trying to assemble at Senonches.

The abrupt slowing of the advance in mid-September (*see Map 11*), while it caused tactical frustration, paradoxically improved the position of the theater medical service by allowing the slower units to close up behind

---

[9] 68th Medical Group Annual Rpt, 1944, pp. 15–16.

[10] Ibid., p. 11; Surg, First U.S. Army, Annual Rpt, 1944, pp. 44 and 60; 177 Medical Battalion Annual Rpt, 1944, pp. 17–20; 13th, 42d, 45th, 47th, and 51st Field Hospitals Annual Rpts, 1944; 57th, 175th, and 176th Medical Battalions Annual Rpts, 1944.

the front line. Colonel Rogers designated Eupen, Belgium, behind the army's center, as a medical concentration area and directed the assemblage there of his supply depot, exhaustion centers, convalescent hospital, gas treatment battalion, and medical group headquarters. He also concentrated around Eupen most of his evacuation hospitals, except for one or two supporting each wing of the army. Moving by truck, and in a few instances by rail over recently rebuilt lines, all the army medical units had arrived within convenient supporting distance of the front by early October.[11]

As the First Army advanced, the point at which it turned casualties over to the Communications Zone shifted eastward, then northward. In the initial stage of the offensive, patients went by ambulance from army hospitals to the OMAHA beach holding unit, now under the Advance Section's control, or to the ADSEC 77th Evacuation Hospital, which opened at St.-Lo on 9 August. The latter unit relieved army installations of an immobilizing burden of lightly wounded, and it sorted casualties of all types for air and sea evacuation. As the army moved farther from the beaches, it sent evacuees successively to an airstrip near Avranches, to ADSEC holding units at Le Mans and Chartres, and to general hospitals and an airfield at Paris. In Belgium, with ADSEC facilities temporarily left far behind, the army turned some of its field and evacuation hospitals, and for a brief period an exhaustion center, into improvised holding units. These units received patients from mobile hospitals nearer the front and retained them until ADSEC ambulances could transfer them to airstrips and railheads near or below the French border.[12]

On 19 September Colonel Rogers again reorganized his medical groups and redefined their missions. Departing from the earlier pattern of specialized functions, Rogers placed each of his three groups in charge of evacuation for a particular corps, from clearing stations to the forwardmost ADSEC element. He reassigned units so as to give each group an identical composition—two battalion headquarters and one clearing, three collecting, and four ambulance companies. Rogers delegated to the groups responsibility for deploying field and evacuation hospitals in their sectors, tasks hitherto performed largely by the army surgeon's office. Directly under Rogers' control, two separate medical battalions evacuated the convalescent hospital and the specialized

[11] Surg, First U.S. Army, Annual Rpt, 1944, pp. 17–19, 42–46, 60, 161–65; Surg, V Corps, Annual Rpt, 1944, pp. 16–18; VII Corps Medical Plan, pp. 69–71, 77–83, 88, encl. 1 to Surg, VII Corps, Annual Rpt, 1944; Surg, XIX Corps, Annual Rpt, 1944, pp. 5–6; 4th Convalescent Hospital Annual Rpt, 1944, pp. 1–2; 1st Medical Depot Company Annual Rpt, 1944, pp. 5–6; Editorial Advisory Board, 1962, p. 142; Memo, Kenner to CofS, SHAEF, 20 Sep 44, sub: Report of Inspection of FUSA Medical Service . . . , in Medical Division, COSSAC/SHAEF, War Diary, September 1944.

[12] 31st Medical Group Annual Rpt, 1944, p. 16 and an. C; 134th Medical Group Annual Rpt, 1944, p. 9; Kenner, 12 (*sic*) Aug 44, sub: Report of Inspection of Medical Troops and Installations . . . , 2–13 Aug 44, and Memo, Kenner to CofS, SHAEF, 20 Sep 44, sub: Report of Inspection of FUSA Medical Service . . . , both in Medical Division, COSSAC/SHAEF, War Diary, August and September 1944; Surg, ADSEC, Daily Activities Rpt, 12 Aug 44, and Operations Division, OofSurg, ADSEC, Weekly Activities Rpt, week ending 19 Aug 44, both in Beasley Papers, MHI.

treatment installations and performed such miscellaneous tasks as overseeing the army's Provisional Medical Department Truck Company, a pool of vehicles used primarily for moving evacuation hospitals. So reorganized, the First Army medical service confidently prepared to care for the casualties of the impending battle for the West Wall.[13]

Third Army Medical Support

For the medical troops of the Third Army, the army's activation on 1 August was the culmination of half a year of planning and preparation. The army surgeon, Colonel Hurley, and his section of twenty-five officers and thirty-five enlisted men had been with the headquarters since its formation at Fort Sam Houston, Texas, and traveled with it to England in March 1944 (*Chart 9*). When General Patton took command of the army, he replaced a number of key officers, including the chief of staff, with veterans of his Mediterranean campaigns. In the surgeon's office he made only one change; he substituted his close friend and personal phsyician, Lt. Col. Charles B. Odom, MC, for the surgical consultant who had come out from the United States. This shift, and general unfamiliarity with the forceful, idiosyncratic Patton, initially caused tension and uncertainty among the Fort Sam Houston contingent. Smooth working relationships soon developed, however, and Odom's combat experience was welcome leavening for a medical staff that had spent the war to this point training troops in the United States.[14]

During the four-month stay at Patton's headquarters in the village of Knutsford, the surgeon's section drew up a Third Army NEPTUNE medical plan and completed the equipment and training of the army's over 100 nondivisional medical units. With the rest of the headquarters, the medical section crossed the Channel in two echelons on 6 and 18 July. Colonel Hurley set up his office near St.-Sauveur-le-Vicomte, in the Cotentin, about 8 miles from what was then the First Army front line. Slightly behind schedule, most of the army medical units disembarked in Normandy between 7 and 31 July. The evacuation hospitals, a field hospital, the auxiliary surgical teams, and a few other units went into operation at once under the First Army's control, most of them in support of the VIII Corps. Other organizations, including the medical groups and battalions, bivouacked in a concentration area around Barneville in the western Cotentin.

During the weeks before commitment to action, the army surgeon, and his corps surgeons, when they arrived, devoted much time to medical contingency planning. Colonel Hurley

[13] The assignments were: 31st Medical Group to support the XIX Corps; the 68th Medical Group, the VII Corps; and the 134th Medical Group, the V Corps. Specialized treatment units were the 618th and 622d Clearing Companies (NP) and the 91st Medical Gas Treatment Battalion (contagious diseases, venereal disease, and self-inflicted wounds). See also Surg, First U.S. Army, Annual Rpt, 1944, pp. 43–46; 31st, 68th and 134th Medical Groups Annual Rpts, 1944; 57th and 177th Medical Battalions Annual Rpts, 1944.

[14] Surg, Third U.S. Army, Annual Rpt, 1944, pp. 1–13, 19, 59–66, ex. VI; Editorial Advisory Board, 1962, pp. 85–90 and 98. The army staff came to the theater expecting to be commanded by General Hodges.

CHART 9—ORGANIZATION OF THE MEDICAL SECTION, THIRD ARMY, 1944

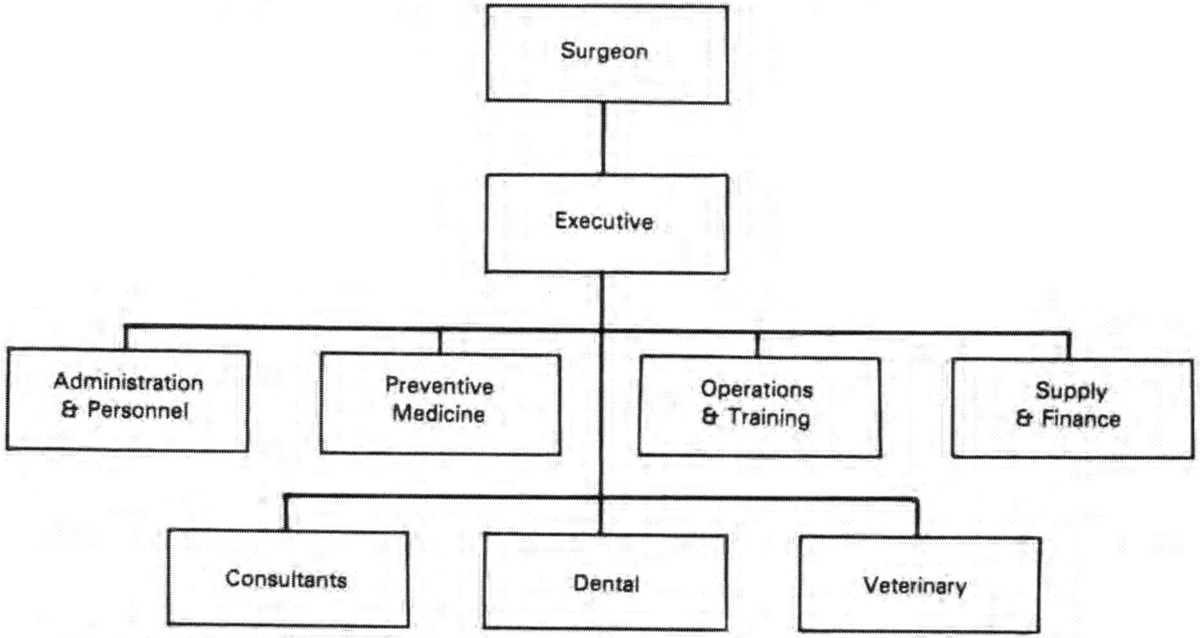

Source: Surg, Third U.S. Army, Annual Rpt, 1944, ex. VI-11a.

and his staff also paid attention to supply. Third Army units, like those of other commands, often crossed the Channel separately from their equipment. To reduce loss and misdirection, Hurley's medical supply officer, in cooperation with his ADSEC counterpart, stationed men on the beaches to watch for incoming Third Army medical gear and to ensure its prompt unloading and delivery. Elements of the two army medical depot companies, the 32d and 33d, had been in Normandy since D-Day, attached to the First Army and ADSEC. Late in July these companies reassembled under the Third Army's control. The 32d, at Bricquebec in the concentration area, replenished supplies and replaced equipment for army medical units. The 33d, at Besneville close behind the VIII Corps, received and stored for the beginning of operations ten medical maintenance units made up by the Advance Section, which contained fifteen days of supplies for 200,000 men.[15]

On 1 August the Third Army went into operation and resumed control of its medical units and surgical teams that had been attached to the First Army. Colonel Hurley at once organized his forces to support simultaneous offensives in Brittany and in the interior of France. He had ample resources with which to work. Compared to the First Army, the Third was lavishly endowed with nondivisional medical support, especially for evacuation. Its initial medical troop allocation, more than double that of the First Army for about the same number of divisions, included five groups, seventeen battalions, and twenty-one ambulance, eighteen collecting, and ten clearing companies.[16]

The Third Army kept the same medical organization throughout the pursuit and the transition to static warfare on the Moselle. Its medical system, like its general method of administration and command, emphasized simplicity, informality, and the assumption of responsibility by lower echelons. The army employed its medical groups solely to control evacuation, assigning to them all of its ambulance companies and also the ambulance platoons of its collecting companies. A different group evacuated the clearing stations of each of the army's varying number of corps—normally two or three in the eastward advance plus the VIII Corps in Brittany. A single group, the 69th, transferred patients between evacuation and convalescent hospitals and holding units. When necessary, it also evacuated casualties from these installations to the Communications Zone. The

[15] Surg, First U.S. Army, Annual Rpt, 1944, p. 15; Surg, Third U.S. Army, Rpt, 1944, pp. 12–25, 99, 103–06, 153–59, ex. III; Third U.S. Army Outline Plan, Operation NEPTUNE, Annex 16: Medical Plan, in CMH; Editorial Advisory Board, 1962, pp. 85–86; Memo, Lt Col H. Reinstein to Surg, Ninth U.S. Army, 9 Sep 44, sub: Observation of Medical Service in Operation, TUSA, Shambora Papers, MHI (in same collection, see Third US Army fldr); Surg, ADSEC, COMZ, Annual Rpt, 1944, p. 26; Surg, XII Corps, Annual Rpt, 1944, p. 3; 67th Medical Group Annual Rpt, 1944, p. 6; Supply Division, OofSurg, ADSEC, Weekly Activities Rpts, weeks ending 30 Jul and 5 Aug 44, Beasley Papers, MHI; 32d Medical Depot Company Annual Rpt, 1944, pp. 4 and 6.

[16] Surg, Third U.S. Army, Annual Rpt, 1944, pp. 15–16. For First Army figures, see Chapter VI of this volume. Even as reorganized in September 1944, the First Army included only three groups, eight battalions, and fourteen ambulance, eleven collecting, and six clearing companies. See Surg, First U.S. Army, Annual Rpt, 1944, pp. 45–46.

group commanders, according to a Ninth Army observer, possessed "an extreme degree of latitude" in directing patient flow from clearing stations to the rear. Army collecting and clearing companies, directly under the surgeon's office, usually reinforced evacuation hospitals; they treated the sick and lightly wounded and stayed behind with nontransportables to free the larger units for forward movement. The army's seven-eight field and eleven-fourteen evacuation hospitals (the numbers varied during the campaign) functioned in what was by now the conventional manner. Corps surgeons controlled the movements of the field hospitals supporting their divisions, and, as the campaign went on, they assumed, in cooperation with the unit commanders, most of the task of deploying evacuation hospitals. The three army gas treatment battalions served at different times as holding units and improvised convalescent hospitals, and they provided trucks to move other organizations.[17]

In Brittany the VIII Corps surgeon, Col. Richard H. Eckhardt, MC, managed an independent medical service for a force separated by a rapidly widening distance from the main body of the army. To support three infantry divisions attacking Brest, another patrolling along the Loire, and an armored division containing the garrison at Lorient, the Third Army attached to the VIII Corps a medical group (the 64th), three medical battalions, one field and four evacuation hospitals, and several ambulance, collecting, and clearing companies. The corps drew medical supplies from a section of the 33d Medical Depot Company at Rostrenen in central Brittany. It maintained a ten-day evacuation policy for combat exhaustion patients, the sick, and the slightly wounded and sent all other casualties directly to England by plane or LST. A clearing company holding unit at Morlaix, on the north shore of the peninsula, received these evacuees from corps hospitals and prepared them for further movement. At the height of the fighting for Brest VIII Corps medical installations handled 300-400 casualties per day.[18]

Medical units supporting the main Third Army drive to the Moselle, like their First Army counterparts, had difficulty keeping up. Field hospitals, by borrowing trucks from divisions and corps, managed to push at least some of their platoons well forward, but in spite of their best efforts distances of as much as 100 miles opened between their leading and rearmost elements. Third Army evacuation hospitals, each of which moved an average of four times during

[17] Quotation from Memo, Reinstein to Surg, Ninth U.S. Army, 9 Sep 44, sub: Observation of Medical Service in Operation, TUSA, Shambora Papers, MHI. See also Surg, Third U.S. Army, Annual Rpt, 1944, pp. 25, 27, 31, 39, 73–78, 87–93; 4th Auxiliary Surgical Group Annual Rpt, 1944, pp. 9–12; Surg, XX Corps, Annual Rpt, 1944, pp. 24–25; 66th Medical Group Annual Rpt, 1944, pp. 4–5 and 9; 67th Medical Group Annual Rpt, 1944, pp. 9–10; 95th Medical Gas Treatment Battalion Annual Rpt, 1944, pp. 3–5. For a well-known summary of Patton's view of command and organization, see George S. Patton, Jr., *War as I Knew It*, an. by Colonel Paul D. Harkins (Boston: Houghton Mifflin Co., 1947), pp. 399–400.

[18] Surg, Third U.S. Army, Annual Rpt, 1944, pp. 27–28 and 160; Surg, VII Corps, Annual Rpt, 1944, pp. 4–7; 64th Medical Group Annual Rpt, 1944, p. 5; 33d Medical Depot Company Annual Rpt, 1944, an. 1; Memo, Kenner to CofS, SHAEF, 4 Sep 44, sub: Inspection Report, Brittany Sector, 3 September 1944, in Medical Division, COSSAC/SHAEF, War Diary, September 1944.

August alone, advanced more rapidly than those of the First Army, although with increasing difficulty. At least a few always were close to the corps rear boundaries, and many had reached or crossed the Meuse by early September. The 32d and 33d Medical Depot Companies leapfrogged their advance and base platoons forward, so as to have issuing facilities open most of the time with convenient reach of the combat units. The 32d Company set up at Verdun on 8 September, and the 33d arrived at Toul twelve days later. The Third Army's convalescent hospital, the 6th, fared less well. It had opened at Vitre on 8 August and then advanced by sections, hampered by the need to carry along patients ready for duty who could not be returned to their units for lack of transportation. By early September the hospital was split into three echelons, the easternmost at St.-Mihiel and the rearmost still at Vitre, almost 500 miles away. As the army halted along the Moselle in September, Colonel Hurley was able to bring his medical units up close behind the front. Instead of concentrating them in a single area, the Third Army surgeon spread his forces out along a line roughly from Verdun to Nancy, with evacuation hospitals paired for alternate movement and a depot company supporting each wing of the army.[19]

In mid-August Colonel Hurley established a fifteen-day evacuation policy for the army, which he extended to thirty days after the front stabilized in late September. To remove casualties requiring longer care, Hurley relied almost entirely on air transportation until the end of the pursuit. On the assumption that COMZ installations would fall behind the advance, the Third Army surgeon organized his own rear holding unit, consisting of the 94th Medical Gas Treatment Battalion reinforced with an ambulance company and a collecting element and with a field hospital platoon attached for emergency surgery. Using six different forward airstrips, this unit evacuated over 9,700 patients, most of them in C–47s of the IX Troop Carrier Command. It stayed at each strip only until an ADSEC unit arrived to take over evacuation there and then moved on. The army holding unit finally settled down at Toul on the eighteenth, sharing the evacuation task with an ADSEC facility at Etain, just east of Verdun. As railheads reached Verdun and Toul, both units sent casualties out by hospital train as well as by plane. These units, supplemented by the army's 750-bed evacuation hospital, the 12th, which had opened at Verdun on the seventh, kept the forward evacuation hospitals continually cleared, even when weather and shortages of aircraft temporarily halted the flow of patients to the Communications Zone and Great Britain.[20]

---

[19] Surg, Thrid U.S. Army, Annual Rpt, 1944, pp. 27–29, 33–36, 94–96, 159–64; Surg, XII Corps, Annual Rpt, 1944, p. 4; Surg, XX Corps, Annual Rpt, 1944, pp. 22–24; 32d and 33d Medical Depot Companies and 6th Convalescent Hospital Annual Rpts, 1944; Memo, Reinstein to Surg, Ninth U.S. Army, 9 Sep 44, sub: Observation of Medical Service in Operation, TUSA, Shambora Papers, MHI. The 12th Army Group surgeon considered the Third Army more effective in pushing up its hospitals than the other armies. See Gorby Interv, 1962, pp. 10–11, CMH.

[20] Surg, Third U.S. Army, Annual Rpt, 1944, pp. 72–73, 77–78, 81–84, 95; Memo, Kenner to CofS,

Continued

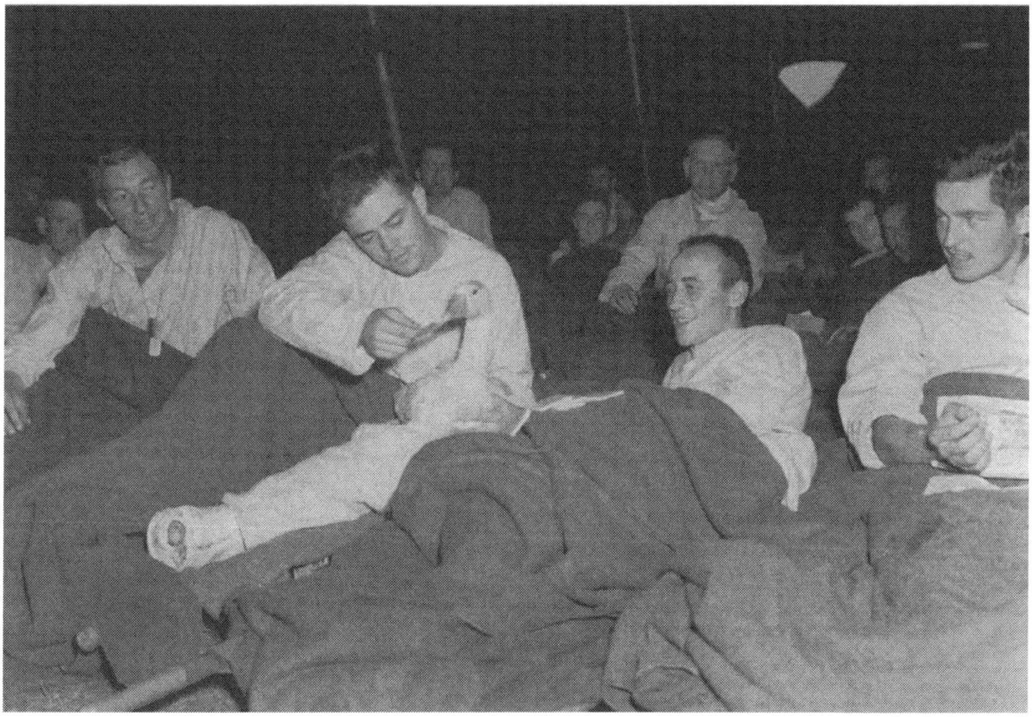

AWAITING EVACUATION FROM THE THIRD ARMY'S AIR HOLDING UNIT AT TOUL

Seventh and Ninth Armies Medical Support

The Seventh and Ninth Army medical departments initially had different tasks. Seventh Army medics participated in an amphibious assault and wide-ranging exploitation. The Ninth Army medical service, in contrast, began its existence supporting a siege and preparing forces for later movement into the front line. By the end of September, as their parent armies joined, or got ready to join, the array facing the West Wall, both army medical services were on the verge of incorporation into a more or less uniform system of support.

On 15 August elements of Maj. Gen. Alexander M. Patch's U.S. Seventh Army and General Jean de Lattre de Tassigny's French Army B (later redesignated the French First Army) assaulted the Riviera beaches in Operation DRAGOON, beginning the long-delayed campaign for southern France. These armies went into action under the Supreme Allied Commander in the Mediterranean and drew their logistical support from NATOUSA headquarters. Overwhelming weak opposition on the beaches, the American VI Corps, the only one under the Seventh Army, pursued the withdrawing German *Army Group G* up the Rhone valley; after securing the

SHAEF, 16 Oct 44, sub: Report of Inspection of TUSA Medical Service, in Medical Division, COSSAC/SHAEF, War Diary, October 1944; 94th Medical Gas Treatment Battalion Annual Rpt, 1944, pp. 2–6.

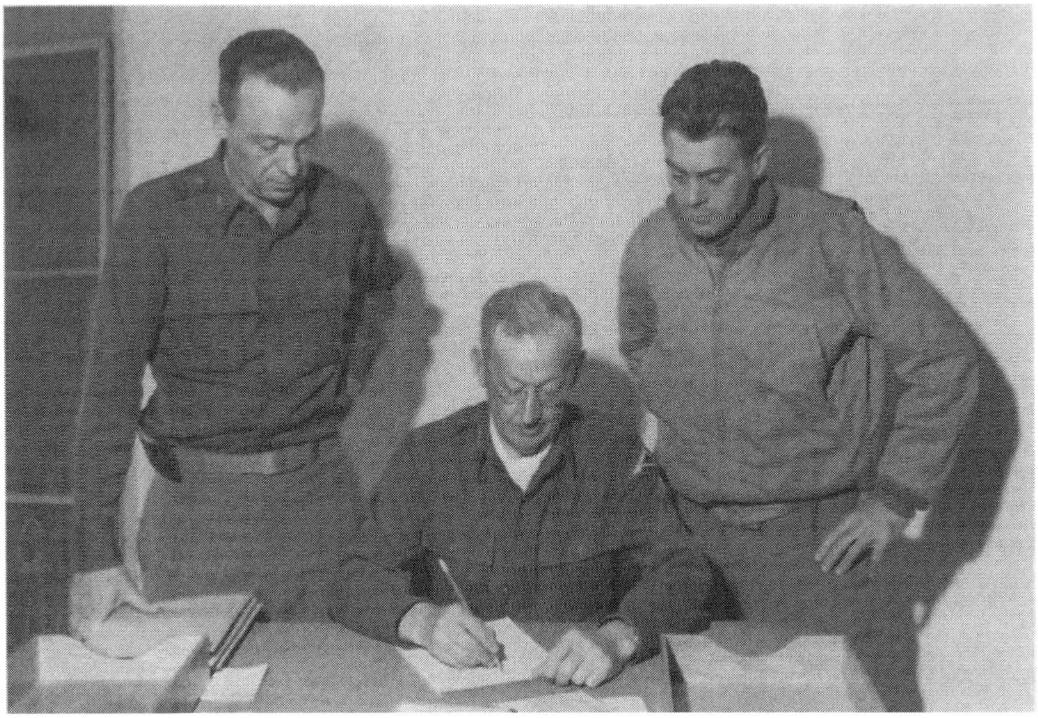

COL. MYRON P. RUDOLPH *(seated), with his evacuation and operation officers*

major ports of Toulon and Marseilles, the French army joined the northward advance. On 3 September the Allies took Lyon and a week later Dijon, near which, on the eleventh, Seventh and Third Army patrols made contact. Four days later the U.S. 6th Army Group, under General Devers, assumed control of the two armies from the Riviera. This army group, in turn, was under the operational control of SHAEF but logistically still tied to the Mediterranean.

Both the Seventh Army surgeon, Col. Myron P. Rudolph, MC, and the VI Corps surgeon, Col. Rollin L. Bauchspies, MC, were veterans of earlier Mediterranean operations, Bauchspies having been with the corps at Anzio. Hence their medical support arrangements were based on well-tried methods and hard-learned lessons. In the landings medical units came ashore in a sequence similar to that in Normandy: divisional elements and a beach support group medical battalion first, followed by field and then evacuation hospitals. Once engaged in mobile operations, the Seventh Army employed its field and evacuation hospitals in the usual manner. Without a medical group, it used one separate battalion to empty division and corps clearing stations and another to move patients to the rear of the evacuation hospitals.

Between 15 August and 29 September Seventh Army medical installations admitted about 28,000 patients, of whom 20,000, including 6,700 battle casualties, were U.S. troops. The army transferred people needing extended care to NATOUSA hospitals in Italy and later in southern France. At the outset most evacuees went by ambulance to the beaches for transfer to landing craft and hospital ships; but, as the distance between army facilities and the coast increased, air evacuation came to predominate. By late September the army was sending most patients by plane from Besancon to a COMZ holding unit at Istres, which in turn dispatched them to fixed hospitals in Naples or around Marseilles. Besides receiving Seventh Army casualties, the North African Theater furnished medical supplies, including whole blood. To control its growing number of facilities in southern France, the theater, as the campaign developed, established two base sections encompassing the Riviera and the Rhone and Saone valleys.[21]

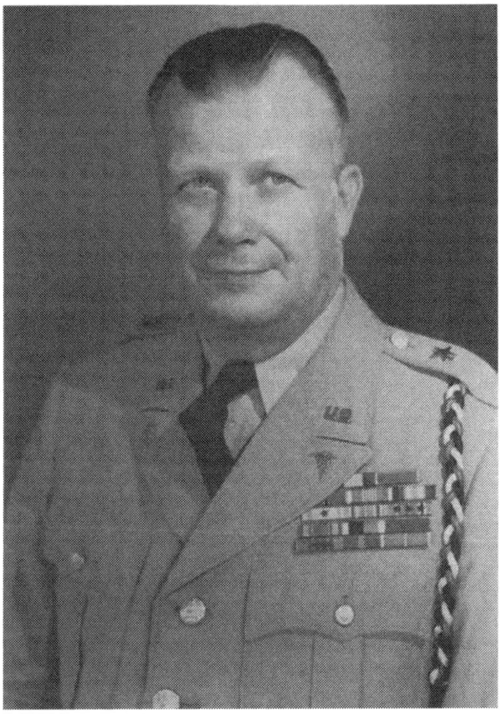
BRIG. GEN. WILLIAM E. SHAMBORA *(1950 photograph)*

In contrast to the veteran Seventh Army medical staff, that of Ninth Army, which arrived in England during May and June 1944 fresh from activation at Fort Sam Houston, lacked operational experience. The army surgeon, Col. William E. Shambora, MC, did have one distinctive qualification for his post: as chief medical officer of the Army Ground Forces, he had helped to develop the types of field medical units he now was to direct in action. At Bristol, awaiting movement to France, Shambora and his section availed themselves at every opportunity of the battle experience of those who had preceded them into the field. They visited the First and Third Armies to observe the medical service in action and COMZ hospitals to study the treatment of casualties, and they incorporated what they learned in their plans and training directives.[22]

[21] This account summarizes the more extensive treatment in Wiltse, *Mediterranean*, ch. X. See also Memo, Col J. K. Davis to CMedOff, SHAEF, 26 Sep 44, sub: Visit to Hq, 6th Army Group, in Medical Division, COSSAC/SHAEF, War Diary, September 1944. The French First Army had its own divisional and corps medical units and, once in its home country, relied for fixed hospitals on local civilian facilities.

[22] In Shambora Papers, MHI, see Surg, Ninth U.S. Army, Daily Journal, 31 Jul 44; Medical Encl to Training Memo No. 1, Ninth U.S. Army, n.d.; Orders, 12th Army Group to CG, Ninth U.S. Army, 28 Jul 44. See also Surg, Ninth U.S. Army, Annual Rpt, 1944, pp. 1-6 and 26; Interv, OSG with Maj Gen William E. Shambora (hereafter cited as Shambora Interv), 8 Oct 62, pp. 5 and 14-17, CMH; Editorial Advisory Board, 1962, pp. 134-35.

The army headquarters enbarked for France on 29 August. After a short period in billets in Normandy, it went into operation on 5 September, at Mi Foret, near Rennes at the base of the Brittany peninsula. During the rest of the month the medical section had relatively little to do. Colonel Shambora left support of the attack on Brest largely to the VIII Corps surgeon, while he oversaw the evacuation of the few sick and injured from the forces patrolling along the Loire. Shambora also arranged for the reception of additional Ninth Army medical units that arrived from England, including two group headquarters, an auxiliary surgical group, and a number of ambulance, collecting, and clearing companies. The army surgeon set up camps for these units, administered by the 95th Medical Gas Treatment Battalion, in the army service troops concentration area at Melun, south of Paris. After Brest surrendered, he supervised the evacuation of over 4,700 sick and wounded Germans from the fortified city's underground hospitals and regrouped VIII Corps medical elements for movement to the north.[23]

During the pursuit the First, Third, and Ninth Army medical services operated under the supervision of the 12th Army Group surgeon, Colonel Gorby. Gorby and his section moved to Normandy late in July with the rest of group headquarters and established themselves initially in "tents and self-dug foxholes" in an apple orchard. Until the 12th Army Group went into operation on 1 August, its surgeon largely confined his activities to establishing communication with the army surgeons and planning for future operations. Thereafter, Colonel Gorby played a gradually expanding role in allocating medical units among the armies, supervising and coordinating their medical services, and assisting them in dealing with the Communications Zone. As the lines of communication lengthened, General Hawley sought Gorby's assistance in coordinating evacuation from the armies. "You are in closer touch with the situation than any officers from my own office," he told Gorby on the eleventh, "and I wish that you would keep them advised of the needs of the two Armies and help them in the solution of the problem." The group surgeon, however, advised army surgeons rather than dictating their policies, and it was the army surgeons who carried the main burden of improvising solutions to the evacuation and hospitalization problems of the pursuit.[24]

Adapting to Mobile Warfare

For all the armies, especially those exploiting the breakout from Nor-

[23] The Ninth Army acquired from the Third, along with the VII Corps, the 64th Medical Group, three medical battalions, four evacuation hospitals, a gas treatment battalion, and four ambulance, four collecting, and three clearing companies. See Surg, Third U.S. Army, Annual Rpt, 1944, pp. 34–35 and 75–76; Surg, Ninth U.S. Army, Annual Rpt, 1944, pp. 1–2 and 6–8; 64th Medical Group Annual Rpt, 1944, p. 6; Surg, Ninth U.S. Army, Daily Journal, 5–30 Sep 44, Shambora Papers, MHI.

[24] First quotation from Comments on Draft Ms by Col Thomas F. Whayne, USA (Ret) (hereafter cited as Whayne Comments), 4 Dec 86, p. 14, CMH. Colonel Whayne was chief of Preventive Medicine and the Medical Intelligence Branch in Gorby's office. Second quotation from Ltr, Hawley to Gorby, 11 Aug 44, file HD 024 ETO CS (Hawley Chron). See also 12th Army Group Report of Operations, vol. XIII (Medical Section), pp. 7–8.

mandy, the German collapse in France created a new set of medical support problems. The strain on certain elements of the treatment and evacuation system eased, but that on other elements increased. In general, as the First Army surgeon put it, the problems of pursuit were "more logistical than medical in nature. . . . Service rendered to battle casualties was regulated to a lesser extent by surgical skill and experience and more by such factors as distance, available transportation, and supply." [25]

A decline in casualty rates accompanied the near-disintegration of German resistance. In the First Army the rate of battle-caused hospital admissions, measured in patients per 1,000 men per year, fell from over 1,100 in July to 890 in August and 445 in September. Similarly, neuropsychiatric admission rates declined from over 230 in July to about 190 in August, and to 100 in September. The statistical trend was evident from day to day in field installations. The VIII Corps surgeon noted as early as 22 August: "Where five or six hundred patients were passing through . . . clearing stations in a single day, not so long ago, now 12 or 15 battle casualties are the maximum." In the Third Army, which had not experienced the hard static fighting of the First, battle casualty rates were moderate throughout August and September, remaining at about 550 per 1,000 men per year. During August Third Army casualties included an unusually high proportion of bullet wounds to those from bomb and shell fragments—another indication of the fluid small-scale character of the fighting. This proportion became more normal in September, as German artillery reinforced the solidifying defense of the Moselle. Nevertheless, the field army medical service in the pursuit still had to handle a significant number of patients. First Army hospitals admitted over 19,000 wounded between 1 August and 12 September, not counting sick and injured. Those of the Third Army received about 23,000 battle casualties in the same period, and another 18,000 from other causes.[26]

In the infantry divisions the pursuit produced no major changes in the medical system. When the advance was rolling ahead, impeded only by feeble rear guards, unit doctors and aidmen, as the 16th Infantry surgeon recalled, often "were along for the ride." At times the only casualties were those Americans bruised by welcoming civilians who, in their enthusiasm, threw fruit, wine bottles, and other solid gifts into fast-moving trucks and jeeps. Aid stations and collecting companies kept most of their men and equipment loaded on their vehicles, dismounting only the minimum needed to care for the few casualties as they occurred. Clearing companies, which lacked trucks to move all their elements at once and had to

[25] Surg, First U.S. Army, Annual Rpt, 1944, p. 64.

[26] Quotation from VII Corps Medical Plan, p. 67, encl. 1 to Surg, VII Corps, Annual Rpt, 1944. Statistics from Surg, First U.S. Army, Annual Rpt, 1944, pp. 169 and 171; First U.S. Army Report of Operations, 1 Aug 44–22 Feb 45, bk. IV, p. 198; and Surg, Third U.S. Army, Annual Rpt, 1944, pp. 37, 87, exs. XIX, XX, XXVII. See also Kenner, 12 (*sic*) Aug 44, sub: Report of Inspection of Medical Troops and Installations . . . , 2–13 Aug 44, in Medical Division, COSSAC/SHAEF, War Diary, August 1944.

shuttle forward by alternate platoons, had difficulty keeping up but managed advances of up to 190 miles in four or five days. First Army division clearing stations dropped off their accompanying field hospital platoons for the pursuit. Third Army field hospital elements, which stayed with the clearing stations, scrambled constantly to obtain trucks from corps medical battalions and evacuation hospitals. In the army's XII and XX Corps provisional holding units, formed from elements of the corps medical battalions, took over postoperative care of nontransportable patients, allowing the field hospital platoons to move promptly with their clearing stations.[27]

When divisions encountered hard fighting, as at Mortain, Falaise, Brest, and the Moselle crossings, their aidmen and medical officers continued to use the treatment and evacuation methods worked out in the hedgerows; however, they had to make adaptations and improvisations to meet the varied tactical and terrain conditions of mobile combat. In the Mortain battle, for instance, the 2d Battalion, 120th Infantry (30th Division), lost its entire aid station, captured by a German armored column, and was surrounded for five days under constant attack. Aidmen with the isolated companies gave the many wounded what treatment they could and placed them in deep slit trenches for protection against fire. To remedy a critical supply shortage, artillery supporting the battalion fired 105-mm. and 155-mm. smoke shells filled with bandages, tape, and morphine into the perimeter. While some of the most severely injured died, the aidmen kept the majority alive until American counterattacks ended the siege.[28]

In the Third Army's battle for bridgeheads east of the Moselle, medics engaged in complicated, dangerous boating of wounded across a wide river under fire, from lodgements often too constricted or too thoroughly swept by German artillery to accommodate battalion aid stations, not to mention collecting and clearing elements. In this intense close-quarters fighting, aidmen and litterbearers suffered heavily. At Dornot, near Metz, where the 5th Infantry Division gained a bridgehead only to be forced out by savage counterattacks, "medics went out after the wounded but the en[emy] would either shoot them down or . . . let the medic get up to the wounded and then shoot the medic and the wounded man." Displays of endurance and valor were common, such as that of William G. Rea, aidman in Company K, 11th Infantry. During the withdrawal from the Dornot bridgehead "Rea crossed the river three times in

[27] Quotation from Tegtmeyer "Diary," bk. II, p. 54. See also Interv, OSG with Capt. E. G. Asherman (hereafter cited as Asherman Interv), 3 Feb 45, box 221, RG 112, NARA; VII Corps Medical Plan, p. 65, encl. 1 to Surg, VII Corps, Annual Rpt, 1944; Surg, XII Corps, Annual Rpt, 1944, p. 4; Surg, XX Corps, Annual Rpt, 1944, p. 22; 30th Field Hospital Annual Rpt, 1944, pp. 14–15. For examples of clearing station movement, see Surgs, 1st, 28th, 30th, and 90th Infantry Divisions Annual Rpts, 1944.

[28] Blumenson, *Breakout and Pursuit*, pp. 488–90; VII Corps Medical Plan, pp. 61 and 63, encl. 1 to Surg, VII Corps, Annual Rpt, 1944; Surg, 30th Infantry Division, Annual Rpt, 1944, p. 4. Bradley, *Aid Man*, describes the capture of the aid station. On the activities of the 120th Infantry during 6–12 August 1944, see 30th Infantry Division Combat Intervs, box 24038, RG 407, NARA.

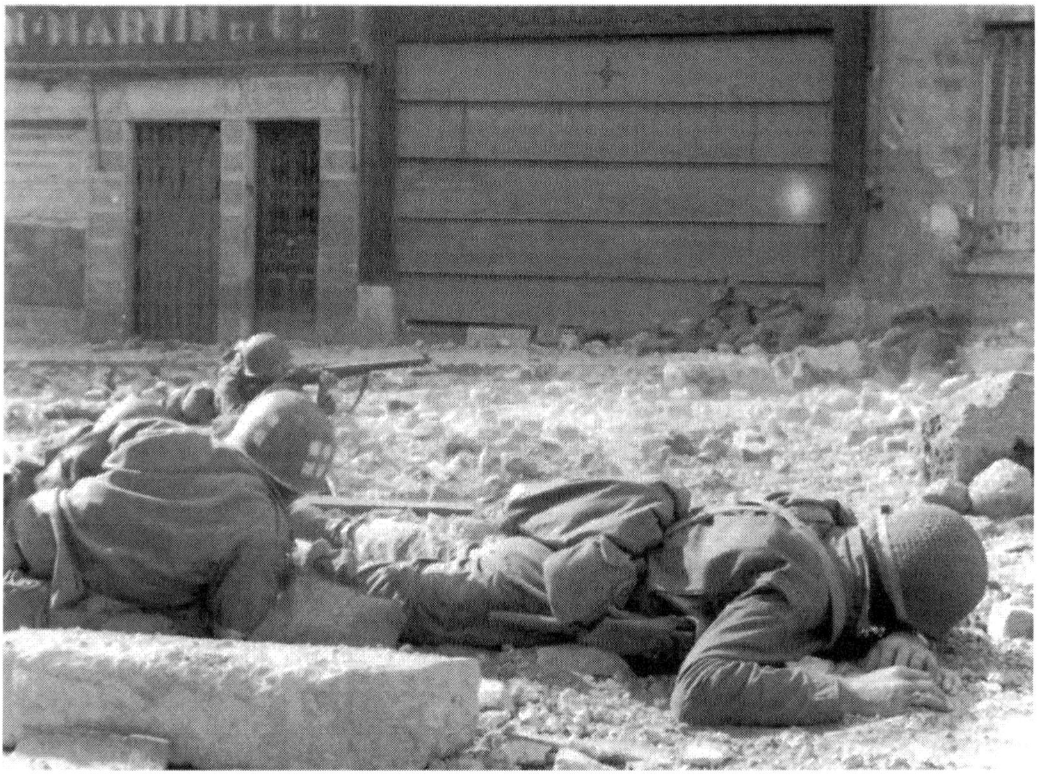

MEDIC AIDING A CASUALTY OF THE MOSELLE FIGHTING

evacuating litter patients. One time he carried a wounded man 300 yards, unaided, walking erect through small arms fire, after having crawled 300 yards to reach the man." Other medics at Dornot were as heroic, but less fortunate. Four men of the 5th Medical Battalion appropriated an abandoned engineer assault boat and crossed the fire-swept Moselle to bring back a couple of casualties, only to be blown out of the water by a tank shell as they began a second trip.[29]

In the breakout and pursuit armored division medical units, for the first time in the campaign, performed the function for which they had been designed: treatment and evacuation of casualties in fast-moving independent combat commands. The armored division medical service, completely motorized and lavishly equipped with radios, worked on the same general principles as that of the infantry, but with variations in organization and procedures. Combat units—except for

[29] First quotation from Narrative by Lt Harry A. Morris. Second quotation from Narrative ("Crossing of the Moselle") by 2d Battalion, 11th Infantry. Both in 5th Infantry Division Combat Intervs, box 24023, RG 407, NARA. See also Surg, 5th Infantry Division, Annual Rpt, 1944, pp. 17–21. Surg, 80th Infantry Division, Annual Rpt, 1944, pp. 6–8, describes medical support of a more successful Moselle crossing.

the armored infantry battalions, which usually secured non-T/O company aidmen from corps or army—concentrated their medical detachments in battalion aid stations, from which men in jeeps and half-tracks went forward to pick up casualties. Each of the three-lettered companies of an armored division medical battalion included both collecting and clearing elements and was capable by itself of providing evacuation and emergency surgery for a combat command. Especially during a rapid deep penetration of enemy lines a combat command medical service, consisting of unit detachments and the attached collecting and clearing company, functioned independently, directed by the command surgeon (selected from the medical battalion or a unit of the command) and the medical company commander.

Tank battalions, for front-line casualty handling, relied on crews thoroughly trained in first aid and in escape and rescue from damaged or burning vehicles. Tankers were often heroic in taking care of their own. A 4th Armored Division bow gunner, Pvt. Theodore T. Liscavage, in combat east of the Moselle, returned twice under fire to his knocked-out tank in an ultimately successful attempt to pull out the injured driver; Liscavage eventually received the Silver Star. In extreme danger, even badly wounded tank crewmen extricated themselves. Near Avranches another division soldier, hurt in both legs and badly burned, still managed to crawl out of his flaming tank and reach a ditch, where he lay in agony until picked up, at some risk to themselves, by a graves registration officer and an enlisted man who happened to be nearby. In the 2d Armored Division, according to the surgeon, the burn casualty rate was unexpectedly low, largely because of the speed with which men piled out of any hit or smoldering tank.

When armored vehicles unloaded casualties, they notified their battalion aid station. The aid station then sent ambulance jeeps or half-tracks to the reported location of the wounded. As observed by Lt. Col. Roosevelt Cafarelli, MC, the 6th Armored Division surgeon, "The litter bearers and medical technicians with their ambulance jeeps, equipped with plasma, morphine, splints, blankets and litters, functioned courageously as finger-like projections of the aid stations. . . . The aid station was brought to the patient, and the dictum 'Splint them where they lie' was fulfilled." These aidmen often drove into danger. During the St.-Lo breakthrough a 2d Armored Division medical half-track advanced along a hedgerow lane to pick up two injured crewmen, removed from a wrecked Sherman by infantrymen. The aidmen, and some assisting riflemen, "were just starting to load [the casualties] into the half-track when a German mortar shell landed right on top of the group. All were wounded, none killed." Especially at night, battalion aidmen often used jeeps in preference to half-tracks for collecting wounded, as the noise of the larger vehicles could draw random fire.[30]

[30] First quotation from Surg, 6th Armored Division, Annual Rpt, 1944, encl. 2. Second quotation from Narrative by Company E, 22d Infantry, 25 Jul–2 Aug 44, in 4th Infantry Division Combat Intervs, box 24021, RG 407, NARA. The other incidents are

Continued

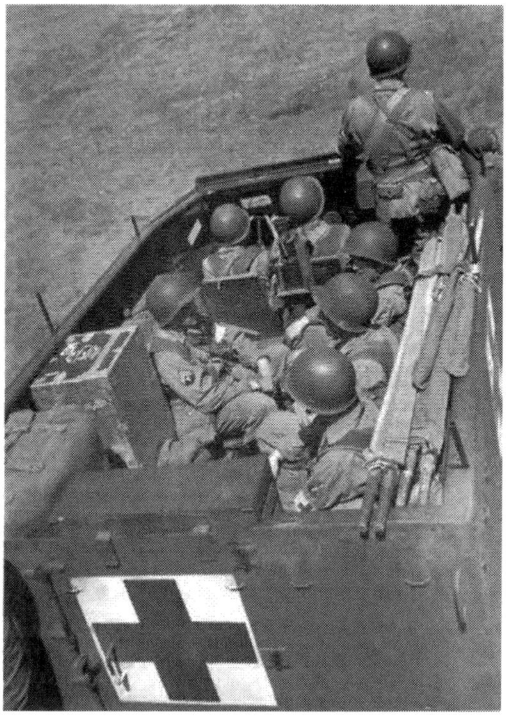

TYPICAL HALF-TRACK

Armored medical company commanders, working with combat commands, used radio and also liaison officers (frequently dentists underemployed in combat) to keep themselves informed of the rapidly changing tactical situation so that they could react promptly to the vicissitudes of mechanized battle. Ambulances of the medical company normally traveled with the armored column, their distribution within it depending on the preferences of the tactical commander and the surgeon. The clearing element, built around a truck-mounted surgical unit, followed close behind—disconcertingly close in the view of an infantry officer who saw an armored treatment station (as clearing stations in these divisions were called) calmly setting up near St.-Lo within 500 yards of a fire fight. Moving too rapidly for field hospital platoons to keep up with them, the treatment elements generally did a minimum of surgery; instead, using attached ambulances from army medical groups, they promptly dispatched even the most severely injured to field or evacuation hospitals often scores of miles behind them. Nevertheless, they could operate when they had to. A 2d Armored Division surgeon recalled

> one instance when we were unable to get ambulances back and had a patient brought in with a partial evisceration, perforated bowel and extensive intra-abdomial hemorrhage. We were able to arrest the hemorrhage, resected a portion of the ileum and gave copious amounts of plasma and blood (from our own men). The next morning the road back was clear and we were moving on so we had to evacuate him. Although we did not actually expect him to survive the operation we got a letter from him the other day from England.[31]

During action, armored medical battalion commanders usually maintained only administrative oversight of their committed companies. If the division, as it usually did, kept a combat command in reserve, the division surgeon often employed that command's attached medical company to hold sick, lightly wounded, and

from 4th Armored Division Combat Intervs, box 24092, RG 407, NARA. See also Surg, 2d Armored Division, Annual Rpt, 1944, pp. 13–14 and 45–54.

[31] Quotation from Ltr, Lt Col J. S. Weire to TSG, 10 Oct 44, file HD:ETO:370.05:Evacuation and Movement of Troops. The armored clearing station episode is in Rpt, 2d Battalion, 2d Infantry, sub: Counterattack on Hill 211, in 4th Infantry Division Combat Intervs, box 24021, RG 407, NARA.

combat exhaustion patients. The medical battalion headquarters companies acted as rolling supply depots; they issued expendable items to active companies, which in turn replenished battalion aid stations. Such was the system that proved itself in action during the breakout from Normandy. Using it, the 6th Armored Division, for example, during its six day 200-mile drive through Brittany, managed to get most of its wounded back to army hospitals, even though the country beyond its immediate lines of march remained in German hands.[32]

During the advance the First and Third Army surgeons, with their executive officers and those in charge of hospitalization, evacuation, and supply, usually accompanied the forward echelon of army headquarters, which kept as close as possible to the front. The rest of the medical section followed, as much as 100 miles behind, with the rear headquarters echelon. Corps and division surgeons similarly divided their staffs. Wherever located, it required constant effort and much improvisation for surgeons to maintain contact with and control over their widespread units. As the pursuit outran the construction of telephone lines and even the range of radios, surgeons had to rely largely on couriers to transmit orders and collect information. In the Third Army the surgeon's executive officer recalled that "individual officers . . . had to go out [and] contact units and find out where they were. The use of ambulances, the use of jeep messengers, all of these things come into play in controlling an army that's moving rapidly." During September, to ensure prompt response to the constantly changing situation, Colonel Rogers of the First Army sent his executive officer with a small advance medical party into Belgium ahead even of the army's forward echelon. These officers, who accompanied the 1st Division much of the time, made on-the-spot decisions on such matters as selection of Eupen for a medical concentration area.[33]

Securing transportation to move evacuation hospitals and larger medical units constantly taxed the ingenuity of army surgeons. These organizations, unlike divisional and corps elements and army medical groups and their subunits, had to obtain extra vehicles to lift all their people and equipment at once. A 400-bed evacuation hospital, for instance, required 30 more trucks than its standard allowance if it were to move in a single convoy. Such units could, and often did, shift position by shuttling in their organic vehicles, but this process was time-consuming and wearing on drivers and machines alike.

Because all other parts of the field armies also were moving and had no

[32] Surgs, 2d, 4th, 5th, and 6th Armored Divisions, Annual Rpts, 1944; Asherman Interv, 3 Feb 45, box 221, RG 112, NARA; Surg, XX Corps, Annual Rpt, 1944, p. 21.

[33] Quotation from Editorial Advisory Board, 1962, pp. 148–49. See also ibid., pp. 143–47 and 150; First U.S. Army Report of Operations, 1 Aug 44–22 Feb 45, bk. IV, pp. 133–34; Surg, Third U.S. Army, Annual Rpt, 1944, pp. 26, 32–33, 69, 74; VII Corps Medical Plan, pp. 54–55, encl. 1 to Surg, VII Corps, Annual Rpt, 1944; Surg, VIII Corps, Annual Rpt, 1944, p. 6; Surg, 5th Infantry Division, Annual Rpt, 1944, pp. 16–17; Briefing (untitled and n.d.), ca. August 1944, and Memo, Reinstein to Surg, Ninth U.S. Army, 9 Sep 44, sub: Observation of Medical Service in Operation, TUSA, both in Shambora Papers, MHI.

vehicles to spare, army medics had to rely on their own transportation. The First Army surgeon, after concentrating his forces at Senonches, formed a Provisional Medical Department Truck Company, composed of over 200 vehicles detached from evacuation hospitals and gas treatment battalions. (The 96 trucks of the latter were an invaluable asset that army surgeons occasionally had to defend against diversion to other uses.) This unit provided a pool of trucks for rapid concentration where needed, but hospital commanders objected to what amounted to the permanent removal of most of their vehicles. The Third Army formed a similar truck pool, also taken from evacuation hospitals and gas treatment battalions, but, in keeping with its more informal organization, left the vehicles with their parent units except when required for army missions. In ordinary movements Third Army evacuation hospitals often simply borrowed trucks from one another, rather than going through army channels. However they obtained vehicles, medical units of both armies had to compete with everyone else for gasoline, especially when forward-area supplies ran short in early September. The army surgeons, by vigorous wheeling and dealing, secured enough fuel for essential transportation and evacuation. Individual units used ingenuity, such as salvaging the residue in discarded jerry cans, to keep their own tanks from running dry.[34]

In both field armies the evacuation hospitals, the large units that moved most frequently, became expert at the process. Typically, once the army directed a hospital to a new general area, the unit sent an advance party to locate and begin preparing a specific site, usually after securing approval for it from the nearest corps headquarters. Veteran location scouts learned to pick high ground, preferably a pasture, because cultivated fields were dusty when dry and a morass of mud when wet. The preparatory parties often worked under fire, as the armies tried to push evacuation hospitals as far forward as possible in anticipation of further advances by the combat elements. The main body, meanwhile, usually stopped receiving patients several days before a movement; turned those left in its wards over to another hospital or a holding unit; and then took down its tents and packed personal and unit equipment. When transportation arrived, often after a frustrating wait, the unit loaded up and set off, the personnel riding in ambulances and jeeps and, occasionally, in the open backs of trucks.

Movement, over crowded roads, often at night under blackout or air attack, produced its share of accidents and lost vehicles and property. Depending on circumstances, army traffic control directions, and the commander's preference, hospitals

---

[34] For unit truck requirements, see Memo, Reinstein to Surg, Ninth U.S. Army, 9 Sep 44, sub: Observation of Medical Service in Operation, TUSA, Shambora Papers, MHI; Surg, First U.S. Army, Annual Rpt, 1944, pp. 59-60; Surg, Third U.S. Army, Annual Rpt, 1944, pp. 34-91; Surg, V Corps, Annual Rpt, 1944, p. 17; VII Corps Medical Plan, p. 79, encl. 1 to Surg, VII Corps, Annual Rpt, 1944; 31st Medical Group Annual Rpt, 1944, p. 16; 68th Medical Group Annual Rpt, pp. 11-12; 12th, 41st, 91st, 106th, and 109th Evacuation Hospitals Annual Rpts, 1944; 57th Medical Battalion Annual Rpt, 1944, pp. 17 and 19-20; Editorial Advisory Board, 1962, pp. 119, 138, 142-43.

traveled either in large convoys or by infiltration, which meant: "Load the vehicles and start them forward toward their destination as single units. Supply each driver with a strip map and leave him to his own skill and determination." At least some hospitals preferred the latter method, as it avoided the difficulties of keeping many trucks together amid the general stream of traffic. Hospitals usually tried to arrive at their new sites around noon, and an experienced unit could unpack, pitch tents, set up equipment, and be ready to receive patients in three-five hours. As did other units, hospitals on the move through liberated France and Belgium encountered an enthusiastic popular welcome. In Belgium, civilians gathered to watch hospitals being put up, brought gifts and food and wine, and at times volunteered to help as workers and guards.[35]

Army medical supply in the pursuit was concerned not only with trying to keep depot companies within practicable distance of the forward hospitals and clearing stations but also with replenishing the depots from COMZ installations that fell steadily farther behind. The army depot companies had to borrow trucks from other units to transport themselves and their supplies—a two- to three-week reserve, including over 2,000 inventory items and weighing between 500 and 1,200 tons. In both field armies the advance sections of the depot companies, normally carrying 50–100 tons of the most frequently issued supplies, leapfrogged ahead close behind the divisions. The base depots moved less often and more laboriously. The First Army's 1st Medical Depot Company had special difficulty, for it had accumulated large stocks during the hedgerow battles. After its first move to St.-Lo early in August, which required three days and 180 trucks to move over 1,300 tons of materiel, the company began stripping down for the pursuit. It issued to units or turned back to the Advance Section hundreds of tons of supplies, including refrigerators and other bulky items. Even with these reductions in load, the company still required large vehicle reinforcements for each advance, as well as additional manpower, borrowed from the medical groups. As supply lines lengthened in spite of such expedients, several corps formed small subdepots in their medical battalions, from which they issued to subordinate units.

The theater medical service was more successful than the other technical services in replenishing its depots in the field armies. Medical supplies were small in tonnage compared to fuel and ammunition, and, with the low casualty rate, issues were limited. In the Third Army, for example, a ten-day reserve, calculated on normal usage, sufficed in the pursuit for twenty or thirty days. Delays and diffi-

---

[35] Quotation from 106th Evacuation Hospital Annual Rpt, 1944, p. 11. See also 12th, 41st, and 91st Evacuations Hospitals Annual Rpts, 1944; Abraham Katz, ed., *Fifth Evac* (Fulda, FRG, 1945), pp. 37–38; A. W. Kuhlmann et al., *A Narrative Style Report of the Activities of the 41st Evacuation Hospital, Semimobile* (Bad Neuheim, FRG, 1945), pp. 89–90 and 94–95; Surg, First U.S. Army, Annual Rpt, 1944, pp. 59–60; Briefing (untitled and n.d.), ca. August 1944, and Memo, Reinstein to Surg, Ninth U.S. Army, 9 Sep 44, sub: Observation of Medical Service in Operation, TUSA, both in Shambora Papers, MHI; 68th Medical Group Annual Rpt, 1944, p. 14; Interv, Medical History Branch, CMH, with Dr. J. A. Gosman, MD (hereafter cited as Gosman Interv), 24 Mar 82, CMH.

culties did occur. Army surgeons had to send their own trucks back to the Communications Zone to pick up requisitioned supplies. Other materiel came forward on replacement vehicles bound for the combat units. In both the First and Third Armies the surgeons arranged special airlifts, directly from the United Kingdom, of such urgently needed items as penicillin, sutures, intravenous solution, and plasma. Early in September both armies suffered from an acute shortage of blankets and litters, as evacuation drained hospitals and clearing stations of these mundane but vital commodities. Emergency shipments from COMZ remedied the deficiency by the end of the month, but at one point the First Army had in reserve only 800 litters and 10,000 blankets, all captured from the Germans.

The armies in fact made up many deficiencies from enemy stocks. As troops overran what had been German logistical support areas, they seized medicines, hospital equipment, and surgical supplies. During August the Third Army alone captured over 100 tons of this materiel. Whenever possible, the armies turned captured supplies over to their depots. There, soldiers translated labels and tried to determine which German items had equivalents in the U.S. supply table; these they added to stock for issue. The residue went to civil affairs units, to meet local civilian needs, or to POW enclosure dispensaries. At times the armies, unable to move captured supplies, simply turned them over to units on a first-come-first-served basis, and divisions also helped themselves to much that their own troops found. In the Third Army rush across France, for instance, the 5th Division supplied itself by capture with, among other things, dental instruments, bandages, gauze, adhesive tape, tetanus antitoxin, bottles, corks, paper bags, cognac, and brandy. The division's attached field hospital picked up rubber sheeting, instrument trays, and plaster of Paris.[36]

The circumstances of mobile warfare that complicated forward movement of medical units and supplies created, if anything, greater difficulties in evacuation, both within and from the field armies. According to General Hawley, in a rapid advance "we may get only one-fifth as many casualties, but it takes five times the effort to get each casualty out." [37]

Within their areas the field armies had to move substantial numbers of helpless men over growing distances. During September alone ambulances of the 68th Medical Group in the First Army made over 20,000 patient-carrying trips, in the course of which the vehicles traveled over 311,000 miles. Evacuation of the wide-ranging armored divisions accounted for a good part of this mileage in both armies. The 6th Armored Division,

---

[36] Surg, First U.S. Army, Annual Rpt, 1944, pp. 16–19 and 59; First U.S. Army Report of Operations, 1 Aug 44–22 Feb 45, bk. IV, pp. 152–54; Surg, Third U.S. Army, Annual Rpt. pp. 159–65; 31st Medical Group Annual Rpt, 1944, pp. 16–17; 68th Medical Group Annual Rpt, 1944, pp. 10 and 14; 32d and 33d Medical Depot Companies Annual Rpts, 1944; Surgs, V, XII, and XIX Corps, Annual Rpts, 1944; Surgs, 1st and 5th Infantry Divisions Annual Rpts, 1944; Medical Division, COSSAC/SHAEF, War Diary, August–September 1944; Editorial Advisory Board, 1962, pp. 151–52; Ruppenthal, *Logistical Support*, 1:519. Supply problems in the Seventh Army were similar. See Wiltse, *Mediterranean*, pp. 405–06.

[37] Notes Taken at Press Conference, Paris, 4 October 1944, . . . by the Chief Surgeon, ETOUSA, in Hawley Papers, MHI.

for example, during its dash across Brittany, within days opened a 100-mile distance between its clearing station and the nearest Third Army hospitals. With no field hospital platoon able to keep up with it and receive nontransportable casualties from small engagements, the division stationed part of an armored medical company at roughly the midpoint of its evacuation route to immobilize emergency cases. Even with this expedient a few men died who might have been saved by earlier surgery; others reached evacuation hospitals in poor condition. Elsewhere, especially in early September, when lines of evacuation were stretched to the utmost, both infantry and armored divisions occasionally left wounded in civilian hospitals rather than risk the patients' lives in long ambulance rides.

Evacuation over long distances tied up army ambulances in numbers out of proportion to the casualties carried. In the 2d Armored Division, according to one surgeon, "the maximum run from our station to the nearest hospital . . . was one hundred forty miles. Travelling those distances over unknown roads, the . . . drivers were able to take their patients to the hospital but were unable to get back to us as they had to find our new location. . . . We considered an ambulance sent to the rear lost to use for one day." Some ambulances were more permanently lost on these runs, which often passed through unsecured areas infested with armed Germans. Ambulances came under fire; others were captured with drivers, attendants, and wounded. Sometimes the Germans left rearward-moving ambulances alone but attacked or detained those returning empty to the front. During the Third Army tank battle at Arracourt in September, the 4th Armored Division lost fourteen drivers, twenty-one patients, and seven ambulances and trucks in a single German ambush on a road erroneously reported safe.[38]

With both clearing stations and evacuation hospitals widely separated and moving frequently, the medical groups perforce adopted new expedients for controlling the flow of patients. They found that the standard fixed ambulance control points were inefficient, because ambulances had to make lengthy detours on already long runs to check in with them. To prevent this waste of time and gasoline, the Third Army's 66th Medical Group sent jeep-mounted liaison teams to reconnoiter every evacuation hospital in its sector twice daily and then distributed instructions for ambulance drivers to each medical battalion and division clearing station. Other medical groups placed traffic control officers at clearing stations or formed mobile regulating teams able to set up and move control points on short notice.[39]

---

[38] Quotation from Asherman Interv, 3 Feb 45, box 221, RG 112, NARA. See also VII Corps Medical Plan, pp. 74–75 and 78–79, encl. 1 to Surg, VII Corps, Annual Rpt, 1944; Surg, 4th Armored Division, Annual Rpt, 1944, p. 9 and encl. 6; Surg, 6th Armored Division, Annual Rpt, 1944, encl. 7; 64th Medical Group Annual Rpt, 1944, p. 2; 66th Medical Group Annual Rpt, 1944, p. 11; 57th Medical Battalion Annual Rpt, 1944, pp. 12 and 16; 4th Armored Division Combat Intervs, box 24092, RG 407, NARA; 104th Evacuation Hospital Annual Rpt, 1944, pp. 7–8.

[39] 66th Medical Group Annual Rpt, 1944, pp. 11–12 and encl. 6; 67th Medical Group Annual Rpt, 1944, p. 9; 57th Medical Battalion Annual Rpt, 1944, pp. 13–14.

In spite of the lengthening distances to be covered and the limited supply of vehicles and fuel, the field armies, thanks to low casualty rates, encountered no major internal evacuation bottlenecks. The only evacuation emergencies of the pursuit involved disposition of large numbers of wounded German prisoners taken in the Falaise and Mons encirclements. Some of these wounded hobbled into the American lines under white flags carried by their own aidmen. U.S. troops overran others in German aid stations and hospitals or found them lying on the battlefield, often suffering from exposure and infection. This sudden flood of enemy casualties (the 90th Infantry Division clearing station at Falaise admitted 1,500 in one week) temporarily overwhelmed and immobilized divisional medical units and the few hospitals not left far to the rear. At the 103d Evacuation Hospital German litter patients from Falaise covered the ground around the tents, reminding the hospital commander of scenes from the Civil War motion picture *Gone with the Wind*. Clearing stations and hospitals pressed captured German doctors and aidmen into service to help care for the prisoners, but the language barrier and general disorganization limited the Germans' usefulness. Under a First Army policy, announced on 12 August, medical units treated only nontransportables and the most severely injured and sick. They sent all the rest on to POW enclosures in vehicles hastily collected by corps surgeons and the 68th Medical Group. In spite of the attenuation of evacuation forces, corps and army medics moved these casualties out rapidly. At Mons, for example, the 68th and the VII Corps relieved the 1st Infantry and 3d Armored Divisions of about 1,500 Germans in three days, although not before the division surgeons had developed a desperation plan for putting the enemy wounded in a French Resistance-run civilian hospital.[40]

The other field armies also had to handle German wounded. The Third Army, while it evacuated no big pockets, hospitalized over 5,400 Germans during August and September and also cared for almost 600 sick and wounded Allied soldiers found in a captured hospital in Rennes. The Ninth Army's VIII Corps evacuated over 4,700 POW casualties and almost 1,000 enemy medical personnel from Brest after the fortress capitulated, and its 83d Infantry Division sent ambulances over 90 miles south of the Loire to bring out the casualties among the 20,000 Germans who, cut off from the rest of their forces in France, had agreed to surrender.[41]

---

[40] On First Army policy, see Surg, First U.S. Army, Annual Rpt, 1944, p. 46; Cir No. 106, HQ, First U.S. Army, 12 Aug 44, file HD 383.6. On Falaise, see Surg, V Corps, Annual Rpt, 1944, p. 14; Surg, 90th Infantry Division, Annual Rpt, 1944, pp. 14–15 and encl. 5; 41st Evacuation Hospital Annual Rpt, 1944, pp. 8–9; 103d Evacuation Hospital Annual Rpt, 1944, p. 14; Narrative ("The Chambois Gap, 15–26 August 1944") by 90th Infantry Division, in 90th Infantry Division Combat Intervs, box 24065, RG 407, NARA. On Mons, see VII Corps Medical Plan, pp. 76–77, encl. 1 to Surg, VII Corps, Annual Rpt, 1944; Surg, 1st Infantry Division, Annual Rpt, 1944, pp. 14–15; 47th Field Hospital Annual Rpt, 1944, p. 5; 57th Medical Battalion Annual Rpt, 1944, p. 17; 177th Medical Battalion Annual Rpt, 1944, pp. 19–20.

[41] Surg, Third U.S. Army, Annual Rpt, 1944, pp. 30–31 and 87; Surg, VIII Corps, Annual Rpt, 1944, p. 7; Surg, 8th Infantry Division, Annual Rpt, 1944, pp. 7 and 11–12; Surg, 83d Infantry Division, Annual Rpt, 1944, p. 5; 64th Medical Group Annual Rpt, 1944, p. 6. For a general discussion of ETO care of POWs, see Chapter XVI of this volume.

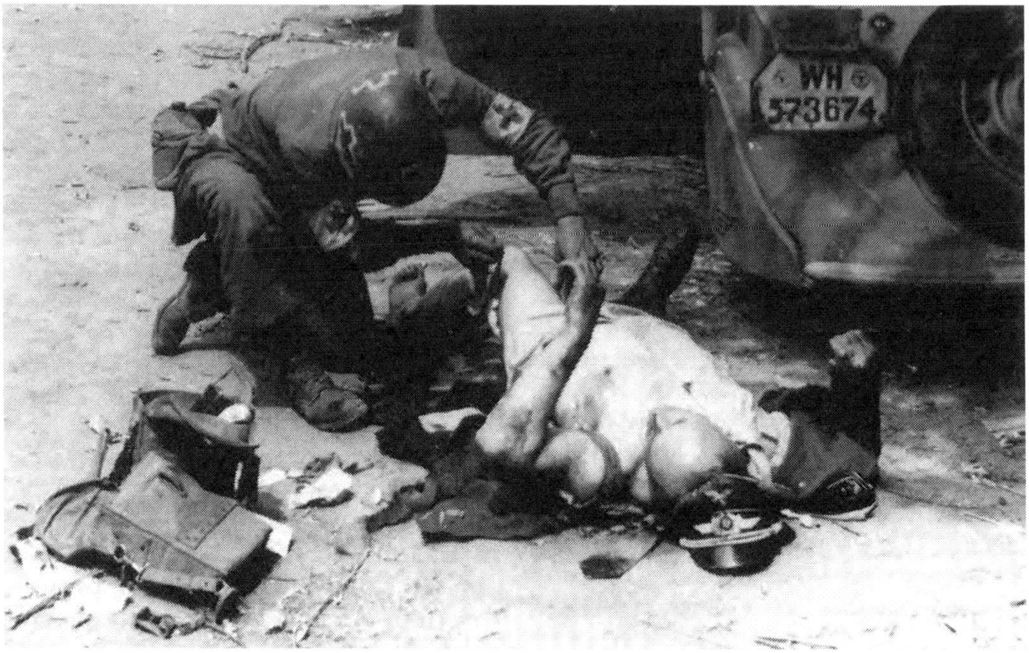

Medics Treating Wounded German Soldiers, *a few of the thousands swept up in the pursuit across France and Belgium*

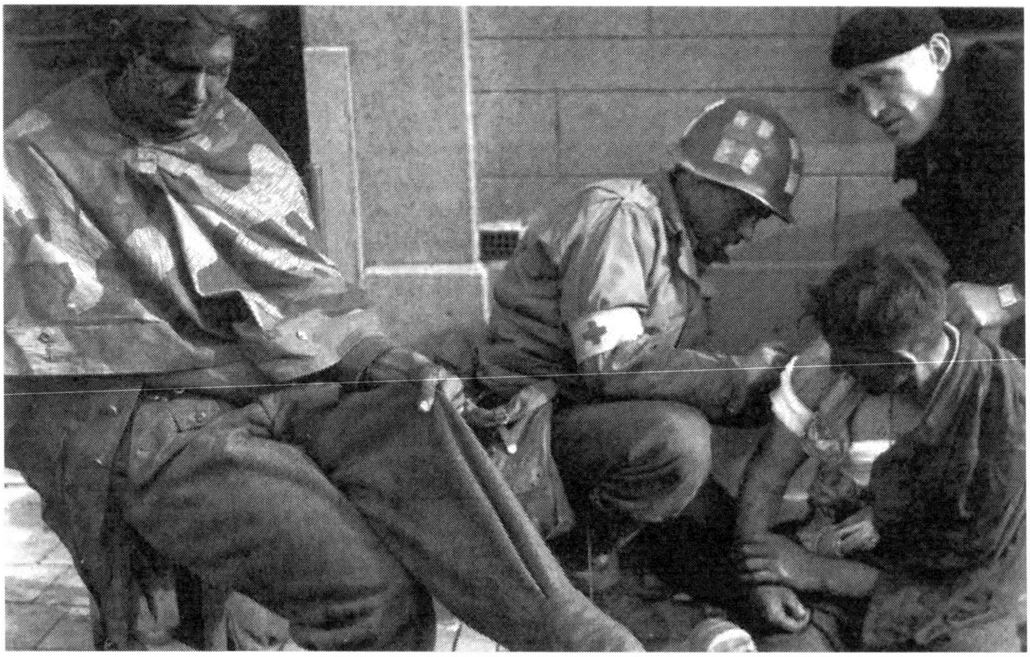

The First and Third Armies both had difficulty clearing their evacuation hospitals of patients destined for the Communications Zone. The problem stemmed from largely unavoidable ADSEC delays in moving up its own medical units and hospitals. Of the two field armies, the Third was the more fortunate in evacuation. Throughout the pursuit it was able regularly to send off patients by air from a succession of forward airstrips, using its own holding unit, and still more through ADSEC facilities once they caught up. The First Army, on the other hand, did not maintain a permanent holding unit and could not arrange for continuous air evacuation until mid-September, when the Advance Section opened a facility within convenient distance. Until then, the army used both its own and ADSEC ambulances to transfer patients to the Communications Zone and also pressed inactive field and evacuation hospitals, and at one point a combat exhaustion center, into use as provisional holding units. Both armies underwent an evacuation crisis during late September, resulting from a spell of bad weather and diversion of transport planes to Operation MARKET-GARDEN. Within a few days the First Army accumulated about 3,000 casualties awaiting evacuation and the Third Army about half that number. Fortunately, a return of clear weather and release of aircraft from the offensive in Holland permitted air evacuation to resume. By the end of September the advance of COMZ railheads to Liege behind the First Army and to Toul and Verdun behind the Third made possible all-weather mass evacuation by hospital train. Nevertheless, the army surgeons—and also General Kenner, who closely followed this situation—were not easy in their minds about evacuation until well into the autumn. In the south the Seventh Army had similar difficulty, also as a consequence of slow development of its communciations zone. By late September its hospitals contained over 1,400 patients awaiting transportation.[42]

Supporting Operation MARKET

In Operation MARKET, the airborne portion of General Montgomery's September breakthrough attempt in Holland,[43] American medics had to provide treatment and evacuation for two divisions landed behind enemy lines and dependent for logistical support on a British army. Medical planning for MARKET, therefore, was a cooperative effort. The American team consisted of the surgeons of the XVIII Airborne Corps and 82d and 101st Airborne Divisions; the British team was composed of senior-ranking medical officers from the Headquarters-Airborne Troops, the Second Army, and the XXX Corps. Under the overall Headquarters-Airborne Troops medical plan, each of the three assault divisions was to be prepared to collect and hold its own wounded and to perform essential

---

[42] Surg, First U.S. Army, Annual Rpt, 1944, pp. 46–47, 162, 165; Surg, Third U.S. Army, Annual Rpt, 1944, pp. 36 and 80–84; Briefing (untitled and n.d.), ca. August 1944, and Memo, Reinstein to Surg, Ninth U.S. Army, 9 Sep 44, sub: Observation of Medical Service in Operation, TUSA, both in Shambora Papers, MHI; Medical Division, COSSAC/SHAEF, War Diary, August–September 1944.

[43] The entire operation was known as MARKET-GARDEN, with the latter portion denoting the ground attack by the British XXX Corps.

life-saving surgery on them until air evacuation became possible or until the ground force, the XXX Corps, reached them in its drive up the corridor that the parachute and glider troops were to open. The XXX Corps was to move medical installations forward and evacuate its own wounded and those of the British 1st Airborne Division. Attached to the British corps, U.S. First Army ambulance, collecting, and clearing companies, and an evacuation hospital, were to handle American casualties.[44]

The U.S. XVIII Airborne Corps and the 82d and 101st Divisions based their medical plans on lessons learned in the D-Day drop. They revamped the equipment and supply allowances of regimental and battalion medical detachments and aid stations, removing items that had proved useless and adding others, such as glider-carried jeeps and trailers, that experience indicated would be of value. Corps and division surgeons paid special attention to increasing the airborne medical companies' capacity for emergency surgery, which had been barely adequate in Normandy. Besides reinforcing each company with an auxiliary surgical team, as had been done in the earlier operation, the airborne corps attached for MARKET a field hospital platoon, to go in by glider with the rest of the company. These platoons came from the 50th Field Hospital, which had been receiving water-evacuated casualties at Weymouth. Attached in August, they had little time for training before MARKET began and flew in gliders for the first time on the way to Holland.[45]

Tactically, the American part of MARKET went generally according to plan (*Map 12*). On D-day, 17 September, the daylight parachute and glider landings were models of precision compared to those in Normandy, with few losses in men and aircraft. The 101st Division, committed farthest south, secured its lodgement area and the bridges around Eindhoven and Veghel. Just north of it, the 82d Division, after a hard fight and a daring cross-river assault, captured intact the vital span over the Waal at Nijmegen. Holding the ground taken was more difficult, and more costly in casualties, as the Germans counterattacked repeatedly and in force to cut the XXX Corps line of communications. By the twenty-fifth the two American divisions had lost a total of 530 dead, 2,038 wounded, and 974 missing—significant casualties but hardly comparable to the more then 6,000 suffered by the British 1st Division.[46]

The airborne division medical elements shared in the general good fortune of the drop, arriving on the ground with almost all their men and with their equipment substantially intact. Unit first aid and evacuation proceeded about as smoothly as such

---

[44] For British planning and arrangements, see Crew, *AMS, Campaigns: North-West Europe*, 4:294 and 299–306; Col Renfro Interv, 10 Oct 44, in 101st Airborne Division Combat Intervs, box 24073, RG 407, NARA; 31st Medical Group Annual Rpt, 1944, p. 18; 134th Medical Group Annual Rpt, 1944, p. 9.

[45] The airborne divisions had been pulled out of Normandy in July and returned to England, where they refitted and planned for operations rendered unnecessary by the speed of the pursuit. See Surg, XVIII Airborne Corps, Annual Rpt, 1944, p. 2; Surg, 82d Airborne Division, Annual Rpt, 1944, an. III; Surg, 101st Airborne Division, Annual Rpt, 1944, p. 8; 50th Field Hospital Annual Rpt, 1944, pp. 1–2; Crandall Interv, 8 Jun 45, box 222, RG 112, NARA.

[46] MacDonald, *Siegfried Line*, chs. VI–VIII. Casualties are tabulated on p. 199.

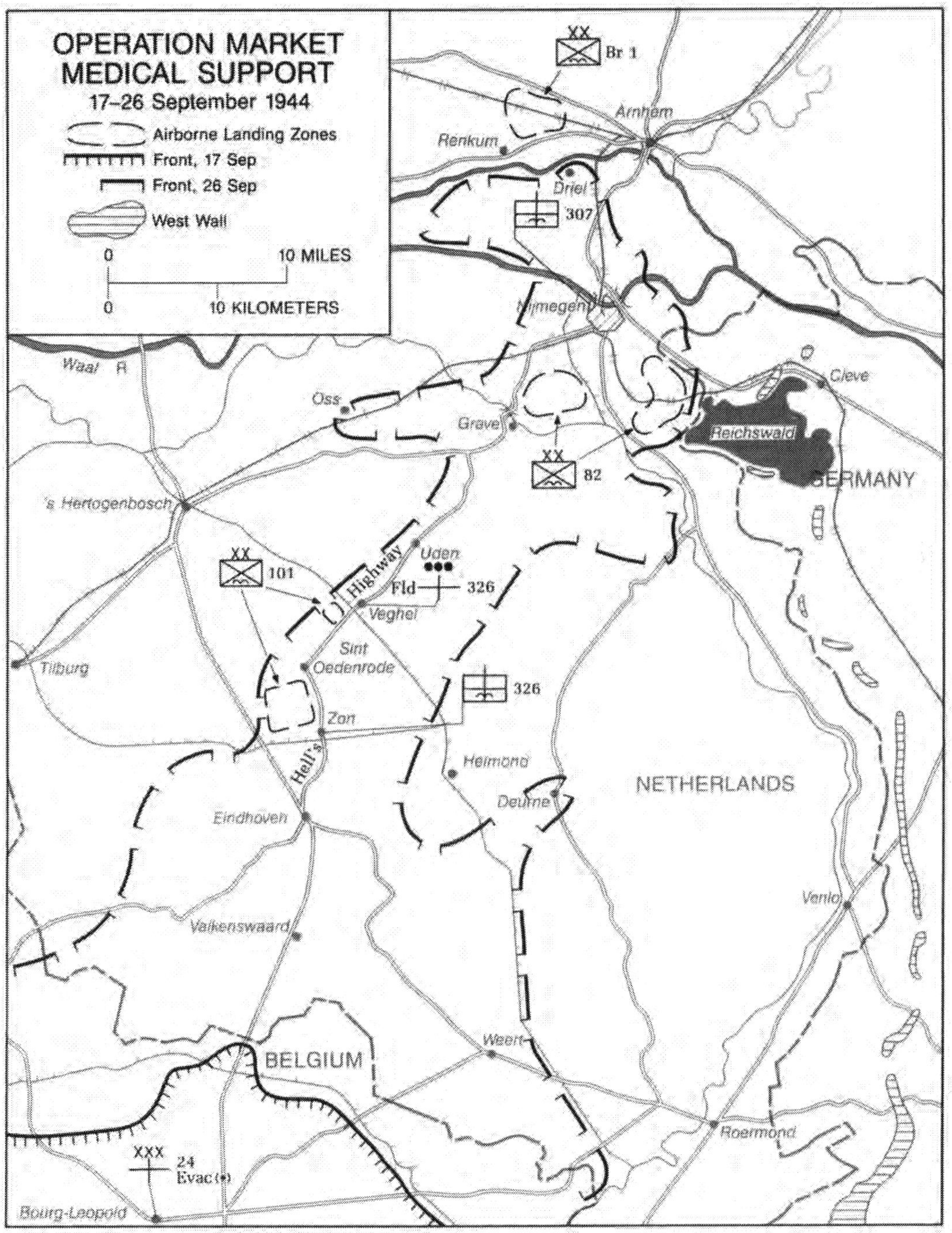

OPERATION MARKET
MEDICAL SUPPORT
17–26 September 1944
Airborne Landing Zones
Front, 17 Sep
Front, 26 Sep
West Wall
0
10 MILES
0
10 KILOMETERS
Br 1
Arnhem
Renkum
Driel
307
Nijmegen
Waal R
Oss
Grave
82
Cleve
Reichswald
GERMANY
's Hertogenbosch
Uden
Highway
101
Fld
326
Veghel
Tilburg
Sint
Oedenrode
326
Zon
Hell's
Helmond
Deurne
NETHERLANDS
Eindhoven
Valkenswaard
Venlo
Weert
BELGIUM
Roermond
XXX
24
Evac
Bourg-Leopold

MAP 12

activities could in actual combat. Nevertheless, in Holland as in Normandy, improvisation and courage came near to being standard procedure for the airborne medics. On 22 September, for example, during one of the major German attempts to cut the corridor in the 101st Division sector, elements of the 3d Battalion, 327th Glider Infantry, made a successful local counterattack and then received orders to fall back and regroup. Before doing so, the battalion had to retrieve its wounded, scattered in buildings and open ground. The battalion commander, Lt. Col. Ray C. Allen, recalled:

> We just couldn't walk off and leave our wounded. That was when our medical detachment under . . . Maj Martin Wisley did its stuff. . . . They had to advance all the way under fire, crawling most of the time in ditches. Not having enough litters to carry out all the wounded at one time, they had to dart from house to house, dodging fire from artillery and mortars and small arms, procuring ladders and tearing doors from houses to use as litters. . . . Several men were evacuated from houses through the windows, because fire on the doorways was too intense. The medics then had to drag each improvised litter down ditches for two or three hundred yards to safety.[47]

As they had in Normandy, the division medical companies landed small advance parties on D-day, to scout clearing station sites and to begin collecting and treating wounded. The main body of the companies, with their attached field hospital platoons, came in by glider during the afternoon of 18 September. Collecting elements moved out to contact the regiments, while the rest of each company, helped by Dutch civilians, set up its clearing and surgical station. The 101st Division's 326th Airborne Medical Company worked at two locations: a commandeered tuberculosis sanitarium in Zon, occupied by the company itself, at the southern end of the division area of responsibility; and a tented facility near Veghel at the northern end, composed of the field hospital platoon and a surgical team. In the 82d Division zone the 307th Airborne Medical Company and its attached forces established a single station south of Nijmegen, in a school that the Germans had converted into an obstetrical hospital for "Hitler Mothers."

The clearing stations treated a steady stream of casualties, mostly American troops and also a few British dropped off by XXX Corps units hurrying toward Arnhem. The 101st Division's medical company accumulated over 400 patients and that of the 82d Division about 300 before ambulances reached them, respectively on 19 and 20 September. Especially when German attacks temporarily stopped road evacuation, the airborne doctors operated on all types of patients, including men with severe chest and abdominal injuries. Working under roofs in relatively favorable conditions, the surgeons obtained satisfactory results. One of them commented: "Only two or three . . . thoracic cases that reached surgery [in the 101st Division] didn't survive. The ones that did not survive were very severe injuries, of the type that

---

[47] Allen quoted in Leonard Rapport and Arthur Norwood, Jr., *Rendezvous with Destiny: A History of the 101st Airborne Division* (Greenville, Tex., 1948), pp. 356–57.

couldn't have been saved anywhere." [48]

Throughout the campaign the divisions received at least adequate medical resupply, initially through air drops and later by road. When American supply deliveries did fall short, the British more than made up the deficiencies. According to the 82d Division surgeon, Lt. Col. William C. Lindstrom, MC, British "generosity and whole hearted cooperation" during the offensive "left nothing to be desired." Overall, the airborne division medical service, as revised after Normandy, proved effective during MARKET, although Colonel Lindstrom recommended at the end of the campaign that the division medical company be enlarged into a small battalion.[49]

As the airborne assault began, the American medical contingent with the British XXX Corps moved into position close behind the line of departure. The 384th Collecting Company (actually an ambulance unit in spite of its designation) established its headquarters at Hechtel and attached platoons to the British evacuation elements scheduled to advance up the corridor. Nearby, at Bourg-Leopold, the 24th Evacuation Hospital opened, reinforced by elements of the 662d Clearing and 493d Collecting Companies.

Ambulances of the 384th and 493d Companies closely followed the XXX Corps' advance. On 19–20 September platoons made contact with the two airborne division clearing stations and relieved them of about 600 casualties. Ambulance evacuation during the following week entailed running the gauntlet on what was aptly called "Hell's Highway," the single two-lane road that was the artery of the advance. Southbound ambulances battled a constant northward flow of British troop and supply trucks; often, they had to take to sidewalks, shoulders, and the fields to get around huge traffic jams. Periodically, German attacks blocked sections of the highway, and the enemy artillery fire posed a never-ending hazard. A 384th Company driver received the Silver Star for pulling an injured British soldier out of an ammunition truck set afire by a shell. The ambulance platoons evacuated over 1,600 patients from the 101st Division to Bourg-Leopold during the first nine days of MARKET-GARDEN; but evacuation over the 75-mile run from the 82d stopped altogether for four days and was sporadic thereafter until SHAEF and the British Second Army arranged late in September for airlifts from Eindhoven and Nijmegen.[50]

Almost all the wounded Americans who traveled "Hell's Highway"

---

[48] Crandall Interv, 8 Jun 45, box 222, RG 112, NARA.

[49] Quotation from Surg, 82d Airborne Division, Annual Rpt, 1944, an. III; Surg, 101st Airborne Division, Annual Rpt, 1944, pp. 5–6, 9, 18; Crew, *AMS, Campaigns: North-West Europe,* 4:233; Memo, Col. J. K. Davis to CMedOff, SHAEF, 28 Sep 44, sub: Visit to British Second Army (hereafter cited as MARKET-GARDEN Rpt), in Medical Division, COSSAC/SHAEF, War Diary, September 1944.

[50] Crew, *AMS, Campaigns: North-West Europe,* 4:294–97; Surg, 82d Airborne Division, 1944, an. III; Davis, MARKET-GARDEN Rpt, 28 Sep 44, in Medical Division, COSSAC/SHAEF, War Diary, September 1944; 493d Collecting Company Annual Rpt, 1944; 384th Collecting Company (956th Ambulance Company) Annual Rpt, 1944, in 57th Medical Battalion Annual Rpt, 1944. Reorganized under the 956th's T/O&E in November 1943, the 384th was not redesignated until after MARKET-GARDEN.

passed through the 24th Evacuation Hospital. This 400-bed unit, commanded by Col. Carl M. Rylander, MC, had been one of the first of its type to go into operation on OMAHA beach. It set up and went to work in Belgium under difficult conditions. The unit's vehicles, moving by infiltration, journeyed from Dijon to Bourg-Leopold through heavy fog and rain, over slippery roads crowded with British tanks and trucks. On 18 September the hospital pitched tents in what the unit historian described as "a marshy field of heather." During the first twenty-four hours of operation the 24th received 512 casualties; during the following week it admitted over 1,600 patients and evacuated about 1,300. In spite of requests by Colonel Rylander, the hospital had no reinforcing surgical teams during its busiest period. Its own surgical staff, working sixteen- and eighteen-hour days, performed over 540 operations, with 26 deaths. Besides caring for patients, the 24th furnished medical supplies to the airborne divisions. To replenish its stocks, the hospital arranged through the British Second Army and 21 Army Group for an emergency resupply flight of eight C-47s from Cherbourg, which brought in enough materiel for a small temporary depot. Using American and British ambulances, the 24th evacuated patients to British general hospitals and a triage unit at Diest, northeast of Brussels. From there, men able to travel went either to the Belgian capital for air evacuation across the Channel or, by train and ambulance, to Dieppe for embarkation on hospital carrriers.[51]

After MARKET-GARDEN ended, the 82d and 101st Airborne Divisions continued fighting in Holland until late November, defending the eastern flank of the salient they had helped to create. The separate medical companies and the 24th Evacuation Hospital, still attached to the British Second Army, remained to support them. During October the 24th moved into Holland. It established itself first in a waterlogged field near Uden and later, to the joy of the staff, took over a modern steel and glass hospital building in Nijmegen. The unit worked there, uncomfortably close to the combat zone and constantly shaken—and occasionally hit—by German shells aimed at the nearby Nijmegen bridge, until the airborne divisions left the line.[52]

At the West Wall

In the period between COBRA and MARKET-GARDEN the field army medical service expanded dramatically in size, geographical extent, and variety of missions. Medical forces of three additional American armies went into operation alongside the veterans of

[51] British general hospitals were much smaller than American units of that designation and performed a variety of tasks, including, as in this instance, a mission more typical of a U.S. evacuation hospital. Quoted words from "Lest We Forget": The 24th Evacuation Hospital (hereafter cited as 24th Evac Hist), October 1945, pp. 56–58, 60–61, 92–94. See also 24th Evacuation Hospital Annual Rpt, 1944, pp. 6–7; Davis, MARKET-GARDEN Rpt, 28 Sep 44, in Medical Division, COSSAC/SHAEF, War Diary, 1944, September 1944.

[52] MacDonald, *Siegfried Line*, ch. VIII; 57th Medical Batallion Annual Rpt, 1944, p. 20; 24th Evac Hist, October 1945, pp. 58–61.

the First. Army medical facilities by late September were spread throughout Holland, Belgium, and northeastern France, from Nijmegen through Eupen, Verdun, and Toul to Besancon. During the advance from Normandy the doctors and aidmen with combat units met and overcame a variety of tactical situations, from the brief meeting engagements of nearly unopposed pursuit to bitterly contested cross-river assaults. Medical groups improvised solutions to the problems of evacuation over long distances. Army hospitals and supply units learned how to move frequently and quickly. Medical units of many types proved able to perform a variety of functions beyond their standard missions, at diffferent points in the evacuation chain. Colonel Rogers summarized one major lesson of the pursuit: "A fixed or standard operational set up of medical units, however efficient for a certain type of warfare, cannot be maintained during all phases of combat. Flexibility and adaptability to the tactical situation are essential." [53]

The field army medical service made the transition from static to mobile warfare, but with difficulty. Its larger units, especially, were far from self-sufficient in transportation and fell behind the general advance. Forward hospitalization and evacuation facilities had become thin on the ground by the end of the pursuit. However, the low casualty rate prevented this circumstance from having noticeably adverse effects on the care of the sick and wounded. By the time revived German resistance began to increase American casualties, most army facilities had closed up behind the new battle line. As the armies prepared to attack the West Wall in force, the principal uncertainty confronting their surgeons was how soon the Communications Zone would overcome its own difficulties in the advance and be ready to provide adequate support.

[53] Surg, First U.S. Army, Annual Rpt, 1944, pp. 64-65.

CHAPTER X

The Expanding COMZ

As the field armies lunged across France and the Low Countries in the summer of 1944, the first task of the Communications Zone was to organize the newly captured territory behind them. For this purpose COMZ established continental base sections, identical in function to those in the United Kingdom. Under plans made before the invasion, each base section headquarters in Great Britain created from its personnel the nucleus of a new section, to be deployed across the Channel as the campaign developed. The parent base sections, at the same time, prepared for a realignment as districts within a single headquarters, known as the United Kingdom Base. Covering all the British Isles, this headquarters was to go into operation as a substantial portion of COMZ moved to France.

During August, after the armies at last had established their rear boundaries on the second, three continental sections went into operation. The Brittany Base Section, with headquarters at Rennes, supported the siege of Brest; the Normandy Base Section, assembled partly from the Advance Section and partly from a base section in Britain, assumed jurisdiction over the Cotentin and the area inland from OMAHA beach; and the Seine Section oversaw U.S. activities in newly liberated Paris. Still more base sections took shape in September, as the continental lodgement expanded and lines of communications lengthened. The Loire Base Section, initially intended to take over the port of Brest, instead set up headquarters at Le Mans; its boundaries encompassed a 130-mile-wide swath of France between the Seine and the Loire. North of the Seine, the Oise Base Section went into operation at Reims, encompassing territory between Paris and the rear boundary of ADSEC. The Channel Base Section took control of U.S. logistical activities at Rouen and Le Havre, major ports in the British communications zone that the Americans had permission to use for disembarking troops and cargo. The Advance Section, meanwhile, moved forward in the wake of the armies, furnishing immediate COMZ support to the combat forces and establishing depots and other facilities that it relinquished to the static sections filling in behind it. By mid-September ADSEC controlled an elongated territory in eastern France and Belgium. In the United Kingdom the Eastern Base Section had reverted to a district of the Western Base Section a month before D-Day; the Northern Ireland Base Section did likewise nine days after the invasion. On 10 September the United Kingdom Base went into operation, with the remaining three original base sections—Southern, Central, and Western—reorganized as subordinate districts (*see Map 13*).[1]

Most of the continental base section surgeons had served in the same capacity in their sections' parent headquarters in Great Britain. As in their previous posts they supervised hospitals, depots, and other medical service units and installations in their areas; they provided hospitalization, evacuation, and medical supplies for troops stationed there; and they advised section commanders on preventive medicine and sanitation. On the Continent several base section surgeons had additional responsibilities at crucial points in the theater chain of evacuation. Lt. Col. Raymond E. Duke, MC, in the Normandy Base Section, had charge of sea evacuation to England, of the disembarkation and storage of most medical supplies reaching the Continent, and of a large group of general hospitals. Because of the importance of this position, General Hawley prevailed on the section commander to appoint Duke, who had been theater hospital inspector on the chief surgeon's staff, to replace a less experienced base surgeon brought from England.

In the Brittany Base Section Col. Robert B. Hill, MC, provided evacuation and medical supply for the forces besieging Brest. The Seine Section surgeon, Lt. Col. Thair B. Rich, MC, left the Central Base Section in London expecting to oversee in Paris only a few hospitals and dispensaries serving headquarters and troops on leave. When he reached France, he found himself in charge of several thousand general hospital beds, a major depot, and rail and air holding units at what rapidly became the medical supply and evacuation center of the entire continental Communications Zone. Rich's staff from the Central Base Section perforce received hasty augmentation from General Hawley's office, 12th Army Group, Advance Section, and a general hospital. In the Channel Base Section Col. Mack M. Green, MC, managed the medical affairs of American enclaves in a British zone, including eventually the great port of Antwerp. Besides caring for the sick and injured of local service units, Green and his assistants set up hospitals and dispensaries for the large RED HORSE troop staging area that COMZ established at Le Havre.[2]

Hawley Moves to Paris

The Office of the Chief Surgeon had begun its move to France in mid-June. At that time an advance element under Colonel Spruit, formerly Hawley's deputy at Cheltenham, crossed the Channel with the headquarters of the abortive Forward Echelon of COMZ and established itself at Va-

[1] Ruppenthal, *Logistical Support*, 1:216–18; ibid., vol. 2, *September 1944–May 1945* (1959), pp. 24 and 32–38; Surg, United Kindgom Base, Annual Rpt, 1944, p. 59.

[2] Surg, Seine Section, and Surgs, Normandy, Brittany, Channel, Loire, and Oise Base Sections, Annual Rpts, 1944. For Duke's appointment, see Ltr, Hawley to Col Theodore Wyman, Jr., 1 Aug 44, file HD 024 ETO CS (Hawley Chron). Rich recalls the expansion of his mission in Editorial Advisory Board, 1962, pp. 123–24.

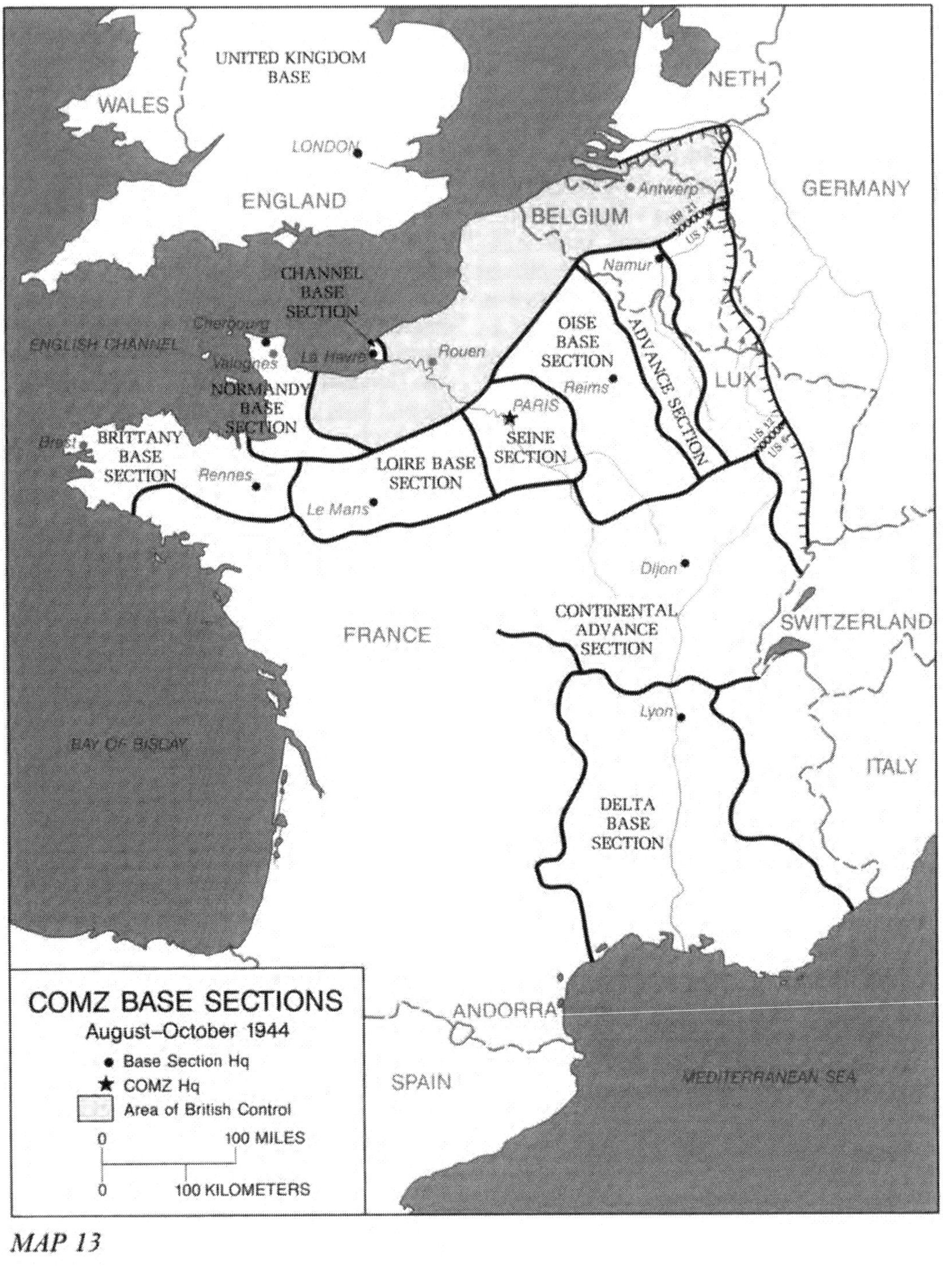
UNITED KINGDOM BASE
WALES
NETH
LONDON
Antwerp
GERMANY
ENGLAND
BELGIUM
Namur
CHANNEL BASE SECTION
Cherbourg
ENGLISH CHANNEL
Valognes
La Havre
Rouen
OISE BASE SECTION
ADVANCE SECTION
Reims
LUX
NORMANDY BASE SECTION
PARIS
SEINE SECTION
Brest
BRITTANY BASE SECTION
Rennes
LOIRE BASE SECTION
Le Mans
Dijon
CONTINENTAL ADVANCE SECTION
SWITZERLAND
FRANCE
Lyon
BAY OF BISCAY
ITALY
DELTA BASE SECTION
COMZ BASE SECTIONS
August–October 1944
Base Section Hq
COMZ Hq
Area of British Control
0
100 MILES
0
100 KILOMETERS
ANDORRA
SPAIN
MEDITERRANEAN SEA

MAP 13

lognes in the central Cotentin, the planned COMZ headquarters site. Awaiting the activation of FECOMZ, Spruit and his group observed medical operations and assisted (and sometimes, at Hawley's behest, pressured) the Advance Section on such matters as setting up general hospitals. FECOMZ never went into operation. Instead, in mid-August, the main COMZ headquarters moved to Valognes so that General Lee could take personal charge of his expanding continental establishment. As part of this movement, General Hawley and his London and Cheltenham staffs—less about 50 officers and 150 enlisted people left behind for the United Kingdom Base—transferred to Valognes in a series of echelons. Spruit and several of his men, much to their disappointment, now went back to England to join the new base headquarters. Housed in a spacious tent and hut camp, in woodlands almost untouched by combat, Hawley and his assistants worked in pleasant surroundings. However, the disruption attendant on uprooting personnel, furniture, and records, and a lack of communications, put the chief surgeon's staff almost completely out of action during the weeks when Paris fell and the armies crossed the Seine.[3]

Hardly had the office settled in at Valognes when it moved again, this time to Paris. As soon as the Allies liberated the French capital, General Lee, without prior SHAEF authorization, and to General Eisenhower's annoyance, precipitately rushed COMZ headquarters into the city. SHAEF reluctantly accepted Lee's fait accompli. Lee acted in order to place his headquarters at what he expected to be the center of continental logistics and, his detractors claimed, in order to secure the most comfortable accommodations available. Hawley was only a few steps behind his commander. A day or two after the liberation, he sent his executive officer and his chiefs of hospitalization and supply into Paris by jeep to secure locations for, respectively, offices, general hospitals, and a major medical depot. All three men accomplished their missions with dispatch and some disregard for formal procedure. Swift action had side benefits: The depot building turned out to be a warehouse for the German officers club's liquor, all of which for medicinal purposes, became U.S. Army property. The main body of the chief surgeon's staff transferred to Paris by truck and hospital train and opened in a requisitioned hotel on the Avenue Kleber on 14 September. By the end of 1944 all divisions of Hawley's establishment were in Paris except Rehabilitation, which remained in London to supervise its extensive facilities in Britain.[4]

---

[3] Administration Division, OofCSurg, HQ, ETOUSA, Annual Rpt, 1944, pp. 8–14 and encls. 5–6; Evacuation Branch, Operations Branch, OofCSurg, HQ, ETOUSA, Annual Rpt, 1944, pp. 6–7; Planning Branch, Operations Division, OofCSurg, HQ, ETOUSA, Annual Rpt, 1944, pp. 12–13; Hospitalization Division, OofCSurg, HQ, ETOUSA, Annual Rpt, 1944, p. 8; Supply Division, OofCSurg, HQ, ETOUSA, Annual Rpt, 1944, sec. I, p. 1. For descriptions of the site at Valognes, see Ltr, Hawley to TSG, 24 Aug 44, file HD 024 ETO O/CS (Hawley-SGO Corresp); Joseph R. Darnall, "Fixed Hospitals Follow the Breakthrough to Paris," *The Military Surgeon* 101 (October 1947): 276–77. Middleton Interv, 1968–69, vol. 1, p. 228, NLM, describes Spruit's disappointment.

[4] Ruppenthal, *Logistical Support*, 2:31–32; Administration Division, OofCSurg, HQ, ETOUSA, Annual Rpt, 1944, pp. 8–14; Evacuation Branch, Operations

Continued

In England the residue of the chief surgeon's staff, reinforced by medical people from the Southern Base Section, formed the United Kingdom Base surgeon's office. Initially, the staff was located at Cheltenham, but it soon took over General Hawley's old London quarters at 9 North Audley Street. The United Kingdom Base medical department, which included over 100 general and station hospitals and scores of other facilities, possessed higher status and more independence of action than those of ordinary base sections. Colonel Spruit, the base surgeon, also served as a deputy chief surgeon, ETO. He exercised within the British Isles most of the chief surgeon's authority over the medical service, including the right, in consultation with base and district authorities, to remove or transfer hospital commanders. Spruit also directed the reception and treatment of casualties from the Continent, as well as air and sea evacuation from the theater to the United States.[5]

Hawley, Spruit, and the base section surgeons, even as they tried to move and reorganize their own staffs, grappled with the conflicting tasks that all elements of the Communications Zone confronted during the rapid advance. On the one hand, COMZ had to furnish to the combat forces enough ammunition, food, and gasoline to enable them to continue their victorious drive as long as possible. Yet at the same time, to sustain the full-scale offensive to the Rhine and beyond, COMZ had to advance its own troops and materiel so as to build a network of intermediate facilities between the armies and, by now, the well-developed Normandy ports and supply dumps. With limited transportation and steadily lengthening distances to overcome, the Communications Zone could not do both jobs at once. Necessarily, it put support of the armies—at a minimal level—first and used what resources were left over to develop its logistical base in northern France and Belgium. The end result was less than satisfactory, tactically and logistically. The armies had to halt for a month at the West Wall, for lack of supplies, affording the Germans invaluable recovery time, while the Communications Zone established at least rudimentary advance facilities. Even then, an underdeveloped structure hampered operations throughout most of the fall and winter. The COMZ medical service shared this dilemma with the rest of COMZ, and it faced the added problem of moving masses of casualties to the rear as well as support units and supplies to the front.[6]

Forging the Evacuation Chain

Until the breakout from Normandy, evacuation from the armies to the

Division, OofCSurg, HQ, ETOUSA, Annual Rpt, 1944, p. 9. Hawley and several other officers recount their entry into Paris in Hawley Interv, 1962, pp. 74–76, CMH, and Editorial Advisory Board, 1962, pp. 120 and 123. See also Carter, ed., *Surgical Consultants*, 2:251, and Middleton Interv, 1968–69, vol. 2, p. 560, NLM.

[5] Surg, United Kingdom Base, Annual Rpt, 1944; Memo, Hawley to Surg, United Kingdom Base, 16 Sep 44, sub: Scope of ETO Medical Operations in UK Base, file HD 024 ETO CS (Hawley Chron); Administration Division, OofCSurg, HQ, ETOUSA, Annual Rpt, 1944, pp. 4 and 14.

[6] Ruppenthal, *Logistical Support*, 1:481–89, summarizes the logistics dilemma.

Communications Zone was a simple matter. ADSEC ambulances transferred patients from army hospitals to beach holding units, the air holding unit at Biniville, and eventually the tented general hospitals at Carentan, La Haye-du-Puits, and Cherbourg. As the distance widened between these facilities and the armies, the Communications Zone confronted its particular version of the general logistics dilemma: how to construct an intermediate chain of hospitals and evacuation facilities across France and Belgium while at the same time daily relieving the armies of their casualties. General Hawley summed up the problem: "How the hell [do] you keep up with the evacuation of three fast-moving armies with absolutely no communications, railroads that operate at two miles per hour, and airplanes that are never to be had when they are needed?" [7]

As transportation became more difficult, triage became more complicated. From the beachhead all sick and wounded not curable in army hospitals had been sent back to England but the opening of COMZ hospitals in Normandy permitted retention of more patients on the French side of the Channel. Accordingly, on 22 August the Communications Zone extended its continental evacuation policy from ten to fifteen days; on 1 September it further extended the policy to thirty days. Army and ADSEC surgeons, under this policy, had to designate early in the evacuation process those patients they deemed returnable to duty on the Continent for transfer to general hospitals in Normandy or elsewhere in France. They continued to dispatch all other casualties to Great Britain, directly by air from forward areas whenever possible and by land through a series of intermediate installations when necessary. These basic sorting principles largely determined the structure of the continental evacuation system as it evolved, in haste and much confusion, during the pursuit.[8]

The task of removing patients from the armies and starting them on their journeys through the Communications Zone belonged primarily to the ADSEC surgeon, Colonel Beasley. Beasley and his staff, who also did much of the initial planning and development of the entire medical COMZ, worked closely with, and under pressure from, General Hawley. The chief surgeon, concerned that the Advance Section was too slow in responding to the changing tactical situation, repeatedly exhorted Beasley to "think mobility, mobility, MOBILITY. You must keep up with the armies." Mobility Beasley's own office certainly possessed. With ADSEC headquarters, it shifted in rapid communications-disrupting succession from Normandy to Le

[7] Quotation from Ltr, Hawley to Brig Gen A. B. Davis, 15 Sep 44, box 2, Hawley Papers, MHI. See also Evacuation Branch, Operations Division, OofCSurg, HQ, ETOUSA, Annual Rpt. 1944, p. 7.

[8] Admin Memo No. 2, Surg, ADSEC, 5 Aug 44, in Essential Technical Medical Data Rpt, HQ, ETOUSA, August 1944 (see also p. 1 of September 1944 report); Evacuation Branch, Operations Division, OofCSurg, HQ, ETOUSA, Annual Rpt, 1944, p. 16; Ltrs, OofCSurg, HQ, ETOUSA, to Base Section and Hospital Cdrs, 22 Aug and 1 Sep 44, sub: Evacuation Policy in the COMZ, file HD:370.05: Evacuation and Troop Movements; Memo, Hawley to G-4, COMZ, 1 Sep 44, sub: Distribution of Patients Among Hospitals in France, file HD:ETO: 370:Evacuation, September-December 1944.

Mans, Etampes, Reims, and finally Namur, which it reached on 22 October. To oversee medical activities throughout the extensive Advance Section, Beasley set up suboffices in Liege and Bar-le-Duc as the armies paused at the West Wall. The ADSEC surgeon maintained direct personal contact with the field army commanders and their surgeons. He also attached medical liaison officers, selected before D-Day for the First and Third Armies, to the army headquarters. These officers transmitted medical support and supply requests and complaints to Beasley; they also reported daily to him the positions of the army medical units and the number of casualties in them awaiting evacuation.[9]

Under Beasley's technical supervision, the medical evacuation sections of the 24th and 25th Regulating Stations controlled the day-to-day movement of sick and wounded across the army rear boundaries. With their parent regulating stations, which managed the flow of traffic into and out of the army areas, the medical sections went into operation late in July, that of the 24th supporting the Third Army and that of the 25th the First. Like the rest of the station personnel, the four officers and four enlisted men of each evacuation section began work with the sketchiest of training, no experience, and only World War I precedents to guide them. They learned on the job and by mid-September had established effective working relations with the armies and ADSEC. This was especially the case after Colonel Beasley obtained field-grade MC officers from COMZ headquarters to command the sections, Lt. Col. Maurice E. Glock for the 25th Regulating Station and Maj. Sidney Blumenthal for the 24th. Glock and Blumenthal and their assistants allocated ADSEC hospital and holding unit beds to the armies and dispatched ambulances to collect patients from army facilities. They also helped select locations for air and rail holding units. They supervised the loading of hospital trains, once these came into use, although dispatch of the trains, contrary to original plans, remained the responsibility of the Evacuation Branch in General Hawley's office. Supplementing the efforts of the ADSEC liaison officers, the medical regulators formed another channel of communications between COMZ and army surgeons.[10]

ADSEC holding units constituted the indispensable link between mobile army evacuation hospitals and the usually distant railheads and airfields. They received sick and wounded by ambulance from the army units, per-

[9] Quotation from Ltr, Hawley to Beasley, 22 Aug 44, file HD 024 ETO CS (Hawley Chron). See also Ltrs, Hawley to TSG, 24 Aug 44, and TSG to Hawley, 1 Sep 44, file HD 024 ETO O/CS (Hawley-SGO Corresp); Surg, ADSEC, COMZ, Annual Rpt, 1944, pp. 5, 8–9, 11; Ltr, Beasley to Col W. E. Shambora, 14 Oct 44, Shambora Papers, MHI; Surg, ADSEC, Daily Activities Rpts, August–October 1944, and Rpts, Liaison Offs, First, Third, and Ninth Armies, August–December 1944, all in Beasley Papers, MHI; Editorial Advisory Board, 1962, pp. 129–30; Interv, OSG with Maj Gen Paul R. Hawley, 18 Apr 50 (hereafter cited as Hawley Interv, 1950), file HD 000.71, CMH.

[10] For general development of regulating stations, see Ruppenthal, *Logistical Support*, 1:497–99; Evacuation Branch, Operations Division, OofCSurg, HQ, ETOUSA, Annual Rpt, 1944, pp. 8–9, and, in file HD 024 ETO, ibid., *Daily Diary*, 31 Aug 44; Surg, ADSEC, COMZ, Annual Rpt, 1944, pp. 17 and 60; Ltr, Lt Col M. E. Glock to Col F. E. Mowrey, 12 Sep 44, file HD:ETO:370:Evacuation, September–December 1944.

mitting the latter to clear out patients promptly and move forward. The holding units provided shelter, food, and minimal supportive and emergency care for a large, rapid turnover of casualties, whom they retained only long enough to accumulate efficient loads for air and rail transportation. These organizations had to be put together in the field; no T/O unit for this purpose existed, and the NEPTUNE planners had not anticipated the size and importance such facilities would assume in a fast-moving mechanized advance. At the outset the theater made the Communications Zone solely responsible for setting up holding units close to the army rear boundaries. However, as COMZ fell behind the pursuit, the armies perforce improvised their own units to function until replaced by those of the Advance Section. The theater in late September formally directed this sharing of the task. In practice, when lines of evacuation were longest, the armies and ADSEC both had holding units in operation, relaying casualties toward the rear.[11]

[11]Operations Division, OofCSurg, HQ, ETOUSA, Annual Rpt, 1944, pp. 3–4; Evacuation Branch, Operations Division, OofCSurg, HQ, ETOUSA, Annual Rpt, 1944, p. 8 and encl. 6; Surg, ADSEC, COMZ, Annual Rpt, 1944, pp. 15 and 56–57; Memo, HQ, 12th Army Group, to Surgs, First and Third Armies, ADSEC, and COMZ, 8 Aug 44, AirEvacCorresp, file HD 580 ETO; Memo, HQ, ETOUSA, to CGs of Air, Ground, and Service Forces, 24 Sep 44, sub: Evacuation of Army Medical Installations, in Planning Branch, Operations Division, OofCSurg, HQ, ETOUSA, Annual Rpt, 1944. In proportion to their strength, the World War II field armies contained fewer hospital beds than did their World War I counterparts; hence, they had almost no long-term patient-holding capacity. See Hospitalization Division, OofCSurg, HQ, ETOUSA, Annual Rpt, 1944, pp. 23–24.

For holding units behind the armies, the Advance Section used the 7th, 9th, 12th, and 28th Field Hospitals; the 77th Evacuation Hospital, its only 750-bed unit; and the 93d Medical Gas Treatment Battalion. The first real holding units, aside from those established earlier on the beaches, went into operation in mid-August. The 77th, succeeded by the 7th, set up near St.-Lo for reception and triage of First Army casualties. At roughly the same time, elements of the 12th and the 93d opened an air evacuation facility for the Third Army at an airstrip near Avranches. From then on, as the Allies overran France and the Low Countries, holding units opened and closed with bewildering frequency. They advanced successively to Le Mans, Chartres, Orleans, and Reims, always trying to stay within something resembling a practicable ambulance haul of the rearmost army hospitals. By late September the holding units serving the First Army were well up into Belgium; those supporting the Third Army had reached Etain and Toul. ADSEC medical battalions, the 428th in support of the First Army and the 425th following the Third, traveled with the holding units. Their attached ambulance companies, under control of the regulating stations, collected patients from the armies and furnished transportation between holding units and airfields. Far to the southwest of the main battlefront, the 29th Field Hospital and 666th Clearing Company, under the Brittany Base Section, evacuated the VIII Corps. With detachments at an airfield and on the beach near Morlaix, these units shipped casualties directly to Great Britain by plane and LST.[12]

Wherever they were set up, holding units built around field hospitals struggled with similar problems. The field hospitals, like their counterparts in the armies, had to scour the countryside for trucks for every movement. Usually expanded to 600 or more beds in the holding role, they found themselves with a surplus of professional staff and shortages of cooks, admission and evacuation clerks, ward attendants, and litterbearers. To remedy this deficiency, ADSEC attached gas treatment and sanitary companies, and occasionally groups of combat exhaustion convalescents, to the field hospitals. Lacking enough mess equipment, tentage, cots, and bedding for their expanded capacity, field hospitals borrowed materiel from other medical units or appropriated captured German supplies. While it accomplished the mission, the field hospital, in the words of the 7th's commander, was "not an ideal unit for holding and mass evacuation of patients. It is necessary to supplement it with personnel from various organizations and the result is a hybrid affair with many complications, frictions, and multiplicities in overhead." [13]

The forward holding units sent off most of their patients by air, long-term cases directly to Great Britain and those falling within the continental time limit to a field near La Haye-du-Puits for transfer to the Normandy general hospitals. For the medical service, during the height of the pursuit, air transport was the only means available for spanning the steadily widening gap between the combat forces and the COMZ treatment and evacuation facilities still clustered near the beaches and in England. During August and September C-47s flying from British bases carried about 54,000 patients across the Channel and another 6,300 to destinations in France. The Advance Section, after it moved out of Normandy, for practical purposes did all its evacuation by air until late September.[14]

While extremely efficient, and beneficial to the patients, air evacuation in the European Theater rested administratively on foundations of sand. Under SHAEF policy, transportation of casualties had no status as a separate mission; instead it was consid-

[12] 7th, 9th, 12th, and 28th Field Hospitals, 77th Evacuation Hospital, 93d Medical Gas Treatment Battalion, and 425th and 428th Medical Battalions Annual Rpts, 1944; Surg, ADSEC, Daily Activities Rpts, August-September 1944, and Operations and Evacuation Divisions, OofSurg, ADSEC, Weekly Activities Rpts, August-September 1944, all in Beasley Papers, MHI; Memo, Evacuation Division, OofSurg, ADSEC, to Surg, ADSEC, 17 Sep 44, sub: Daily Situation and Activities Rpts, file HD:ETO:370: Evacuation, September-December 1944; Evacuation Branch, Operations Division, OofCSurg, HQ, ETOUSA, Annual Rpt, 1944, p. 9; Surg, Brittany Base Section, Annual Rpt, 1944, pp. 2-3; 29th Field Hospital Annual Rpt, 1944, pp. 13-16.

[13] Quotation from 7th Field Hospital Annual Rpt, 1944, p. 3. See also Surg, ADSEC, COMZ, Annual Rpt, 1944, p. 65; 8th Field Hospital Annual Rpt, 1944, p. 7; 9th Field Hospital Annual Rpt, 1944, pp. 9-14 and 19-20.

[14] Msgs, HQ, COMZ (FWD), to 24th and 25th Regulating Stations, 29 Aug 44, EvacCorresp, 1942-44, file HD 024 ETO; Memo, Hawley to G-4, COMZ, 1 Sep 44, sub: Distribution of Patients Among Hospitals in France, file HD:ETO:370: Evacuation, September-December 1944; Essential Technical Medical Data Rpt, HQ, ETOUSA, September 1944, p. 2; Evacuation Branch, Operations Division, OofCSurg, HQ, ETOUSA, Annual Rpt, 1944, pp. 7-8; Link and Coleman, *AAF Medical Support*, p. 609; Surg, ADSEC, COMZ, Annual Rpt, 1944, ex. H.

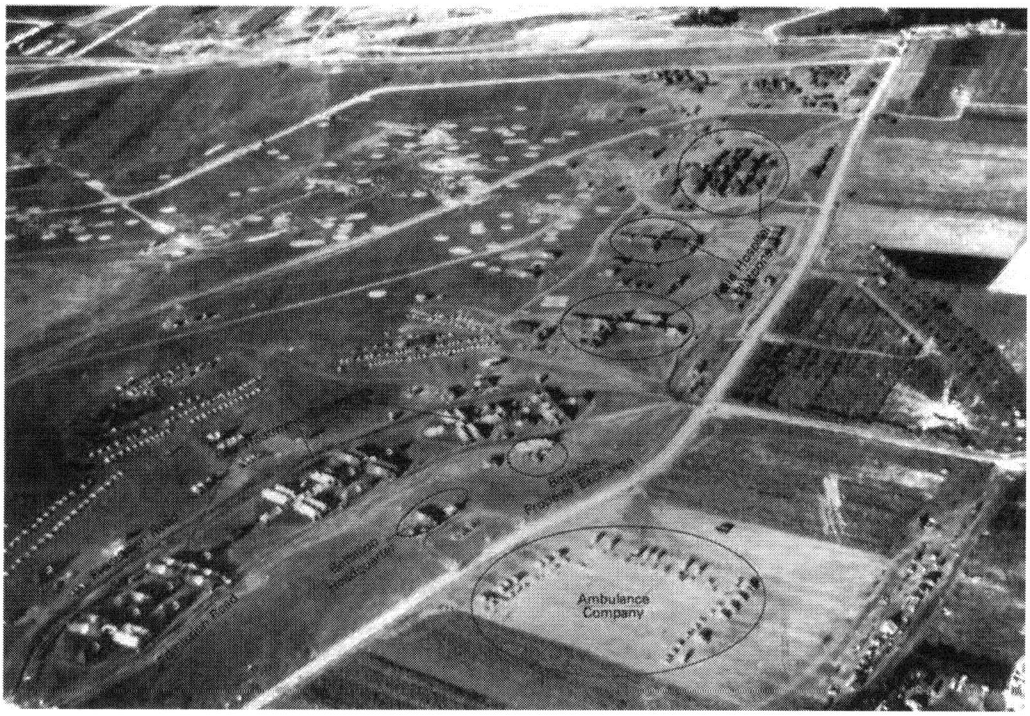

INSTALLATION OF AIR HOLDING UNIT AT TOUL, *consisting of elements of a gas treatment battalion and two field hospitals*

ered strictly a side benefit of emergency resupply. If transport planes carried cargo for the armies to forward airstrips, they could take out wounded and sick on their emtpy return flights. But as Hawley succinctly summarized, "Where there is no supply by air, there is no evacuation by air." [15]

Air resupply itself possessed uncertain priority, and responsibility for it was divided. Two separate air headquarters, each with other primary missions than logistical supply of the ground forces, controlled most ETO transport planes. Under the Ninth Air Force the IX Troop Carrier Command, with over 1,400 aircraft, flew supply missions and also was formally in charge of air evacuation. However, its principal task was transporting airborne troops; SHAEF withdrew its planes from supply and evacuation whenever a major air drop was in prospect. The other command, the 302d Air Transport Wing, directly under USSTAF, had about 180 aircraft and did a disproportionately large share of both supply and evacuation, even though its main mission was logistical support of the air forces. SHAEF assigned tasks to both these commands through the Combined Air Transport Operations

[15] Memo, Hawley to Kenner, 30 Aug 44, sub: Evacuation by Air, file HD:ETO:370:Evacuation, September–December 1944.

Room (CATOR), an agency of the Allied Expeditionary Air Forces. Located at Stanmore, England, CATOR received transport mission requests from the Allied armies and allocated British or American aircraft to them. However, it had little authority over the operating air headquarters and no capacity to plan and coordinate transport activities. Further, CATOR worked under a SHAEF policy of minimizing nonemergency air resupply of ground forces whenever alternative means were available.[16]

The IX Troop Carrier Command was responsible for coordinating air evacuation with the armies and Communications Zone. For this purpose the command assigned an air evacuation officer to General Hawley's staff and maintained liaison with the principal ground force headquarters. Early in the pursuit, for example, IX Troop Carrier Command and the Third Army directly negotiated evacuation and air supply arrangements. However, no means existed by which Hawley, as theater chief surgeon, could assemble the total daily evacuation requirements of the armies and the Advance Section and present them to CATOR for matching with the day's planned resupply flights, except by impossibly time-consuming transmission through several intermediate headquarters. His air evacuation officer, Hawley complained, "has no authority to act and is able to get air evacuation only through personal contacts, and then only when resupply is in operation. He has been unable to obtain much information in advance." Late in August Hawley began a campaign for the establishment of air evacuation as a separate mission independent of resupply and for a direct channel of communications between his office and the authorities controlling the planes. He also suggested the assignment of C–47s exclusively to medical evacuation and supply. On the latter proposal Hawley received support from General Grow, the USSTAF surgeon, and from General Kenner, who called for the placement of "a certain number of C–47s . . . under the immediate control of the Medical Department . . . organized as a medical air unit, marked with the Red Cross and employed only for medical missions." SHAEF and USSTAF took no immediate action on these recommendations.[17]

General Hawley, aware as he was of the fragility of his long air-dependent evacuation chain, worked diligently during the pursuit to implement preinvasion plans for using hospital trains, running on repaired continental lines, as the primary means of mass long-distance casualty move-

[16] The Ninth Air Force provided tactical and logistical support to the U.S. armies. Air transport organization and problems are summarized in Craven and Cates, eds., *AAF*, 3:554–62. See also Ruppenthal, *Logistical Support*, 1:572–73.

[17] First quotation from Memo, Hawley to CG, COMZ, 15 Sep 44, sub: Status of Means for Evacuation, file HD 024 ETO CS (Hawley Chron). Second quotation from Memo, Kenner to ACofS, G–4, SHAEF, 2 Sep 44, sub: Evacuation by Air, in Medical Division, COSSAC/SHAEF, War Diary, September 1944. See also MFR, 28 Aug 44, sub: Conference Between Representatives of Third Army and Troop Carrier Command at HQ, TUSA, EvacCorresp, 1942–44, file HD 024 ETO; Memo, Hawley to Kenner, 30 Aug 44, sub: Evacuation by Air, file HD:ETO:370:Evacuation, September–December 1944; Memo, Hawley to CofS, COMZ, 8 Sep 44, sub: Request for Planes, and endorsements, AirEvacCorresp, file HD 580 ETO; Link and Coleman, *AAF Medical Support*, pp. 599–604.

ment. Early in July, accordingly, SHAEF, the 12th Army Group, and the Communications Zone worked out a schedule for cross-Channel ferrying of the British-built overseas hospital trains that the medical service had been using in England, but the delayed opening of the Cherbourg docks and marshaling yards prevented early movement of the equipment. Meanwhile, the Transportation Corps by the end of the month had restored most of the Cotentin rail network. Taking advantage of this circumstance, the Advance Section on 4 August put a locally improvised ambulance train into service. The train, with the 11th Hospital Train personnel as staff, consisted of French freight cars fitted with litter brackets, with openings cut in the ends of the boxcars to permit movement between them during runs, and with one car converted into a primitive kitchen. It carried loads of about 100 stretcher and 125 ambulatory patients from St.-Lo and the Normandy general hosptials to Cherbourg. On 14 August, with Cherbourg now open, the first overseas train to reach the Continent, Number 27, carrying the 43d Hospital Train, rolled off a British car ferry onto French tracks. Three days later it made its inaugural trip from Lison Junction to Cherbourg.[18]

Outside Normandy, the deficiencies of hastily repaired railroads, and even more a shortage of rolling stock, restricted rail evacuation throughout the pursuit. The lines between Normandy and Paris, never the most highly developed part of the French system, had been heavily bombed before D-Day to keep German reinforcements out of the invasion battle; they had suffered also from German demolitions as the enemy retreated. Engineer units, nevertheless, opened a circuitous route into Paris on 30 August and had portions of the much more extensive but less damaged network north and east of the capital usable as far as Liege, Verdun, and Toul by late September. On 2 September the first hospital train, Number 27, with the 203d General Hospital crowded on board as passengers, entered Paris. It arrived after an eighty-hour journey by way of St.-Lo, Coutances, Avranches, Folligny, Mayenne, Le Mans, Dreux, Chartres, Rambouillet, and Versailles, which included a day spent waiting for a derailed train to be cleared off the tracks and also other halts to reconnoiter the ramshackle line ahead. Based on the Gare St.-Lazare, the train at once began a grueling series of runs between the forward railheads and Paris, alternating with slow bumpy trips to Cherbourg. On the Normandy runs it carried casualties back and medical units, usually general hospitals, forward.[19]

[18] For preinvasion plans, see An. 9—Medical, p. 14, to FECOMZ Plan, 14 May 44, file HD 370 ETO. Ruppenthal, *Logistical Support*, 1:544–53, traces the restoration of continental trackage. See also Surg, ADSEC, Daily Activities Rpts, 26, 29 July and 4, 17 Aug 44, and Evacuation and Hospitalization Divisions, OofSurg, ADSEC, Weekly Activities Rpts, weeks ending 5 and 19 Aug 44, all in Beasley Papers, MHI; Evacuation Branch, Operations Division, OofCSurg, HQ, ETOUSA, Annual Rpt, 1944, encl. 4, and, in file HD 024 ETO, ibid., Daily Diary, 3, 5, 11, and 31 Jul 44; Memo, Col F. H. Mowrey to Surg, Southern Base Section, 6 Jul 44, sub: Hospital Trains, EvacCorresp, 1944–45, file HD 370.05 ETO; Surg, ADSEC, COMZ, Annual Rpt, 1944, p. 17; 11th Hospital Train Annual Rpt, 1944; 43d Hospital Train Hist, 1944, pp. 2–3.

[19] 43d Hospital Train Hist, 1944, pp. 3–5.

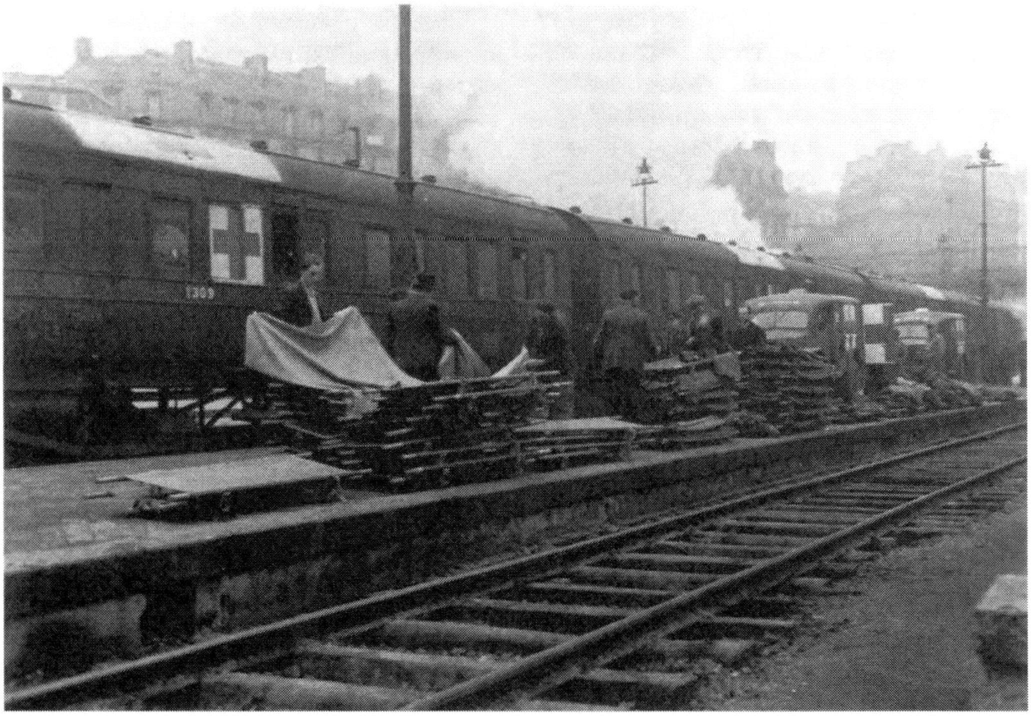

FRENCH CIVILIAN LITTERBEARERS PREPARING TO UNLOAD A HOSPITAL TRAIN AT GARE ST.-LAZARE

In spite of urging by General Hawley, few additional trains crossed the Channel during August and early September. The high-roofed passenger cars of the overseas trains had to compete for space on the few rail ferries that could carry them with even more urgently needed locomotives, and the locomotive shortage in France often idled what trains were available. As late as 18 September the medical service had only five hospital trains in continental operation, two in Normandy and three stabled in Paris. With a capacity of about 300 patients each, these trains could make no more than one round trip to the front or Cherbourg every couple of days. Hence, they could not begin to met the evacuation needs of the armies.[20]

Besides trying to reduce his dependency on air transportation, Hawley attempted to shorten his lines of evaucation, and secure more flexibility in distributing patients, by aggressively pushing forward his general hospitals. Under preinvasion plans the twenty-five general hospitals ear-

[20] Memos, Hawley to G–4, ETO, 5 Aug 44, and Hawley to CG, COMZ, 18 Sep 44, sub: Status of Evacuation as of 1200 Hours, file HD 024 ETO CS (Hawley Chron); Memo, Hawley to Kenner, 30 Aug 44, sub: Evacuation by Air, file HD:ETO:370: Evacuation, September–December 1944; Ltr, Hawley to TSG, 24 Aug 44, file HD 024 ETO O/CS (Hawley-SGO Corresp); Editorial Advisory Board, 1962, p. 188; Essential Technical Medical Data Rpt, HQ, ETOUSA, September 1944, p. 2.

marked for early continental deployment were to have been located well south of the Seine, with the largest clusters at Rennes, Vitre, Laval, and Le Mans. The course of the campaign nullified these plans. Hawley, as the pursuit accelerated, started advancing general hospitals as far toward the front as possible for the purpose of opening the maximum number of continental fixed beds within convenient supporting distance of the armies (*see Map 14*). Because the cumbersome 1,000-bed units took time to move and prepare for operation, whether in tents or taken-over buildings, they had to occupy their chosen sites almost before the infantry had driven out the last Germans. The chief surgeon was willing to risk losing units in order to have them in the right places at the right time. He told Beasley: "There are uncommitted general hospitals in the C[OM]Z. You should ask my office to send them forward to you so that you can, in turn, establish them as far forward as possible. But you should commit no more of these in any one place than is absolutely necessary. . . . Save some to move forward to other sites." To the surgeon general, Hawley declared: "We are throwing general hospitals forward as fast as we can get transport to move them." [21]

In late August, besides the six general hospitals established in the Cotentin, Hawley had about a dozen others in bivouac near the beaches awaiting plant assignments, the landing of their equipment, or both. At the chief surgeon's instructions ADSEC on 20 August opened the 127th General Hospital in Rennes and the 19th in Le Mans, both in former French civilian hospital buildings. Hawley devoted his main effort to establishing several thousand fixed beds in newly liberated Paris. His Hospitalization Division chief, Colonel Darnall, entered the capital as Allied troops still were mopping up German resistance. Darnall secured from the Gaullist authorities options on most of the city's largest hospitals, many of them only recently evacuated by the Germans. The chief surgeon rushed units forward from Normandy by every available conveyance to occupy these plants. Advance elements of the 108th General Hospital, the first to begin operations, took possession of Beaujon Hospital on 31 August; the unit opened 400 beds on 2 September, so near the fighting that patients came in directly from division clearing stations. Two more general hospitals, the 203d and 217th, went into limited operation within the next couple of days. By the third week of September a total of six hospitals (five general and one station) were in place and functioning. Officers of Hawley's and Beasley's staffs were

[21] First quotation from Ltr, Hawley to Beasley, 22 Aug 44, file HD 024 ETO CS (Hawley Chron). Second quotation from Ltr, Hawley to TSG, 24 Aug 44, file HD 024 ETO O/CS (Hawley-SGO Corresp). See also Memo, Hawley to G-4, COMZ (Fwd), 15 Aug 44, EvacCorresp, 1942-44, file HD 024 ETO; Surg, ADSEC, COMZ, Annual Rpt, 1944, p. 23; Operations Division, OofCSurg, HQ, ETOUSA, Annual Rpt, 1944, p. 4; Darnall, "Breakthrough to Paris," pp. 276-77; Hawley Interv, 1962, p. 82, CMH.

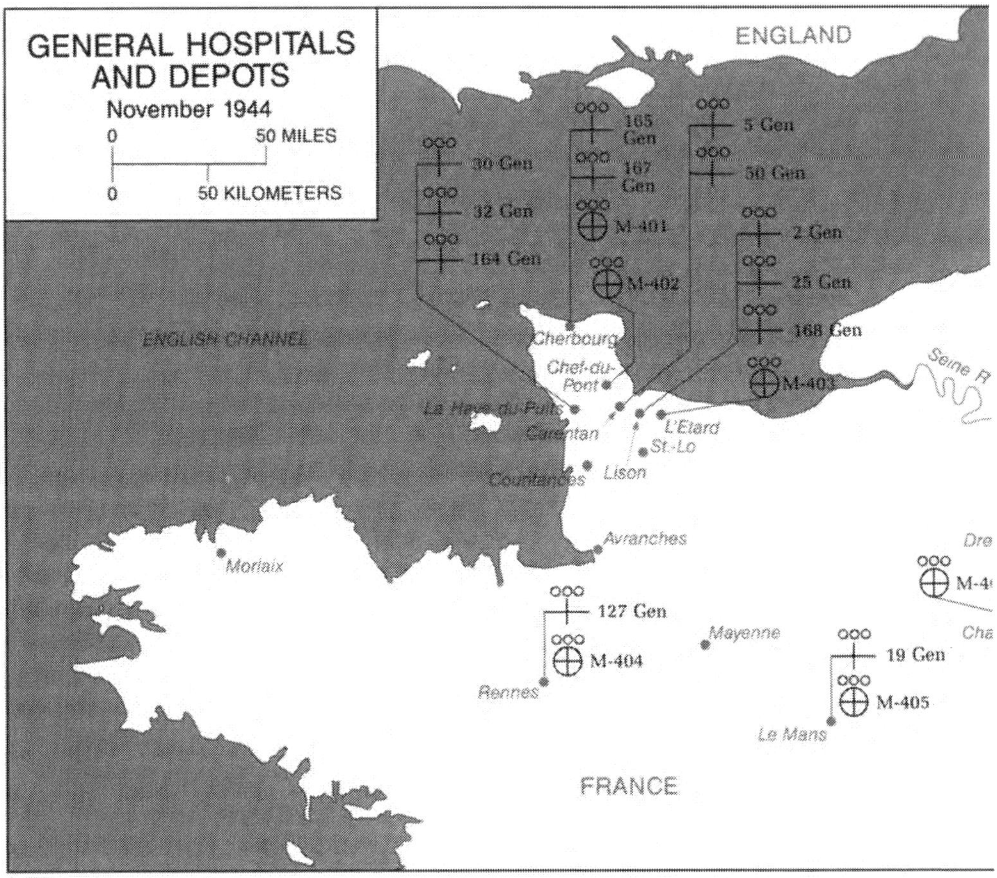
GENERAL HOSPITALS
AND DEPOTS
November 1944
0
50 MILES
0
50 KILOMETERS
ENGLAND
30 Gen
32 Gen
164 Gen
165 Gen
167 Gen
M-401
M-402
5 Gen
50 Gen
2 Gen
25 Gen
168 Gen
M-403
Seine R
ENGLISH CHANNEL
Cherbourg
Chef-du-Pont
La Haye-du-Puits
Carentan
L'Etard
St.-Lo
Lison
Countances
Avranches
Moriaix
127 Gen
M-404
Rennes
Mayenne
19 Gen
M-405
Le Mans
FRANCE

MAP 14

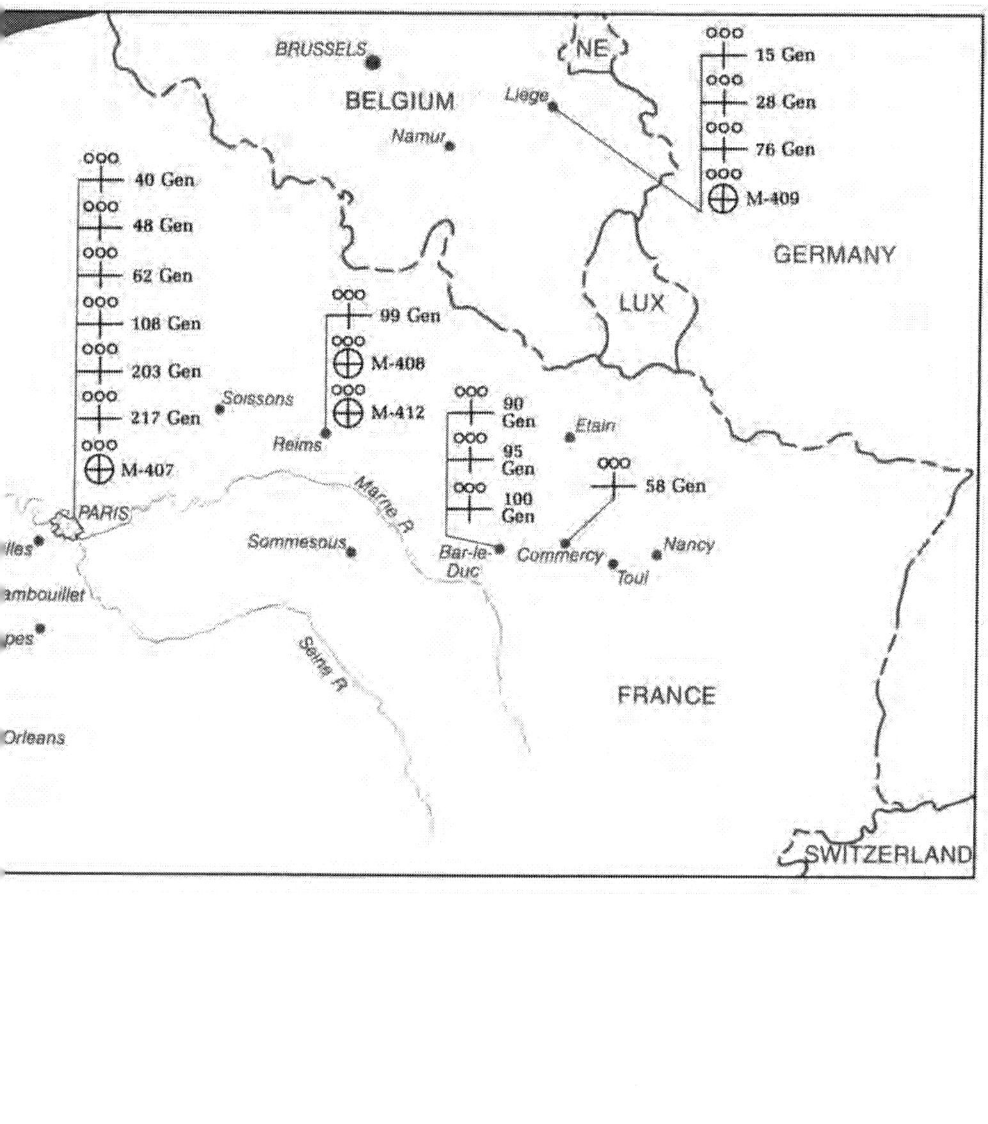
BRUSSELS
NE
BELGIUM
Liege
Namur
15 Gen
28 Gen
76 Gen
M-409
GERMANY
LUX
40 Gen
48 Gen
62 Gen
108 Gen
203 Gen
217 Gen
M-407
99 Gen
M-408
M-412
Soissons
Reims
90 Gen
95 Gen
100 Gen
Etain
58 Gen
PARIS
Marne R.
Sommesous
Bar-le-Duc
Commercy
Toul
Nancy
ambouillet
Seine R.
FRANCE
Orleans
SWITZERLAND

scouting for additional sites around Paris and in northern France and Belgium.[22]

Paris, as the stabling of hospital trains and the concentration of general hospitals there indicated, rapidly became the hub of the continental evacuation system. The principal rail lines from Belgium and eastern France converged at the capital, and it possessed two major airports. On 5 September representatives of the chief surgeon and the surgeons of ADSEC, Seine Section, and the armies initialed an evacuation plan under which most casualties not flown directly from the Advance Section to Britain and Normandy would pass through Paris. An air holding unit and ambulance directing point at Le Bourget field in the northern outskirts was to receive and sort patients from ADSEC and the armies—then only a short distance away. The unit was to send over-30-day patients directly to England by air and those destined for COMZ either by plane to Normandy or by ambulance to the Paris general hospitals. Those hospitals, in turn, were to evacuate by air to the United Kingdom through Le Bourget and, as trains became available, by rail to the Normandy Base Section.[23]

Two companies of Advance Section's 93d Medical Gas Treatment Battalion opened the Le Bourget holding unit on 5 September; ten days later, they turned it over to the 8th Field Hospital, which the gas treatment battalion's trucks had hauled up from Normandy. As the Paris evacuation system went into full operation, the hospital soon found itself running one of the busiest holding units on the Continent. Housed in tents near the runways and later in a converted school building, the 8th, with the 426th Medical Ambulance and 706th Medical Sanitary Companies attached, routinely handled over 1,000 patients a day—incoming casualties from the First and Third Armies and outgoing evacuees from the Paris general hospitals.[24]

The Paris hospitals and holding unit were barely in place when the need for them became urgent. Throughout the first couple of weeks after the armies crossed the Seine, SHAEF had committed most of its transport planes to their resupply; hence, the medical service had been able to rely almost entirely on air evacuation. On 15 September this situation abruptly changed. Supreme Allied Headquarters, without advance warning to the medical service, withdrew the IX Troop Carrier Command from logistical missions to prepare for

[22] The five general hospitals were the 108th (Beaujon), 217th (La Pitie), 203d (Garches), 40th (Le Vesinet), and 62d (Eaubonne); the station hospital was the 365th (American Hospital of Paris). See Hospitalization Division, OofCSurg, HQ, ETOUSA, Annual Rpt, 1944, pp. 10–11. See also Essential Technical Medical Data Rpt, HQ, ETOUSA, August 1944, encl. 1; Surg, ADSEC, Daily Activites Rpts, August–September 1944, Beasley Papers, MHI; Surg, Seine Section, Annual Rpt, 1944, p. 27; 108th General Hospital Annual Rpt, 1944, p. 14; 127th General Hospital Annual Rpt, 1944, p. 3; Ltrs, Hawley to TSG, 24 Aug and 14 Sep 44, file HD 024 ETO O/CS (Hawley–SGO Coresp); Darnall, "Breakthrough to Paris," pp. 280–81.

[23] Memo, Maj D. J. Twohig to DepCSurg, HQ, COMZ (Fwd), 5 Sep 44, sub: Plan for Evacuation Through Paris Area, file HD:ETO:370:Evacuation, September–December 1944; Surg, Seine Section, Annual Rpt, 1944, p. 26.

[24] 8th Field Hospital Hist, 1943–44, pp. 7–8; 93d Medical Gas Treatment Battalion Hist, 1943–44, pp. 10–11.

MARKET-GARDEN, just as the first attacks on the West Wall increased combat casualties. For the next couple of weeks the airborne operation tied up most Allied transport planes when bad weather did not ground them. Patients, many needing early definitive treatment, filled army and ADSEC holding units and then backed up into the evacuation hospitals. By the twentieth at least 5,000 sick and wounded were awaiting evacuation in and just to the rear of the armies, and the Advance Section was removing them at a rate of only 1,500 a day.

COMZ evacuation officers improvised frantically to compensate for the near-total loss of air transport. What hospital trains were available shuttled continuously between the forward areas and Paris. The ADSEC holding units behind the First Army sent casualties all the way from Belgium to the French capital by ambulance. These expedients, however, quickly filled the Paris general hospitals, which themselves had few means of sending off patients. From the 302d Transport Wing, General Hawley obtained some evacuation planes, no more than a quarter of those he needed. He finally resolved the immediate crisis by arranging informally, through General Grow, for an indeterminate but substantial number of off-the-record IX Troop Carrier Command evacuation flights.[25]

Hawley took the evacuation crisis as an occasion to bring to a head his campaign for more reliable, responsive air support. Through General Lee, he asked SHAEF immediately to assign 200 C–47s daily to evacuation until the patient backlog was cleared up, which should take about three days. Thereafter, Hawley wanted 50 planes a day, which would give him a daily capacity of about 2,000 casualties. SHAEF rejected this proposal. On 21 September Lt. Gen. Walter Bedell Smith, Eisenhower's chief of staff, informed General Lee that airborne operations then in progress ruled out the proposed medical airlift and that "in any event, your medical evacuation plans must not be predicated on any fixed air evacuation. Rather, air evacuation must be considered as a bonus to be available from time to time as conditions permit." Smith held firm even in the face of an appeal from General Bradley. He explained to the army group commander that C–47s for the medical service would have to come from air commands "created to meet specific operational needs, and their permanent diversion to another mission could only be accomplished at the expense of their original purpose." In place of improved air evacuation Smith, after consulting with Kenner and Hawley, gave the medical service high priority for transportation and other support so that it could set up more general hospitals north and east

[25] Memo, Evacuation Division, OofSurg, ADSEC, to Surg, ADSEC, 17 Sep 44, sub: Daily Situation and Activities Report, file HD:ETO:370:Evacuation, September–December 1944; various memos, September 1944, in file HD 024 ETO CS (Hawley Chron); Evacuation Branch, Operations Division, OofCSurg, HQ, ETOUSA, Daily Diary, 3, 16, and 22 Sep 44, file HD 024 ETO; 428th Medical Battalion Annual Rpt, 1944, p. 4; Gorby Interv, 1962, pp. 90–93, CMH; Ltr, Hawley to Col E. L. Bergquist, 28 Sep 44, box 2, Hawley Papers, MHI; Surg, ADSEC, COMZ, Annual Rpt, 1944, p. 18.

of Paris and put additional ambulance trains in operation.[26]

Taking advantage of SHAEF interest and support, Hawley lost no time in strengthening his ground evacuation system. He quickly pushed general hospitals across the Seine. By mid-September he already had two of these units bivouacked at Reims and three more at Paris, ready for assignment. Five more general hospitals in Normandy awaited disembarkation of their equipment. Hawley obtained a speedup in landing the latter units' assemblies at Cherbourg. He deployed the hospitals already in northern France, and others as soon as they came up, in positions close behind the First and Third Armies. To provide more beds for the First Army, the 15th General Hospital opened in Liege on the twenty-first in a former Belgian military hospital and the 28th General Hospital went into operation in the same city about two weeks later. In Paris, meanwhile, a sixth general hospital, the 48th, began admitting patients on the twenty-third and the 99th General Hospital opened in Reims on the twenty-ninth. However, an effort to move three general hospitals into Nancy and another into Verdun ran afoul of the Third Army, which still had those cities within its area and refused to turn over hospitals and other structures occupied by its own medical units. The Advance Section finally opened three general hospitals (the 90th, 95th, and 100th) in Bar-le-Duc, considerably to the west of Nancy, between 18 and 28 October. Wherever located, these and the previously established continental general hospitals functioned essentially as large professionally well-endowed holding and transit facilities. The hospitals in and to the north of Paris gave definitive treatment only to very short-term patients; they evacuated all others as soon as transportable. The Normandy general hospitals retained casualties returnable to duty within thirty days. This was an inefficient use of general hospitals. But a shortage of evacuation hospitals in the COMZ troop basis, and the seemingly limitless demand for holding beds, made it necessary *(see Map 14)*.[27]

The medical service and the Transportation Corps cooperated to put more hospital trains in service. Maj. Gen. Frank S. Ross, the theater chief

[26] First quotation from Memo, Smith to Lee, 21 Sep 44, sub: Medical Evacuation, file HD: 370.05:Evacuation and Movement of Troops. Second quotation from Ltr, Smith to CG, 12th Army Group, 30 Sep 44, sub: Evacuation of Casualties, file HD:ETO:370:Evacuation, September–December 1944. See also September 1944 correspondence in file HD 024 ETO CS (Hawley Chron); Memo, Col V. A. Rapport to Lee, 20 Sep 44, sub: Air Evacuation of Casualties, AirEvacCorresp, file HD 580 ETO; Medical Division, COSSAC/SHAEF, War Diary, September 1944; Link and Coleman, *AAF Medical Support*, p. 606.

[27] Ltrs, Hawley to TSG, 14 Sep 44, and Hawley to Inspector General, WD, 10 Oct 44, file HD 024 ETO O/CS (Hawley-SGO Corresp); September–October 1944 correspondence in file HD 024 ETO CS (Hawley Chron); Surg, ADSEC, Daily Activities Rpts, September–October 1944, Beasley Papers, MHI; Memo, Hawley to G–4, ETO, 21 Sep 44, AirEvacCorresp, file HD 580 ETO; Ltr, Brig Gen H. R. Gay to Hawley, 1 Oct 44, box 2 Hawley Papers, MHI; Essential Technical Medical Data Rpt, HQ, ETOUSA, September 1944, pp. 7–8 and encl. 1; Operations Division, OofCSurg, HQ, ETOUSA, Annual Rpt, 1944, p. 4; Hospitalization Division, OofCSurg, HQ, ETOUSA, Annual Rpt, 1944, p. 12; Surg, ADSEC, COMZ, Annual Rpt, 1944, p. 68; Surg, Normandy Base Section, Annual Rpt, 1944, pp. 8–9; 15th General Hospital Annual Rpt, 1944, pp. 3–4 and 16–17; 76th General Hospital Annual Rpt, 1944, p. 34.

TABLE 8—TRENDS IN EVACUATION FROM THE ARMIES AND ADVANCE SECTION

1944	Sea		Air		Air & Sea	Rail		Total	
	Weekly	Cumulative	Weekly	Cumulative	Cumulative	Weekly	Cumulative	Weekly	Cumulative
June									
12	8,559	8,559	122	122	8,681			8,681	8,681
19	6,249	14,808	1,855	1,977	16,785			8,104	16,785
26	1,592	16,400	3,753	5,730	22,130			5,345	22,130
July									
3	4,544	20,944	1,821	7,551	28,495			6,365	28,495
10	5,601	26,545	2,725	10,276	36,821			8,326	36,821
17	6,372	32,917	5,586	15,862	48,779			11,958	48,779
24	2,644	35,561	4,142	20,004	55,565			6,786	55,565
31	1,668	37,229	7,938	27,942	65,171			9,606	65,171
August									
7	3,982	41,211	7,338	35,280	76,491	529	529	11,849	77,020
14	2,703	43,914	8,699	43,979	87,893	389	918	11,791	88,811
21	304	44,218	3,059	47,038	91,256	364	1,282	3,727	92,538
28			2,377	49,415	93,633		1,282	2,377	94,915
September									
4			2,089	51,504	95,722		1,282	2,089	97,004
11			3,404	54,908	99,126	212	1,494	3,616	100,620
18			1,143	56,051	100,269	1,332	2,826	2,475	103,095
25			5,693	61,744	105,962	2,348	5,174	8,041	111,136
October									
2			5,641	67,385	111,603	1,776	6,950	7,417	118,553
9			1,527	68,912	113,130	5,529	12,479	7,056	125,609
16			2,082	70,994	115,212	5,788	18,267	7,870	133,479
23			716	71,710	115,928	5,130	23,397	5,846	139,325
30			189	71,899	116,117	3,996	27,393	4,185	143,510

Source: Surg, ADSEC, COMZ, Annual Rpt, 1944, ex. H.

of Transportation, spurred by SHAEF and COMZ and by direct appeals from Hawley, within twenty-one days moved seventeen trains across the Channel. Ross also improvised expedients, such as coupling empty hospital trains to those hauling supplies and ammunition, to move this vitally needed equipment forward from Cherbourg to Paris. At Paris the Transportation Corps, late in September, assembled three additional improvised trains from French hospital and passenger cars, with medical equipment cobbled together from American and captured German stocks. By the end of October the medical service had twenty-five hospital trains running on the Continent—enough by themselves, Hawley estimated, to meet the armies' daily evacuation requirements. The chief surgeon arranged with the railway scheduling authorities for daily high-priority runs between Paris and the front and from the capital to Cherbourg. With the means thus enlarged, rail evacuation attained its originally intended predominance (*Table 8*). The number of patients transported by train grew from less than 1,400 in August to 13,700 in September and 35,000 in October. In September six hospital trains from Paris entered the

Normandy Base Section; in October the base section received thirty-five. Other evacuation elements redeployed to take maximum advantage of the railroads. At Paris an entire medical ambulance company, the 552d, went into operation late in September, transferring patients between railway stations and general hospitals. The Advance Section relocated its holding units for easier access to the railheads and, beginning early in October, consistently evacuated more casualties by rail than by air.[28]

While rail evacuation increased in scale and effectiveness, air evacuation remained for the medical service an important and, in many respects, a preferred alternative. General Hawley, for example, considered air movement of casualties less costly, in terms of cargo space taken up, than rail transportation. Surgeons still favored air evacuation for the most severely wounded. By that method a man could go from the Advance Section to his place of definitive treatment within a few hours, whereas evacuation by rail through Paris to Cherbourg and then by ship across the Channel took about four days. With such considerations in mind, the medical service and the air forces during the autumn worked to make air evacuation more efficient and continuously available.[29]

Late in September the chief surgeon acquired an air evacuation unit of his own, the 320th Squadron, 302d Transport Wing. This squadron, based at Le Bourget, flew twenty UC-64s, single-engine high-wing monoplanes designed for freight and passenger service in the Canadian arctic and purchased by the Army for observation, liaison, and light cargo-carrying. The UC-64s had not proved particularly satisfactory for any of their intended missions. Hence, USSTAF was willing to place the aircraft, and their underemployed, bored crews, at the disposal of General Hawley, in partial compensation for the C-47s it could not give him. The chief surgeon employed the UC-64s, each of which could accommodate three litter and a couple of sitting patients, not only for emergency evacuation from the armies to Paris but also to haul forward urgently needed medical supplies. In their first three months of service the "Grow Escadrille," as the pilots nicknamed themselves, transported 1,100 casualties, 30,000 pints of blood, and about 460 tons of other medical supplies.[30]

---

[28] September–October 1944 correspondence in file HD 024 ETO CS (Hawley Chron); Evacuation Branch, Operations Division, OofCSurg, HQ, ETOUSA, Annual Rpt, 1944, encls. 4 and 9, and, in file HD 024 ETO, ibid., Daily Diary, 3, 5, 6, and 9 Oct 44; Essential Technical Medical Data Rpt, HQ, ETOUSA, September 1944, p. 2, and October 1944, p. 2; Troop Movements and Training Branch, Operations Division, OofCSurg, HQ, ETOUSA, Annual Rpt, 1944, p. 15; Surg, ADSEC, COMZ, Annual Rpt, 1944, p. 57 and ex. H; Surg, Normandy Base Section, Annual Rpt, 1944, pp. 6–7; Surg, Seine Section, Annual Rpt, 1944, p. 27; 552d Ambulance Company Annual Rpt, 1944, pp. 9–11; 12th Field Hospital Annual Rpt, 1944, pp. 8–9; 77th Evacuation Hospital Annual Rpt, 1944, p. 7; Hawley Interv, 1950, file HD 000.71, CMH; Hawley Interv, 1962, pp. 84–85, CMH.

[29] Ltr, Hawley to CG, COMZ, 4 Oct 44, sub: The Effect of Rail Evacuation Upon Rail Cargo Capacities, file HD 024 ETO CS (Hawley Chron); Essential Technical Medical Data Rpt, HQ, ETOUSA, October 1944, p. 2.

[30] Memo, Hawley to Operations Division, OofCSurg, HQ, ETOUSA, 28 Sep 44, sub: Policies Governing Use of UC-64 Planes, file HD 024 ETO CS (Hawley Chron); Memos, Col K. R. Bendetsen to G-4, COMZ, 2 Oct 44, sub: Supplemental Air Evac-

Continued

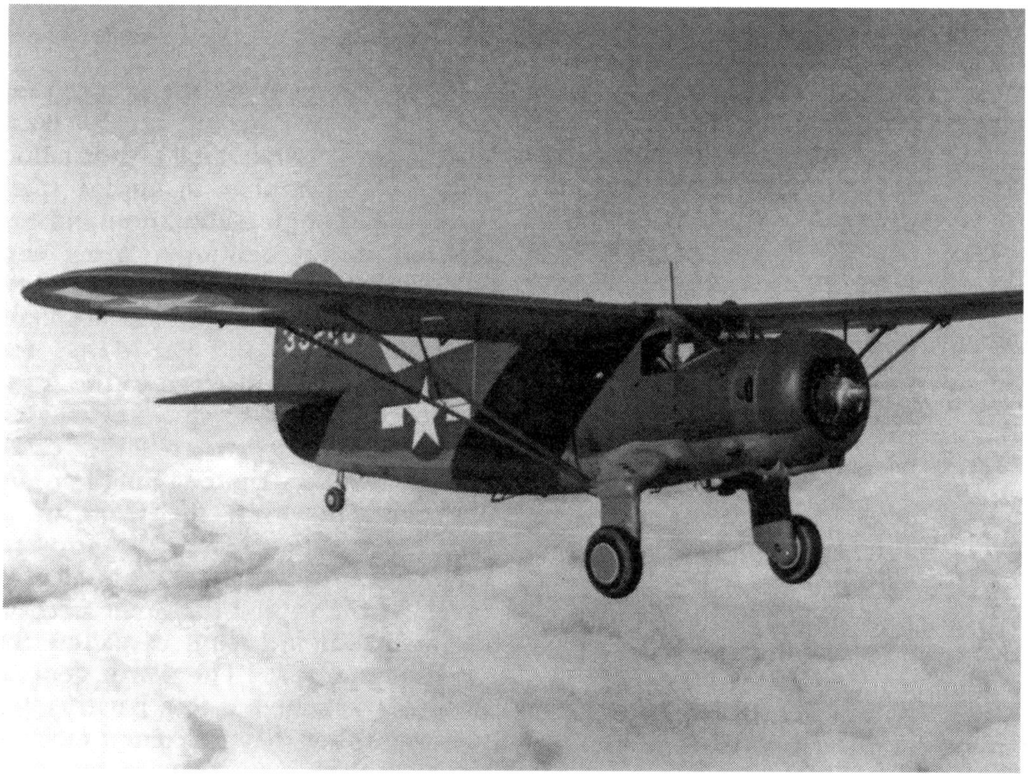

UC-64 OF THE "GROW ESCADRILLE"

During the autumn the theater significantly improved its procedures for requesting C-47s for evacuation. On 8 September SHAEF transferred oversight of U.S. air evacuation from the Ninth Air Force to USSTAF, thereby elevating responsibility for the task to the senior theater air headquarters. The IX Troop Carrier Command remained the principal implementing agency. At General Smith's suggestion the air forces, armies, and Communications Zone early in October revamped their medical evacuation liaison and communications systems. As a result of this effort General Hawley's office at last could collect daily reports of the number and locations of casualties awaiting evacuation and transmit the information to CATOR in time for the transport agency to correlate it with the next day's supply flights. Evacuation still had no status as a separate mission and remained dependent on aerial resupply, but cooperative officers in the IX Troop Carrier Command and the 302d Transport

uation Service, and Maj R. S. Gilfilian to CSurg, ETO, 13 Dec 44, sub: Inter-Continental Evacuation by UC-64s, AirEvacCorresp, file HD 580 ETO; Kendrick, *Blood Program*, pp. 535-36; Link and Coleman, *AAF Medical Support*, p. 607. Medical use of UC-64s was contemplated well before D-Day. See Summary of Gen Kenner-Gen Grow Conference, 4 Apr 44, in Medical Division, COSSAC/SHAEF, War Diary, April 1944.

Wing often evaded this restriction, to the benefit of the medical service. When the medics desperately needed planes, their aviation colleagues, with a little ingenuity, usually could discover an urgent requirement for cargo somewhere, or they could send a replacement aircraft just arrived in the theater on an extra mission before it reported to its assigned squadron. By such formal and informal means the Army Air Forces, within the confines of SHAEF policy, always made at least some evacuation aircraft available to the medical service.[31]

The medical service rapidly eliminated its late September evacuation backlog, assisted by the almost daily arrival of additional hospital trains; by the resumption of large-scale air resupply after MARKET-GARDEN; and, above all, by a lull in combat and its attendant reduction in casualties. At the end of September no more than 800 patients were awaiting evacuation in the armies and ADSEC, and the Paris hospitals were clearing out their own accumulations by air and rail. Evacuation continued to improve during October. On the nineteenth the Evacuation Branch of Hawley's office reported that the situation was "excellent in forward areas" and that the Paris hospitals had 2,000 empty beds.[32]

By late October, as the armies prepared for a new assault on the West Wall, the continental evacuation system was complete in outline (*Diagram 3*), although elaboration and expansion would continue. Army and ADSEC holding units sent very short-term patients to the general hospitals at Liege, Reims, and Bar-le-Duc, for definitive treatment close to the front and early return to duty. Whenever possible, they dispatched severe cases directly to the United Kingdom by air. Now, however, the majority of long-term patients left the forward area by hospital train, bound for Paris. At the capital the Seine Section detrained all incoming casualties for sorting and rest. The Paris general hospitals retained a few patients for treatment, but they evacuated most as soon as they were able to travel in order to maintain large reserves of empty beds for sudden surges of casualties from the front. Evacuees from Paris might go by ambulance to Le Bourget, for loading on United Kingdom-bound aircraft. More likely, they would be taken to the Gare St.-Lazare and placed on trains again, for the up to three-day run to the Normandy Base Section general hospitals or to Cherbourg and embarkation on hospital carriers for the voyage to Southampton. While surgeons continued to prefer air evacuation whenever they

---

[31] Ltr, Smith to CG, 12th Army Group, 30 Sep 44, sub: Evacuation of Casualties, file HD:ETO:370:Evacuation, September-December 1944; Evacuation Branch, Operations Division, OofCSurg, HQ, ETOUSA, Annual Rpt, 1944, pp. 13-14, and, in file HD 024 ETO, ibid., Daily Diary, 18 Sep and 1, 2, 4, 6 Oct 44; Link and Coleman, *AAF Medical Support*, pp. 606-07 and 616. See also Memo, Col F. H. Mowrey to G-4, ETO, 4 Oct 44, sub: Communications for Air Evacuation; SOP, IX Troop Carrier Command, 18 Oct 44, sub: Medical Air Evacuation of Casualties; Ltr, Col F. H. Mowrey to CSurg, ETO, 22 Nov 44, sub: Air Evacuation. All in AirEvacCorresp, file HD 580 ETO.

[32] Quoted words from Evacuation Branch, Operations Division, OofCSurg, HQ, ETOUSA, Daily Dairy, 19 Oct 44, file HD 024 ETO. See also ibid., entries for 29 Sep-31 Oct 44, same file; Memos, Hawley to Kenner, 26 and 29 Sep 44, file HD 024 ETO CS (Hawley Chron); Essential Technical Medical Data Rpt, HQ, ETOUSA, October 1944, p. 1.

DIAGRAM 3—ETO EVACUATION SYSTEM, LATE 1944

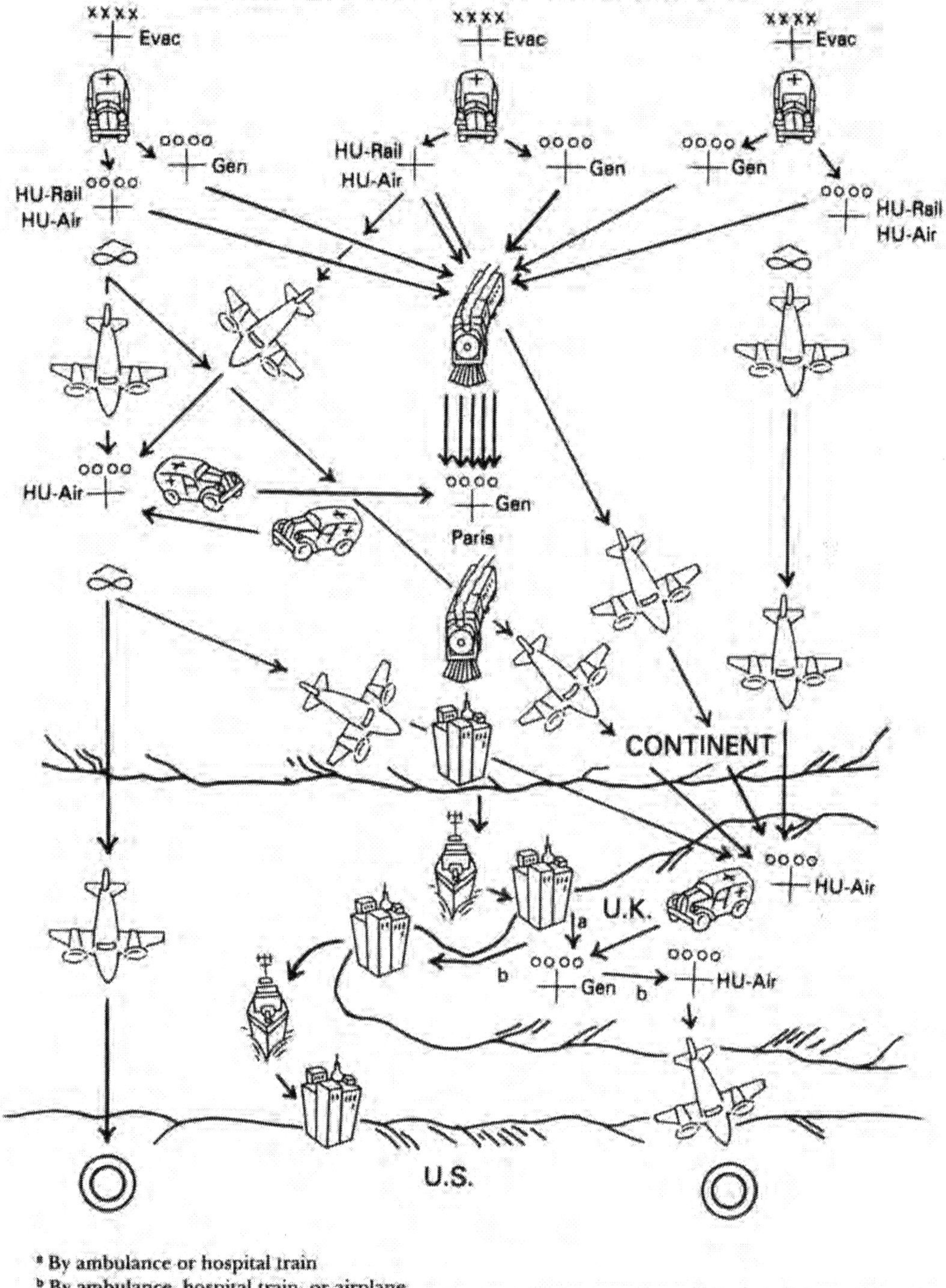

[a] By ambulance or hospital train
[b] By ambulance, hospital train, or airplane
Source: Evacuation Branch, Operations Branch, OofCSurg, HQ, ETOUSA, Annual Rpt, 1944, encl. 3.

could obtain it, the medical service on the Continent now appeared to possess the resources and flexibility to get along without it.[33]

General Hospitals to the Front

Between the St.-Lo breakout and the end of October the medical service placed 18,000 general hospital beds in operation on the Continent. The majority of these were in units hastily moved forward and established in northern France and Belgium, to help relieve army facilities and hold patients for air and rail evacuation. Deploying these large, cumbersome hospitals was a complicated task, involving inter-Allied politics as well as American logistics. The hospitals themselves, besides overcoming the problems of movement, had to adapt to new, often unsuitable quarters and to take on functions different from those usually performed by general hospitals.[34]

Several divisions of the chief surgeon's office had a hand in setting up general hospitals. The Operations Division selected the areas in which they were to be established and oversaw the entire deployment procedure to ensure that hospitals opened where they were supposed to more or less on time. The Hospitalization Division located, and secured permission to use, particular buildings or pieces of land and directed the movement and setting up of units. The Supply Division put together and shipped the bulky unit equipment assemblies, trying, not altogether successfully, to bring them together in France with the people who were to use them.[35]

Colonel Darnall did much of the site reconnaissance in person, assisted by Lt. Col. Irving A. Marshall, the head of his Construction Branch, and by officers from the Advance Section and the newly formed Allied governments. During August Darnall selected hospital locations around Rennes and then entered Paris in the first days of liberation to stake medical service claims there. Early in September he traveled eastward from the capital over the old American World War I battlefields, where he himself had worked in an evacuation hospital, to choose sites close behind the Third Army. As the pursuit ended at the West Wall, he made a four-day 800-mile swing through Belgium and Luxemburg. Riding in jeeps and equipped, Darnall recalled, "with maps, K-rations, full canteens, and jerricans of gasoline," the hospital reconnaissance parties kept up with the forward combat troops and occasionally, in the confusion, entered towns ahead of them. Darnall and his assistants inspected dozens of buildings and tramped over acres of pasture and cultivated land, marking usable locations on maps to guide subsequent planning. Whenever possible, they selected sites grouped together on roads and railways, for organization later into hospital centers.[36]

[33] Memo, Col. F. H. Mowrey to DepCSurg, ETO, 8 Nov 44, AirEvacCorresp, file HD 580 ETO; Evacuation Branch, Operations Division, OofCSurg, HQ, ETOUSA, Annual Rpt, 1944, pp. 9–11; Essential Technical Medical Data Rpt, HQ, ETOUSA, October 1944, p. 2.

[34] The number of beds is from Ltr, Hawley to Inspector General, WD, 10 Oct 44, file HD 024 ETO O/CS (Hawley-SGO Corresp).

[35] Operations Division, OofCSurg, HQ, ETOUSA, Annual Rpt, 1944, p. 4.

[36] Quotation from Joseph R. Darnall, "Hunting Hospital Sites beyond Paris, September 1944," *The*

Continued

Once Darnall and his associates found suitable locations, they negotiated with COMZ and army headquarters, and with Allied civil authorities, for permission to occupy them. Under theater policy, hospitals had first claim on existing buildings, which the medical service, for obvious reasons of patient comfort and operating convenience, preferred to use whenever available. Nevertheless, in the army areas COMZ general hospitals at times took second place to medical units of the organization in control of the ground, as in the case of the Third Army's exclusion of general hospitals from Verdun and Nancy. In liberated towns and cities the medics had to deal, through SHAEF, with reestablished French or Belgian civil administrations. These governments, understandably, often put their own peoples' health and social needs ahead of U.S. Army requirements, and SHAEF frequently deferred to their wishes. Fortunately for the medical service, the overrunning of much of France and the Low Countries without heavy fighting left a larger than anticipated stock of intact structures. In most places the Hospitalization Division simply took over facilities formerly appropriated by the Germans. The division thereby avoided any new displacement of civilians and at the same time made it politically awkward for local officials to deny to the Allies what they previously had yielded to the enemy. As an added benefit, this policy provided the Americans with many of the best hospitals, because those were precisely the buildings the Germans had seized.[37]

When Darnall and Marshall entered Paris in the last days of August seeking hospital buildings, they made immediate, beneficial contact with the newly installed acting French minister of health, Dr. Pasteur Vallery Radot. According to Darnall, Radot, a Resistance member and grandson of the famous scientist Louis Pasteur, "realized that the salvation of France lay not in quickly grabbing back the properties vacated by the retreating Germans, but in helping the Americans to acquire and utilize these facilities until the war was won." The Americans, with Radot's help, within days secured five of the largest and best-equipped civilian hospitals, all of which had been occupied by the Germans until the liberation. During the late September evacuation crisis Radot's successor unhesitatingly evicted a recently installed French staff from a sixth facility, Lariboisiere, to make room for the 48th General Hospital. The Count de Chambrun, the German-appointed French administrator of the American Hospital of Paris, an American-financed private institution, was less accommodating. A suspected collaborator, as were many of

Military Surgeon 103 (August 1948): 85–93. See also ibid., "Breakthrough to Paris," pp. 271–81; Hospitalization Division, OofCSurg, HQ, ETOUSA, Annual Rpt, 1944, pp. 3 and 10–12; Surg, ADSEC, Daily Activities Rpts, August–September 1944, Beasley Papers, MHI.

[37] For hospital priority, see An. 8–Medical, pp. 5–6, to ADSEC Plan, 30 Apr 44, and An. 9–Medical, pp. 39–40, to FECOMZ Plan, 14 May 44, file HD 370 ETO; Operations Division, OofCSurg, HQ, ETOUSA, Annual Rpt, 1944, p. 5; ADSEC Hist, pp. 73–74; Darnall, "Breakthrough to Paris," pp. 273–74; Hospitalization Division, OofCSurg, HQ, ETOUSA, Semiannual Rpt, January–June 1945. Ltr, Hawley to Kenner, 3 Nov 44, file HD 024 ETO CS (Hawley Chron), illustrates difficulties with civilian authorities.

his staff, Chambrun first appealed to General Hawley not to take over his well-appointed 150-bed facility. That failing, Chambrun asked Hawley to let the existing international staff stay on as U.S. Army employees. Hawley refused both requests and took the hospital, less because he absolutely needed it than as a symbolic compensation to the French for the expropriation of so many of their facilities. The chief surgeon installed the 350th Station Hospital in the plant, where it cared for officer and female patients from the U.S. headquarters in the capital.[38]

As it secured buildings and open-field sites, the Hospitalization Division moved units forward to occupy them. To achieve this, the division first coordinated with medical service channels and then forwarded a request to the COMZ G-4 to issue directives to the appropriate base sections, which actually conducted the movement. Most general hospitals that went into operation during the pursuit came to the Continent from the United Kingdom, although late in September units began arriving directly from the United States. All the hospitals spent varying lengths of time encamped in Normandy, in hedgerow fields that still bore the scars and debris of battle. Most staging hospitals sent doctors and nurses off on detached service, usually with auxiliary surgical teams. The rest of their people whiled away the time in training, physical conditioning, and bargaining with neighboring civilians for Calvados and souvenirs.[39] Two of the first hospitals into Paris, the 108th and 203d, were preparing to open tented plants near Cherbourg when they received orders to stop work and pack again for movement.

The personnel of hospitals bound for Paris and points north and east of it usually traveled on empty hospital trains, except for detachments driving the unit vehicles. For the nearly 1,000 men and women of a general hospital, crowded into a single train along with the on-board medical unit, it was an uncomfortable trip, memorable for the shortage of seats, berths, toilets, and cooking facilities and for the interminable delays. Inevitably, units became separated from their equipment assemblies; the 48th General Hospital, for example, went to Paris while its outfit went to Liege. Hospitals arriving early in newly captured cities underwent a variety of adventures. The 62d General Hospital, which entered Paris on 30 August, spent three days trying to find a headquarters to assign it a location and then—without maps—the locations itself. Bivouacked at a chateau south of the capital, unit personnel heard nightly rifle shots as Free Frenchmen rounded up German stragglers in the nearby woods. They also found several Germans living in their own attic on stolen American rations. With no

[38] Hospitalization Division, OofCSurg, HQ, ETOUSA, Annual Rpt, 1944, p. 11; Darnall, "Breakthrough to Paris," pp. 277–81 (quotation on p. 281); ibid., "Sidelights," p. 26; Surg, Seine Section, Annual Rpt, 1944, pp. 16–17; Ltr, Hawley to General Purchasing Agent, ETO, 24 Sep 44, file HD 024 ETO CS (Hawley Chron); Editorial Advisory Board, 1962, pp. 123–124 and 192–93; Hawley Interv, 1962, pp. 77–79; CMH. The 350th Station Hospital in fact employed many of the nurses, clerical people, and general laborers of the American Hospital. See 350th Station Hospital Annual Rpt, 1944.

[39] Calvados was a French brandy from the Department of Calvados.

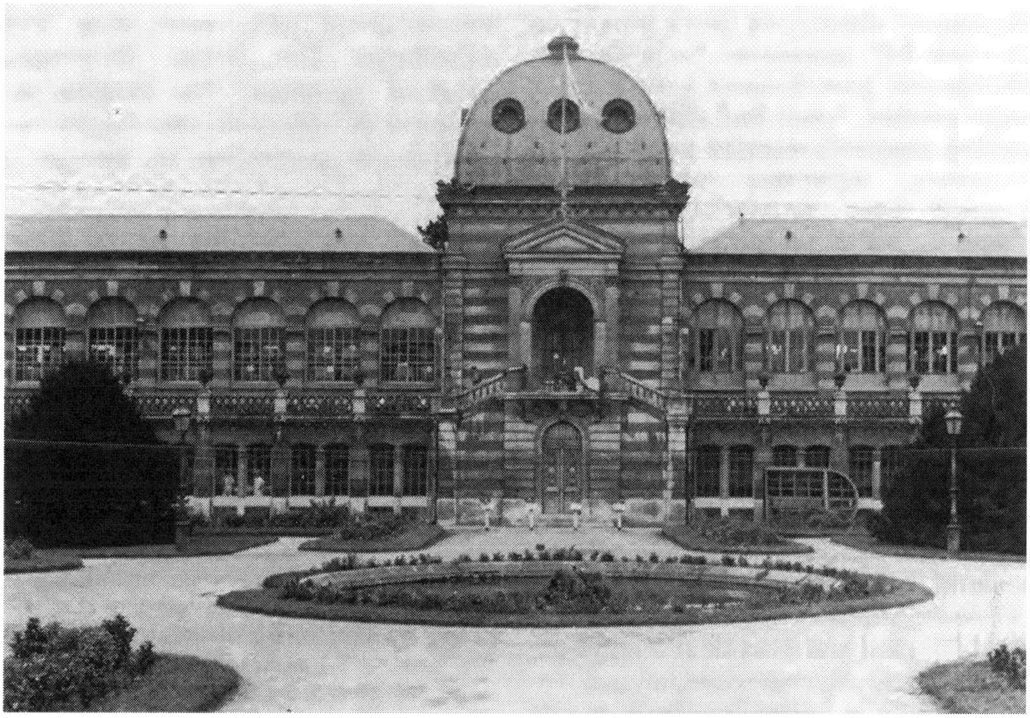

CIVILIAN HOSPITAL IN PARIS VACATED BY RETREATING GERMANS

supply depots yet in operation, the hospital sent its own trucks back to the beaches for food and gasoline, only to have several cargoes hijacked on the return trip, reportedly by Third Army troops.[40]

Whether in buildings or tented camps, general hospitals labored to place their facilities in operation in the shortest possible time. Units occupying existing hospitals often had to contend with the results of German vandalism. In many of the large Paris hospitals the departing enemy ripped out wiring, plugged toilets, sabotaged plumbing, carried off or smashed furnishings and equipment, and created a revolting welter of rotten garbage, soiled dressings, and overflowing urinals and bedpans. Yet the Germans left other plants almost undamaged, with furniture, instruments, and X-ray and other machines in good order, ready for use. In a few instances the Americans found well-stocked pharmacies. Even in the more severely vandalized premises, general hospitals could begin receiving patients within days of moving in, after a thorough cleanup and limited repairs.

Units that had to remodel barracks and schools or construct expedition-

[40] Troop Movements and Training Branch, Operations Division, OofCSurg, HQ, ETOUSA, Annual Rpt, 1944, pp. 14–15; Surg. Normandy Base Section, Annual Rpt, 1944, pp. 2–4 and 16–17; Surg, ADSEC, Daily Activities Rpt, 17 Aug 44, Beasley Papers, MHI; 15th, 40th, 48th, 62d, 95th, 99th, 108th, and 203d General Hospitals Annual Rpts, 1944; 15th General Hospital Unofficial Hist, 1943–44; Brown Interv, 1979, CMH.

ary tented plants took much longer to go into full operation. Even though the theater gave hospital construction high priority, units had difficulty obtaining engineer support and building materials, especially when hard-pressed base section commanders chose to put other projects ahead of those for the medical service. Torrential rains, which began in mid-October, turned open-field sites into seas of mud, further slowing the work. General hospitals facing long construction delays concentrated on getting their people and equipment under shelter and opening wards for emergency care and holding purposes. To speed the opening of the general hospitals at Bar-le-Duc, the Advance Section temporarily attached field hospital platoons to them. These platoons set up tented operating facilities for the larger hospitals, which otherwise could not have performed surgery until the engineers finished extensive renovation of their plants.[41]

The forward general hospitals, accustomed to providing comparatively leisurely long-term treatment, had to reorganize on the job for mass casualty reception, emergency care, and evacuation. The first hospitals to open were inundated with wounded, many fresh from division clearing stations. In Paris the 108th General Hospital admitted about 1,000 patients—the majority German prisoners who had received little more than first aid—during its initial forty-eight hours of operation. The hospital responded to the crisis with rapid improvisation. According to the unit's report:

> Our own U.S.A. supplies had not come up from Le Mans, many of our surgeons and shock teams . . . were still away on detached service, no penicillin was available, the hospital communications systems had been destroyed by the retreating Germans, and we had no practical experience as a group in handling large numbers of casualties as an evacuation hospital. We used German paper dressings and other material they had left behind. . . . We put dentists, chemists and bacteriologists to work in the wards with the medical men who were not giving anesthetics or assisting in surgery. We worked 36 hours straight, hoping to catch up, but were still 500 cases, needing operation, behind schedule. We then organized 12-hour day and night shifts and operated only upon the most severely wounded. . . .

For the 108th, and the other hospitals that followed it into operation, the flow of casualties directly from aid and clearing stations soon ended. Nevertheless, most general hospitals on the Continent continued to give only the simplest of care to a rapid turnover of patients. Only those farthest to the rear, in the Normandy, Brittany, and Loire Base Sections, performed anything like their textbook functions.[42]

---

[41] Surg, ADSEC, COMZ, Annual Rpt. 1944, pp. 49–50; Surg, Brittany Base Section, Annual Rpt, 1944, p. 2; 15th, 40th, 62d, 76th, 99th, 100th, 203d, and 217th General Hospitals Annual Rpts, 1944; Darnall, "Breakthrough to Paris," pp. 279–80; Hawley Interv, 1962, pp. 76–77, CMH; Memo, Hawley to G–4, ETO, 5 Oct 44, sub: Hospital Construction—Le Mans, file HD 024 ETO CS (Hawley Chron); 58th Field Hospital Annual Rpt, 1944, pp. 11–18.

[42] 108th General Hospital Annual Rpt, 1944, pp. 19–20 and 24–25; 127th General Hospital Annual Rpt, 1944, p. 4. These units also acted as station hospitals for neighboring COMZ troops. See Surg, Oise Base Section, Annual Rpt, 1944, pp. 4–5 and 8–9.

Medical Supply in the Pursuit

The unanticipated rapidity of the advance upset COMZ plans for an orderly flow of supplies from the coast through intermediate depots to the Advance Section and from the latter to the armies. The Communications Zone disembarked sufficient stores at Cherbourg, at the minor Normandy ports, and at OMAHA and UTAH beaches, all of which, thanks to the hard work and ingenuity of engineer and port troops, greatly exceeded their expected cargo-handling capacity. The difficulty lay in establishing and stocking depots in the widening distance between the initial lodgement area and the front. The Advance Section projected, then abandoned, several logistical support areas as the armies left them far behind. Supreme Allied Headquarters, anticipating an early Rhine crossing, temporarily delayed the setting up of depots in Paris so that development of this key logistical center began only as the offensive slowed down in mid-September.

When the Advance Section did open forward depots, the trailing base sections lacked transportation to move goods to them. With the railroads, especially those south and west of Paris, able to carry only a fraction of the required tonnage, and with air transport limited in capacity and uncertain of availability, the Communications Zone had to rely on trucks for most long-distance hauling until well into the autumn. Its vehicle complement, not intended for such use, was barely adequate for the task. To make the most of what they had, COMZ and ADSEC late in August assembled most of their own truck companies and others borrowed from the armies—over 120 in all—for the Red Ball Express. Running around the clock on specially marked highways closed to all other traffic, Red Ball vehicles carried supplies from the Normandy dumps to a terminal area near Chartres, and later to forward transfer points at Soissons behind the First Army and at Sommesous in the rear of the Third. In a month of strenuous operation Red Ball convoys moved forward over 135,000 tons of freight and aircraft perhaps another 13,000. These deliveries, however, fell short of the amounts the armies needed to fight at full effectiveness. The 12th Army Group, and later SHAEF, in mid-September began allocating the daily tonnage that reached the front among the armies and ADSEC so as to maintain at least a limited offensive and ensure balanced distribution on the basis of tactical plans. Most of the time the higher headquarters gave priority to the First Army. The tonnage allocation system, although plagued by confused record-keeping, duplicate requisitions, disputes between the armies and COMZ about who was receiving how much, and occasional unauthorized appropriation of shipments, more or less met minimum operational requirements. However, it did not allow the Communications Zone to build up forward reserves. Only in October and November, when the railroads at last started hauling significant tonnage, did the depots north and east of the Seine begin to fill.[43]

---

[43] Ruppenthal, *Logistical Support*, 1:488–99 and 553–83; ibid., 2:3–8, 17–21, 53, 57, 88, 134–41, 169–80, 355–57; ADSEC Hist, pp. 74–75 and 102–03.

Medical supplies accounted for only a small proportion of the tonnage handled by the Communications Zone. In mid-August, for example, out of 395,000 long tons of stores in ADSEC dumps, only 5,100 tons belonged to the medical service. Nevertheless, the medical service encountered its full share of supply problems. As did the other technical services, it set up a string of depots across France and Belgium and then, with limited transportation and under constant pressure of time, tried to stock them while still meeting the day-to-day needs of field army and COMZ units.[44]

The Advance Section established medical supply depots in the track of the armies in a network radiating from the pre-breakthrough facilities at Cherbourg, Chef-du-Pont, and L'Etard. During late August medical depot companies successively opened Depots M-404 and M-405. Located in a factory building and warehouses in Rennes, M-404 supplied the troops in Brittany; located in Le Mans but never fully stocked, M-405 served mainly local COMZ units. Supplies initially intended for Le Mans, which was to be part of a major logistical support area but was never completed as the advance left it far behind, went instead to Depot M-406T, set up on 26 August in stubble fields near Chartres. Part of a major Red Ball Express terminal, M-406T received and distributed about 4,000 tons of medical supplies before closing on 29 September. On 6 September the 31st Medical Depot Company moved into two large warehouses formerly belonging to the Paris Chamber of Commerce and transformed them into Depot M-407. Conveniently located alongside a rail spur and a canal, M-407 became the single most important continental medical supply facility. It received materiel from Normandy and from M-406T at Chartres, shipped supplies forward to the armies and ADSEC, and supported the hospitals and holding units in Paris. Beyond the Seine, Depot M-408 began operations in a taken-over warehouse in Reims on the twentieth, issuing to the armies and to neighboring COMZ units. Finally, as the Advance Section established a forward logistical base at Liege, Depot M-409 opened on 27 October in a Belgian customs warehouse and nearby garages to serve the First and Ninth Armies. Depots farther to the rear, meanwhile, closed down, M-401 at Cherbourg in late August, M-404 at Rennes in mid-October, and M-403 at L'Etard in mid-November. Depot M-402 at Chef-du-Pont expanded into the main Normandy receiving point for supplies arriving on the Continent from England and America.[45]

The continental depots labored under handicaps (*see Map 14*). As had been true in Great Britain, T/O depot companies seldom had enough men to operate large COMZ installations. They augmented their strength with German prisoners (who, howev-

[44] ADSEC Hist, p. 75.

[45] Supply Division, OofCSurg, HQ, ETOUSA, Annual Rpt, 1944, sec. II, pp. 8-15; Surg, ADSEC, COMZ, Annual Rpt, 1944, pp. 27-29 and ex. K; Surg, Brittany Base Section, Annual Rpt, 1944, pp. 4-5; Surg, Seine Section, Annual Rpt, 1944, pp. 40-42; 13th and 30th Medical Depot Companies Annual Rpts, 1944. Medical depots exclusively had an "M" prefix, while general depots, which might have medical sections, carried a "G" prefix.

er, required depot company men to guard them), with enlisted men detailed from staging medical units, and with French civilians. At M–407 the 31st Company eventually employed over 200 Parisians. The depot companies needed all the manpower they could obtain because, except for M–407, they were short of cranes, forklifts, and other machinery for moving heavy weights. Much of their initial stock arrived on the massive sled-like skids intended for beach disembarkation and open-air storage. Lacking equipment for lifting these skids, depot troops often had to unpack them on the trucks that brought them, thereby delaying the release of scarce vehicles. At Le Mans and Chartres they hit upon the expedient of digging pits into which trucks could back, bringing the decks of their cargo compartments level with the ground and permitting other vehicles, or men with ropes, to drag off the skids. Open-field depots dissolved into quagmires, as heavy traffic destroyed the surfaces of dirt roads and as the fall rains soaked the countryside. The mud became so deep at M–406T that Red Ball trucks at times simply unloaded where they bogged down. After much effort, the 30th Company, which operated this depot, managed to pave two roads with gravel and obtained a portable conveyor to move freight from trucks to the fields, where it rested on dunnage made of brush and timber from the nearby woods. At busy M–402, deepening mud finally defeated the efforts of the 11th Medical Depot Company to keep supplies moving, even though the company reconditioned several abandoned French and German tractors to free mired vehicles. During November the depot shifted operations to Carentan, where it obtained buildings and hard-surfaced open storage on an abandoned airstrip.[46]

Control of depot operations and supply issues changed as the lines of communications lengthened. At the start of the pursuit the ADSEC and FECOMZ surgeons supervised all medical supply functions, including reception of incoming goods and issues to the Communications Zone and the armies. The ADSEC medical supply division processed all requisitions from the armies, either filling them from its own dumps or calling for emergency shipments from Great Britain. As it moved away from the coast, the Advance Section turned over its beach installations to the Normandy Base Section, the surgeon of which thereafter oversaw reception and forwarding of medical supplies that arrived by sea. The Advance Section set up the depots at Rennes, Le Mans, Chartres, and Reims, and then left them to other base sections as it continued to follow the armies. From mid-August on, the Supply Division of the chief surgeon's office assumed direct technical supervision of receiving, storage, stock control, and issuing by all COMZ depots. The armies then requisitioned directly from the depots through the regulating stations, entirely bypassing the ADSEC surgeon.[47]

---

[46] Surg, ADSEC, COMZ, Annual Rpt, 1944, p. 29; Surg, Normandy Base Section, Annual Rpt, 1944, p. 19; Surg, Seine Section, Annual Rpt, 1944, pp. 40–41; 11th, 13th, and 30th Medical Depot Companies Annual Rpts, 1944.

[47] Surg, ADSEC, COMZ, Annual Rpt, 1944, p. 27 and ex. K; Supply Division, OofSurg, ADSEC, Weekly Activities Rpt, week ending 19 Aug 44,

Continued

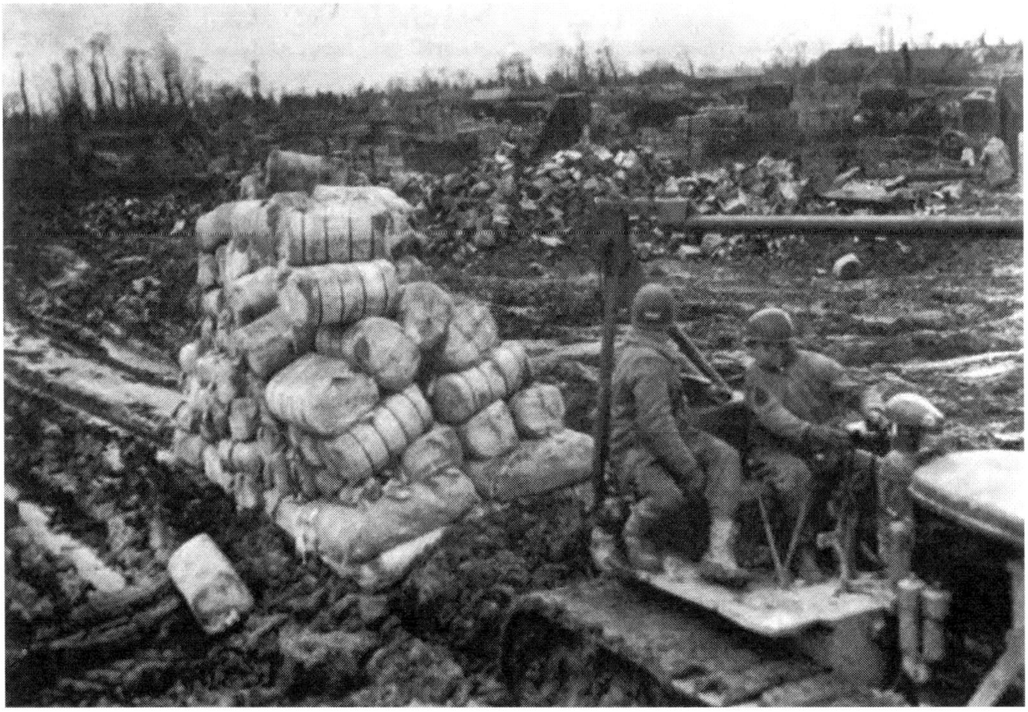

MANEUVERING A CAPTURED GERMAN TRACTOR THROUGH THE MUD AT MEDICAL DEPOT M-402

Beginning in September the 12th Army Group-SHAEF tonnage allocation systems dominated medical supply of the armies and ADSEC. Under these systems each army and the Advance Section received a daily allowance of supplies, which they divided among their own technical services as the basis for their requisitions. For the medical service First Army, Third Army, and ADSEC allotments together varied from 20 to 90 tons a day, depending on the period of the pursuit. At COMZ headquarters medical supply officers, working with the G-4, reconciled army and ADSEC requisitions with the Red Ball space assigned to the medical service for that day. The Normandy Base Section loaded the supplies and started them forward, initially to the Chartres terminal area and later to Soissons and Sommesous. At the latter two places ADSEC medical in-transit storage points (MISPs), manned by detachments from the regulating stations, checked incoming Red Ball trucks for medical service freight and either directed the drivers to final destinations or unloaded the cargo and held it for pickup by the armies.

Through tonnage allocation and the Red Ball Express, the medical service was guaranteed transportation

Beasley Papers, MHI; Surg, Normandy Base Section, Annual Rpt, 1944, pp. 18-19; Fenton Interv, 7 Jun 45, box 222, RG 112, NARA.

for a limited amount of its supplies, but the systems had their drawbacks. Tonnage allocation, while it worked well for uniform bulk shipments, such as rations, ammunition, and POL, was ill-adapted to the variety of small items the medics had to move. The daily transportation allowance, measured in total weight and volume, did not always match the day's requisitions, forcing the Supply Division to leave out some articles while including others, not wanted by the armies, to fill the assigned space. Stock control broke down in both the armies and Communications Zone. The Supply Division chief, Colonel Hays, reported that the "armies were constantly in a quandary as to the quantities yet due in and had difficulty in preparing their requisitions." Medical service supplies, seldom enough on a given day to fill an entire convoy, usually went forward in single truckloads. In spite of the best efforts of the MISPs, shipments often disappeared en route, as the vehicles carrying them broke down or were misdirected. The Red Ball system as a whole suffered from deficiencies in convoy control so that the Supply Division rarely could trace missing cargoes.[48]

During the pursuit air transport played as vital a role in medical supply of the armies as it did in evacuating casualties, and in the supply function it was more reliable. Unlike evacuation, aerial resupply of ground forces possessed status as a recognized mission, which the chief surgeon could request through a liaison officer at CATOR. In addition, before D-Day, General Hawley persuaded the theater to assign one C–47, reinforced in late June by a second, exclusively to the medical service each day to fly whole blood, biologicals, and emergency cargoes across the Channel. These aircraft picked up their loads at Greenham Common airstrip, conveniently close to Depot G–45 at Thatcham, a major medical supply facility, and to the ETO blood bank at Salisbury. They discharged freight at army and ADSEC fields, and also at Le Bourget, for transfer to the UC–64s. During August, September, and October the regularly assigned transports, and others on occasional missions, hauled several hundred thousand pounds of medical supplies each week. According to Lt. Col. Robert R. Kelley, MC, one of Hays' assistants, "During nip-and-tuck phases of the operations, we were able in all instances to adequately make supplies available through . . . air lift." Airlift, however, also had its disruptive aspects. Most air shipments, particularly emergency ones, duplicated supplies previously requisitioned and delayed somewhere in the line of communications, thereby contributing to record-keeping confusion and to the misallocation of materiel.[49]

---

[48] Quotation from Supply Division, OofCSurg, HQ, ETOUSA, Annual Rpt, 1944, sec. II, ex. III (Memo, Col S. B. Hays to Hawley, 24 Dec 44, sub: Difficulties in Moving Medical Supplies and Equipment), pp. 1, 8–9, 11. See also Surg, ADSEC, COMZ, Annual Rpt, 1944, pp. 28 and 59–60; Surg, ADSEC, Daily Activities Rpt, 13 Sep 44, Beasley Papers, MHI; ADSEC Hist, pp. 75–76.

[49] Quotation from Kelley Interv, 27 Jan 45, box 221, RG 112, NARA. See also Supply Division, OofCSurg, HQ, ETOUSA, Annual Rpt, 1944, sec. II, pp. 20–22 and exs. X and XI; Kendrick, *Blood Program*, p. 533.

While the Red Ball Express and aerial resupply kept army and COMZ medical units going from day to day, they were no substitute for full, balanced continental stocks, properly distributed among rear, intermediate, and forward depots. The Supply Division, before the invasion, had made detailed plans for establishing such stocks, initially by pre-scheduled shipments from Great Britain and, after about 1 September, by deliveries directly from the United States to France. The army's delay in opening Cherbourg, and its failure to open the Brittany ports at all, caused the entire supply buildup to fall behind schedule. In Britain, goods intended for cross-Channel movement backed up in ports and depots; cargoes from the United States had to be diverted to England from Normandy added to the congestion. Other medical supplies remained unreachable for weeks, even months, on vessels anchored offshore awaiting access to limited unloading facilities. One ship from New York, which arrived in French waters on 17 August, did not begin discharging her cargo until 10 December. Because the New York Port of Embarkation usually placed all of a given shipment of a particular item on only a few vessels, such diversions and unloading delays totally upset the effort to accumulate balanced stocks. Reserves never reached the desired D+180 level of sixty days, and surpluses in some categories were matched by persistent shortages in others. The Supply Division repeatedly had to make emergency requisitions upon the United Kingdom Base to replace continental stores or meet immediate needs.[50]

The difficulties of landing supplies on the Continent were minor compared with those of moving goods forward, especially for the purpose of filling COMZ depots. With the Red Ball Express and air transport almost entirely employed in day-to-day support of operations, medical supply officers and depot commanders relied on improvisation and the seizure of every random opportunity to build up their advance reserves. To stock Depot M-404 at Rennes, Colonel Hays and his staff collected trucks from the Normandy Base Section general hospitals for a shuttle from Chef-du-Pont. In late September the Supply Division transferred about 800 tons of freight from Normandy to Paris in over 560 replacement jeeps, trucks, and weapons carriers destined for the armies. Hays provided drivers, detailed from staging medical units, for these vehicles, in return for Ordnance service permission to fill them with medical cargo for a one-way trip. When closing M-406T, the commander of the 30th Depot Company, unable to round up trucks to shift supplies to Paris and Reims, finally secured 17 tank retrievers. A single one of these large flatbeds could haul over 30 tons at a time, either directly to a destination depot or to a railhead. As hospital trains began running out of Paris, the depot there

[50] Ltr, Hawley to TSG, 14 Sep 44, file HD 024 ETO O/CS (Hawley-SGO Corresp); An. 9—Medical, p. 4 and encl. 1, to FECOMZ Plan, 14 May 44, file HD 370 ETO; Wiltse, ed., *Medical Supply*, pp. 265-390; Kelley Interv, 27 Jan 45, box 221, RG 112, NARA; Supply Division, OofCSurg, HQ, ETOUSA, Annual Rpt, 1944, sec. II, ex. III, pp. 1 and 3-4, and sec. V. p. 4.

hitched loaded freight cars onto them for their forward trips. The Advance Section, early in October, set up a medical in-transit storage point at Liege to receive cargoes thus transported; the same installation sent emergency requisitions back to Paris on southbound trains. Use of such expedients declined as the railroads carried increasing tonnages, but the struggle adequately to stock the depots continued throughout the rest of 1944.[51]

Like the field armies, the Communications Zone augmented its supplies and overcame some temporary scarcities with captured German instruments, dressings, hospital equipment, and drugs. In Paris alone the Seine Section discovered 127 separate caches of enemy medical materiel—in warehouses, office buildings, tunnels, barracks, barges, railroad cars, and hospitals. The American collected these supplies, made inventories, checked medicines for safety and correct labeling, and separated out items already in the medical service catalog or which could substitute for standard Army goods. They issued the rest of the materiel to civil affairs units, local health authorities, and POW camp dispensaries. In September, elements of the 13th Medical Depot Company set up in Reims a central collecting point for captured supplies in what had been a major German medical depot. This facility, designated Depot M-412, received enemy medical materiel from throughout the theater and prepared it for American and Allied use. It eventually helped to equip and supply twenty-eight U.S. Army hospitals, fourteen POW enclosure dispensaries, and eighteen displaced person camps, as well as sent selected articles to the Medical Field Service School at Carlisle Barracks, Pennsylvania, for study. For Army medical units, captured goods alleviated some shortages and provided supplementary items. Hospital trains, for example, used German aluminum milk cans and mess equipment for feeding patients during runs.[52]

During the pursuit the Communications Zone kept supplies flowing to the armies at a rate sufficient to meet the fortunately reduced requirements of a period of mobile warfare with light casualties. It also filled the day-to-day needs of its own holding units, general hospitals, and other installations. Only COMZ medical units in army areas reported difficulty in securing supplies; not permitted to draw for expendables on scanty army stocks, these organizations had to send their own trucks long distances back to ADSEC or the beaches, or to call for emergency air shipments. Medical supply officers, by loading stores on anything they could find that was moving forward, made at least a start on building reserves close

[51] Supply Division, OofCSurg, HQ, ETOUSA, Annual Rpt, 1944, sec. II, ex. III, pp. 1–2 and 14–15; Fenton Interv, 7 Jun 45, box 222, RG 112, NARA; Surg, Normandy Base Section, Annual Rpt, 1944, pp. 20–21; Surg. Seine Section, Annual Rpt, 1944, pp. 39–40; Surg, ADSEC, COMZ, Annual Rpt, 1944, p. 29; Surg, ADSEC, Daily Activities Rpt, 31 Aug 44, Beasley Papers, MHI; 30th and 66th Medical Depot Companies Annual Rpts, 1944.

[52] Surg, ADSEC, COMZ, Annual Rpt, 1944, p. 28 and ex. K; Supply Division, OofCSurg, HQ, ETOUSA, Annual Rpt, 1944, sec. II, pp. 16–17; Surg, Seine Section, Annual Rpt, 1944, pp. 38–39; Surg, Oise Base Section, Annual Rpt, 1944, pp. 3–4; 13th Medical Depot Company Annual Rpt, 1944, pp. 15–16.

to the front. As was true for evacuation, the framework of a continental medical supply system was in place by the end of October.[53]

Supplying Whole Blood

The European Theater whole blood distribution system, carefully planned and organized before D-Day, was in full operation by the time of the St.-Lo breakout. Behind each of the armies, an ADSEC blood bank detachment, located at a resupply airfield, received daily planeloads of blood from the Salisbury bank, which sent it across the Channel packed in ice in insulated Marmite cans designed originally as Quartermaster food containers. Refrigerator trucks of the ADSEC detachments delivered the blood to counterpart units with the First and Third Armies; the army detachments in turn distributed the precious fluid to evacuation hospitals and clearing stations. Colonel Beasley's deputy surgeon, Colonel Mason, who had helped set up the system, now directed its operation, working closely with the army group and army surgeons. The blood supply service encountered typical difficulties of the pursuit, such as diversion of its vehicles to other missions and inability of truck drivers to find rapidly moving evacuation and field hospitals. In general, though, the whole blood system worked smoothly, even as supply lines lengthened and one ADSEC detachment was taken away from support of the main advance to supply the VIII Corps in Brittany.[54]

For General Hawley and his assistants, the question late in July was whether the detachments would have enough blood to distribute. The first two months of combat surgery in evacuation and field hospitals confirmed what medical officers had anticipated before D-Day: that the rate of blood usage would be high and that the theater, from its own sources, would not be able to meet the demand. Whereas the writers of the *Manual of Therapy* envisioned surgeons administering approximately 1 pint of whole blood to every 2 of plasma, the actual ratio was nearer 1 to 1. Surgeons in Normandy used an average of 1 pint of whole blood for every 4 casualties. On visits to the forward hospitals Hawley and his consultants, after careful observation, concluded not only that such lavish (as they thought) transfusion of whole blood was clinically justified, especially in combating shock, but that patients probably would benefit from even more blood than surgeons were administering. At first sceptical, Hawley was later to recall that doctors in the Normandy evacuation hospitals

[53] For COMZ unit supply problems, see 9th Field Hospital Annual Rpt, 1944, p. 13; 15th General Hospital Annual Rpt, 1944, p. 8; and 127th General Hospital Annual Rpt, 1944, p. 7.

[54] Assignments were: First Army - Detachment A, with Detachment B in COMZ; Third Army - Detachment C, with Detachment D in COMZ. See Kendrick, *Blood Program*, pp. 518–21, 532–35, 549–51; Supply Division, OofCSurg, HQ, ETOUSA, Annual Rpt, 1944, sec. II, p. 20; Surg, ADSEC, COMZ, Annual Rpt, 1944, pp. 55–56; Surg, ADSEC, Daily Activities Rpts, 22 Jul and 16 Aug 44, Beasley Papers, MHI; Surg, Brittany Base Section, Annual Rpt, 1944, p. 5. On operating difficulties, see Ltr, Hawley to Col J. A. Rogers, 19 Jul 44, file HD 024 ETO CS (Hawley Chron); Surg, XII Corps, Annual Rpt, 1944, p. 6; Surg, XX Corps, Annual Rpt, 1944, p. 24; Joseph B. Mason, "The Role of ADSEC in the Supply of Whole Blood to the Twelfth Army Group," *The Military Surgeon* 103 (July 1948): 9–14.

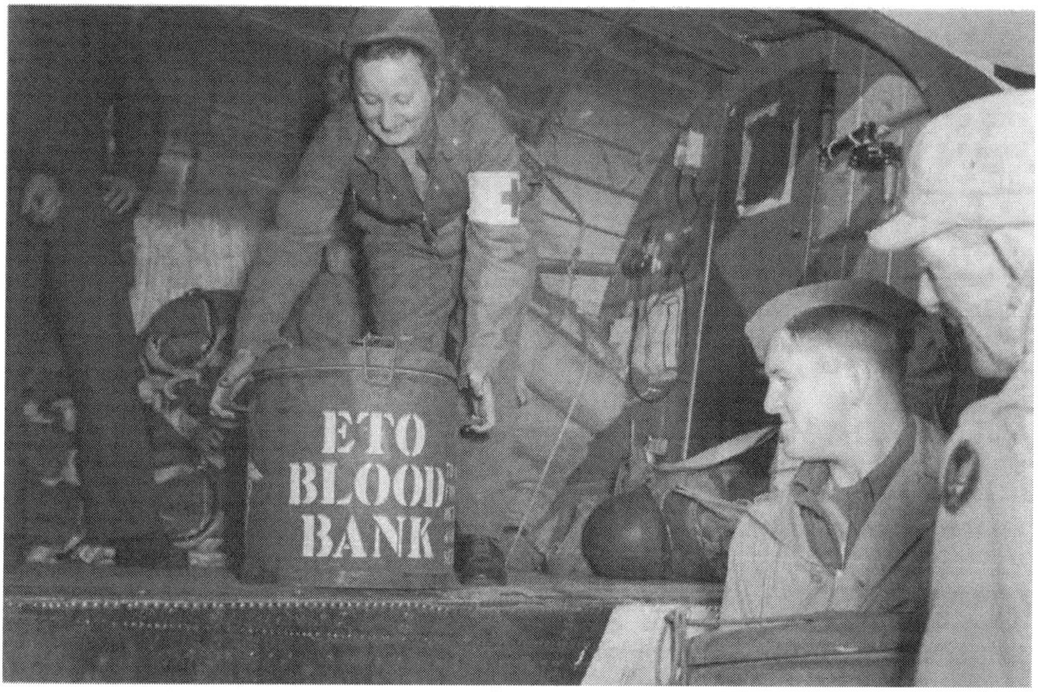

Flight Nurse Lifting Marmite Can of ETO Blood Onto a Continent-Bound C-47

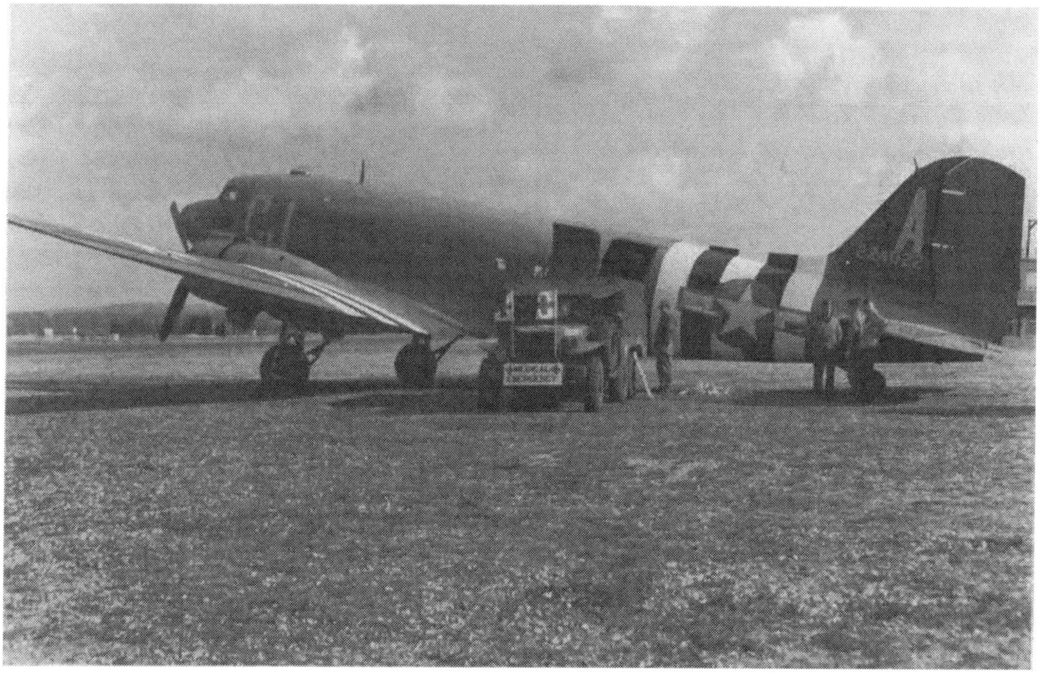

"made a Christian out of me. They convinced me." Accordingly, army blood requirements increased. By the end of June the First Army was consuming about 500 pints a day, in effect the entire production capacity of the Salisbury bank. The Third Army, as it prepared to go into action, requested 300 pints a day initially, to be increased to 550 as its front expanded, an amount that the theater blood bank, with its donor pool of COMZ troops shrinking as units moved to France, could not possibly furnish. With a shortage imminent, the 12th Army Group surgeon early in August began daily allocation of the available blood to the armies to ensure its most efficient use. Evacuation and general hospitals set up their own blood banks, drawing from their personnel and the lightly wounded. They used German POWs as donors for their injured countrymen.[55]

These expedients, however, were but stopgaps. Hawley and his assistants realized that the theater needed an additional source of whole blood and that the only possible one was the United States. Surgeon General Kirk, before the invasion, had rejected as unnecessary and impractical a theater proposal to fly blood across the Atlantic. Nevertheless, under pressure of necessity, Hawley revived it, even though he himself feared that, given the time required for shipment, blood from the United States would have only a short usable life in the European Theater. After a final conference with his consultants on 28 July, Hawley four days later radioed to General Kirk a request for a daily transatlantic blood airlift of up to 1,000 pints. In a follow-up letter he informed the surgeon general that the Air Transport Command had agreed to provide long-range C–54s for the mission, and insisted that blood was being used economically and that it was "saving lives and hastening recovery of patients." [56] Hawley also arranged to fly Colonel Cutler, his chief surgical consultant, Major Hardin, officer in charge of the ETO blood bank, and Col. William F. MacFee, MC, a veteran evacuation hospital commander, to Washington to plead the theater case in person. The three men left Prestwick on 12 August.

Even as the delegation was airborne, the issue was all but settled. In early August General Kirk, on the basis of additional study and of firsthand observation on a trip to the Mediterranean Theater in July 1944, reversed his earlier decision against shipping blood overseas and put his Surgery Division to work on tentative plans for a blood airlift to Europe. By the time Cutler and his colleagues landed in Washington, Kirk's consultants already had worked out a method for shipping blood and had tested it by flying sample lots to Prestwick, Bermuda, Los Angeles, and Hawaii. All that remained for the

[55] Quotation from Editorial Advisory Board, 1962, pp. 107–08. See also Kendrick, *Blood Program*, pp. 484–87 and 556–65; Surg, ADSEC, COMZ, Annual Rpt, 1944, pp. 53–54; Admin Memo No. 2, Surg, ADSEC, 5 Aug 44, in Essential Technical Medical Data Rpt, HQ, ETOUSA, August 1944; Medical Division, COSSAC/SHAEF, War Diary, August 1944; Ltr, Hawley to Rogers, 19 Jul 44, file HD 024 ETO CS (Hawley Chron). For a dissenting view of blood use, see Keeler Interv, 17 Jul 45, box 223, RG 112, NARA.

[56] Ltr, Hawley to TSG, 5 Aug 44, file HD 024 ETO O/CS (Hawley-SGO Corresp).

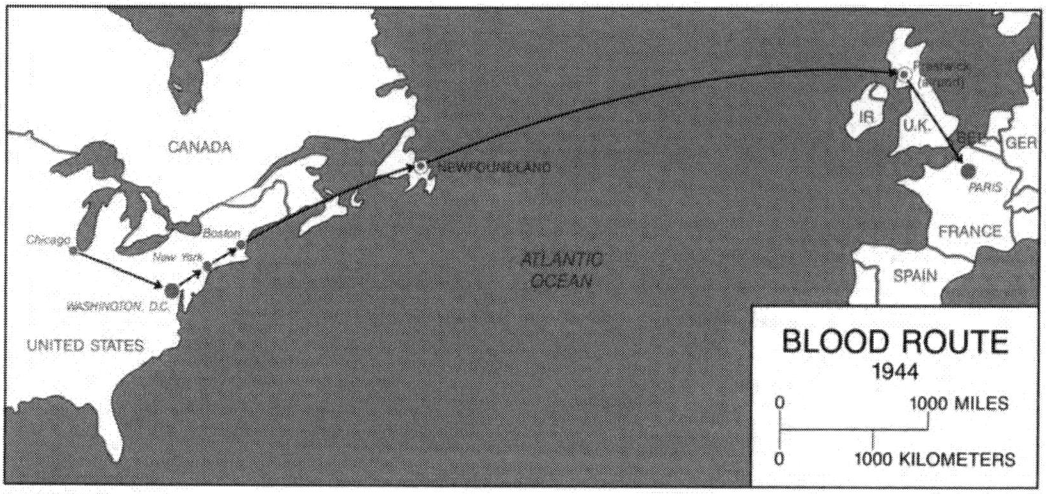

MAP 15

ETO representatives to do was to help work out detailed arrangements, which they promptly did.[57]

Blood flights began on 21 August, with a shipment of 258 pints from New York, via Newfoundland, to Prestwick (*Map 15*). Under the formula worked out by Cutler in Washington, the daily amounts were to increase to 500 pints on 28 August and 1,000 by 11 September. Actual deliveries reached a little over 500 pints per day in late October, the reduction from the scheduled goal resulting from a decrease in demand. The Red Cross collected the fresh blood at centers on the East Coast and in the Midwest, processed it, and put it up for shipment in 1,000 cc. bottles containing equal amounts of blood and Alsever's solution, a preservative. So prepared, the blood could be flown without refrigeration, which saved weight. Air Transport Command C-54s unloaded the blood at Prestwick, for movement by truck to Salisbury and transfer to C-47s for the cross-Channel flight. Late in October transatlantic planes carrying blood began landing at Orly Field, near Paris, eliminating the time-consuming extra handling in Great Britain. Kept refrigerated except while actually on the airplane, the preserved American blood could be used safely for at least eight or nine days after it reached the theater. Blood from the United States soon predominated in ETO stocks. During September, for example, the armies received about 11,000 pints from America and only 5,600 from within the theater. Ironically, the beginning of shipments from the United States coincided with a decline in casualty rates. In late September the medical service possessed a surplus of about 6,000 pints and made special efforts to use up the oldest blood before it had to be discarded.[58]

[57] Kendrick, *Blood Program*, pp. 487–93; Ltrs, TSG to Hawley, 11 Aug and 1 Sep 44, file HD 024 ETO O/CS (Hawley-SGO Corresp); Hawley Interv, 1962, p. 62, CMH.

[58] Unlike ETO blood, which contained no preservative and was shipped in food cans packed with ice,

Continued

The theater blood bank reorganized and expanded for continental operations. Under plans made back in April, the medical service converted the newly arrived 127th Station Hospital into a second blood bank unit. On 26 August the 127th took over the Salisbury collection and processing plant. The veteran 152d Station Hospital then moved to Paris, first to temporary quarters at the 203d General Hospital and then to a permanent facility at Vitry. This unit, beginning early in November, received all blood sent to the Continent from Britain and the United States and distributed it to ADSEC detachments. It also collected blood locally from COMZ troops. At the front the four detachments serving the First and Third Armies were augmented on 1 November by Detachments A and B of the 127th Station Hospital, which supported the recently deployed Ninth Army. Refrigerator trucks of these units regularly distributed as many as 20,000 pints of blood a month, with losses of less than 10 percent from breakage, refrigerator failure, and deterioration from lack of use. The latter wastage was unavoidable, for army medical units requisitioned daily on the basis of casualty estimates and thus preferred to err on the high side. Clearly, the whole blood service, with its supplies now assured, had proved to be one of the ETO medical service's major logistical successes.[59]

On the Eve of New Battles

During the three months following the breakout from Normandy, the medical service, like the other technical services, saw its preinvasion plans for orderly development of the Communications Zone swept aside by events. The chief surgeon and his assistants constructed evacuation, hospitalization, and medical supply systems on the run, while trying to meet the daily needs of the armies and to push people and equipment forward along the axes of advance. By late October they had completed the framework of a medical Communications Zone stretching from the beaches to the army rear boundaries. General hospitals were in operation at key points in France and Belgium, supply depots were being stocked, and rail and air evacuation channels were increasing in variety and efficiency.

Nevertheless, the medical support system gave evidence of its hurried, disorderly origins. It incorporated major inefficiencies, such as employment of many of the theater's best staffed general hospitals as holding and transit units. Air evacuation, the most rapid and clinically beneficial means of moving patients, remained at the mercy of weather and administrative uncertainties. There existed

American blood traveled all the way to the front in cardboard containers, each holding six bottles. See Kendrick, *Blood Program*, pp. 208–10, 493–96, 538–41, 554–55; Essential Technical Medical Data Rpts, HQ, ETOUSA, August 1944, pp. 13–14, September 1944, p. 13, and October 1944, p. 4; Supply Division, OofCSurg, HQ, ETOUSA, Annual Rpt, 1944, sec. II, p. 22; Medical Bulletin No. 25, OofCSurg, HQ, ETOUSA, 1 Nov 44, sub: The Supply of Preserved Blood From the Zone of Interior to the European Theater of Operations; Ltr, Hawley to TSG, 14 Sep 44, file HD 024 ETO O/CS (Hawley-SGO Corresp).

[59] Kendrick, *Blood Program*, pp. 513–17 and 566–67; Surg, ADSEC, COMZ, Annual Rpt, 1944, pp. 54–56; Essential Technical Medical Data Rpt, HQ, ETOUSA, October 1944, p. 4.

within the medical service, also, other organizational weaknesses and personnel and materiel shortages largely overlooked in the triumphant forward rush of the summer. The effects of all these deficiencies would become apparent, and provoke vigorous efforts to overcome them, during the winter of hard, costly fighting that lay ahead at the West Wall.

CHAPTER XI

Hard Fighting at the West Wall

During the autumn and early winter of 1944 the Allied armies reorganized and drove forward all along a front that now extended from the Channel to the Swiss border. They collided with a revived and reinforced Wehrmacht in what became at many points a bitter, costly battle of attrition. In this battle the European Theater field army medical service, taking the strain of a continuous high casualty rate, reached full development in organization and technique.

By mid-September the U.S. 12th and 6th Army Groups formed respectively the center and right of the Allied line. They included twenty-seven of the forty-nine divisions then at the disposal of SHAEF on the Continent. Americans—in the army groups and their supporting air and service forces—made up about half of the 2 million men under Eisenhower's command. The American army groups paused at the West Wall and the Moselle, to build up their attenuated supply system and to reorganize for the new offensive. When these troop rearrangements were completed late in October, the 12th Army Group had three armies on line—from left to right, the Ninth, First, and Third. To the right of the 12th Army Group General Devers' 6th Army Group, which came under SHAEF's operational control on 15 September, placed the two corps of the French First Army on its right wing and the U.S. Seventh Army, composed only of the three-division VI Corps, on its left. SHAEF, late in September, reinforced the Seventh Army with the rightmost corps of the Third Army and also with new divisions shipped directly from America to southern France.[1]

The American and French armies, and the British and Canadian elements of Montgomery's 21 Army Group on the Allied left, launched their new attacks between 8 and 16 November. SHAEF, still reflecting some of the optimism of the summer, when hopes for an early German collapse had run high, set ambitious objectives for this drive: reaching the Rhine, destroying the German armies west of that river, and perhaps securing bridgeheads across it. At the minimum, a continued fall-winter offensive would deny the enemy leisure to rebuild his armies, strengthen his for-

[1] The Ninth Army brought the VIII Corps up from Brittany early in October and initially entered the line in the Ardennes. It shifted to the 12th Army Group's left after relinquishing the corps to the First Army and in turn taking over the latter's left-most corps, the XIX.

tifications, and introduce new weapons. The Germans, however, had used all too well what breathing space the September and October pause in Allied attacks had given them. By the time the new offensive started, their desperate late-summer mobilization had produced enough troops to contain the Allied advance while accumulating a 25-division reserve for Hitler's projected grand counterattack. Gone were the days of swift breakthroughs and hell-for-leather armor exploitation. The battle became one of attrition, as British, French, and American divisions crawled forward against tenacious resistance. The Germans drew upon the hard-learned defensive experience of five years of war and made lavish, effective use of mines and artillery; they exacted a fearful price in men and time for every town, village, ridgeline, river crossing, and pillbox. The rain, snow, and freezing temperatures of one of the earliest and severest winters on record in that part of Europe reduced Allied mobility and air support and added to the misery of the combatants on both sides.

Nevertheless, through hard pounding and steady pressure the Allies made limited territorial gains. On their left wing the British Second and Canadian First Armies conquered the German forces blocking the seaward approaches to Antwerp, thus opening that great port to shorten Allied supply lines; then they liberated most of southern Holland. The U.S. Ninth and First Armies, attacking side by side, forced their way well inside the German frontier and drove almost to the Roer River, the last major water barrier between them and the Rhine.

On the southern flank of this attack the First Army fought possibly the bitterest battle of the campaign for the Huertgen Forest, a gloomy roadless tangle of fir trees, hills, and ravines. Although the Americans cleared the woodlands in the end, combat for the infantrymen of five divisions who battled there was a nightmare of endless minefields, treetop shellbursts, hidden pillboxes and machine-gun nests, and fierce German counterattacks. A rifle company in the Huertgen Forest could lose 100–200 percent of its original strength in a week's fighting; battalion and company officers and NCOs were killed and wounded or broke down in near-disastrous proportions. A 4th Infantry Division soldier summed it up:

> You can't get all of the dead because you can't find them, and they stay there to remind the guys advancing as to what might hit them. You can't get protection. You can't see. You can't get fields of fire. The trees are slashed like a scythe by artillery. Everything is tangled. You can scarcely walk. Everybody is cold and wet, and the mixture of cold rain and sleet keeps falling. Then they jump off again and soon there is only a handful of the old men left.[2]

South of the Ardennes the enemy defended with similar tenacity, but American troops gained more ground. Patton's Third Army crossed the rain-swollen Moselle in force; took Metz on 22 November; and a month later, after liberating 5,000 square miles of Lorraine, reached the German border at the Saar River. On the right of the Third Army the 6th

[2] Interv, T5g George Morgan, 1st Battalion, 22d Infantry, in 4th Infantry Division Combat Intervs, box 24021, RG 407, NARA.

Army Group cleared the west bank of the Rhine from the Swiss border to Strasbourg, except for a German-held bridgehead around Colmar. While the French First Army battered at this pocket, the U.S. Seventh Army in early December pushed northeastward though the old Maginot Line fortifications and prepared to assault the West Wall. The American armies thus captured significant territory, though less than their commanders had hoped to secure. In addition, they inflicted tens of thousands of German casualties, destroyed large quantities of equipment, and took almost 200,000 prisoners.[3]

The four American armies paid a high price for this ground and the wearing down of German forces. Between them, they suffered over 140,000 battle casualties, more than 85 percent of them in the infantry rifle companies. Among the approximately 100,000 wounded, the pattern of cause and location of injury resembled that in earlier phases of the campaign. About 65 percent fell victim to shell, bomb, and grenade fragments, and a similar proportion were hit in the arms and legs. Besides combat casualties, army hospitals during November and December admitted another 150,000 cases of injury, sickness, and combat fatigue. The cold damp weather increased the incidence of respiratory ailments. An epidemic of trenchfoot crowded clearing stations and evacuation hospitals with crippled soldiers, many permanently incapacitated for combat duty, and further diminished the already casualty-thinned ranks of the infantry.[4]

Organizing for the Offensive

Redeployments and exchange of medical units accompanied the reorganization of the American armies for the November offensive. New ground force medical formations continued to arrive in the theater, increasing the number of medical personnel in the armies to over 65,000 by mid-December. The 12th and 6th Army Group surgeons, in consultation with those of the armies and with Generals Kenner and Hawley, distributed the new arrivals and reshuffled the forces already on the ground to give each army a medical complement proportional to its strength.[5]

The Ninth Army, for example, initially entered the line in the Ardennes with the 64th Medical Group, sup-

[3] This account is based on MacDonald, *Siegfried Line*, passim; Cole, *Lorraine Campaign*, passim; Robert R. Smith and Jeffrey J. Clarke, *The Riviera to the Rhine* (Washington, D.C.: U.S. Army Center of Military History, forthcoming), chs. XVI–XXVI; Seventh U.S. Army Report of Operations, France and Germany, 1944–1945, vol. II, pp. 456–94, 505–13, 529.

[4] MacDonald, *Siegfried Line*, p. 617; Cole, *Lorraine Campaign*, pp. 592–93; Surg, First U.S. Army, Annual Rpt, 1944, pp. 5–6; First U.S. Army Report of Operations, 1 Aug 44–22 Feb 45, bk. IV, pp. 139, 179, 201, 205; Surg, Third U.S. Army, Annual Rpt, 1944, pp. 43–44, 104, 108, ex XXVII; Surg, Seventh U.S. Army, Annual Rpt, 1944, pp. 29–32 and 37d–37f; Seventh U.S. Army Report of Operations, 1944–1945, vol. III, p. 1,029; Surg, Ninth U.S. Army, Annual Report, 1944, pp. 20–22; Surg, Ninth U.S. Army, Combat Experience Tables of Casualties, Ninth U.S. Army, October–December 1944 (hereafter cited as Combat Experience Rpt, with month), file HD 319.1–2. For typical casualty distribution among arms, see Surg, XIX Corps, Annual Rpt, 1944, encl. 20.

[5] Ground forces medical personnel amounted to about 32–38 percent of the total theater medical strength of over 212,000 in late December. See Personnel Division, OofCSurg, HQ, ETOUSA, Annual Rpt, 1944, app. D. MFR, Col B. A. Holtzworth, 8 Jan 45, sub: Notes on Service Troops, Moses Papers, MHI, gives 12th Army Group standards for field army medical troop strength.

porting the VIII Corps, as well as several former Third Army field and evacuation hospitals and other units taken over in Brittany. When it moved to Holland and joined the 12th Army Group's left wing, the army relinquished these organizations, except for two field hospitals, to the First Army and assumed command in turn of the 31st Medical Group, which supported the XIX Corps (taken over from the First Army) and three evacuation hospitals. The new army also inherited several evacuation hospitals and field hospital platoons serving American divisions, including the 82d and 101st, which were fighting in Holland under 21 Army Group in the aftermath of MARKET-GARDEN. Other Ninth Army medical units, arriving from the United States and Great Britain, assembled at concentration areas in France and Belgium and then moved into Holland to support the army's second corps, the XIII, when it began operations late in November.[6]

The Seventh Army came ashore on the Riviera with a complement of medical battalions, of ambulance, clearing, and collecting companies, and of field and evacuation hospitals sufficient only for a single corps. As SHAEF added to that army's combat strength, it also reinforced the medical service—a process involving multilateral consultations among the surgeons of the two army groups, four field armies, and two separate communications zones. During September the Seventh Army acquired from the Third Army an additional medical battalion headquarters, three collecting companies, a clearing company, and a field hospital, as well as the Third's XV Corps. SHAEF at the same time directed the European Theater and 12th Army Group to provide the southern army with three additional ambulance companies, three evacuation hospitals, a depot company, and part of an auxiliary surgical group. Both headquarters complied, in part by transferring units already in France to the 6th Army Group and in part by diverting new units then still in the continuing flow of troops across the Atlantic. Late in November, with planning under way to expand Seventh Army to three corps and nine divisions, SHAEF called on the northern forces for still more field medical units, and they again responded with redeployments, to include, whenever possible, redirecting reinforcements already at sea to the French Mediterranean ports.

Augmentation of the Seventh Army medical service did not go altogther smoothly. Colonel Gorby, the 12th's surgeon, resisted turning over an auxiliary surgical group, insisting he needed it for his own still expanding army group, but in the end he complied with SHAEF directions. The 6th Army Group surgeon, Col. Oscar S. Reeder, MC, and the Seventh Army surgeon, Colonel Rudolph, at times disagreed in estimating their requirements. Reeder, for example, accepted a medical group headquarters, taken from the Third Army, for which the Seventh Army surgeon had no use, but withdrew a request for a gas treatment battalion that Rudolph wanted. The medical units assigned

---

[6] Surg, Ninth U.S. Army, Annual Rpt, 1944, pp. 8–9 and 11–13; Surg, First U.S. Army, Annual Rpt, 1944, p. 48; First U.S. Army Report of Operations, 1 Aug 44–22 Feb 45, bk. IV, p. 136.

to the Seventh Army took a while to arrive. Those allocated in September, for instance, joined only in late November. The three evacuation hospitals that arrived immediately after being activated in the United States needed additional training before they could become operational. While the unwanted medical group headquarters, the 67th, waited for a new assignment, the Seventh Army conducted most of the autumn campaign with a shortage of field and evacuation hospitals, only partially alleviated by borrowing from the southern communications zone. These difficulties, however, were only temporary. By late December the Seventh Army included ten evacuation and four field hospitals, a convalescent hospital, portions of two auxiliary surgical groups, six separate medical battalions with attached collecting and clearing companies, six ambulance companies, a depot company, and assorted laboratory and veterinary units (the latter loaned to the French First Army to care for its pack animals).[7]

The French First Army, the other major component of the 6th Army Group, possessed its own separate medical service. This army, organized and equipped in North Africa with American assistance, included a full complement of ground forces medical units with American tables of organization and equipment and with French personnel. Its hospitalization and evacuation system closely resembled those of the U.S. field armies. By late 1944 the French had about 7,000 field and evacuation hospital beds in operation for their two corps and seven divisions; up to that point in the campaign they had cared for about 23,000 casualties. They evacuated their long-term patients by rail to fixed hospitals, many of them civilian, in liberated southern France and had their own supporting communications zone organization, Base 901, in the same area. The French relied heavily on American medical supplies, which they delivered to their forward units through their own depot system. General Kenner, after a mid-December inspection, pronounced the French First Army medical situation "quite satisfactory, sufficient medical units are available, and civilian facilities and personnel augment them throughout the area."[8]

Except in allocating medical units, the army group surgeons—Colonel Gorby of the 12th and Colonel Reeder of the 6th—guided their subordinate army surgeons with a loose rein. The group surgeons confined their activities largely to keeping informed about operations, collecting medical reports and statistics, disseminating and interpreting SHAEF

[7] Surg, Seventh U.S. Army, Annual Rpt, 1944, pp. 15-17, 19-22, 112-14; 12th Army Group Report of Operations, vol. VIII (Medical Section), pp. 57 and 116; Troop Movements and Training Branch, Operations Division, OofCSurg, HQ, ETOUSA, Annual Rpt, 1944, pp. 8 and 11; Gorby Interv, 1962, pp. 54-55, CMH; 67th Medical Group Annual Rpt, 1944, p. 17. For negotiations on medical reinforcements for the Seventh Army, see correspondence in DRAGOON 1944 file, CMH.

[8] Quotation from Medical Division, COSSAC/SHAEF, War Diary, December 1944. See also Surg, Seventh U.S. Army, Annual Rpt, 1944, pp. 6-7; MFR, Lt Col J. H. Voegtly, 29 Sep 44, sub: Organization of Sixth Army Group and Medical Services of Sixth Army Group, in Surg, 6th Army Group, Annual Rpt, 1944-1945. For a general account of the formation of the French First Army, see Marcel Vigneras, *Rearming the French*, United States Army in World War II (Washington, D.C.: Office of the Chief of Military History, Department of the Army, 1957), chs. X and XI.

and theater medical directives, and occasionally assisting the army surgeons in dealing with COMZ. However, they encouraged the armies to work directly with the Communications Zone whenever possible on evacuation and supply matters, and most of the time the army surgeons did so. Colonel Reeder's small (two officers and three enlisted men) medical section was especially limited in functions and influence. It had only one American army to oversee and, until May 1945, was submerged within the group G-4 office instead of constituting a separate special staff section.[9]

Day-to-day direction of activities, both administrative and clinical, rested primarily with the army surgeons and their fifty- to sixty-person staffs. The surgeons of all four armies had satisfactory working relationships with their army commanders, who generally paid little attention to the medical service except on the exceedingly rare occasions when something went drastically wrong. Usually located with the forward, or tactical, echelon of army headquarters, the surgeons participated in all stages of operational planning. For practical purposes, they had operational control of nondivisional medical units, although the formal definition of this authority varied from army to army. Their medical and surgical consultants supervised patient care and enforced the principles of the ETO *Manual of Therapy*, as well as apportioning auxiliary surgical teams among army hospitals. Army surgeons spent much effort on communications. In the 12th Army Group they maintained liaison officers at group headquarters, and they had attached to them liaison officers from the Advance Section. Army surgeons kept in touch with their own medical units by telephone and courier. The Third Army surgeon at Nancy, for example, had eleven telephones in his office and nineteen drivers and vehicles at his disposal, all in constant use.[10]

For the army surgeons, and for those at corps and division levels, planning and coordinating medical support for the November-December offensive was a comparatively straightforward task. The surgeons confronted a problem similar to that in the hedgerow battles: evacuation of a large but steady volume of casualties over relatively short distances from slowly advancing combat units. Until the German Ardennes counterstroke, the Allies held the tactical initiative; hence, surgeons generally could forecast accurately the rates and locations of casualties and the supply and evacuation requirements of each stage of the attack. The absence of major breakthroughs, although disappointing to tactical com-

[9]Gorby Interv, 1962, p. 5, CMH; Hartford Interv, 7-8 Oct 80, tape 1, side 2, CMH; Surg, 6th Army Group, Annual Rpt, 1944-1945, pp. 1-3.

[10]First U.S. Army Report of Operations, 20 Oct 43-1 Aug 44, bk. 1, pp. 16-17; Surg, Third U.S. Army, Annual Rpt, 1944, pp. 37-38 and 68-70; Surg, Ninth U.S. Army, Annual Rpt, 1944, pp. 3 and 6; Surg, Seventh U.S. Army, Annual Rpt, 1944, pp. 116 and 129; Hartford Interv, 7-8 Oct 80, tape 1, side 2, CMH; Editorial Advisory Board, 1962, pp. 97-98. In Shambora Papers, MHI, see Surg, Ninth U.S. Army, Daily Journal, 1 Nov 44; Memo, Col W. E. Shambora to ACofS, G-4, Ninth U.S. Army, 12 Jun 45, sub: Organization of the Medical Section, HQ, NUSA; Memo. Reinstein to Surg, Ninth U.S. Army, 9 Sep 44, sub: Observation of Medical Service in Operation, TUSA; and Memo, HQ, ADSEC, COMZ, to Surg, Ninth U.S. Army, 28 Sep 44, sub: Liaison Officer.

manders, simplified the army medical service's task by reducing the need to move large installations. Third Army evacuation hospitals, for example, changed position an average of slightly more than once each month during this offensive; in the pursuit they had moved three times as often.

The army medical service, accordingly, readily took the strain of the hard autumn and winter fighting. Army medical people at each link in the evacuation chain elaborated upon the expedients and adaptations of standard procedure introduced earlier in the campaign; they relearned old lessons and occasionally learned new ones. Above all, for army medics at every echelon the November and early December battles meant long hours of hard labor, physical and emotional stress, and—for some—deadly danger.[11]

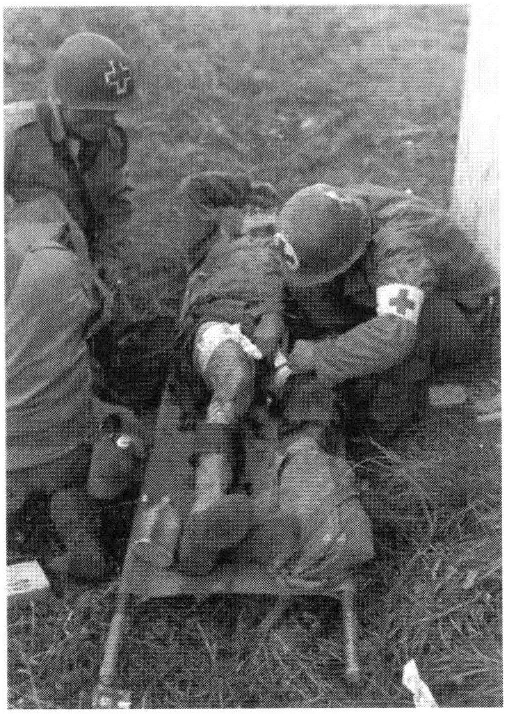

MEDICS ON THE LINE

Medics on the Line

Divisional unit detachments and medical battalions at the forward end of the entire evacuation chain collected casualties under fire, stabilized their condition, and started them toward safety and healing in the rear. Increasingly, by late 1944, the latter function—evacuation—was becoming the primary one for all medical personnel forward of the clearing stations. By army policy medics confined treatment to the bare minimum needed to fit casualties for immediate further transportation: controlling bleeding, pain, and infection; immobilizing broken limbs; and administering plasma.[12]

First Aid

Medical treatment of wounded soldiers began even before they reached their battalion aid stations. Casualties received first aid at or near the spot on the battlefield where they were injured, administered either by themselves and their buddies or, much more often, by their company aidmen. Each soldier carried an indi-

[11] Surg, Third U.S. Army, Annual Rpt, 1944, pp. 46 and 91–92, gives hospital movement statistics; for offensive plans and preparations, see p. 38. For an example of corps-level assault medical planning, see VII Corps Medical Plan, pp. 93–95, encl. 1 to Surg, VII Corps, Annual Rpt, 1944.

[12] For examples of army policy, see First U.S. Army Report of Operations, 1 Aug 44–22 Feb 45, bk. IV, pp. 166–67, and Cir Ltr No. 2, Surg, Seventh U.S. Army, 18 Jul 44, sub: Surgery, in Surg, Seventh U.S. Army, Annual Rpt, 1944.

vidual first aid packet, containing field dressings and sulfa powder and tablets, and was supposed to know how to improvise and apply splints and tourniquets. First aid procedures called for a wounded man, if able, to seek protection from fire, examine his injury and assess its severity, sprinkle it with sulfa powder, apply a dressing, and swallow his sulfa tablets. Then he was to get back to the aid station on his own or call for the aidman.

In practice, a large proportion of the wounded forgot to do, or could not do, any number of these things. Of casualties polled in COMZ general hospitals, for example, about one-third did not take their sulfa pills before they reached the aid station, claiming that they lacked water to wash them down; doubted the tablets' usefulness; or were incapacitated by their injuries. Soldiers often did not have their belt first aid packets on their persons when hit. "They'd take them off," an aidman reported, "for example to be more comfortable in a fox hole, and we'll usually find the belts [and packets] lying close by." Hurt, frightened soldiers yelled frantically for the aidman even when only slightly wounded and capable of leaving the field under their own power. Many, in panic, further injured themselves, at times fatally. A company aidman recalled the actions of

> a lieutenant. He got hit and just had a little bit of gut hanging out and he sits up and lies down and hollers and thinks he is going to die and we fix him up but he's still excited and pretty soon air gets in and he dies. That same day there's a Jerry with all his guts hanging out. He puts his hand down there and holds it in. We get him to the aid station and we hear later that the son-of-a-bitch still lives. He just held it there and didn't get excited.[13]

Fortunately, comparatively few wounded men—only one in five, according to one hospital survey—had to give themselves first aid. Most found a company aidman at their sides within less than half an hour of being hit. Besides bandaging, splinting, applying tourniquets, administering sulfa powder and tablets, and injecting morphine, aidmen were supposed to fill out an emergency medical tag (EMT) for each casualty, providing the basic record of his identity and initial treatment. Many divisions in practice transferred this chore to the battalion aid stations, for the company medics, amid the urgency and danger of combat, were hardly in an ideal position to do paper work. Company aidmen had a deserved reputation for bravery but they complained that some of their heroics were unnecessary, the result of panic calls for help by the slightly injured or of poor judgment by line officers in sending out their medics under fire. One medic commented: "If a man is hit, he's hit, and it may be better to leave him there for a while than to send the aid man to him on a suicide job—for example, I've seen it done when mortars were pounding the area and every foot was covered with [machine-gun] fire." [14]

---

[13] Rpt No. E–81, Research Branch, Special Services Division, ETO, September 1944, sub: Opinions of Wounded Combat Veterans on Battlefield First Aid Treatment (hereafter cited as ETO, Battlefield First Aid Rpt, 1944), pp. 2–5, file HD:ETO: 350.07:Battle Experiences. Quotations from app., pp. ii and iii.

[14] Quotation from ETO, Battlefield First Aid Rpt, 1944, app., p. ii, file HD:ETO:350.07:Battle Experi-

Continued

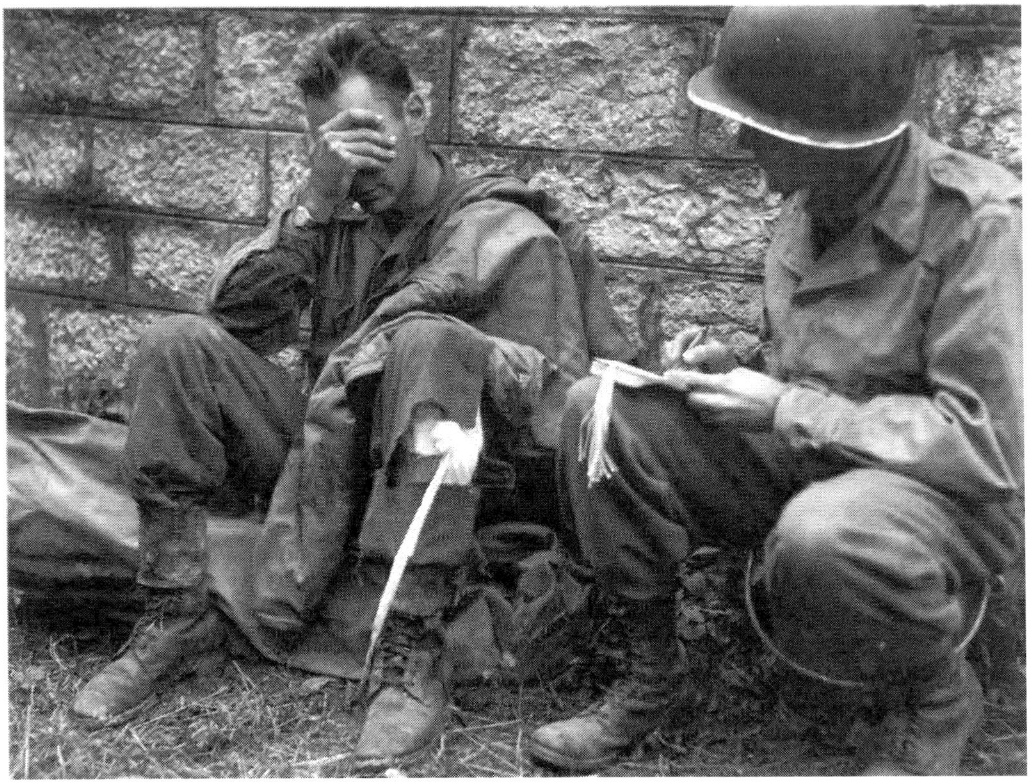

PREPARING AN EMERGENCY MEDICAL TAG

Most demands for courage on the par of aidmen, however, were legitimate and essential to their mission, and the medics responded with dedication and self-sacrifice. During the Third Army fighting along the Moselle, for example, Technician 5th Class Alfred L. Wilson, a company aidman in the 328th Infantry, moved about under heavy shelling treating his unit's many wounded until badly hurt himself. He refused evacuation and, in great pain and slowly bleeding to death, continued dragging himself from one casualty to the next. Finally too weak to move, he instructed other soldiers in giving first aid until unconsciousness overcame him. His unit credited Wilson, who received a posthumous Medal of Honor, with helping to save the lives of at least ten men. A 4th Division captain reported of another aidman in the Huertgen Forest who similarly stayed on duty after being injured: "This man was perhaps an even greater morale aid than a physical aid" to the hard-pressed riflemen around him.[15]

ences. On EMTs, see Surg, 5th Infantry Division, Annual Rpt, 1944, pp. 34–35, and Rpt No. 368, Army Ground Forces Board, 18 Nov 44, sub: Medical Information, 8th Infantry Division, p. 4.

[15] Quotation from Interv, Capt D. Faulkner, in 4th Infantry Division Combat Intervs, box 24021, RG 407, NARA. Wilson's citation is in U.S. Congress, Continued

Not surprisingly, in the light of such performance, aidmen were among the most popular and respected soldiers in their companies. Aidmen and infantry troops alike bitterly resented the War Department refusal—based on the need to maintain the medics' Geneva Convention noncombatant status—to grant eligible enlisted medics the Combat Infantryman Badge and the ten dollars a month extra pay that went with it. In some ETO divisions riflemen collected money from their own wages to give their aidmen the combat bonus. The War Department, however, did not remedy this inequity until barely two months before V–E Day. Medical Department soldiers—mostly aidmen and litterbearers—did collect their share of decorations for valor. Four ETO enlisted medics besides Wilson received Medals of Honor; hundreds of others won Silver or Bronze Stars.[16]

In the judgment of doctors farther to the rear, aidmen and front-line troops gave generally competent first aid, although they made a few persistent errors. Soldiers—whether medical or nonmedical—regularly misused tourniquets. They applied them unnecessarily; left them unloosened for too long; and occasionally evacuated patients with tourniquets concealed by blankets or clothing, and hence not discovered until the limb was doomed. Trying to prevent such abuses, the Seventh Army surgeon directed that the "sole indication" for applying a tourniquet should be "active spurting hemorrhage from a major artery" and that medics in the field or at battalion aid stations should note the presence of a tourniquet on a patient's EMT in capital letters. With the morphine Syrette then in use, aidmen easily could overdose casualties, especially in cold weather when slow blood circulation delayed absorption of the initial shot and the patient received more at an aid or collecting station. To guard against such mistakes, front-line medics who did not fill out EMTs often attached their used morphine Syrettes to soldiers' clothing before evacuating them. In the First Army the surgeon, Colonel Rogers, recommended abandonment of the practice of sprinkling sulfa powder on open fresh wounds as an anti-infection precaution. Combined with the taking of sulfa pills, this treatment resulted in excessive doses, and it also made wounds generally dirtier without reaching the deepest portions most in need of prophylaxis.[17]

Senate, Committee on Veterans' Affairs, *Medal of Honor Recipients, 1863–1978* (hereafter cited as *MOH Recipients*), 96th Cong., 1st Sess. (Washington, D.C.: U.S. Government Printing Office, 1979), pp. 715–16. Surg, XIX Corps, Annual Rpt, 1944, an. E, contains a typical tribute to company aidmen.

[16] The General Staff, on 1 March 1945, authorized a special combat medical badge and ten dollars extra pay a month for Medical Department personnel "daily sharing with the infantry the hazards and hardships of combat." See McMinn and Levin, *Personnel*, pp. 337–38. For views of field troops, see Medical Division, COSSAC/SHAEF, War Diary, December 1944, and ETO, Battlefield First Aid Rpt, 1944, app., p. v, file HD:ETO:350.07:Battle Experiences. For an example of awards received, see Surg, XII Corps, Annual Rpt, 1944, p. 11.

[17] Quotation from Cir Ltr No. 2, Surg, Seventh U.S. Army, 18 Jul 44, sub: Surgery, in Surg, Seventh U.S. Army, Annual Rpt, 1944. See also First U.S. Army Report of Operations, 1 Aug 44–22 Feb 45, bk. IV, pp. 166–67; ETO, Battlefield First Aid Rpt, 1944, app., p. iii, file HD:ETO:350.07:Battle Experiences; Rpt. No. 368, Army Ground Forces Board, 18 Nov 44, Medical Information, 8th Infantry Division, p. 4.

Evacuation

From the place on the battlefield where the aidmen treated a casualty and marked his position, ETO divisional medical installations—and hence the chain of evacuation—stretched rearward over a considerable distance. By late 1944 battalion aid stations typically set up at least a mile behind the engaged infantry and armor elements, to reduce losses from artillery and mortar fire among essential, hard-to-replace doctors and technicians. Collecting stations usually took position about a mile back of the aid stations. Clearing stations remained 3 to as many as 15 miles behind the fighting line, to be free of the patient-disturbing noise and counterbattery fire danger or their own corps and division artillery.[18]

Mass movement of patients over these distances was possible largely because the divisions, by late 1944, in effect had motorized their entire chain of evacuation. Since the Battle of the Hedgerows they had used collecting company ambulances, supplemented by trucks for walking wounded, to evacuate their battalion aid stations. By late autumn they routinely extended motor transport forward of the aid stations as well, whenever possible right to the place where casualties lay on the battlefield. Medics now used jeeps, belonging to battalion aid stations and collecting companies, in preference to litter-bearers, for moving wounded in the forward areas. Fitted with brackets for carrying litters, these small sturdy vehicles could go most places men on foot could; they could accommodate two or three litters each, and as many ambulatory patients as ingenious drivers could crowd on board. One 4th Division litter platoon commander claimed to have hauled fourteen walking wounded on a single trip. On more typical runs, he recalled, "there would be . . . two litter cases side by side on the rear half of the jeep, then usually one across the hood, and then I would have sitting beside me a severely wounded man, or a couple of them, who could . . . sit up."[19]

When their jeeps bogged down in mud and snow, medics often switched to the M-29 Weasel, a small tracked cargo vehicle that had about the same litter capacity as the jeep. Armored division surgeons used light tanks and tank retrievers to move their wounded over ground impassable to jeeps and regular ambulances. On one occasion the 5th Armored Division picked up casualties on the field in medium tanks when heavy shelling prevented any other approach to them. The Shermans maneuvered astride the wounded men; then the crews drew the casualties up inside the tanks through the escape hatches in the bottoms of the hulls. During the Third Army attack on Metz the 95th Infantry Division temporarily pressed an artillery spotter plane into service to fly wounded directly off the battlefield from a point where minefields and enemy fire blocked evacuation by any other means. The aircraft, with a regimental surgeon riding with the pilot to select cases,

[18] For examples of divisional evacuation systems, see Surg, XIX Corps, Annual Rpt, 1944, ans. C and E; Surg, XX Corps, Annual Rpt, 1944, pp. 18–19; and Surg, 10th Armored Division, Annual Rpt, 1944, pp. 30–32 and encl. 14.

[19] Richardson Interv, tape 1, side 2, CMH.

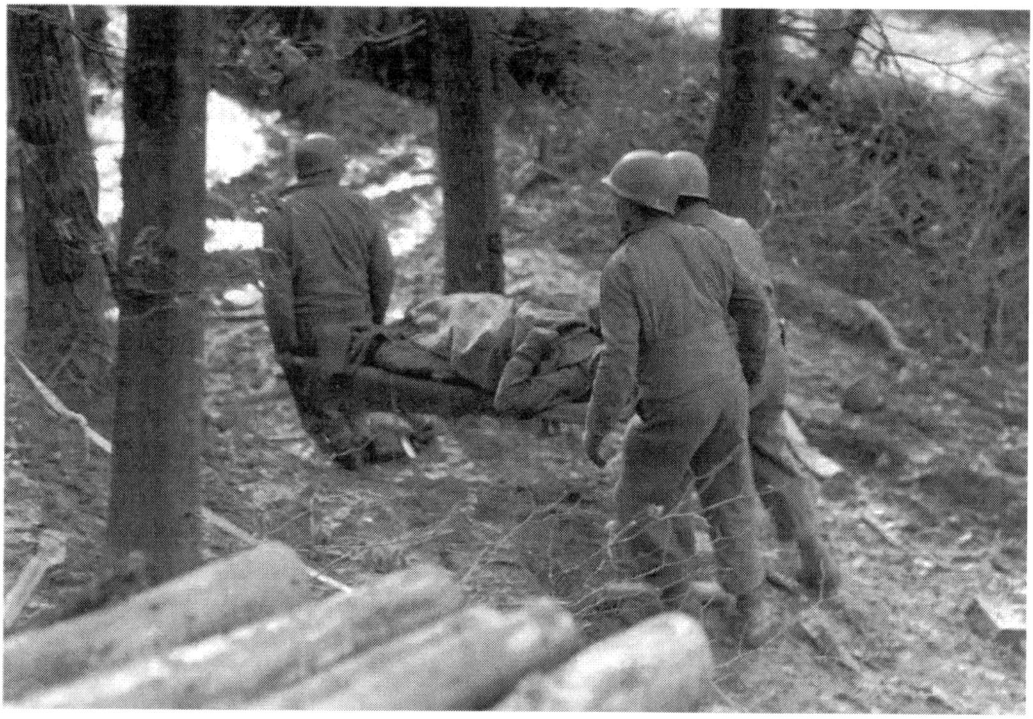

LITTERBEARERS MEETING THE CHALLENGE OF THE HUERTGEN FIGHTING

lifted out nine men in the same number of trips. Clearly, machines rather than human muscle now were moving most casualties most of the time.[20]

Divisions were insatiable consumers of medical manpower, especially when weather and terrain forced them to rely extensively on litterbearers forward of battalion aid stations. The task of litter-bearing in such circumstances was both dangerous and exhausting, for the distances litterbearers had to traverse—often over rugged, wooded country—ranged from 1,000 yards to 4 miles. In the Huertgen Forest 16th Infantry bearers, according to the regimental surgeon, "would work until they were exhausted and then drop. A twelve hour relief and they'd be off on another seventy-two hour shift." Bearers displayed dedication comparable to that of the aidmen with whom they closely cooperated. A 4th Division enlisted medic made two 1,000-yard hauls after a glancing blow from a shell fragment had fractured his skull. Yet even the bravest and strongest men needed frequent rest, and litterbearers suffered a steady drain of casualties from enemy fire and mines. A few broke down emotionally. Another 4th Division litterbearer, after carry-

[20] Surg, 1st Infantry Division, Annual Rpt, 1944, pp. 22 and 32; Surg, 90th Infantry Division, Annual Rpt, 1944, pp. 20–23; Medical Bulletin, 95th Infantry Division, 1–30 Nov 44, pt. II, in Surg, 95th Infantry Division, Annual Rpt, 1944; Surg, 4th Armored Division, Annual Rpt, 1944, p. 11; Surg, 5th Armored Division, Annual Rpt, 1944, p. 54.

ing to the rear on his back two men from an infantry company with which he had worked for some time and to which he had grown closely attached, began muttering, "They're killing my boys; they're killing my boys." He tried to find a rifle with which to fight back and "had to be evacuated for combat exhaustion." [21]

Infantry battalion and collecting company litterbearers (the latter all but supplanted by ambulances for work to the rear of the aid stations) customarily combined forces to remove wounded from the battlefield. They were far too few for the job during intense combat and when weather, terrain, or the tactical situation prevented vehicles from assisting them. The Huertgen fighting, in particular, absorbed bearers at an almost intolerable rate. The 1st Infantry Division, during its time in the forest, used 240 additional litterbearers; the 4th Division employed 140. Under prearranged procedures division surgeons obtained these extra men, and also casualty replacements, from their corps medical battalions and the army medical groups. These units drafted bearers from their own attached organizations and, in emergencies, drew upon any other medical personnel within reach. The 68th Medical Group, for example, which supported the VII Corps, provided infantry divisions in the Huertgen Forest with over 450 reinforcement bearers, including the enlisted personnel of two entire collecting companies. Running out of spare medical troops, the group obtained 190 nonmedical infantry replacements from one of the depots. It issued them Red Cross brassards; sketchily trained them in first aid, evacuation, and Geneva Convention rights and duties; and threw them into the line for several weeks. On another occasion the Advance Section sent the First Army a contingent of litterbearers combed out of staging general hospitals. Even with all this extra help, the rifle companies often had to draft combat soldiers from their own thin ranks to carry wounded at least part of the way to their battalion aid stations. These expedients met the immediate requirements. The necessity for them, however, pointed up the inadequacy of the existing division complement of bearers and also underscored how indispensable, under the prevailing conditions, evacuation by vehicle had become.[22]

With so much first aid being performed on the field, battalion aid stations concentrated more on evacuating casualties than on treating them. The aid stations, by the time the November offensive began, had honed and perfected their operational tech-

---

[21] Quotation from Tegtmeyer "Diary," pt. II, p. 90. Second and third quotations from Intervs, Assistant Surgeon and Aidmen, 1st Battalion, 22d Infantry, in 4th Infantry Division Combat Intervs, box 24021, RG 407, NARA. See also Richardson Interv, tape 1, sides 1 and 2, CMH.

[22] First U.S. Army Report of Operations, 1 Aug 44–22 Feb 45, bk. IV, pp. 130–40 and 144; Surg, V Corps, Annual Rpt, 1944, p. 19; VII Corps Medical Plan, pp. 89–91 and 97–98, encl. 1 to Surg, VII Corps, Annual Rpt, 1944; 68th Medical Group Annual Rpt, 1944, pp. 16, 19–21, 25; 134th Medical Group Annual Rpt, 1944, p. 19; Surg, 1st Infantry Division, Annual Rpt, 1944, pp. 22–23; Surg, 3d Infantry Division, Annual Rpt, 1944, encl. 1; Surg, 4th Infantry Division, Annual Rpt, 1944, p. 3; Surg, 8th Infantry Division, Annual Rpt, 1944, pp. 14–16; Surg, 28th Infantry Division, Annual Rpt, 1944, encl. 5; Intervs, Company G, 22 Infantry, in 4th Infantry Division Combat Intervs, box 24021, RG 407, NARA.

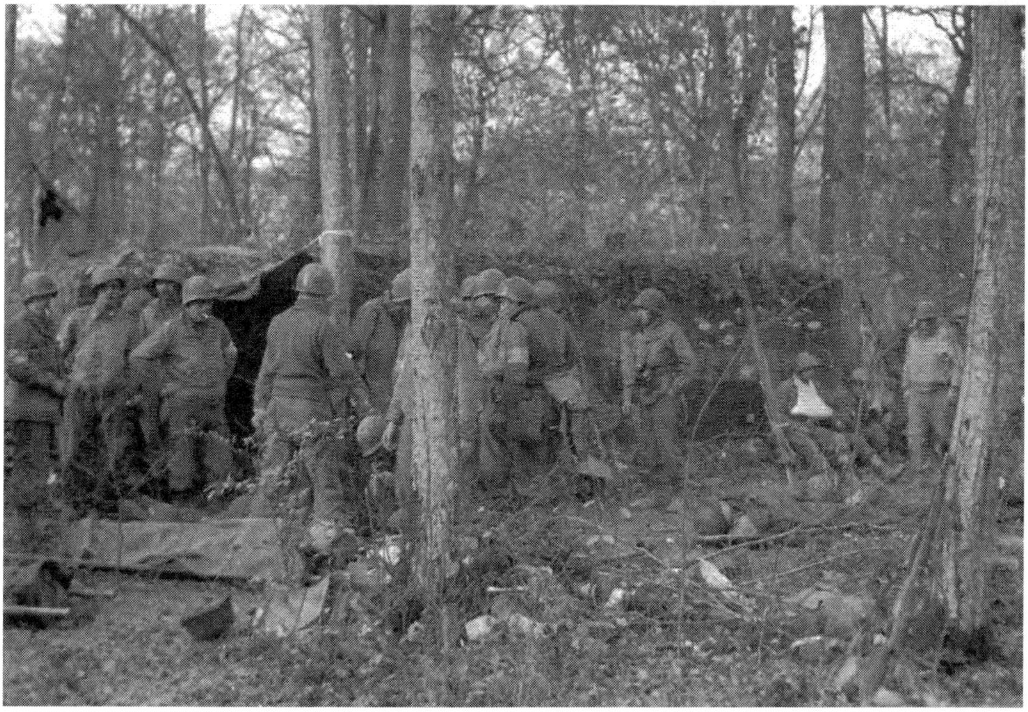

BATTALION AID STATION PERSONNEL READYING CASUALTIES *for the next stage of their rearward evacuation*

niques. Because the stations, for safety reasons, had to keep their distance from the rifle companies, battalion surgeons often established small advance collecting points nearer the infantry. These typically consisted of an officer (frequently the assistant battalion surgeon), a few litter teams, and a couple of jeep ambulances. They gathered casualties and evacuated them to the main aid stations. The latter almost invariably found shelter under roofs and preferably underground, in solidly constructed cellars or abandoned dugouts, which afforded protection from shelling as well as the elements. To better direct evacuation, battalion surgeons, whenever they could, established telephone or radio contact with the company command posts. At night the telephone wires, and sometimes white tape stretched along the ground, guided the rearward traffic of litterbearers and walking wounded. When casualties reached them, the surgeons and their enlisted technicians checked and replaced dressings, splints, and tourniquets and dispensed additional morphine. They filled out EMTs if company aidmen had not done so. They normally administered the first plasma the wounded received. When casualties came through in large numbers, the aid stations, to get patients out quickly, suspended tagging the wounded and limited transfusion and resuscitation to the minimum required to keep injured men alive during the next stage of their rearward journeys. In the First Army, especially, "the rule was to sacrifice full resuscitation for early evacuation." [23]

By the time the autumn battles began, most battalions had Medical Administrative Corps (MAC) officers as assistant surgeons. Usually sent in to replace Medical Corps (MC) casualties, the MAC lieutenants, by most accounts, performed creditably. The regimental surgeon of the 16th Infantry, for example, commented: "The doctors could take care of the wounded and the [MAC] lieutenants could keep the evacuation going. . . . They had been well taught in first aid and were skillful in bandaging and splinting and were able to assist the surgeons in their work." At least one battalion surgeon, in the 3d Infantry Division, proposed replacing all MCs at battalion level with MACs. He argued that little actual need existed in the battalions for the doctors' professional skills and that regimental surgeons, if necessary, could assist their aid stations in diagnosing and treating difficult cases. The armies, nevertheless, retained their MC battalion surgeons.[24]

Divisional collecting companies worked closely in evacuation with the regimental and battalion detachments, often pooling men and equipment with them, as in litter-bearing forward of the aid stations. A collecting company normally operated continuously with the same infantry regiment. During action the company set up its station as close to the regimental command post as safety and the maintenance of noncombatant status allowed and also tied into the regimental telephone system for direct communications with the battalion surgeons. Many companies found it convenient to divide their ambulances into two groups. One, dispatched by an advance loading post, shuttled between aid stations and the collecting station; the second ambulance element picked up patients at the collecting station for the usually longer run to the clearing company and field hospital platoon. Under this arrangement, drivers in the forward contingent gained familiarity with the frequently tortuous, hazardous routes to the aid stations. Collecting station personnel at the same time gave patients whatever refreshment and stabilizing treatment they needed and grouped them into efficient ambulance loads for the next stage of their journey.[25]

In especially difficult tactical situations, infantry battalion and collecting company medics resorted to all manner of expedients to keep evacuation going. Such was the case during

[23] Quotation from First U.S. Army Report of Operations, 1 Aug 44–22 Feb 45, bk. IV, p. 166; see also p. 164. For examples of aid station operations, see Surg, 3d Infantry Division, Annual Rpt, 1944, encl. 2; AGF Rpt No. 892, War Department Observers Board, ETO, 30 Apr 45, sub: Combat Experiences (hereafter cited as AGF, Combat Experiences Rpt, 1945), pp. 9–10, file HD:ETO:350.07:Battle Experiences; Interv, Assistant Surgeon and Aidmen, 1st Battalion, 22d Infantry, in 4th Infantry Division Combat Intervs, box 24021, RG 407, NARA.

[24] Quotation from Tegtmeyer "Diary," pt. II, pp. 90–91. For the recommendation to replace MCs with MACs, see Surg, 3d Infantry Division, Annual Rpt, 1944, encl. 2. Richardson Interv, tape 1, side 2, CMH, describes the role of MACs in evacuation.

[25] Surg, 3d Infantry Division, Annual Rpt, 1944, encls. 1 and 2; Surg, 5th Infantry Division, Annual Rpt, 1944, pp. 35–36; AGF, Combat Experiences Rpt, 1945, pp. 9–11, file HD:ETO:350.07:Battle Experiences.

the disastrous attack of the 28th Infantry Division in the Huertgen Forest early in November. In this operation the 1st and 3d Battalions of the 112th Infantry seized a salient of key high ground around the villages of Schmidt and Kommerscheidt, deep in German-held territory, and then came under heavy infantry, tank, and artillery counterattack from three sides. The battalions' route of supply and evacuation consisted of a narrow trail, muddy from the incessant rain, which wound its way down into the gorge of the Kall River and then up another ridge to the American-held town of Vossenack, some 2 miles northwest of Kommerscheidt. Vossenack itself was under intense German infantry attack, as well as artillery bombardment from high ground to its northeast.

The battalion surgeons, Captains Paschal A. Linguiti, MC, of the 1st and Michael De Marco, MC, of the 3d, faced a difficult evacuation problem. Ambulances from their supporting collecting company—C, 103d Medical Battalion, which had its station near Vossenack—could not negotiate the trail across the Kall. Hence, the battalions had to send casualties back in jeeps and weasels (the division had large numbers of the latter attached for this operation) to an ambulance loading point near the top of the ridge at Vossenack. Linguiti initially set up his 1st Battalion aid station in a basement in Kommerscheidt; De Marco, with his 3d Battalion station, took position about a mile farther to the rear, west of the Kall, sheltered in a cave-like 18-by-12-foot dugout built into the steep hillside that bordered the trail. The station in Kommerscheidt in effect functioned as an advance collecting point; it sent wounded in whatever vehicles were available to the 3d Battalion installation for relay on up the hill to the ambulance loading point.

As the American position at Schmidt and Kommerscheidt deteriorated, so did the evacuation situation. Linguiti and De Marco consolidated their two aid stations in the dugout. Disabled American tanks and other vehicles along the trail and German shelling of the ambulance loading point effectively halted evacuation of all but walking wounded, whom the surgeons sent to the rear in parties led by medical troops. Litter patients, eventually about sixty-five of them, accumulated in and around the dugout. Linguiti and De Marco cared for them as best they could, helped by their MAC assistant surgeons, the battalion chaplains, a dwindling contingent of enlisted medics, and infantry stragglers whom the surgeons disarmed and pressed into service as attendants and litterbearers. The medics had adequate food for their patients and enough medical supplies for what little treatment they were attempting, but they were short of blankets and shelter. The dugout could accommodate only about twenty-five patients. The remainder, wrapped in what coverings were available, lay along the trail in the cold, rain, and snow, protected by soldiers holding Red Cross flags. This protection was needed because, during the final days of the battle, German troops infiltrating behind the 1st and 3d Battalions periodically visited the aid station. However, except for announcing that the medics were captured and making sure that no armed Americans were present, the Germans left the facility unmolested. They allowed American walking wounded from Kommerscheidt to reach the station and at one point offered Linguiti and De Marco food and medicine, which the surgeons declined. Nevertheless, the Germans did confiscate the aid station's few vehicles.

After the survivors of the 1st and 3d Battalions withdrew from Kommerscheidt on the night of 8–9 November, in the process inundating the aid station with a final stream of walking and litter-borne casualties, Linguiti and De Marco and their staff and patients remained within German lines. The enemy evidently had neither the means nor the inclination to remove the American doctors and wounded. The local German commander agreed to a truce, proposed by the 112th Infantry's surgeon, Maj. Albert L. Berndt, MC, for removal of both sides' casualties from the Kall valley. Under this arrangement the battalion surgeons, after further adventures with a German unit not party to the truce, eventually managed to assemble a makeshift truck and weasel convoy to carry themselves, the other medical officers and men, the chaplains, and the severely wounded back to American lines. However, they had to surrender the lightly wounded and their nonmedical personnel as prisoners of war.[26]

The experience of Captains Linguiti and De Marco, besides illustrating the vicissitudes of forward area evacuation, pointed up another circumstance of the campaign very important to Army medics: the enemy's continued adherence to the international laws and customs of war affecting wounded and those who cared for them on the battlefield. As had been true since Normandy, German troops, at least until the Ardennes offensive, rarely engaged in aimed fire at aidmen, litterbearers, or Red Cross–marked medical facilities. Infantry of both sides, on many occasions, temporarily ceased fire or made short local truces to allow their medics to clear casualties from the field. During a counterattack in the Huertgen Forest the Germans captured a 22d Infantry, 4th Division, aidman. They put him to work caring for American casualties and then employed him, and a German medical soldier, to carry the wounded GIs to a point near American lines while both sides held their fire. American units provided reciprocal courtesies. During an attack at Frenzerburg Castle on the fringes of the Huertgen Forest, for instance, elements of the 47th Infantry, 9th Division, observed a three-hour truce so that a German ambulance could remove thirty severely wounded enemy defenders. On the other hand, the 47th Infantry took prisoner eight less seriously injured Germans who would have been able to return to combat.[27]

[26] This narrative is based on reports of Major Berndt, Captains Linguiti and De Marco, 2d Lt. A. J. Muglia, and 1st Lt. L. C. Johnson, all in 28th Infantry Division Combat Intervs, box 24032, RG 407, NARA. For tactical and logistical details of this battle, see MacDonald, *Siegfried Line*, ch. XV, and Charles B. MacDonald and Sidney T. Mathews, *Three Battles: Arnaville, Altuzzo, and Schmidt*, United States Army in World War II (Washington, D.C.: Office of the Chief of Military History, Department of the Army, 1952), pp. 251–418.

[27] Intervs, Assistant Surgeon and Aidmen, 1st Battalion, 22d Infantry, in 4th Infantry Division Combat Intervs, box 24021; Intervs, Lt Col Lewis E. Maness and Capt W. L. McWaters, in 9th Infantry

Continued

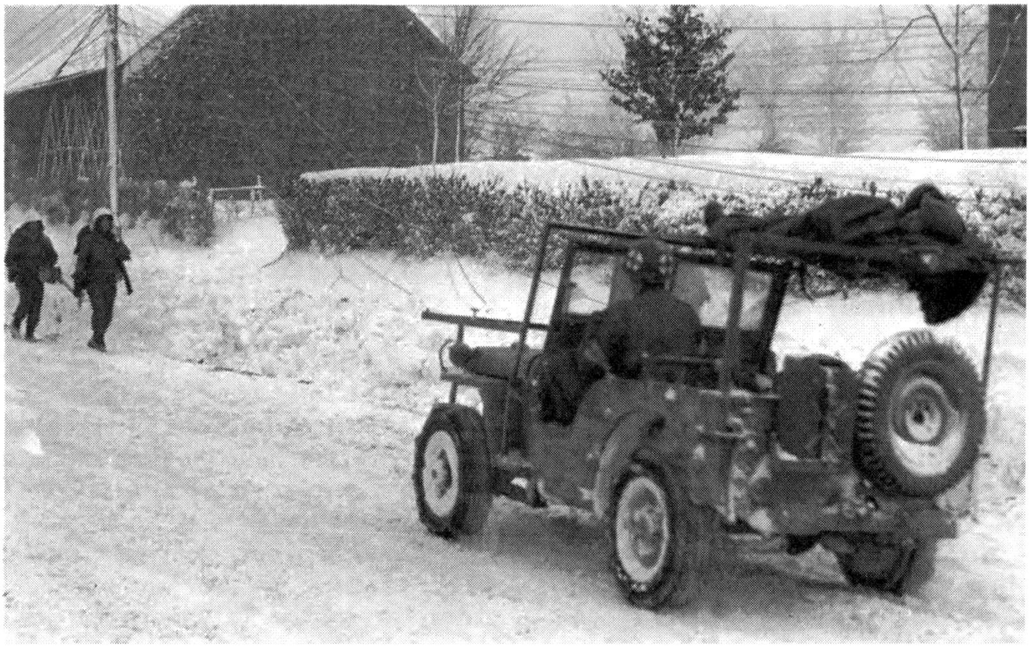

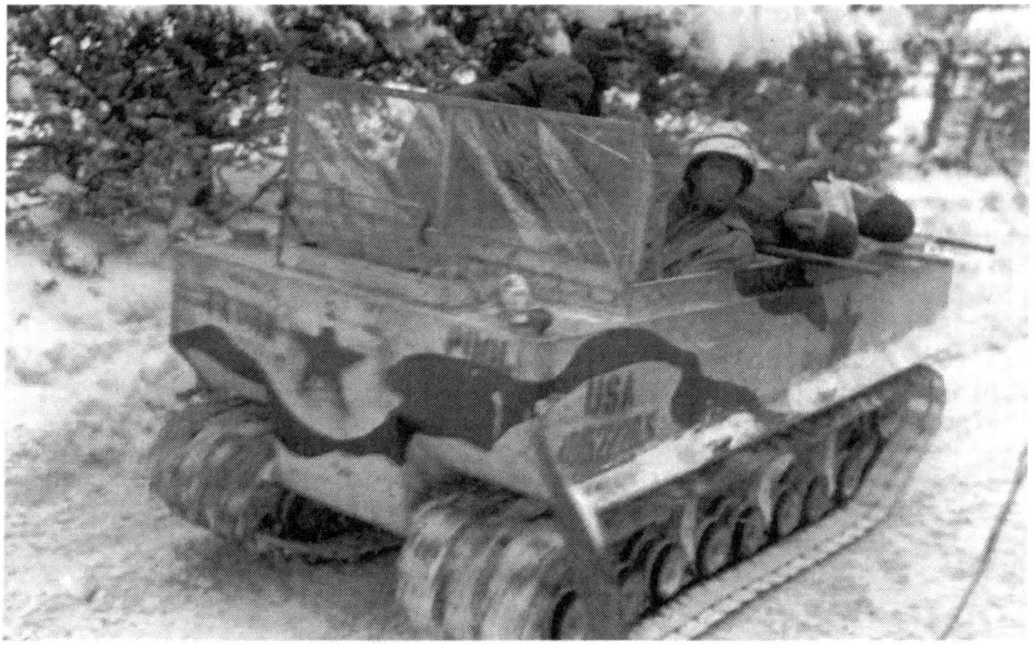

WORKHORSES OF BATTLEFIELD EVACUATION. *Much of the work for transporting casualties fell to the jeep, fitted with brackets for carrying litters. When these sturdy vehicles bogged down in mud and heavy snow, medics switched to the tracked M–29 Weasel.*

In response to repeated claims by German prisoners that they often could not see the Red Cross arm brassard on the battlefield, the army medical service adopted more conspicuous Geneva Convention markings. Late in November the 12th Army Group, at the request of Colonel Shambora, the Ninth Army surgeon, formally authorized medical troops to paint large red crosses in white fields on their helmets, a practice already widespread among aidmen and litterbearers. The 7th Armored Division determined in tests that men so marked stood out from other soldiers at distances of up to 750 yards. Medics in some divisions either carried Red Cross flags with which to signal their identity when moving under fire or wore improvised Red Cross tabards and vests modeled on those of German aidmen. The army medical service also scrupulously guarded its noncombatant status against encroachment by its own side. Division surgeons and other medical officers registered vehement protest against use of Red Cross–marked vehicles for nonmedical purposes and against the placing of artillery, tanks, and combat-related supplies too close to their aid stations. More conspicuous Geneva Convention insignia probably saved the lives of many front-line medics in the mud, snow, and mist of the autumn and winter battlefields, and mutual respect for international usage diminished somewhat the dangers they faced. Hazards, however, remained in plenty. As one medical soldier put it, "Artillery and mortars don't know the difference between a rifleman and a guy with a red cross brassard on his arm." [28]

From Battle Line to Hospitals

To the rear of the divisions the medical organizations of the different armies retained the varying forms they had assumed at the end of the pursuit. The First Army, and the Ninth Army following its example, attached most nondivisional medical units except hospitals to their medical groups; the First Army also attached to its groups the field hospitals working with the division clearing stations. These armies placed one medical group in charge of evacuation and various other support activities for each of their corps, with an area of responsibility extending from the division rear boundaries to that of the army. The Third Army, by contrast, employed all but one of its medical groups strictly for evacuation, attaching only ambulance units to them; one group evacuated the division clearing stations of each corps and an additional group transferred patients among and to the rear of evacuation and convalescent hospitals. The Third Army's employment of its medical groups seemed to General Hawley and others to be inefficient. Indeed,

Division Combat Intervs, box 24027. For other comments, see also reports of Linguiti and De Marco, in 28th Infantry Division Combat Intervs, box 24032, All in RG 407, NARA.

[28] Quotation from ETO, Battlefield First Aid Rpt, 1944, app., p. v, file HD:ETO:350.07:Battle Experiences. On markings, see Surg, Ninth U.S. Army, Daily Journal, 13, 21 and 25 Nov 44, Shambora Papers, MHI, and Surg, 95th Infantry Division, Annual Rpt, 1944, pp. 11–12. For examples of protests, see Surg, 101st Airborne Division, Annual Rpt, 1944, p. 19, and Memo, Capt P. A. Linguiti to Surg, 112th Infantry, 16 Nov 44, sub: Misuse of Aid Station Site, in 28th Infantry Division Combat Intervs, box 24032, RG 407, NARA.

the commander of one of the army's groups pointed out that his headquarters, with two medical battalions attached, during most of the campaign controlled only four ambulance companies. The Seventh Army got along without medical groups altogether. Separate medical battalions, often with as many as eight companies attached, evacuated its corps, and the army surgeon directly controlled hospitals and other facilities. Offered a medical group from the Third Army, the Seventh Army surgeon, Colonel Rudolph, refused it. He declared that "no necessity existed for such a unit since the functions of . . . a group could be and were being performed either by the battalion clearing corps or by the Operations Section of the Surgeon's Office." Whatever their differences and drawbacks, all these systems worked well enough that neither theater nor army group surgeons considered it necessary to interfere with them.[29]

Especially in the First and Ninth Armies, medical groups performed a number of miscellaneous but vital functions. They operated dispensaries and prophylactic stations for nondivisional army troops. They deployed collecting and clearing companies to reinforce evacuation hospitals; provided additional litterbearers to the divisions; and collected trucks to move the larger army medical units. Because the groups' role in evacuation required constant liaison with tactical headquarters, these units served as communications centers and intelligence clearinghouses for other army medical service organizations. The commander of the 68th Medical Group in the First Army, for example, opened up his morning staff briefing on the military situation and evacuation plans to all medical unit commanders in his area of operations. Other groups distributed periodical news and information bulletins, one inevitably entitled "Poop from Group." The 69th Medical Group in the Third Army ran a daily courier service, which collected statistical reports from all the hospitals for the army surgeon and distributed his messages and circulars to every medical facility. Similarly, in the Seventh Army the medical battalions also augmented hospitals and reinforced the division medical service, as well as operated a neuropsychiatric treatment facility for each corps.[30]

Whatever their subsidiary activities, the principal function of the medical groups, and of the battalions that substituted for them in the Seventh Army, was evacuation of the division clearing stations. At the height of the offensive the groups transported wounded in large numbers. During November, for example, the Third Army's 66th Medical Group handled over 12,000 XX Corps patients; its

[29] Quotation from Surg, Seventh U.S. Army, Annual Rpt, 1944, pp. 17, 20–21, 115–16. See also Surg, Third U.S. Army, Annual Rpt, 1944, pp. 75–76; Surg, Ninth U.S. Army, Annual Rpt, 1944, p. 17; Surg, Ninth U.S. Army, Daily Journal, 1 Nov 44, Shambora Papers, MHI; 1st, 31st, 67th, 68th, 69th, and 134th Medical Groups Annual Rpts, 1944. For additional detail on group functions and organization, see Chapter IX of this volume. Hawley's concern about the Third Army's use of groups is in Ltr, Hawley to Col A. L. Gorby, 23 Nov 44, file HD 024 ETO CS (Hawley Chron). Gorby Interv, 1962, pp. 36–37, CMH, expresses general satisfaction with army employment of groups.

[30] 1st, 66th, 67th, 68th, 69th, and 134th Medical Groups Annual Rpts, 1944; Surg, Seventh U.S. Army, Annual Rpt, 1944, p. 116

67th Medical Group, in the same period, evacuated over 19,000 XII Corps casualties. The groups' attached battalions, each of which usually supported one or more divisions, normally placed a platoon of ten ambulances at each active infantry clearing or armored treatment station while holding other vehicles in a reserve pool to meet sudden casualty surges. The battalions set up ambulance control points at key road junctions to direct the flow of patients to particular evacuation hospitals. The 66th tried to avoid detouring ambulances through these points. It established an elaborate system for issuing frequent evacuation plans to its battalions, on the basis of which the battalions could send ambulances directly from clearing stations to their final destinations. This system, however, never achieved full acceptance by army authorities. In December, when the group shifted position to help evacuate Third Army forces in the Ardennes, army headquarters ordered it to establish a standard regulating post.

The groups by late 1944 had learned to control casualty flow with increasing sophistication, seeking to shorten as much as possible each patient's time on the road while not overloading any evacuation hospitals. Most of the groups distributed wounded primarily on the basis of what they called "surgical lag" or "surgical backlog," which the Seventh Army typically defined as "the time, expressed in hours, required for a hospital to complete the surgery required on all moderately to severely wounded . . . casualties then present." Medical groups found from experience that this figure, although subject to inconsistencies in the estimating methods of individual chiefs of surgical service, indicated more reliably than did the simple number of empty beds the actual remaining capacity of a hospital. Depending on the situation and army directives, medical groups at times sorted casualties by type or severity, for example, sending surgical cases needing early operation to evacuation hospitals nearest the front. As hospitals moved into buildings during the autumn, groups had to take into account such details as the limited capacity of receiving wards no longer expandable by pitching more tents. When they could, groups deferred to the wishes of hospital commanders; some wanted a steady stream of new patients, while others preferred to receive them in periodic batches. Juggling such factors and considerations in constantly changing patterns, the groups kept the evacuation system within the armies operating with few interruptions, even in the face of deteriorating weather and road surfaces. They suffered late in the year from a shortage of ambulances and ambulance companies, but General Hawley remedied this by speeding up the transatlantic flow of machines and units and by stripping ambulances from the Communications Zone for the field armies.[31]

Each army established an evacuation policy that governed the movement of casualties from its hospitals to those of the Communications Zone

[31] Quotation from Surg, Seventh U.S. Army, Annual Rpt, 1944, pp. 126–28. See also ibid., pp. 16 and 116–17; 1st, 66th, 67th, 68th, and 134th Medical Groups Annual Rpts, 1944. On the ambulance shortage, see 12th Army Group Report of Operations, vol. XIII (Medical Section), p. 57, and correspondence in file HD ETO 451.8 (Amb), 1942–44.

(*see Diagram 4*). Normally, the armies evacuated all patients who needed more than 10 days, on the average, of hospitalization. But they varied this limit in response to the incidence of casualties and the number of empty beds, with an eye always to keeping as many salvageable men as possible within army boundaries until they returned to duty. Accordingly, during the October lull in combat, the First and Third Armies adopted, respectively, 20- and 21-day evacuation policies. Under these they could retain the increasing number of soldiers who came down with respiratory ailments as the weather turned cold and wet, as well as their lightly wounded, their venereal disease cases, and many neuropsychiatric patients. As casualties increased again in November, the armies reverted to 14-day, 10-day, and even shorter policies. The Ninth Army at one point ordered the daily evacuation of all its transportable patients, to clear beds for fresh wounded from the front. At various times during the offensive the First, Third, and Ninth Armies, their evacuation hospitals rapidly filling to capacity, all resorted to "bypassing." When this policy was in effect, evacuation hospitals stopped performing surgery on all but the most severe and urgent cases. They sent other surgical patients, after brief stabilizing treatment, immediately to COMZ general hospitals close in rear of the armies. By this means the army installations reduced their own surgical backlogs, while low-priority patients actually reached the operating table sooner than they would have in the evacuation hospitals. First Army hospitals, at the height of the offensive, bypassed well over 50 percent of the battle casualties they admitted.[32]

As the front stabilized, so did the locations at which patients passed from the armies to the Communications Zone. The First and Ninth Armies, during the fall and winter, sent casualties to ADSEC holding units and general hospitals at Liege and to a holding unit at Verviers. The Third Army evacuated through Toul, Etain, Nancy, and, as it approached the German border, Thionville. The Seventh Army, which continued to rely on the separate Southern Line of Communications (SOLOC) for evacuation and long-term hospitalization, evacuated through Luxeuil and Besancon to Marseilles and Naples. Later in the campaign its holding units shifted northward to Bayon and Tantonville, about 10 miles south of Nancy. With SOLOC slow to build up and short of hospital beds, the Seventh Army sent limited numbers of patients by air and rail to northern COMZ general hospitals in Paris, the Oise Base Section, and the United Kingdom. Increasingly, during late 1944, ADSEC and its southern counterpart, Continental Advance Section (CONAD), took over the operation of holding units in rear of the armies and the ambulance evacuation of casualties from army hospitals. Only the Third Army continued to maintain

[32] First U.S. Army Report of Operations, 1 Aug 44–22 Feb 45, bk. IV, pp. 137 and 163–64; Surg, Third U.S. Army, Annual Rpt, 1944, pp. 45 and 79; Surg, Ninth U.S. Army, Annual Rpt, 1944, p. 28; Surg, Ninth U.S. Army, Combat Experience Rpt, November 1944, file HD 319.1-2; Memo, Kenner to CofS, SHAEF, 5 Dec 44, sub: Report of Inspection, Medical Service, First and Ninth U.S. Armies, Inclusive Period 20–30 Nov 44, in Medical Division, COSSAC/SHAEF, War Diary, December 1944.

DIAGRAM 4—FIELD ARMIES AND COMZ EVACUATION RESPONSIBILITY

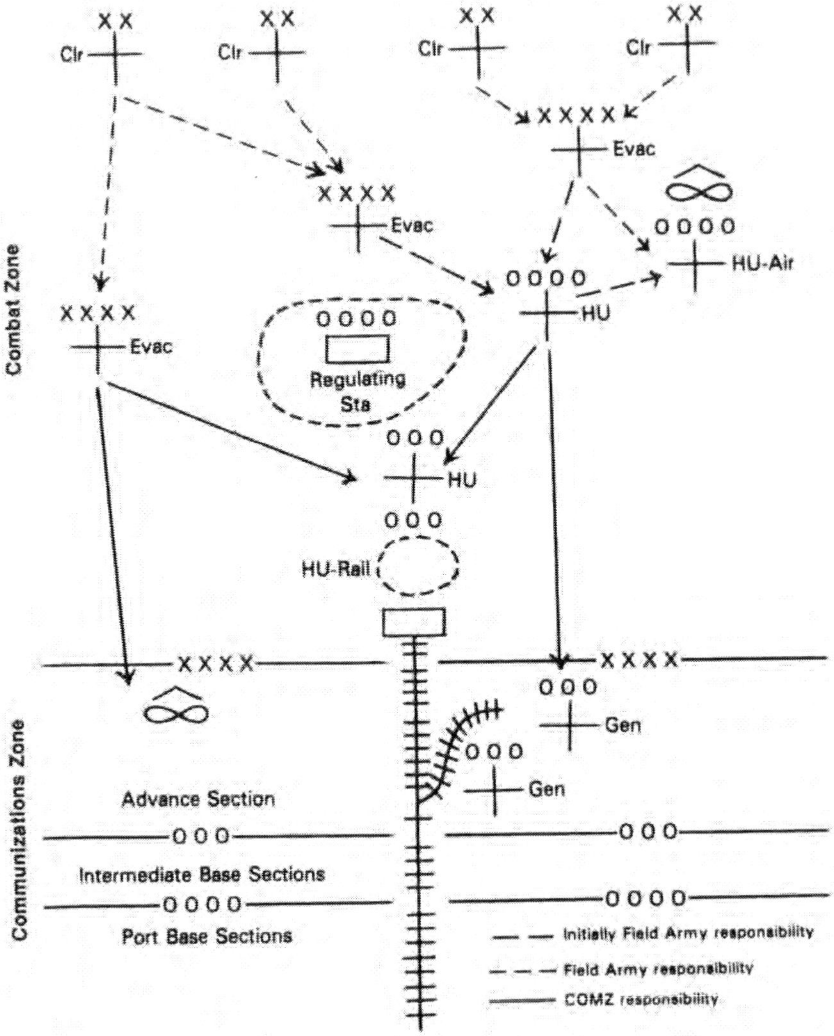

Source: Evacuation Branch, Operations Division, OofCSurg, HQ, ETOUSA, Annual Rpt, 1944, encl. 5.

its own air-rail holding unit, and its 69th Medical Group shared with ADSEC the work of transporting patients to the Communications Zone (*see Map 16*).

All the armies continued to evacuate their severely wounded by air from forward fields whenever possible. However, as flying weather worsened and rail service steadily expanded, hospital trains carried the greater proportion of patients leaving the army areas. On the whole, the flow of casualties from the armies went smoothly during the November and December battles. Interruptions of evacuation, such as had clogged army facilities at the end of the pursuit, became increasingly rare as ADSEC and CONAD enlarged the quantity and variety of their means of transportation, and as the slow progress of the offensive reduced the need to move forward holding units and extend rail lines. In evacuation, as in other aspects of medical support, bad news for the tactician was, paradoxically, good news—in terms of operational efficiency—for the logistician.[33]

Army Hospitals at Work

In each field army, during late 1944, the hospital system reached full development. Field hospital platoons attached to division clearing stations worked on the most urgent emergency surgical cases. Evacuation hospitals handled the transportable severely wounded, the patients with minor injuries, and most of the sick. A convalescent hospital in each army relieved the evacuation hospitals of nearly recovered patients and reconditioned them for return to duty. Improvised special facilities cared for soldiers with contagious or communicable diseases and venereal infections, as well as for neuropsychiatric casualties.

Surgical work in the armies centered in the field and evacuation hospitals. Field hospital surgeons spent most of their time operating on men with massive chest and abdominal injuries, severe compound fractures, and traumatic amputations. Their principal objective was to keep their patients alive and to place them in condition for further evacuation. Postoperative death rates in these installations ran between 12 and 25 percent, higher than in any other type of hospital, and reflected the all but hopeless condition of many of the wounded who arrived on their operating tables. All too common were cases such as the Ninth Army soldier who died twenty-four hours after surgery in the 2d Platoon, 53d Field Hospital: "S[hell] F[ragment] W[ound] multiple with complete amputation right foot; C[ompound]

---

[33] Medical Division, COSSAC/SHAEF, War Diary, October–December 1944; First U.S. Army Report of Operations, 1 Aug 44–22 Feb 45, bk. IV, pp. 136–37 and 140; Surg, Third U.S. Army, Annual Rpt, 1944, pp. 80–85; Surg, Ninth U.S. Army, Annual Rpt, 1944, pp. 12–13; 69th Medical Group Annual Rpt, 1944, pp. 11–12 and 16–17; 134th Medical Group Annual Rpt, 1944, p. 12; 41st Evacuation Hospital Annual Rpt, 1944, pp. 59–60, which gives a hospital view on improving evacuation; HQ, SOLOC, History of the Medical Section, Headquarters, Southern Line of Communications, ETO, U.S. Army, 20 November 1944–1 January 1945 (hereafter cited as SOLOC Medical Hist), pp. 20–26; Surg, CONAD, Annual Rpt, 1944, pp. 8–10; MFR, Col J. H. Voegtly, 16 Nov 44, sub: Medical Service, Southern Group of Armies, and Memo, Anon. to Col Peyton, 18 Nov 44, sub: Notes Taken at Conference on Medical Service for Southern Group of Armies, both in DRAGOON 1944 file, CMH. See also appropriate pages in Chapter XIX of Smith and Clarke, *Riviera to the Rhine*.

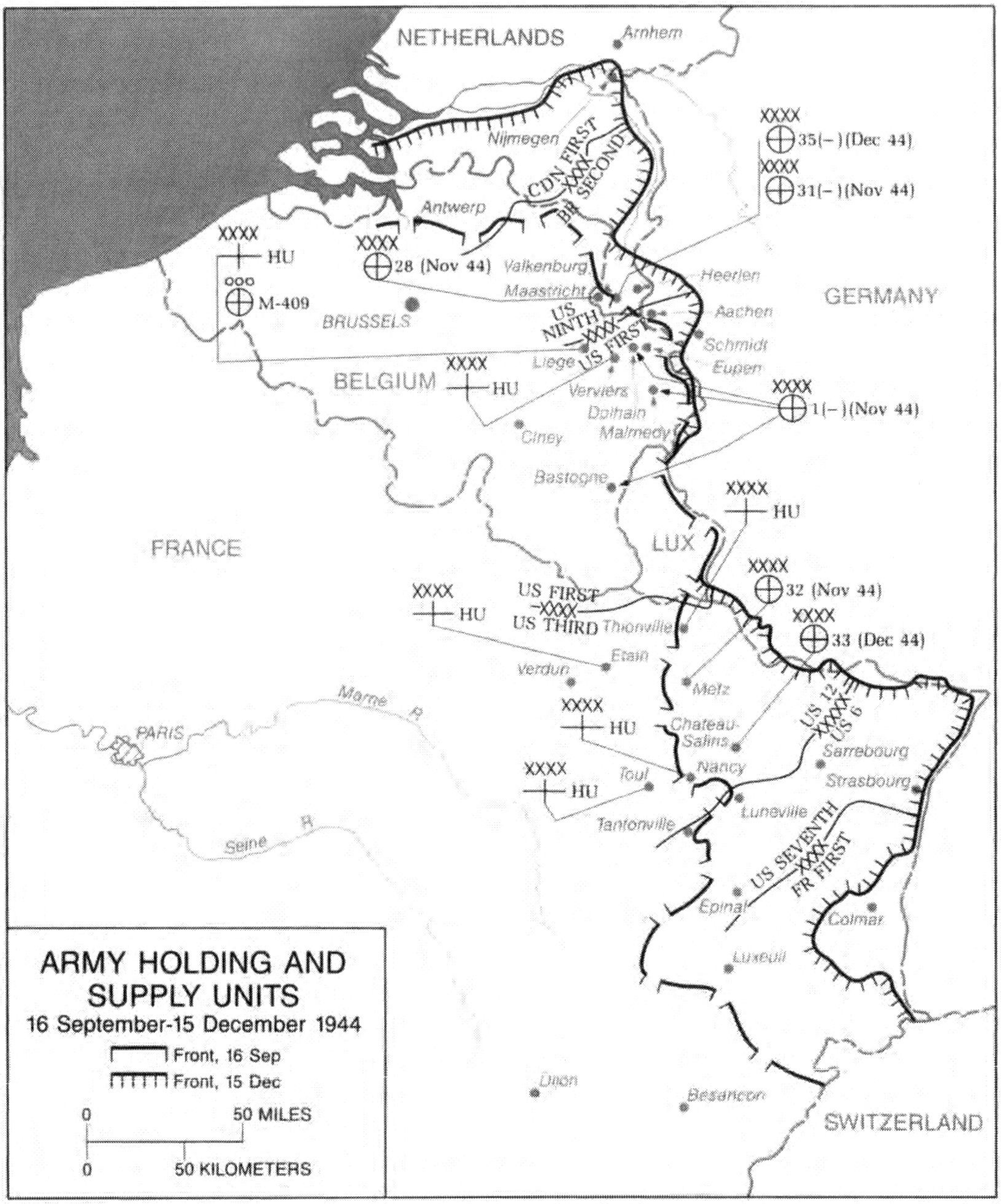
NETHERLANDS
Arnhem
Nijmegen
CDN FIRST
XXXX
BR SECOND
Antwerp
XXXX
35(–)(Dec 44)
XXXX
31(–)(Nov 44)
XXXX
HU
XXXX
28 (Nov 44)
Valkenburg
Heerlen
M-409
Maastricht
GERMANY
BRUSSELS
US NINTH
XXXX
US FIRST
Aachen
Schmidt
Liege
Eupen
XXXX
BELGIUM
HU
XXXX
Verviers
1(–)(Nov 44)
Dolhain
Malmedy
Ciney
Bastogne
XXXX
HU
FRANCE
LUX
XXXX
32 (Nov 44)
XXXX
HU
US FIRST
XXXX
US THIRD
Thionville
XXXX
33 (Dec 44)
Etain
Verdun
Metz
Marne R
US 12
XXXX
US 6
XXXX
HU
Chateau-Salins
PARIS
Sarrebourg
Nancy
XXXX
HU
Toul
Strasbourg
Luneville
Tantonville
Seine R
US SEVENTH
XXXX
FR FIRST
Epinal
Colmar
Luxeuil
Dijon
Besancon
SWITZERLAND
ARMY HOLDING AND
SUPPLY UNITS
16 September-15 December 1944
Front, 16 Sep
Front, 15 Dec
0
50 MILES
0
50 KILOMETERS

MAP 16

F[racture] left fibula, soft tissue wounds [right] thigh and left leg; . . . severe muscle damage both legs. . . ." [34]

Evacuation hospital surgeons operated on the great majority of orthopedic patients, who usually were transportable enough to bypass the field hospital platoons. By debridement and the application of plaster casts, the surgeons prepared these casualties for further transportation and laid the groundwork for definitive treatment in COMZ general hospitals. In compound fractures, according to a Third Army surgeon, "what we had to do was create a clean, organizable wound out of an indiscriminately smeared up, messed up situation." Evacuation hospital surgeons, while they handled a large number of minor and moderately severe injuries, also encountered massive wounds, some of which gruesomely illustrated the macabre mischances of modern combat. The same Third Army surgeon recalled:

The French manure pile . . . came into the operating room. An infantryman had hidden next to one when the shell blew up in the pile filling his thigh from knee to buttocks with manure, all tightly packed in as into a sausage, [and] smashing muscle and femur bone. He was in critical condition. . . . I started debriding after the second set of bottles of blood was partly in. . . . After a major debridement, pockets containing manure kept appearing in deeper and deeper layers in all directions until there was not much left of the limb. Reluctantly I had to disarticulate [amputate] the limb at the hip and debride the buttock. This man developed kidney failure and died on the ninth day. . . .[35]

Field and evacuation hospitals alike depended for surgical reinforcements upon teams from the auxiliary surgical groups; indeed such teams made up the entire operating room staff of the field hospital platoons. The European Theater by late 1944 possessed five complete auxiliary groups, attached to the field armies and army groups, and the equivalent of half of another, assigned to COMZ. Each group included about twenty-five teams of doctors, nurses, and enlisted technicians, the majority organized for general surgery and the rest for neurosurgery, maxillofacial work, X-ray, and dental prosthetics. These teams contained an impressive array of professional talent, and the theater took pains to maintain the quality of their personnel. Accordingly, when the Ninth Army's 5th Auxiliary Surgical Group arrived in France with a substantial number of young, inexperienced medical officers, the army had no difficulty restaffing it with better qualified men transferred from the Communications Zone and the ground forces. Besides the teams, the auxiliary groups included varying

[34] Quotation from Surg, Ninth U.S. Army, Daily Journal, 9 Nov 44, Shambora Papers, MHI. For other statistics, see Surg, Seventh U.S. Army, Annual Rpt, 1944, pp. 118–20; 11th Field Hospital Annual Rpt, 1944, app. B; 13th Field Hospital Annual Rpt, encls. 4–5; 48th Field Hospital Semiannual Rpt, January-June 1945, p. 15; 51st Field Hospital Annual Rpt, 1944, p. 13; and Memo, Kenner to CofS, SHAEF, 5 Dec 44, sub: Report of Inspection, Medical Service, First and Ninth U.S. Armies, in Medical Division, COSSAC/SHAEF, War Diary, December 1944.

[35] First quotation from Gosman Interv, 24 Mar 82. Second quotation from Joseph A. Gosman, MD, "War without Blood" (1982), p. 150. Both in CMH. For other examples of evacuation hospital work, see 3d Auxiliary Surgical Group Annual Rpt, 1944, pp. 33–35; 5th Evacuation Hospital Annual Rpt, 1944, pp. 12–13; and 41st Evacuation Hospital Annual Rpt, 1944, p. 11.

numbers of truck-mounted mobile operating rooms and X-ray facilities, designed for temporary expansion of busy hospitals. The operating trucks proved to be of only limited use, as the hospitals' capacity for surgery was restricted more by shortages of nurses and other postoperative support than by a lack of theater space. The X-ray units, however, effectively reinforced roentgenological departments swamped by sudden floods of patients.

Auxiliary groups normally attached most of their general teams, heavily weighted with thoracic and abdominal specialists, to field hospital platoons. Maxillofacial, neurosurgical, and other specialized teams went to evacuation hospitals, which received most of the type of patients they treated. During heavy fighting a single auxiliary group could not meet an army's demand for extra surgeons. At such times evacuation hospitals, especially, drew additional temporary teams from staging COMZ units, an arrangement that at once solved the armies' surgical manpower problem and gave useful experience to the fixed hospital personnel.[36]

The presence in units of doctors, nurses, and technicians who administratively and in part professionally answered to another organization created problems of command and human relations. This was especially true in field hospital platoons. The commander of the 3d Auxiliary Surgical Group summed up: "Platoon commanders are irked that teams create awkward problems of supply and transportation, that teams do not come under the administrative control of the hospital, and that teams are neither fish nor fowl." On their side, team members "feel that they are always last in line, that they get second-best, and that they are the unwanted children." Permanent unit staff also resented being relegated to routine ward duties, while auxiliary teams did all the surgery and ran the operating theaters. Even in evacuation hospitals, where the auxiliary teams worked under the unit chiefs of surgical service, the reinforcements had an aura of elitism and professional independence that set them apart. An officer in the 109th Evacuation Hospital observed: "The 'Aux' teams acted like doctors and nurses doing their job, but in uniform. The Evac teams . . . were more members of a military echelon, heirarchy, order . . . in the lower rank of such an order. . . ." Auxiliary surgical group commanders devoted much effort and diplomacy to smoothing out these undercurrents of conflict. Aided by a shared sense of a common professional mission, they usually succeeded.[37]

[36] First U.S. Army Report of Operations, 1 Aug 44–22 Feb 45, bk. IV, pp. 168–69; 3d Auxiliary Surgical Group Annual Rpt, 1944, pp. 33, 35–36, 40, 44–46; 4th Auxiliary Surgical Group Annual Rpt, 1944, p. 7; Surg, Third U.S. Army, Annual Rpt, 1944, pp. 99–102; Surg, Ninth U.S. Army, Annual Rpt, 1944, p. 28.

[37] First and second quotations from 3d Auxiliary Surgical Group Annual Rpt, p. 34. Third quotation from Gosman, "War without Blood," p. 143, CMH. For typical auxiliary team control arrangements, see Medical News No. 1, Ninth U.S. Army, 30 Oct 44, file HD:ETO:300.41, and Cir Ltr No. 7, Surg, Seventh U.S. Army, 28 Sep 44, sub: SOP for the Use and Control of Surgical and Allied Teams of an Auxiliary Surgical Group, in Surg, Seventh U.S. Army, Annual Rpt, 1944. Surg, Ninth U.S. Army, Annual Rpt, 1944, pp. 36–37, and 48th Field Hospital Semiannual Rpt, January–June 1945, p. 17, typify some of the conflicts and complaints.

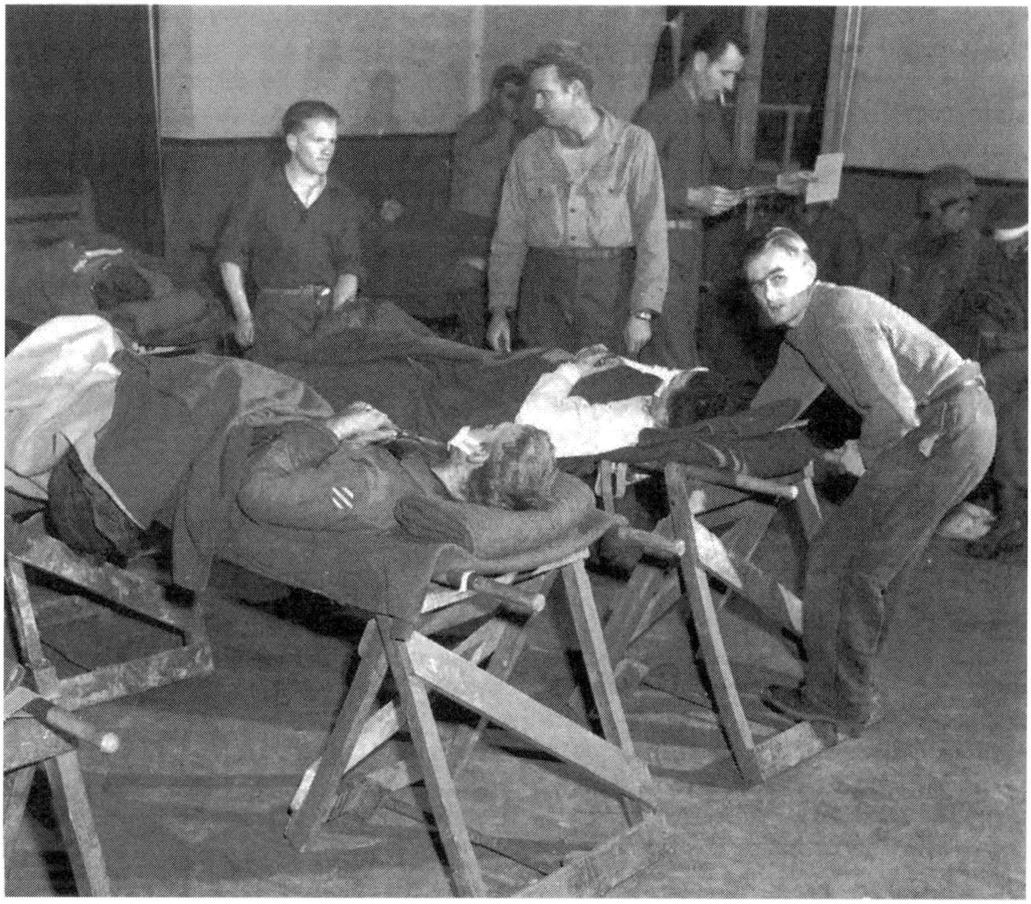

EVACUATION HOSPITAL RECEIVING WARD

Field and evacuation hospitals alike arranged their physical plants and streamlined their procedures for rapid reception, sorting, and treatment of a large volume of patients. Most units, whether in tents or buildings, tried to lay out their facilities so that a casualty would move in a more or less straight line from receiving through surgery to postoperative care and evacuation. Many, by converting cots to work stands for litters, were able to keep a patient on the same stretcher from the time he came off the ambulance until he reached the postoperative ward. Hospitals, after initial episodes of confusion, learned to put their most capable officers in charge of reception and triage. These officers quickly examined each arriving casualty and dispatched him to the shock, preoperative, medical, or immediate evacuation wards. In the shock and preoperative wards, doctors, nurses, and enlisted technicians, working with all possible speed, took the necessary resuscitation and stabilization measures and moved the patient to and from X-ray. Roentgenology constituted a perennial bottleneck when casualties were coming in rapidly, and hospital technicians taxed their ingenuity to the limit to expedite the taking and development of pictures. One unit, the 107th Evacuation Hospital, sent patients in shock to X-ray before resuscitation, in the belief that a slight delay in starting the latter process would be less harmful to the casualty than a subsequent interruption of it. Using such expedients, hospitals could process masses of casualties. On the night of 16 November, for example, the 111th Evacuation Hospital, located at Heerlen, Holland, behind the Ninth Army, admitted 272 patients in four hours; its people examined, sorted, and placed under shelter more that 1 wounded man each minute.[38]

Field and evacuation hospitals organized their surgical staffs to operate on the maximum number of cases within the shortest possible time. In field hospital platoons the attached surgical teams, and in evacuation hospitals normally the chiefs of surgical service or the senior surgeons on shift, scheduled patients for operation. While each army set general guidelines for establishing surgical priority, the officers actually managing the traffic applied these rules with great flexibility, their aim being to keep all available surgeons and tables continually busy. Surgeons, nurses, and technicians worked in more or less permanent teams. A field hospital platoon with two attached teams could complete perhaps twenty major operations a day. A 400-bed evacuation hospital could keep eight to ten operating tables in action around the clock; the number of cases they turned out depended on the severity of the casualties then being received. In theory, surgical teams working twelve hours and resting twelve hours could keep up this pace almost indefinitely; in practice, the regimen quickly took its toll. During periods of heavy action the 9th Evacuation Hospital reported that "the staff was nearly always tired and too often lacking in sleep." A surgeon in the 109th Evacuation Hospital recalled: "I began to tire physically and psychologically from the twelve hour operating stretch every day; then, eating after the last surgery, writing letters and going to sleep. . . . I worked on instinct when tired." [39]

[38] First U.S. Army Report of Operations, 1 Aug 44–22 Feb 45, bk. IV, pp. 161–63, gives a general view of triage and resuscitation in that army. For examples of hospital operations, see 48th Field Hospital Semiannual Rpt, January-June 1945, pp. 5, 8, 11–12; 91st Evacuation Hospital Annual Rpt, 1944, pp. 56–57 and 69; 107th Evacuation Hospital Annual Rpt, 1944, pp. 10–12; and 111th Evacuation Hospital Annual Rpt, 1944, pp. 11 and 13–14.

[39] First quotation from 9th Evacuation Hospital Annual Rpt, 1944, p. 16. Second quotation from Gosman, "War without Blood," pp. 151–52, CMH. See also Gosman Interv, 24 Mar 82, CMH; First U.S. Army Report of Operations, 1 Aug 44–22 Feb 45, bk. IV, p. 162; Surg, Third U.S. Army, Annual Rpt, 1944, pp. 102–03; 3d Auxiliary Surgical Group Annual Rpt, 1944, pp. 33–34. For examples of surgical organization and operations, see 47th Field Hospital Annual Rpt, 1944, pp. 9 and 11; 48th Field Hospital Semiannual Rpt, January-June 1945, p. 8; 59th Field Hospital Annual Rpt, 1944, pp. 10–11; 11th Evacuation Hospital Annual Rpt, 1944, p. 4; 59th Evacuation Hospital Annual Rpt, 1944, p. 4 and sec. III, p. 8; 91st Evacuation Hospital Annual Rpt, 1944, pp. 59–61; 107th Evacuation Hospital Annual Rpt, 1944, p. 16; 111th Evacuation Hospital Annual Rpt, 1944, pp. 15–16; and 24th Evac Hist, October 1945, p. 93.

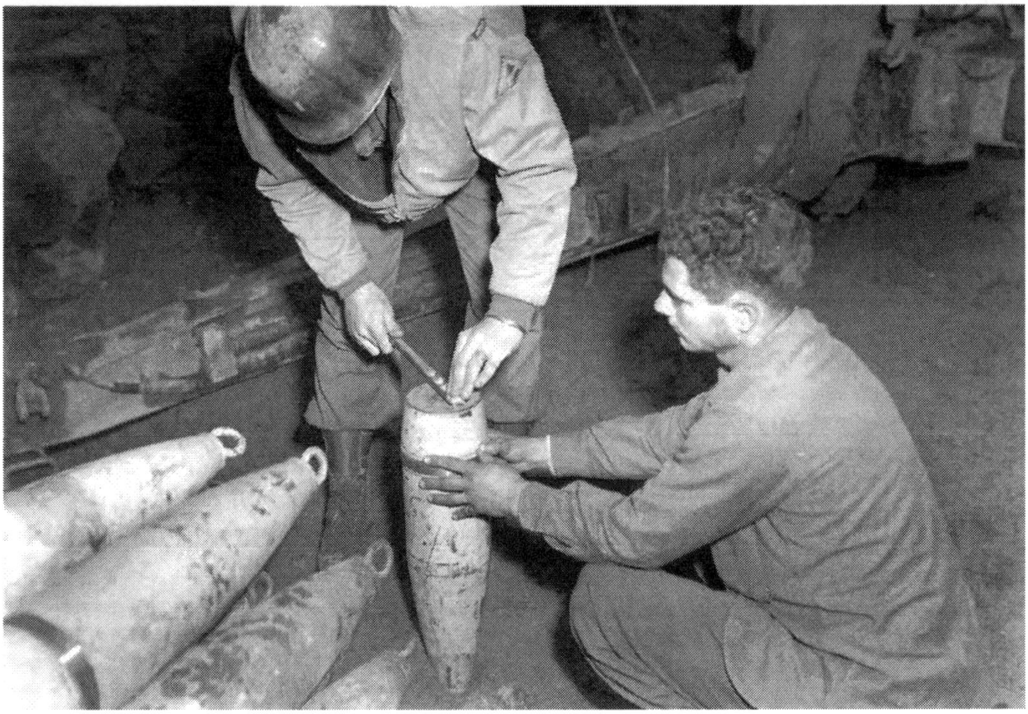

PACKING MEDICAL SUPPLIES IN A 155-MM. HOWITZER SHELL, *to be fired to troops cut off by the Germans*

Inevitably, with surgery being done under forced draft, errors occurred. Surgeons, especially in hospitals newly placed in operation, debrided wounds improperly or inadequately. They neglected to split casts to allow for swelling and permitted too early evacuation of patients with abdominal wounds or severe vascular damage. The army surgeons and their consultants, who kept close watch on the quality of professional practice in their hospitals, labored continually to reduce the incidence of such mistakes. The First Army temporarily stationed medical officers in ADSEC general hospitals, to check on the condition of patients arriving from the army. On the basis of these officers' reports Colonel Rogers, the army surgeon, among other changes revised his evacuation policies for men with chest and vascular injuries. Hospitals constantly reviewed their own surgical practice, for example, by conducting autopsies whenever possible in cases of postoperative death. In general, the quality of field and evacuation hospital surgery stood the test of review farther to the rear. During October, at a Paris meeting of Allied medical officers to discuss battle casualty treatment, COMZ surgeons, with only minor reservations, pronounced themselves satisfied with the condition of the patients reaching them from the armies. Colonel Cutler, the ETO chief surgical consultant, declared that earlier and more effective surgery—combined with widespread use of whole blood and antibiotics and the generally more robust physical condition of the troops—accounted for the higher recovery rate of the wounded in this war as compared to World War I.[40]

Mobile army hospitals tried to evacuate patients within as short a time as possible after their condition was stabilized, the minor postoperative cases almost as soon as they recovered from the effects of anesthesia. The operating surgeon normally had the final say in determining when his patient was transportable, but he had to take into consideration available beds, how many new casualties were arriving, and army policies. The armies, usually in response to COMZ complaints about evacuating too early, required their hospitals to hold certain postoperative patients—notably chest, abdominal, and neurosurgical cases and men with severe extremity wounds involving vascular damage—for a fixed number of days. Hospitals set up separate wards, with surgeons in charge, for such patients and placed the rest in wards designated for immediate evacuation, usually staffed by officers of their medical services. Evacuation hospitals sent off the majority of their patients within less than ten days; field hospitals, because of the severity and complicated nature of their cases, had to retain theirs for longer periods, a requirement that perennially conflicted with their need for mobility. The Third Army attached thirty-man holding units, drawn from collecting and gas treatment companies, to its field hospital platoons to stay behind with nontransportable patients when the main units moved.[41]

Getting a patient out of a hospital was itself a complicated task. The commander of the 110th Evacuation Hospital pointed out:

> When a patient is said to be ready for evacuation, it is not just a matter of putting him in an ambulance. . . . The patient must be made ready as far as clothing is concerned, then there [are] his valuables, and his x-rays. The problem is increased when you have from one hundred . . . to two hundred patients, spread all over the hospital, ready for evacuation.

Each hospital developed its own system for sending off patients. The 110th, for example, used two enlisted men as evacuation clerks, with four litterbearers to collect evacuees from

[40] First U.S. Army Report of Operations, 1 Aug 44–22 Feb 45, bk. IV, pp. 138 and 158; Surg, Ninth U.S. Army, Annual Rpt, 1944, pp. 28–32; Surg, Third U.S. Army, Annual Rpt, 1944, p. 41; Ltr, Hawley to Brig Gen J. A. Rogers, 9 Dec 44, file HD 024 ETO CS (Hawley Chron); Memo, Kenner to CofS, SHAEF, 24 Dec 44, sub: Report of Inspection of 3d US Army Medical Service and Supporting CZ Installations . . . , in Medical Division, COSSAC/SHAEF, War Diary, December 1944. For an example of hospital policy on autopsies, see 48th Field Hospital Semiannual Rpt, January–June 1945, pp. 10–11. Cutler's remarks are in Notes Taken at Press Conference, Paris, 4 Oct 44, . . . by the Chief Surgeon, ETOUSA, in Hawley Papers, MHI.

[41] For typical war operations and evacuation policies, see 48th Field Hospital Semiannual Rpt, January–June 1945; 110th Evacuation Hospital Semiannual Rpt, January–June 1945; 54th Field and 91st and 111th Evacuation Hospitals Annual Rpts, 1944; and Surg, Ninth U.S. Army, Daily Journal, 31 Dec 44, Shambora Papers, MHI. For army policies, see First U.S. Army Report of Operations, 1 Aug 44–22 Feb 45, bk. IV, pp. 163–64; Medical News No. 1, Ninth U.S. Army, 30 Oct 44, file HD:ETO:300.41; and Cir Ltr No. 2, Surg, Seventh U.S. Army, 18 Jul 44, sub: Surgery, in Surg, Seventh U.S. Army, Annual Rpt, 1944. On holding units, see Surg, Third U.S. Army, Annual Rpt, 1944, p. 89; 30th and 60th Field Hospitals Annual Rpts, 1944.

the wards. When the time came to move patients, the registrar alerted the clerks and bearers and the affected wards and sent the evacuation list to the offices in charge of patient valuables and X-ray files. Those offices packed up the appropriate items for each man for attachment, with his records, to his litter when the bearers brought him to a central point in the hospital. After a Red Cross worker made sure that each soldier had cigarettes, candy, and toilet articles, then litter teams began manhandling their charges into waiting ambulances.[42]

By late 1944 each army had a full system of specialized medical facilities in operation, designed to relieve clearing stations and field and evacuation hospitals of certain categories of nonsurgical patients and to keep as many salvageable soldiers as possible within army boundaries and out of the COMZ replacement system. Convalescent hospitals—T/O 3,000-bed units in the First, Third, and Seventh Armies and a 400-bed facility improvised from a gas treatment company in the Ninth—admitted ambulatory patients transferred from evacuation hospitals. They put these men through usually about ten days of physical therapy and reconditioning before sending them back to line units. Other facilities treated men with specific ailments who came to them directly from division clearing stations. The First Army used two clearing companies as 500-bed treatment centers for soldiers with combat fatigue; its gas treatment battalion operated hospitals for malaria, communicable and contagious disease, and self-inflicted-wound patients. The Third Army established venereal disease and neuropsychiatric sections in its 6th Convalescent Hospital, and the Ninth Army employed its gas treatment battalion to care for these casualties and also malaria cases. In the Seventh Army one clearing company and a platoon of another treated neuropsychiatric patients; another clearing company—reorganized for the purpose before the DRAGOON invasion—operated a 250-bed venereal disease hospital. These facilities, besides caring for many nonbattle casualties, helped the armies conserve manpower. In four months, for example, Third and Seventh Army convalescent hospitals returned to duty respectively 11,000 and 10,000 veteran troops.[43]

All the armies made special efforts to salvage as many as possible of their neuropsychiatric casualties—soldiers who suffered emotional breakdowns, of varying symptoms and severity, under the stress of battle. The incidence of such casualties fluctuated, as did that of physical wounding, with the intensity and nature of combat. During heavy fighting, such as that of

[42] Quotation from 110th Evacuation Hospital Semiannual Rpt, January-June 1945, p. 8. For other examples of evacuation systems, see 91st and 107th Evacuation Hospitals Annual Rpts, 1944.

[43] Convalescent hospitals were the 2d (Seventh Army), the 4th (First Army), and the 6th (Third Army). See Surg, First U.S. Army, Annual Rpt, 1944, p. 5; First U.S. Army Report of Operations, 1 Aug 44–22 Feb 45, bk. IV, pp. 134 and 185; Surg, Third U.S. Army, Annual Rpt, 1944, pp. 36, 79–80, 95–97, 111; Surg, Ninth U.S. Army, Annual Rpt, 1944, pp. 12–14 and 18; Surg, Ninth U.S. Army, Combat Experience Rpt, November 1944, file HD 319.1-2; Surg, Seventh U.S. Army, Annual Rpt, 1944, pp. 18–19, 21, 49, 51, 122–25; 2d, 4th, and 6th Convalescent Hospitals Annual Rpts, 1944; 92d and 95th Medical Gas Treatment Battalions Annual Rpts, 1944.

the autumn and winter offensive, neuropsychiatric cases accounted for between 9 and 25 percent of total monthly hospital admissions.

The armies, taking advantage of lessons learned in North Africa and Italy and of the First Army's early experience in Normandy, treated the emotional casualties of battle as temporarily disabled soldiers rather than mental patients, normally categorizing them with the neutral diagnosis "exhaustion." For the sake of both prevention and cure they attempted to treat such patients as close as possible to the fighting line. Typically, infantry battalion surgeons, trained in this work and supervised by their division psychiatrists, held all but the most severely disturbed men at their aid stations for up to twenty-four hours of rest (often under sedation), hot food, a change of clothing, and rudimentary individual and group therapy. Such treatment sufficed for an unrecorded but very high proportion of men with combat reactions, allowing their immediate return to their units.

Men needing a longer period to rest and more intensive therapy were evacuated to their division clearing stations. There, the division psychiatrist, with a pickup staff and improvised facilities, operated an "exhaustion center" that could hold patients for up to seventy-two hours of treatment. The clearing stations also returned to duty a substantial portion of the men they received. The rest went to the various specialized army facilities mentioned above and, in the Third Army, to the neuropsychiatric wards of regular evacuation hospitals, for periods of up to seven days of therapy and reconditioning, ending in a period of refresher training in a military camp rather than a hospital environment. The Third Army used a section of its convalescent hospital as still another echelon of army-level treatment that could hold patients for as long as two or three weeks. However, the other armies evacuated men still unfit for duty directly from their neuropsychiatric hospitals to the Communications Zone.

In the United Kingdom Base most general and station hosptials maintained fully staffed and equipped psychiatric services. In addition, the 312th Station Hospital (NP) and the 96th General Hospital (NP), specialized psychiatric facilities, received the most severely disturbed soldiers from other installations for prolonged, intensive treatment and rehabilitation. The 96th also selected mental patients for evacuation to the United States. On the Continent the Communications Zone attempted to set up neuropsychiatric hospitals close behind the armies to take patients from their exhaustion centers and to complete their treatment so that they could reenter the replacement system. For this purpose ADSEC in mid-November opened the 1,000-bed 130th General Hospital (NP) at Ciney, Belgium, to serve the First and Ninth Armies. At about the same time CONAD established the 500-bed 51st Station Hospital (NP) at Luneville to support the Third and Seventh Armies. However, given the shortage of forward general hospitals, both units were pressed into service to care for medical and surgical patients during the American offensive and the German December counterattacks. They began functioning primarily as neuropsychiatric facilities only during the last weeks of hostilities. Even without them, the armies and COMZ made an impressive record of success in rehabilitating emotionally damaged soldiers. According to a later estimate, out of every 100 psychiatric casualties in the theater, the armies and the Communications Zone restored 90 to some form of duty.[44]

Army hospitals, of whatever type, coped daily with manpower and equipment deficiencies. Ingenuity and improvisation facilitated their overcoming innumerable logistical and operational problems. Field hospitals made do with standard allowances of people and equipment intended for a very different function from the one they were performing. They had a constant battle to secure transportation for their many moves. The six nurses in each platoon were stretched to the limit of their endurance, caring for as many as sixty-five postoperative patients any of whom, in a civilian institution, would have required the exclusive attention of one or more nurses. The Seventh Army, in an attempt to alleviate these problems, reduced the bed capacity of each of its field hospital platoons to 60 and increased the nurse complement to eight with ANC officers borrowed from the Communications Zone. This army also issued additional trucks, trailers, and weapons carriers to each field hospital, giving the unit enough vehicles to move a platoon without outside help. All the armies employed collecting and clearing company elements, POWs, and French and Belgian civilians to meet the insatiable requirements of their evacuation hospitals for additional attendants and laborers. By late 1944 the typical 400-bed evacuation hospital had between fifty and eighty prisoners or civilians attached to it. Civilians replaced the German POWs as units neared the borders of the Reich.[45]

Mud, rain, cold, and snow became major adversaries for army medical installations as the harsh winter closed in. Frequent downpours transformed hosptial areas into seas of mud, in spite of the best efforts of engineers and medical troops with gravel and bulldozers. In one Third Army hospital "a plow came in and scraped mud into piles as if it were dealing with snow." As the days and nights grew colder, steam rose from abdominal incisions in unheated surgical tents. One unit resorted for warmth to potbelly stoves placed close to its operating tables. "Probably due to the closed system of anesthesia and good outdoor ventilation," a surgeon recalled, "and adding a

[44] The foregoing discussion is based on Albert J. Glass, ed., *The Overseas Theaters*, Medical Department, United States Army in World War II (Washington, D.C.: Office of the Surgeon General, Department of the Army, 1973), chs. VIII and IX; restoration-to-duty estimate is on pp. 273–74. See also Surg, Ninth U.S. Army, Annual Rpt, 1944, pp. 32–33. The 130th General Hospital was caught up in the German Ardennes counteroffensive. See Chapter XII of this volume.

[45] Surg, Third U.S. Army, Annual Rpt, 1944, pp. 92–93, 101, 124; Surg, Ninth U.S. Army, Annual Rpt, 1944, p. 19; Surg, Seventh U.S. Army, Annual Rpt, 1944, pp. 43 and 46; 68th Medical Group Annual Rpt, 1944, p. 21; 134th Medical Group Annual Rpt, 1944, pp. 11–12; Surg, XX Corps, Annual Rpt, 1944, pp. 22–23; 48th Field Hospital Semiannual Rpt, January–June 1945; 47th Field Hospital Annual Rpt, 1944; 9th, 11th, 41st, 59th, 91st, 104th, and 111th Evacuation Hospitals Annual Rpts, 1944; Memo, Lt Col A. W. Shiflet to CG, AGF, 11 Nov 44, sub: AGF Report No. 364—Medical Information.

factor of luck, there were no ether explosions." With wind and snow came additional tribulations. Work details swept accumulated snow off tents to keep them from collapsing, and they struggled to secure stovepipes and tent pegs against battering gusts.[46]

To remove staffs and patients from such hardships, the armies during November and December gave their hospitals and other medical units first claim on requisitioned buildings. Hospitals under roofs—in casernes, schools, hotels, monasteries, and even a former German slave labor camp—encountered new problems. Unlike tents, buildings could not be moved to the most convenient points on the routes of evacuation. Thus field hospital platoons, for the sake of shelter, often perforce set up some distance away from the clearing stations they supported. Hospitals usually had to do extensive cleaning and disinfecting to make their quarters habitable. Enlisted medics of one evacuation hospital jokingly suggested that the letters "SM" (Semimobile) in their unit designation really meant "Scrubbing and Mopping." In nonmedical structures floor plans left much to be desired from the hospital point of view. Dispersal of patients among many small rooms, for example, as in schools, meant harder work for nurses, ward attendants, and litterbearers. Units required additional people and equipment, not included in T/O&Es designed for tented operation, to perform plant maintenance and engineering. With these augmentations, evacuation hospitals, especially, needed still more transportation to move them.[47]

As army hospitals acquired campaigning experience, their medics became adept at improvising, and at obtaining—by one means or another—what they needed. Each unit developed its own individual plan for setting up. Colonel Gorby declared: "I don't think I had a field hospital commander, or an evac hospital commander, that would set [up] his operating pavillion and his ward tents and pre-ops and post-ops and receiving and all that in exactly the same way. . . . We indicated that as long as it was effective it was all right." Foraging, as one hospital report put it, "by now had become instinctive." Medics regularly turned the refuse of war into objects that saved their patients' lives or enhanced their own comfort. In the 59th Field Hospital discarded 5-gallon food tins, cut in half, became operating room light fixtures, their polished interiors ready-made reflectors. A large box, a 20-gallon gasoline tank, two faucets, a length of pipe, and a galvanized trough, all salvaged, became a surgeon's scrub sink. Scrap lumber went into back rests for chest-wound pa-

[46] Gosman, "War without Blood," pp. 121 and 130, CMH.

[47] Quotation from 111th Evacuation Hospital Annual Rpt, 1944, p. 10. For hospital problems from the army viewpoint, see An. 6—Medical Plan, p. 14, to FUSA Plan, 25 Feb 44, file HD 370 ETO; First U.S. Army Report of Operations, 1 Aug 44–22 Feb 45, bk. IV, pp. 139 and 155; Surg, Third U.S. Army Annual Rpt, 1944, pp. 39, 91, 122, 167; Surg, Seventh U.S. Army, Annual Rpt, 1944, p. 23; and Surg, Ninth U.S. Army, Annual Rpt, 1944, pp. 19–20 and 23. For examples of unit difficulties, see Surg, XX Corps, Annual Rpt, 1944, p. 23; 48th Field Hospital Semiannual Rpt, January–June 1945; 93d Evacuation Hospital Unit Hist, 1944; 110th Evacuation Hospital Semiannual Rpt, January–June 1945; and 5th, 51st, and 104th Evacuation Hospitals Annual Rpts, 1944.

tients. Other hospitals built their own suction apparatus, as well as ward desks and tables, folding water towers, and portable showers. They mounted their generators on captured enemy trucks and appropriated whatever other usable German materiel came their way, including in one unit a couple of truckloads of liquor seized in Cherbourg and carried across France. Hospitals followed the campaign philosophy: "Take what you can get and hang onto it; each set-up will be a little different, a little better than the last; make your comfort and your amusements now—who knows when you can again?" [48]

Sources of Supply

By the time the offensive began in November, the army supply depots had settled into positions within convenient supporting distance of the front. They gradually edged forward as the attacking divisions gained ground. The Ninth Army brought with it from Brittany a single medical supply unit, the advance section of the 33d Medical Depot Company, temporarily attached from the Third Army. This supply element, which established itself at Valkenburg, Holland, taking over stock of a former First Army dump, distributed supplies to all of the Ninth Army until the last days of December, when the advance section of the 35th Medical Depot Company relieved it. Beginning in late November, another Ninth Army depot company, the 28th, located at Maastricht, assumed the task of receiving supplies from the Communications Zone and forwarding them to the advance element at Valkenburg. Elsewhere in the 12th Army Group, army depots underwent little change. The 1st Medical Depot Company, in the First Army, shifted its base to Dolhain, just west of its former site at Eupen, in order to find suitable buildings. Advance sections of this company operated medical supply points at Malmedy and Bastogne. The Third Army's 32d and 33d Medical Depot Companies, located respectively at Verdun and Toul when the offensive started, moved eastward, the 32d to Metz in late November and the 33d to Chateau-Salins in mid-December.[49]

The Seventh Army had its own separate line of medical supply. Its 7th Medical Depot Company followed the army across the Riviera beaches and up the Rhone valley successively to Epinal, Luneville, and Sarrebourg. Throughout the summer and early fall this company bore most of the burden of hauling supplies the entire distance from the Mediterranean coast. During November the Southern Line of Communications finally relieved the 7th Company of that task

[48] First quotation from Gorby Interv, 1962, pp. 28–29, CMH. Second quotation from 106th Evacuation Hospital Annual Rpt, 1944, pp. 14–15. Third quotation from 8th Field Hospital Annual Rpt, 1944, p. 4, attributing the words to the 91st Evacuation Hospital. See also 59th Field Hospital Annual Rpt, 1944, p. 10. For other comments on improvisations, see Surg, Third U.S. Army, Annual Rpt, 1944, pp. 126–27; remarks of evacuation hospital commanders in file HD:ETO:350.07:Battle Experiences; and 91st, 105th, 106th, and 111th Evacuation Hospitals Annual Rpts, 1944. On liquor supply, see Gosman Interv, 24 Mar 82, CMH.

[49] First U.S. Army Report of Operations, 1 Aug 44–22 Feb 45, bk. IV, pp. 154–55; Surg, Third U.S. Army, Annual Rpt, 1944, pp. 165 and 168–69; Surg, Ninth U.S. Army, Annual Rpt, 1944, p. 12; Surg, XIX Corps, Annual Rpt, 1944, encl. 19; 32d Medical Depot Company Annual Rpt, 1944, pp. 2–3; 33d Medical Depot Company Annual Rpt, 1944, p. 7 and an. 1.

by setting up an intermediate medical depot at Dijon, which in turn was replenished from a base facility at Marseilles. Materiel to stock these depots came from the Mediterranean Theater during the first sixty days of the southern France campaign and thereafter directly from the United States. The Seventh Army also possessed an independent blood service, provided by the 6703d Blood Transfusion Unit. An advance element of this unit distributed blood, initially flown in from Naples and, after 29 October, drawn from service troops at Marseilles and forwarded, via rail, to field and evacuation hospitals. Late in October, as demand exceeded the capacity of the 6703d, the army also began receiving shipments of ETO blood from Paris.[50]

Within the armies, medical supply distribution presented few difficulties beyond those inherent in the conditions of combat. Divisional and corps medical units and detachments drew expendable items on informal requisition from the nearest army supply point, usually an advance section of the depot company or a small dump maintained by the corps. Hospitals, depending on their locations, requisitioned either from the advance points or from the main army depots. Among their liaison functions, the medical groups often assisted hospitals and other nondivisional units in obtaining supplies and resolving logistical difficulties. Divisions employed all types of vehicles and resorted to every conceivable expedient to keep battalion aid stations and front-line medics supplied. They delivered plasma, dressings, and other urgently needed items to temporarily cut-off units by parachute and on a couple of occasions fired materiel to them in specially refilled artillery shells. The 90th Infantry Division, which had several units isolated during its battle for a Saar River bridgehead in December, sent medical supplies to them in remodeled aircraft wing tanks. Fighter-bombers, flying in at treetop level, dropped the tanks accurately into the infantry perimeter.[51]

When the offensive began, the flow of medical supplies from both communications zones into the army depots was still, from the armies' standpoint, less than satisfactory. In the 12th Army Group medical supply deliveries to the armies regularly fell short of the daily SHAEF tonnage allocations. The army depots constantly reported shortages; those of the First Army at one point had zero balances in over 400 inventory items. The

[50] Surg, Seventh U.S. Army, Annual Rpt, 1944, pp. 7–8, 48–49, 117; Surg, CONAD, Annual Rpt, 1944, pp. 13–14; Surg, Delta Base Section, Annual Rpt, 1944, p. 1; Kendrick, *Blood Program,* pp. 447–52; Wiltse, *Mediterranean,* p. 409; Memo, Kenner to CofS, SHAEF, 12 Oct 44, sub: Report of Inspection of Medical Service of 6th US Army Group . . . , in Medical Division, COSSAC/SHAEF, War Diary, October 1944; 7th Medical Depot Company Combat Supply Operations Rpt, [1944], pp. 3–5. For details on the development of SOLOC, see Chapters IX and XIII of this volume.

[51] Surg, Third U.S. Army, Annual Rpt, p. 169; Surg, Seventh U.S. Army, Annual Rpt, 1944, pp. 48–49; Surg, Ninth U.S. Army, Annual Rpt, 1944, p. 38; Surg, Ninth U.S. Army, Daily Journal, 1 Nov 44, Shambora Papers, MHI; 7th Medical Depot Company Combat Supply Operations Rpt, [1944], p. 9. For examples of corps supply points, see Surg, XII Corps, Annual Rpt, 1944, p. 6, and Surg, XIX Corps, Annual Rpt, 1944, p, 19. For group supply activities, see 68th Medical Group Annual Rpt, 1944, p. 28. On wing tanks, see Surg, XX Corps, Annual Rpt, 1944, pp. 7–8; Surg, 90th Infantry Division, Annual Rpt, 1944, pp. 18–19.

Ninth Army during November had to rely entirely on salvage for spare parts for its medical equipment. In spite of these conditions, all the armies kept their operating units supplied with enough of the things they immediately needed to perform their missions. Army surgeons usually could obtain air shipments to meet emergencies, for example, to remedy the drain of litters and blankets caused by evacuation. They regularly employed their own trucks to haul additional materiel forward from COMZ depots. In the 12th Army Group the army surgeons worked continually with the ADSEC regulating stations and the chief surgeon's Supply Division to speed up the processing of requisitions and to trace lost or misdirected cargo. The northern and southern communications zones steadily improved rail transportation and built up their advance depot stocks. In the north the opening of the port of Antwerp late in November drastically shortened American supply lines and permitted full use of ADSEC medical depot M-409 at Liege, close behind the First and Ninth Armies. Signaling the end of the long supply famine, SHAEF on 9 December abolished its tonnage allocation system. By that time the army depots, although still short of some items, were well on the way to accumulating their planned fourteen-day reserves.[52]

The System in Full Stride

The medical service of the American field armies reached a high level of efficiency and effectiveness during the November-December offensive. The armies had perfected their evacuation systems to the point where most battle casualties arrived at division clearing stations or their attached field hospital platoons within one or at most two hours of being injured. Transportable patients usually reached evacuation hospitals no more than eight hours after they suffered their wounds. Men who entered the army hospitals had an excellent chance of surviving. In all four armies less than 3 percent of the battle casualties admitted to medical facilities died, with the majority of the fatalities occurring in the field hospital platoons. Counting nonbattle as well as combat casualties, the death rate in army clearing stations and hospitals amounted to some 1.5 percent of admissions. The armies evacuated their patients to the Communications Zone in generally good condition. The 28th General Hospital at Liege, for example, reported only 2 deaths among 4,000 surgical patients it received from the First and Ninth Armies and only 1 man with gas gangrene, who recovered. Following one of his many

[52] First U.S. Army Report of Operations, 1 Aug 44-22 Feb 45, bk. IV, pp. 154-55; Surg, Third U.S. Army, Annual Rpt, 1944, pp. 163-66 and 168-70; Surg, Seventh U.S. Army, Annual Rpt, 1944, p. 118; Surg, Ninth U.S. Army, Annual Rpt, 1944, pp. 37-38; Surg, Ninth U.S. Army, Daily Journal, 1, 24, 30 Nov and 22 Dec 44, Shambora Papers, MHI; Surg, Delta Base Section, Annual Rpt, 1944, pp. 1-2; 7th Medical Depot Company Combat Supply Operations Rpt, [1944], pp. 3-4. For armies hauling their own supplies, see 32d Medical Depot Company Annual Rpt, 1944, p. 5. Medical Division, COSSAC/SHAEF, War Diary, October-December 1944, contains numerous inspection reports illustrating gradual supply improvement. For details on COMZ supply efforts, see Chapters IX and XIII of this volume.

inspections, General Kenner declared flatly: "The medical service in the forward area has been excellent." [53]

[53] Quotation from Memo, Kenner to CofS, SHAEF, 5 Dec 44, sub: Report of Inspection, Medical Service, First and Ninth US Armies . . . , in Medical Division, COSSAC/SHAEF, War Diary, December 1944. This document also gives the 28th General Hospital statistics. On evacuation times, see Kenner memo previously cited and his other reports in ibid., as well as Surg, 4th Armored Division Annual Rpt, 1944, pp. 21–22. On army death rates, see First U.S. Army Report of Operations, 1 Aug 44–22 Feb 45, bk. IV, pp. 199–200 and 204; Surg, Third U.S. Army, Annual Rpt, 1944, pp. 97–99; Surg, Seventh U.S. Army, Annual Rpt, 1944, p. 28; and Surg, Ninth U.S. Army, Combat Experience Rpts, October–December 1944, file HD 319.1–2.

Thus far in the campaign the field armies possessed the tactical initiative, but in mid-December that condition abruptly changed. Ground force medics were about to undergo what was, for most of them, a new experience: that of retreat before an enemy temporarily and locally superior in numbers and firepower and enjoying the advantage of surprise. The army medical service had proved its ability to support forces engaged in set-piece battles and headlong pursuit. Now its adaptability was to be tested in withdrawal, encirclement, and hastily improvised counterattack.

CHAPTER XII

A Time of Adversity

In the early morning darkness and fog of 16 December 1944 three painstakingly marshaled German field armies attacked the weakly defended Ardennes sector of the First Army front in Belgium and Luxembourg. Over 250,000 troops with 1,000 armored fighting vehicles and 1,900 artillery pieces, in 25 armored and infantry divisions, took part in this desperate counterstroke, for which Hitler and his military advisers had been planning and preparing since the late summer. The Germans intended to pierce the thin American line in the Ardennes, a wooded, hilly sector used by the First Army, with most of its strength concentrated farther north for a drive toward the Roer River, to rest battle-worn divisions and to introduce green ones to combat. Mechanized columns then were to cross the Meuse River and capture Liege and Antwerp. If successful, their drive would destroy many Allied units; disrupt supply lines; and, Hitler optimistically believed, induce the British and Americans to break their "unnatural" alliance with Communist Russia and make peace on terms acceptable to Germany.[1]

The enemy achieved complete surprise. Aided by several days of fog, rain, and snow, which kept the Allied air forces out of the battle, and by unorthodox tactics, including the use of special commando units disguised in American uniforms and civilian clothing, the Germans made their initial breakthrough and gained considerable ground. They destroyed one American infantry division, effectively crippled two others, and eliminated an armored combat command; and they killed, wounded, and captured thousands of American soldiers. Nevertheless, the German advance almost at once fell behind schedule, slowed by the narrow roads and difficult terrain and by the tenacious resistance of the American front-line units.

On the northern wing of the offensive the *Sixth Panzer Army*, with a substantial component of SS troops, supposedly the main breakthrough force, pushed back but failed to rout the 2d and 99th Infantry Divisions on the right flank of the American V Corps. These divisions, rapidly reinforced by

[1] The following summary of operations is drawn from Hugh M. Cole, *The Ardennes: Battle of the Bulge*, United States Army in World War II (Washington, D.C.: Office of the Chief of Military History, Department of the Army, 1965), passim, and Ruppenthal, *Logistical Support*, 2:25–26. The German plan, in fact, was overambitious and even under the best of conditions could not have been carried to success with the available forces.

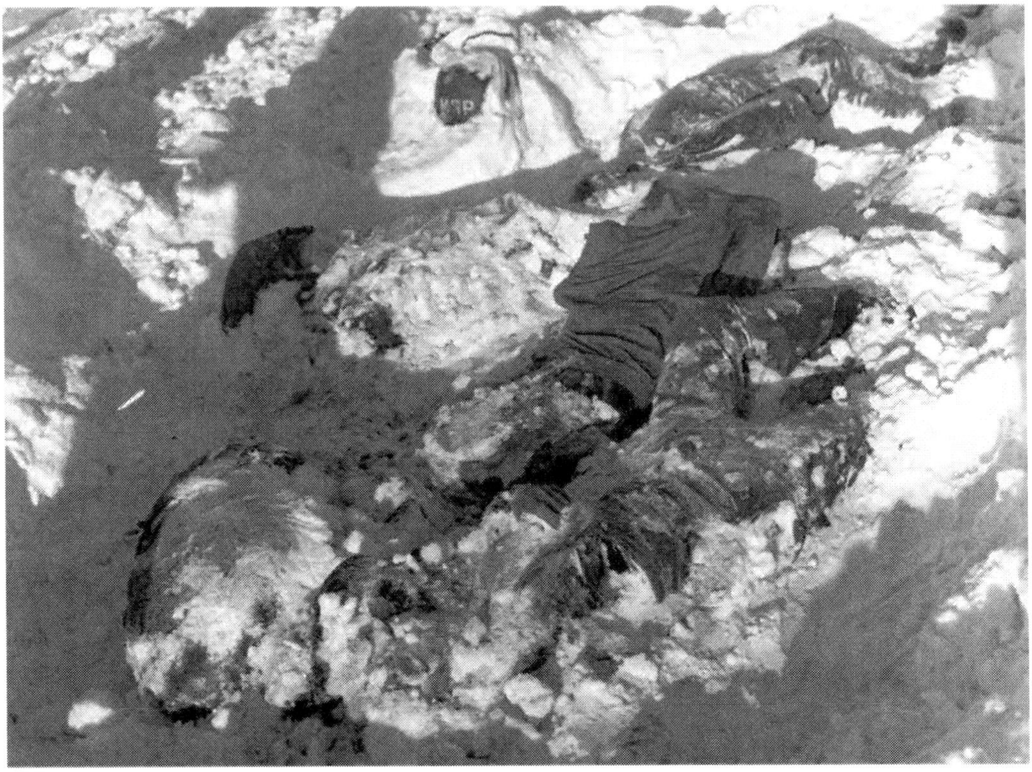

AMERICAN VICTIMS OF THE MALMEDY MASSACRE

others, held firm around Elsenborn and fixed the northern shoulder of the developing "Bulge." *Kampfgruppe Peiper,* an advance element of the *1st SS Panzer Division,* extricated itself from this fighting early on 17 December and drove 20 miles into First Army territory, in the process massacring over 100 American prisoners near Malmedy, but the U.S. 7th Armored Division came in behind *Kampfgruppe Peiper* to hold the St.-Vith road junction for six crucial days. This division and the units that rallied around it held up the advance of most of the *Sixth Panzer Army,* while other American elements isolated the *Peiper* force and broke it up.

The *Seventh Army,* on the far southern wing of the German attack, soon was brought to a standstill by the rightmost VIII Corps formations, which held the longer portion of the American line in the Ardennes. In the center of the VIII Corps front, however, the *Fifth Panzer Army* enveloped the green 106th Infantry Division, awkwardly deployed in a salient in the *Schnee Eiffel* (the extension of the Ardennes into Germany), capturing two American regiments, and broke through the 28th Infantry Division, a battered Huertgen Forest veteran, which was spread thin along the Our River. The *Fifth Panzer Army* now was in position to roll northwestward toward the Meuse. Fortunately for the Americans, the 101st Airborne Division, released from SHAEF reserve, came into the gap on 19 December, just in time to deny to the onrushing Germans the important road junction of Bastogne. Completely encircled for the better part of a week, the airborne troops, aided by elements of two armored combat commands and a miscellany of artillery and support units that had straggled into Bastogne, held the town and further restricted German maneuver.

The Allied high command, although surprised by the initial German onslaught, reacted to it swiftly and effectively. SHAEF early committed its main ground troop reserve, the XVIII Airborne Corps, then recuperating after leaving the line in Holland. While the 101st Division of this corps secured Bastogne, the corps headquarters, with the 82d Airborne Division, helped extend the American line to the right of the V Corps, along the northern flank of the German salient. On 20 December, to improve coordination of the forces on both sides of the breakthrough, General Eisenhower temporarily gave operational control of the First and Ninth Armies to Field Marshal Montgomery's 21 Army Group. Montgomery was to redeploy British and U.S. divisions to stop the Germans at or in front of the Meuse and then counterattack. South of the Bulge, the Third Army took over VIII Corps and prepared to push forward to relieve Bastogne and help pinch off the salient.

The Allies gradually regained the tactical initiative, assisted mightily by a period of clear weather after 23 December, which allowed their air forces to intervene with decisive effect. The First Army shifted divisions from its left flank to its right to check the continuing German advance, bringing the *Fifth* and *Sixth Panzer Armies* to a stop well short of the Meuse. The Third Army, in a remarkable display of tactical and logistical flexibility, within days turned its axis of advance 90 degrees and attacked the enemy's southern flank. On the twenty-seventh, elements of Patton's army opened a corridor to the besieged 101st Division. The Germans had driven a wedge into the First Army front that was 60 miles deep and 50 miles wide at the base, but they had fallen hopelessly short of their ambitious objectives. During the first weeks of 1945 the First and Third Armies counterattacked in bitter cold and snow. They steadily forced back the by now exhausted, dispirited enemy. The Wehrmacht in mid-February was fighting on or behind its 16 December start line. It had left behind on the ground so briefly won over 100,000 men and uncounted quantities of equipment, and it had lost its ability ever again to resume the offensive.

For the American armies the human cost of the Battle of the Ardennes was substantial but difficult to determine exactly, due to the number of commands involved and the reporting of casualties by unit and time period rather than by engagement. According to one authoritative estimate, American combat losses in the period of the German attack, 16 December to 2 January, amounted to at least 41,000 officers and men, including some 4,100 known killed in action, 20,200 wounded, and over 16,900 missing. Many of the missing likely were wounded who fell into enemy hands. First Army hospitals, between 16 December and 22 February, admitted over 78,000 patients, 24,000 of them wounded. Third Army hospitals reported some 70,000 admissions in December and January, including almost 30,000 battle casualties.[2]

For the field army medical service that treated and evacuated these casualties, the Battle of the Ardennes posed some unaccustomed challenges. First Army medics in units and detachments directly in the path of the German assault underwent the new and unwelcome experiences of retreat and, in some instances, capture. Medical units outside the immediate breakthrough area had to relocate in haste as the army fell back before the onslaught and then shifted forces to hold and counterattack. Surgeons with the surrounded 101st Airborne Division at Bastogne resorted to improvisation to provide emergency treatment for the growing accumulation of wounded within the perimeter, trying to keep their patients alive until they could be evacuated. Other medics with the relieving forces attempted to reinforce and resupply their besieged colleagues. The Third Army medical service, besides managing the relief of Bastogne, redeployed dozens of units and rearranged its lines of evacuation as the army swung around and attacked into the Bulge.

Medics in Retreat

The German attack for the most part missed the heaviest concentration of First Army medical units and overran few even of those in its direct path. Most of the large, relatively immobile facilities, such as the convalescent hospital and the base supply depot, were located well to the north of the breakthrough, positioned to support a renewed advance toward the Roer River. The hitherto quiet Ardennes sector held only the installations required for immediate support of the V and VIII Corps. Those installations, due to the previous inactivity of that part of the front, had a very light patient load when the assault began, a circumstance that facilitated their evacuation and withdrawal. In addition, the Germans' mechanized exploitation of their breakthrough started much more slowly than planned; enemy armored columns did not push any distance into the American rear during the first twenty-four hours or so of the battle. This delay, besides contributing to the Germans' ultimate tactical failure, gave many First Army medical units just enough time to escape the blitzkrieg.[3]

Some medical units, nevertheless, suffered severely during the first few days of the offensive, notably those of the infantry divisions that absorbed the initial shock. On the northern shoulder of the Bulge the 99th Division and elements of the 2d fought a bitter three-day battle in woods and

[2] Cole, *Ardennes*, p. 674; First U.S. Army Report of Operations, 1 Aug 44–22 Feb 45, bk. IV, p. 202; Surg, Third U.S. Army, Annual Rpt, 1944, ex. XXVII, and Semiannual Rpt, January–June 1945, an. XIX.

[3] For an example of the light patient load, see Intervs, sub: Medical Units in vic Clervaux, in 28th Infantry Division Combat Intervs, box 24033, RG 407, NARA. Cole, *Ardennes*, pp. 668–71, analyzes the Germans' delay in exploitation.

villages, losing men and ground but denying the *Sixth Panzer Army* a clean breakthrough. The infantry regiments, their thin lines repeatedly infiltrated by enemy troops and tanks, their battalions at times temporarily surrounded, fell back in often chaotic combat. Their surgeons and aidmen, those of the 99th experiencing their first major action, had to cope with a number of difficulties. The cold caused even slightly injured men to go into shock so that litter squads had to carry extra blankets and aid stations had to administer larger than usual amounts of plasma. Battalion aid stations, sheltered in the crossroads villages that were a principal enemy objective, came under intense artillery and mortar bombardment. At times, medics worked on the wounded while tank and infantry firefights raged in the streets around them. The Germans, who included many SS troops, displayed less regard than hitherto for the niceties of civilized warfare. According to the 99th Division surgeon,

> Medical Department soldiers were deliberately killed in spite of Red Cross brassards on both arms and four red crosses on white, circular backgrounds . . . on the helmets. It is further known that vehicles transporting wounded and plainly marked with Geneva Red Cross flags were deliberately riddled by enemy small arms fire and in one instance, a tank at close range fired an armor-piercing shell through an ambulance. . . .[4]

The infantry battalions struggled to evacuate their wounded even as they fell back from position to position. As waves of attacking Germans inundated the foxhole lines, aidmen and litterbearers risked their lives to rescue every injured GI they could reach. Inevitably, wounded men were overrun or had to be abandoned; in some instances, medics voluntarily stayed behind to care for them. Most withdrawing battalions managed to bring their aid stations and their accumulated patients back with them. Battalion medical officers had first call on the available vehicles; they loaded casualties on everything that would roll and sent them out near the front of the retreating columns that groped their way, usually in darkness, along firebreaks and winding roads. Surgeons and aidmen brought up the rear, to collect casualties of the troops covering the retreat. Losses of medics, patients, and station equipment did occur. One regimental aid station, short of transportation, abandoned its equipment to fill its truck with patients. A 99th Division infantry battalion, withdrawing from a nearly surrounded position on 17 December, discovered that it had a dozen or so more casualties than its vehicles could carry. The battalion surgeon, Capt. Frederick J. McIntyre, MC, and his detachment remained in place with these wounded men. According to the regimental surgeon, the aid station "when last seen that day . . . was being overrun by the enemy and was operating under a Geneva flag and a white flag." [5]

[4] Surg, 99th Infantry Division, Annual Rpt, 1944, p. 17.

[5] Quotation from ibid., app. VIa. See also ibid., pp. 15–16 and apps. VIb–VIc; Intervs, Capt R. C. McElroy, Capt R. R. McGee, and 1st Battalion, 394th Infantry, in 99th Infantry Division Combat Intervs, box 24069, RG 407, NARA, which provide additional medical support details; and Medical Bulletin, 2d Infantry Division, December 1944, in Surg, 2d Infantry Division, Annual Rpt, 1944.

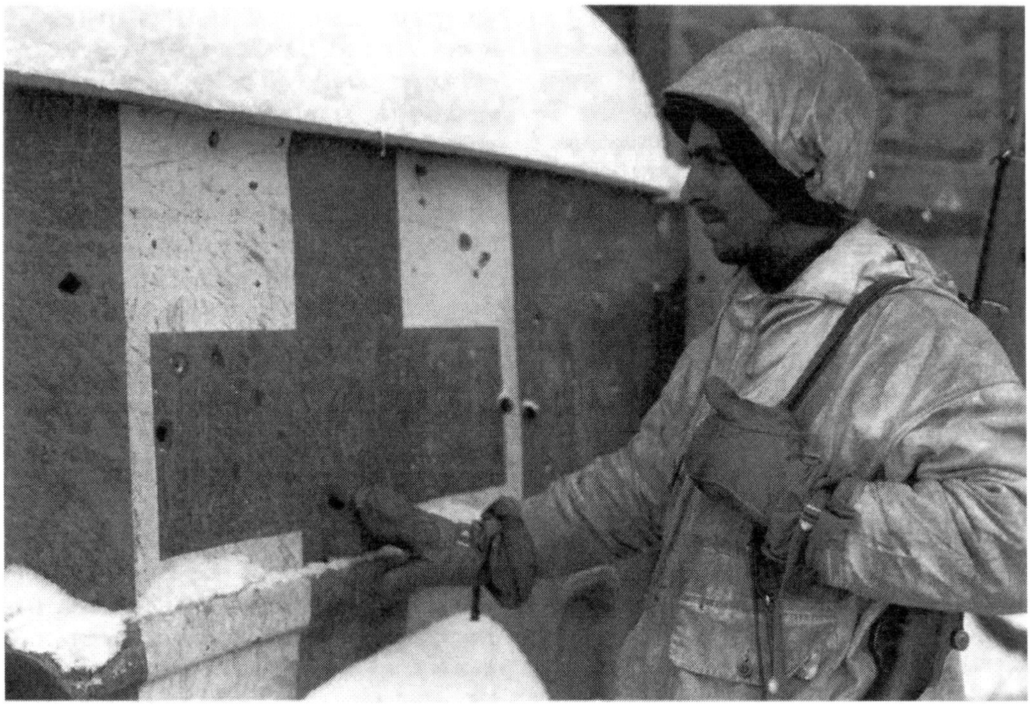

BULLET-RIDDLED ARMY AMBULANCE, *a casualty of the Ardennes fighting*

Although forced to retreat, the 2d and 99th Divisions held together a solid enough line to permit their medical battalions (respectively, the 2d and 324th) to maintain more or less continuous evacuation of their battalion and regimental aid stations. Nevertheless, the first days of the battle were hectic, at times desperate ones, especially for the collecting companies. The companies sandbagged their stations against the point-blank fire of infiltrating German tanks; they prepared to hold wounded for extended periods if evacuation were blocked; they hauled casualties over constantly changing, endangered routes; and they made precipitate retreats with losses in men and materiel. One company of the 324th Medical Battalion had to abandon its entire station equipment; the battalion as a whole reported eighteen men wounded or missing in December. Less heavily engaged, the 2d Medical Batallion had one of its collecting companies put out of action by materiel losses.

As division frontages contracted, the 324th Medical Battalion consolidated elements of its battered collecting companies into a single provisional unit, which evacuated all three infantry regiments. Both division clearing stations pulled back in leapfrogging sections, that of the 2d Division's medical battalion leaving behind a significant amount of equipment. As the divisions reoriented their main supply routes from an east-west to a north-south axis, the clearing companies temporarily had difficulty obtaining army medical group ambulances for evacuation. On several occasions they sent wounded to the rear in trucks. On 19 December, as the front stabilized, the 134th Medical Group reestablished reliable ambulance service between the clearing stations, now located near Elsenborn, and the army hospitals at Eupen. Thereafter, the medical services of the 2d and 99th Divisions, and of the others reinforcing the northern shoulder of the Bulge, rapidly returned to normal.[6]

The medical service of the 106th Infantry Division was engulfed in the catastrophe that befell that inexperienced, exposed unit. During the first four days of the offensive the entire medical complements of the 422d and 423d Infantry, the 589th and 590th Field Artillery Battalions, two engineer companies, and a reconnaissance troop—encircled in the *Schnee Eiffel*—fell into German hands, along with their wounded, numbering in the hundreds. Details of the fate of these surgeons and aidmen are fragmentary, as are those of the entire action. The infantry regiments apparently left behind many of their aid stations, filled with nontransportable patients, during abortive breakout attempts. In the final encirclements the presence of untended wounded, and a lack of people and supplies for their care, probably hastened the surrender of the main body of the 422d Infantry and contributed to the decisions of other isolated American groups to give up.[7]

The 331st Medical Battalion, 106th Division, came off better. On the first day of the attack the battalion's collecting companies kept casualties moving rearward from all three regiments, although Company A, supporting the 422d Infantry, was forced to make an early retreat by one of the encircling German columns. The following day, the extent of the disaster became apparent. Company A lost contact with the 422d and withdrew to St.-Vith. Company B, with the 423d Infantry, was surrounded and eventually captured; Company C, retreating with the division's only surviving regiment, the 424th, evacuated its casualties during its participation in the defense of St.-Vith. The division surgeon and clearing company moved westward from their original position at St.-Vith to Vielsalm, where they handled casualties of a number of divisions blocking the advance of the *Sixth Panzer Army*. As the Germans gradually worked around to the westward of the St.-Vith defenders, the clearing company, on 19 December, shifted a platoon farther west to La Roche, only to have it overrun by an enemy column. The remaining 106th Division medical elements withdrew from Vielsalm on the twenty-second, as American forces under orders re-

[6] For tactical developments, see Cole, *Ardennes*, chs. V and VI; Surg, 99th Infantry Division, Annual Rpt, app. VId; Medical Bulletin, 2d Infantry Division, December 1944, in Surg, 2d Infantry Division, Annual Rpt, 1944.

[7] For accounts of this disaster, see Cole, *Ardennes*, ch. VII, and Richard E. Dupuy, *St. Vith: Lion in the Way. The 106th Infantry Division in World War II* (hereafter cited as *The 106th*) (Washington, D.C.: Infantry Journal Press, 1949), passim. For medical details, see pp. 129–30, 143–44, and 148–50 of the latter work. See also Surg, 106th Infantry Division, Annual Rpt, 1944, p. 4. Other medical details are in the 106th Infantry Division Combat Intervs, box 24081, RG 407, NARA.

luctantly gave up their St.-Vith salient.[8]

The 28th Division, stretched thinly over a 20-mile front immediately to the right of the 106th, gave way under the full weight of the *Fifth Panzer Army* assault. During the first three days of the battle the division's two flank regiments, the 112th Infantry on the north and the 109th on the south, pulled back in reasonably good order and joined the American forces rallying on the shoulders of the breakthrough. Their surgeons and aid stations accompanied them and maintained more or less normal operations throughout the offensive. In the division center, however, the 110th Infantry was all but destroyed in delaying the enemy advance on Bastogne. Its surgeon, Maj. L. S. Frogner, MC, located with the regimental command post at Clervaux, lost all contact with his battalion aid stations during the afternoon of 16 December, as those installations were overrun or cut off in the general wreck. Frogner and his aid station were captured late the following day, after German tanks and infantry overwhelmed the patchwork of headquarters and service elements defending Clervaux.[9]

The division's 103d Medical Battalion, during the quiet period before the attack, had split its clearing company into three separate detachments, each of which handled casualties of a single regiment. This arrangement, adopted to save time and transportation in evacuating sick and wounded from the extended division front, fortuitously was of benefit during the German offensive. It ensured continuous clearing company support of the flanking regiments even as they became separated from the division and were attached for a time to other commands. The 103d Battalion managed to extricate all of its elements, although it lost twenty-one men captured in the retreat. Company B, the collecting company behind the 110th Infantry, had to abandon much of its equipment, as did one platoon of the clearing company. Battalion headquarters withdrew with the division command post from Wiltz to a position near Neufchateau, southwest of Bastogne.[10]

The V and VIII Corps surgeons reacted quickly to the emergency. They tried to extricate their corps medical battalions from danger while keeping contact with their divisions and coordinating evacuation. Colonel Brenn, the V Corps surgeon, and his medical section remained at Eupen throughout the battle, under intermittent German shelling and for a time threatened by enemy paratroopers. The headquarters, the clearing company, and one collecting company of the corps' 53d Medical Battalion—the rear elements, ironically, as the battalion was oriented to support an American attack toward the northeast—

[8] Surg, 106th Infantry Division, Annual Rpt, pp. 4–5 and encl. 7; Dupuy, *The 106th*, pp. 61, 89–90, 98–99. Surg, 7th Armored Division, Annual Rpt, 1944, pp. 21–22, gives additional details of evacuation from St.-Vith.

[9] Cole, *Ardennes*, ch. VIII; Surg, 28th Infantry Division, Annual Rpt, 1944, p. 4; History of the 110th Infantry Regiment (hereafter cited as 110th Infantry Hist), sec. III, pp. 61–74, box 8596, RG 407, NARA; Intervs, sub: Medical Units in vic Clervaux, in 28th Infantry Division Combat Intervs, box 24033, RG 407, NARA.

[10] Surg, 28th Infantry Division, Annual Rpt, 1944, encls. 5–6; Col D. B. Strickler, Action Report of Germans' Ardennes Breakthrough, . . . in 110th Infantry Hist, app., box 8596, RG 407, NARA.

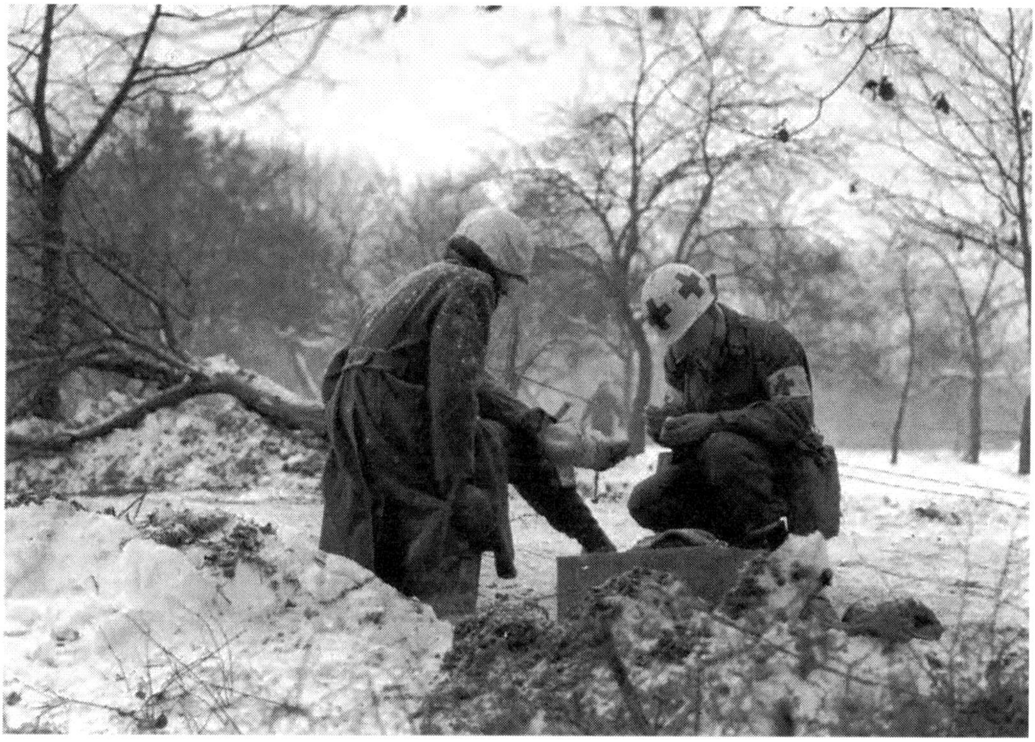

CARING FOR AN INFANTRYMAN INJURED IN THE ARDENNES FIGHTING

were in more danger; their location at Heppenbach was in the middle of the 99th Division battlefield. On 17 December the battalion, by making two trips using all available vehicles, evacuated its personnel, its 180 patients, and about 95 percent of its equipment to Eupen. The trucks had to travel over roads already under German observation, but the enemy did not interfere with them. The battalion, however, did lose three ambulances and five men in an apparent ambush during a separate evacuation mission. With his medical battalion safely repositioned, Brenn concentrated during the rest of the battle on supervising evacuation and trying to determine how many medical personnel and how much equipment his divisions had lost.[11]

The VIII Corps surgeon, Colonel Eckhardt, lost contact early with the flank divisions of his hard-hit corps. His own section, with the corps headquarters, moved in haste from Bastogne to Neufchateau on 18 December and then on the twenty-first to Florenville, still further south. There, "a very unmerry christmas was faintly observed and a not very joyous New Year was welcomed." The corps' 169th Medical Battalion, which had its

[11] Surg, V Corps, Annual Rpt, 1944, pp. 21-22; 53d Medical Battalion Annual Rpt, 1944, p. 14.

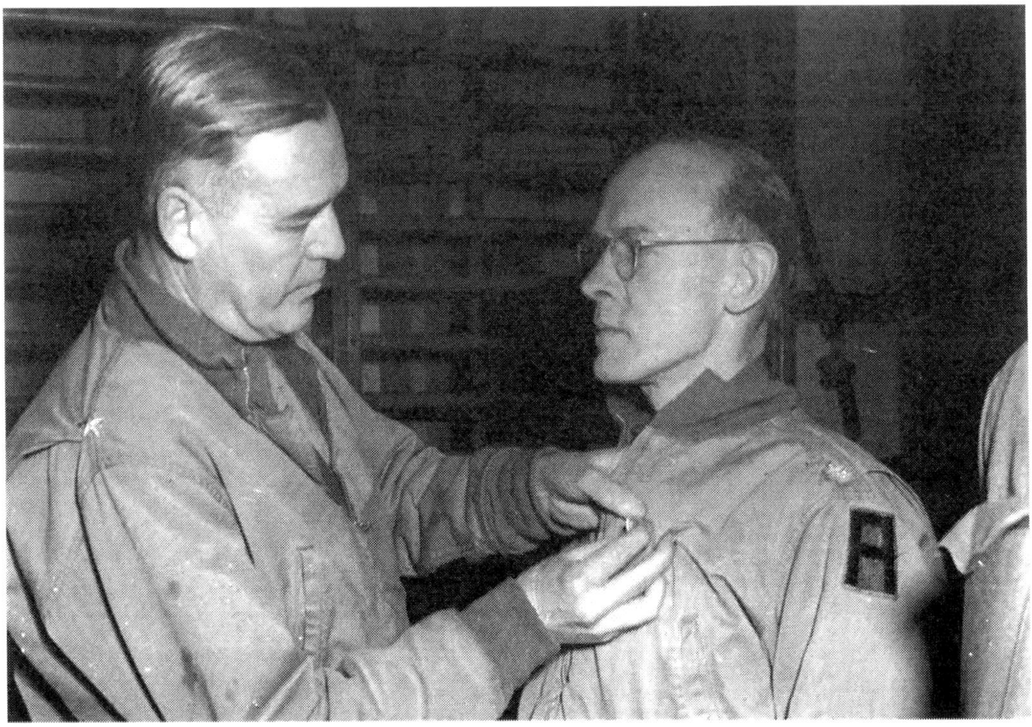

BRIG. GEN. JOHN A. ROGERS, *decorating a field hospital medic*

headquarters and clearing station at Troisvierges, close behind the center of the corps front, and its collecting companies widely spread out, withdrew relatively intact and eventually reassembled near Florenville. This battalion, besides supporting the remaining units of the VIII Corps, also served the 101st Airborne Division after it moved into Bastogne.[12]

In addition to divisional and corps units, the breakthrough area contained a number of First Army medical installations. They included the headquarters and attached battalions of two medical groups: the 134th, located at Malmedy, which evacuated the V Corps; and the 64th, at Troisvierges, supporting the VIII Corps. Platoons of two field hospitals, the 42d and 47th, were spread across the front, receiving nontransportable casualties from the infantry divisions. Evacuation hospitals were clustered on the northern and southern fringes of the Bulge. In the north the 44th and 67th, at Malmedy, were receiving wounded from a local attack by the left-wing divisions of the V Corps. Behind the VIII Corps the 107th Evacuation Hospital, as the German offensive began, had just ceased operations at Clervaux and was preparing to move. The 102d at Echternach and

[12] Quotation from Surg, VIII Corps, Annual Rpt, 1944, p. 8. See also 169th Medical Battalion Annual Rpt, 1944, pp. 10–12.

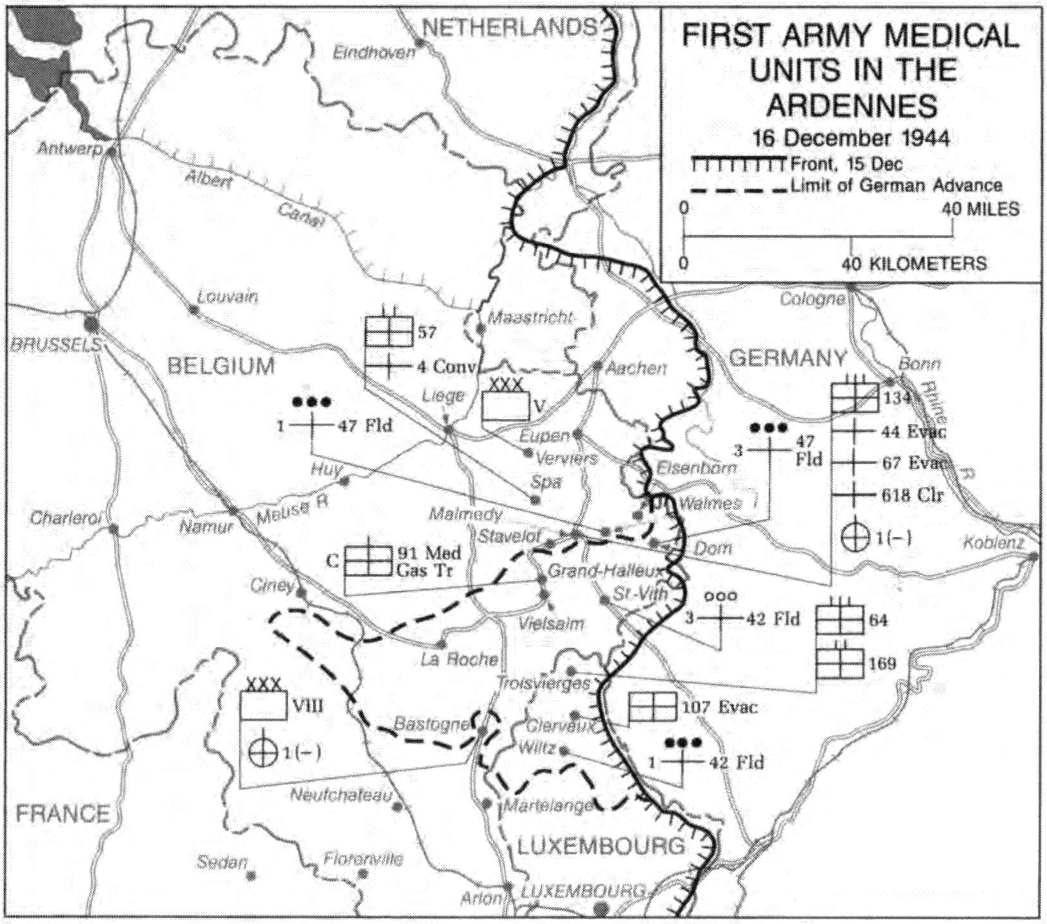

MAP 17

the 110th at Esch were open for patients from the VIII Corps right wing. The Bulge also contained a couple of specialized army hospitals. At Malmedy the 618th Clearing Company operated a center for treatment of combat exhaustion casualties; at Grand-Halleux, west of St.-Vith, Company C, 91st Medical Gas Treatment Battalion, cared for malaria, contagious disease, and self-inflicted wound patients. Advance sections of the 1st Medical Depot Company maintained supply dumps at Malmedy and Bastogne.[13]

The First Army surgeon, Brig. Gen. John A. Rogers, MC, located at army headquarters at Spa, north of the breakthrough area, received his first hint of the enemy offensive early in the morning of 16 December (*Map 17*). It came in the form of reports of heavy shelling from the evacuation

[13] This section is based on the annual reports, 1944, of the units mentioned.

hospitals at Eupen and Malmedy. Around 1900 Rogers learned that the Germans during the day had made "some penetration" of the VIII Corps line and along the boundary between it and V Corps. "A request for information to the army G-3 elicited the response that the action was thought to be local, and the penetration not considered serious." Three hours later, however, the G-3 indicated to Rogers that the Germans attacking the VIII Corps were gaining ground. On the basis of this information Rogers gave orders for the withdrawal of the platoon of the 42d Field Hospital at Wiltz and of the 102d and 107th Evacuation Hospitals, his most exposed units in the rear of the VIII Corps. The next day, as word came of growing pressure on the V Corps, the army surgeon also began sending retreat orders to medical units in the path of the *Sixth Panzer Army*."[14]

Most immediately threatened by the German breakthrough were four field hospital platoons. In the V Corps area the 1st and 3d Platoons of the 47th Field Hospital, located respectively at Waimes and Dom Butgenbach, received wounded from the 2d and 99th Divisions. Behind the VIII Corps the 1st Platoon of the 42d Field Hospital at Wiltz supported the 28th Division clearing station; the 3d Platoon, in St.-Vith, served the 106th Division. These units, unlike the division clearing stations with which they were located, did not possess organic transportation for rapid withdrawals. Further, although working closely with the divisions, the platoons were under the command of the medical groups. In the confusion of the first days of the battle they had difficulty in obtaining timely orders and information; their movements were not always well coordinated with those of the divisions. Surgeons with the platoon at St.-Vith, for example, learned of the offensive only when the hospital was engulfed by 106th Division wounded, by which time, according to them, the division clearing station already had left for Vielsalm. The division surgeon, on the other hand, claimed that the platoon "took off" without warning, leaving him with no emergency surgical capability. On 17 December all these units extricated themselves from their exposed positions, but with a nearly total loss of equipment and, in some instances, with casualties among patients and staff. Regrouped in rear areas, they were out of action for the rest of the battle, their personnel in bivouac or temporarily attached to other medical units.[15]

Two platoons, the 1st of the 47th Field Hospital at Waimes and the 1st of the 42d at Wiltz, had particularly dramatic and, in the latter case, tragic experiences. The 1st Platoon at Waimes continued working throughout the morning of the seventeenth, the staff increasingly agitated by the stories told by incoming wounded of

[14] Rogers was promoted to brigadier general effective 10 November 1944. Surg, First U.S. Army, Annual Rpt, 1944, pp. 53–54, gives a chronology of the surgeon's initial decisions.

[15] 42d Field Hospital Annual Rpt, 1944, pp. 4–5 and encl. 1; 47th Field Hospital Annual Rpt, 1944, ans. 7–8; 64th Medical Group Annual Rpt, 1944, p. 8. On the platoon at St.-Vith, see Clifford L. Graves, *Front Line Surgeons: A History of the Third Auxiliary Surgical Group* (San Diego, Calif.: Frye & Smith, 1950), p. 242, and Interv (source of quotation), Lt Col Carl Belzer, 6 Jan 45, in 106th Infantry Division Combat Intervs, box 24081, RG 407, NARA.

overwhelming German attacks. Orders to evacuate patients and nurses preparatory to withdrawal arrived from the 134th Medical Group around midday. Early in the afternoon, the unit sent its eighteen patients off to the 67th Evacuation Hospital at Malmedy. However, when the nurses, a short time later, tried to follow the same road to the rear, they found it blocked by artillery fire and the proximity of *Kampfgruppe Peiper*. The women, forced by the shelling to leave the ambulance in which they had been riding, walked and hitchhiked back to Waimes. Trucks dispatched by the 134th to transport the platoon failed to arrive; but ambulances from the front, filled with wounded, did.

The 1st Platoon medics, who had packed their equipment for movement, unpacked it again, set up operating theater and wards, and went back to work. They continued treating patients until about 1100 the next day. At that time two armed Germans, one in an American uniform, appeared and announced that the hospital, and a large number of nonmedical stragglers who had collected there during the night, were prisoners. Also caught were the commanding officer of the 180th Medical Battalion, his S–3, and his driver. They had stayed behind in Waimes to help evacuate the hospital after the battalion, a 134th Medical Group unit, had withdrawn from the town. Armed Americans at the hospital considerably outnumbered the enemy, but they made no resistance for fear of compromising the installation's Geneva Convention protection. The hospital platoon commander, Maj. Earl E. Laird, MC, talked the Germans into leaving thirty-six patients where they were, along with the nurses, four medical officers, and a few enlisted technicians to care for them. The enemy lined up everyone else to wait for trucks to carry them into captivity. Fortunately, an alert battalion ambulance driver managed to escape in his vehicle. He brought back troops from a nearby American unit, who chased away the Germans in a brief firefight. With a road to the rear now open, the 1st Platoon evacuated its patients. The personnel then headed for Spa, leaving behind all their hospital equipment but the kitchen. When the unit members reached the First Army rear, they were dispersed among several general and field hospitals for work and lodging.[16]

At Wiltz the 1st Platoon of the 42d Field Hospital, directly in the path of the enemy drive toward Bastogne, received no definite information or order until the afternoon of 18 December. Toward evening, with German columns already threatening to encircle the town, the 28th division passed word that the platoon should prepare for evacuation by a 64th Medical Group truck convoy that was on the way. The hospital confronted a dilemma. It had twenty-two patients whose condition was such that, under the regulations, they should not be moved. Maj. Charles A. Serbst, MC, the senior auxiliary surgical team leader, urged that these wounded men be evacuated anyway, because German captivity would be more hazardous to their survival than a truck

---

[16] 47th Field Hospital Annual Rpt, 1944, an. 7; Graves, *Front Line Surgeons*, pp. 247–49; 180th Medical Battalion Annual Rpt, 1944, p. 3; 575th Ambulance Company Annual Rpt, 1944, p. 9.

ride. The hospital platoon commander, Major Huber, however, insisted that these patients had to stay put. According to the auxiliary surgical group historian, "Serbst was right but Huber prevailed." If patients stayed, it was First Army policy that medical personnel must remain to care for them. Huber, to his credit, adhered to the letter of this regulation also. He, with another officer and sixteen men of the platoon, and with Serbst and his auxiliary team, remained with the casualties and went into captivity early on the nineteenth, when German troops entered Wiltz. The rest of the personnel, with several truckloads of hospital equipment, left during the night of the eighteenth. The medics, running a gauntlet of American roadblocks and German fire, made their way back to VIII Corps lines. However, the trucks carrying the equipment, diverted to another mission, unloaded their cargo in Bastogne, an occurrence for which 101st Airborne Division medics soon would have cause to be grateful.[17]

Both medical groups moved hurriedly to escape the attack. The 134th Medical Group, which evacuated the V Corps, retreated to Spa during the afternoon of the seventeenth. This group lost several ambulance crewmen killed in the Malmedy massacre. Nevertheless, its 179th and 180th Medical Battalions withdrew generally intact and continued evacuating, respectively, the left and right flank divisions of the corps. The 64th Medical Group, supporting the VIII Corps, pulled out of Troisvierges early on the seventeenth. While an advance group command post remained with the corps surgeon at Bastogne, the balance of the unit continued on farther south to Martelange. Several more retreats followed until the group, on the twenty-first, finally reached Sedan. Four days later, as the VIII Corps front at last stabilized, the 64th Group moved to Gerouville, on the Franco-Belgian border east of Sedan, more centrally located for control of evacuation. Throughout the crisis of the battle the attached ambulance and collecting companies of these groups, in spite of frequent displacements and bewilderingly rapid changes in the divisions to be supported, managed to keep casualties moving back from the clearing stations. The groups also did much of the work of mustering trucks to move field hospital platoons and other less mobile organizations.[18]

On the northern edge of the Bulge the westward drive of *Kampfgruppe Peiper* compelled a series of medical unit withdrawals. On 17 December the 44th and 67th Evacuation Hospi-

[17] The First Army considered the decision on removal of patients from an endangered hospital to be "a command function," but insisted that "from a medical viewpoint, if patients are not evacuated, sufficient medical personnel must stay behind to care for the patients even at the risk of capture." See Surg, First U.S. Army, Annual Rpt, 1944, p. 70. Quotation from Graves, *Front Line Surgeons*, p. 259. See also ibid., pp. 258 and 260–61; 42d Field Hospital Annual Rpt, 1944, pp. 4–5; 64th Medical Group Annual Rpt, 1944, p. 8; Surg, Third U.S. Army, Annual Rpt, 1944, pp. 55–56; 110th Evacuation Hospital Semiannual Rpt, January–June 1945, p. 12; 240th Medical Battalion Annual Rpt, 1944, p. 7.

[18] 134th Medical Group Annual Rpt, 1944, pp. 14–17; 64th Medical Group Annual Rpt, 1944, and Semiannual Rpt, January–June 1945, p. 1. For examples of the work of attached medical battalions, see 180th Medical Battalion Annual Rpt, 1944, p. 3, and 240th Medical Battalion Annual Rpt, 1944, pp. 7–10.

tals, the 618th Clearing Company exhaustion center, and the 2d Advance Section, 1st Medical Depot Company, retreated in haste from Malmedy, generally heading for Spa. The following day, the contagious disease and malaria hospital, Company C, 91st Medical Gas Treatment Battalion, pulled out of Grand-Halleux. All these units removed their personnel and patients, most of them in ambulances and trucks provided by the 134th Medical Group and the First Army Provisional Medical Department Truck Company. They also made much use of self-help. The 618th Company, for instance, secured rides for about half of its 200 patients by flagging down passing trucks. For lack of time and transportation, the units for the most part left in place their equipment and, in the case of the depot section, their stock. On the twenty-first and twenty-second, after the battle line stabilized just south of Malmedy, the 134th Medical Group, using vehicles and men of several evacuation hospitals, retrieved most of the outfit of the units withdrawn from that town. The depot section, by sending in a few trucks at a time, managed to haul its stores back to the base depot at Dolhain. A salvage detachment of the gas treatment company, on the other hand, came under German fire at Grand-Halleux and only secured a portion of that unit's equipment. Regardless of how much of their equipment was recovered, the withdrawn hospitals effectively were out of action for the rest of the battle. Most had to retreat a couple of times more as the First Army regrouped. Their people remained in billets or were detailed to work in other medical installations.[19]

By midmorning on 18 December elements of *Kampfgruppe Peiper's* SS armored force had reached Stavelot, less than 10 miles by road from Spa. Few American troops then were between the Germans and First Army headquarters with its cluster of service installations. The army, accordingly, directed all logistical units in Spa, including those of its medical service, to withdraw to Huy, a city on the Meuse about 25 miles to the west, where they would be well situated either to support a new defense line or for further retreat. Army headquarters at the same time moved to the environs of Liege.

This withdrawal involved a number of working medical units and others earlier displaced from farther south. The 134th Medical Group, previously pushed out of Malmedy, joined the new exodus. So did the 57th Medical Battalion, heretofore located at Spa, which constituted the army reserve of collecting and ambulance companies and controlled the now heavily committed Provisional Truck Company. The commander of the 57th prudently had stationed liaison officers at

[19] Surg, First U.S. Army, Annual Rpt, 1944, pp. 22 and 53–54; First U.S. Army Report of Operations, 1 Aug 44–22 Feb 45, bk. IV, p. 156; 134th Medical Group Annual Rpt, 1944, pp. 14–15; Surg, V Corps, Annual Rpt, 1944, p. 22; 44th Evacuation Hospital Annual Rpt, 1944; 67th Evacuation Hospital Annual Rpt, 1944, and Semiannual Rpt, January–June 1945; 618th Clearing Company Annual Rpt, 1944, pp. 5–6; 91st Medical Gas Treatment Battalion Annual Rpt, 1944, p. 5; 1st Medical Depot Company Annual Rpt, 1944, p. 7. For an example of trucks used in equipment recovery, see 45th Evacuation Hospital Annual Rpt, 1944, p. 175. For the origin of the First Army Provisional Medical Department Truck Company, see Chapter IX of this volume.

General Rogers' office and at other headquarters in Spa, to ensure that he would receive up-to-date intelligence and timely orders. He started his battalion off as soon as the enemy was reported at Stavelot. Most important of these new displacements was that of the 4th Convalescent Hospital at Spa. Since the offensive this large installation, besides performing its main mission of patient reconditioning, had housed and fed the personnel of withdrawing medical units. Within less than twenty-four hours the 4th disposed of its 1,400 patients, either returning them to duty or transferring them to COMZ facilities. Then the staff packed up their essential records and unit housekeeping equipment and took the road to Huy. How they managed all this in so short a time, the commanding officer, Col. John W. Claiborne, Jr., MC, was not sure; apparently, he wrote later, it was "a case of team work with all players clicking." At first bivouacked at Huy and later at Tirlemont, the 4th could not resume operations for lack of a suitable site. Its removal from action was a crippling blow to the entire First Army hospitalization and evacuation system.[20]

In the VIII Corps area the 1st Advance Section, 1st Medical Depot Company, pulled out of Bastogne on 18 December. The unit was able to take along only a portion of its stock, even though it commandeered empty ambulances and the trucks that had brought the 42d Field Hospital equipment from Wiltz. A four-man detachment stayed behind with the rest of the supplies. The main body of the unit halted briefly at Libin, some 20 miles west of Bastogne, then retreated again southwestward to Carlsbourg on the twenty-first. Five days later, after the Third Army had taken over medical support of the southern flank of the Bulge, the section moved north and rejoined the base depot at Dolhain.[21]

Of the three evacuation hospitals in the rear of VIII Corps, two were displaced by the German attack. On 16 December the 102d Evacuation Hospital relinquished its position at Echternach, only 6 miles from the front lines, and made a long march right across the battle area to Huy, which it reached on the eighteenth. "A withdrawal of this nature," the unit report declared, "is an experience that all the personnel will long remember." This unit brought along all of its equipment and opened for patients on the twenty-first. The 107th Evacuation Hospital, which had been closed when the offensive started, worked while withdrawing. It first fell back from Clervaux to Libin, where it admitted over 780 patients in eighty-two hours. Assisted by a platoon of the 92d Medical Gas Treatment Battalion, the hospital evacuated 300 patients on the twenty-first, then moved with 100 more to Carlsbourg, where it partially set up again. The next day it retreated for a final time to Sedan. There, after hasty reconnaissance, the

[20] Quotation from 4th Convalescent Hospital Annual Rpt, 1944, pp. 2 and 8. See also First U.S. Army Report of Operations, 1 Aug 44–22 Feb 45, bk. II, p. 120; Surg; First U.S. Army, Annual Rpt, 1944, p. 54; 134th Medical Group Annual Rpt, 1944, p. 15; 57th Medical Battalion Annual Rpt, 1944, pp. 22–24.

[21] First U.S. Army Report of Operations, 1 Aug 44–22 Feb 45, bk. IV, p. 156; 1st Medical Depot Company Annual Rpt, 1944, p. 7.

unit found shelter in a former vocational school and resumed operations on Christmas Eve. During the following week, it handled over 1,000 patients.[22]

The remaining evacuation hospital in rear of the VIII Corps, the 110th at Esch, well south of the breakthrough, stayed in place. During the first week of the German offensive this 400-bed hospital received most of the American casualties from the southern flank of the Bulge, and in addition it fed and temporarily sheltered thousands of troops separated from their units. Patients arrived at a rate of about 300 a day. The surgical backlog at one time also exceeded 300. As no field hospitals any longer were in front of the 110th, these surgical patients included many men with severe chest and abdominal injuries. To cope with this influx, the hospital pitched tents in the paved courtyard of its building to house the sick and lightly wounded. The receiving section culled all the immediately transportable patients from among the incoming casualties, filled out the basic medical forms on them, and at once placed them in ambulances and sent them toward the rear. By such expedients, and by strenuous round-the-clock effort, the staff, heavily reinforced with auxiliary surgical teams, coped with the overload. The 110th handled over 5,000 patients within a month, with a mortality rate of a little less than 1.5 percent among the over 2,200 admitted for surgery.[23]

Medical Realignments

Even as the last medical units extricated themselves from the breakthrough area, the First and Ninth Armies were shifting forces to build a solid line between the Germans and the Meuse. The Ninth Army relinquished four infantry and two armored divisions to its southern neighbor. At the same time its XIX Corps extended to its right to take over most of the territory and several divisions of the First Army's VII Corps, freeing the latter headquarters and its corps troops for commitment on the northern flank of the Bulge. The First Army on 19 December transferred the VIII Corps, with which its headquarters no longer had effective communication, to the Third Army for both operational control and logistical support. At the same time the First Army acquired the XVIII Airborne Corps, which went into line immediately to the right of the V Corps controlling the 82d Airborne Division and others from the Ninth Army and VIII Corps. Finally, on the twenty-fourth, the VII Corps shifted its headquarters from Aachen to Huy. With one armored and two infantry divisions it formed the right wing of an army front anchored on Elsenborn Ridge, and extending from there generally southwestward.

Medical rearrangements accompanied this reorganization. In the Ninth Army the 31st Medical Group and

[22] Quotation from 102d Evacuation Hospital Annual Rpt, 1944, p. 2. See also 107th Evacuation Hospital Annual Rpt, 1944, pp. 6–8; 92d Medical Gas Treatment Battalion Annual Rpt, 1944, pp. 6–7; Surg, Third U.S. Army, Annual Rpt, 1944, p. 56.

[23] 110th Evacuation Hospital Semiannual Rpt, January–June 1945, pp. 3, 18, 42 and encl. 3.

several field and evacuation hospitals changed position to support the southward extension of the XIX Corps and to evacuate casualties of divisions formerly under the First Army. At the same time the Ninth Army surgeon, Colonel Shambora, and his staff made preparations for withdrawal in the event that the Germans extended their offensive to their army's hitherto quiet front or broke clear through the First Army and crossed the Meuse. Shambora selected an alternate medical concentration area just east of Brussels. He redeployed two evacuation hospitals, and platoons of two field hospitals closed and pulled back. Shambora also had his forward evacuation hospitals send all their unused heavy equipment, such as tentage, back to the 35th Medical Depot Company for storage, thereby reducing the transportation requirements in any retreat. The Ninth Army front, however, remained largely inactive.[24]

The First Army, in addition to relinquishing its VIII Corps to the Third Army, transferred its 64th Medical Group (to include its two battalion headquarters, a collecting company, four ambulance companies, and a clearing company) and the corps' medical battalion and one field and three evacuation hospitals. In return, on 21 December, the First Army picked up from the Ninth Army a medical battalion, the 187th, with one ambulance and three collecting companies. The companies went to reinforce the 134th Medical Group, now responsible for evacuating both the V and XVIII Airborne Corps. The army used the additional battalion headquarters, with a collecting company and a clearing company platoon attached, as a provisional medical battalion for the airborne corps, which hitherto had lacked one. During the VII Corps redeployment the 68th Medical Group, which supported the corps, moved its headquarters 50 miles; disengaged from support of five divisions and as many evacuation hospitals; and assumed responsibility for eight new divisions, belonging to the VII and XVIII Airborne Corps, as well as two evacuation hospitals. The group commander observed: "Probably at no previous time had the flexibility and ease of adaptability of a Medical Group been more clearly illustrated than during this emergency. . . ."[25]

To the rear of the fighting line General Rogers attempted to put back together an army evacuation and hospitalization system disrupted by the rapid movement of the front and the displacement of so many medical units. Even though most threatened installations, or at least their personnel, escaped the advancing Germans, Rogers within forty-eight hours of the start of the attack no longer had enough beds in operation for normal hospitalization and evacuation of his

[24] Surg, Ninth U.S. Army, Annual Rpt, 1944, pp. 10–11 and 13–16; 31st Medical Group Annual Rpt, 1944, pp. 19–20.

[25] Quotation from 68th Medical Group Annual Rpt, 1944, p. 22. On 21 December the 134th Medical Group moved forward from Huy to Verviers to be closer to the V Corps. See 134th Medical Group Annual Rpt, 1944, pp. 15–16. See also Surg, First U.S. Army, Annual Rpt, 1944, pp. 54–55 and 57–78; VII Corps Medical Plan, pp. 103–04, encl. 1 to Surg, VII Corps, Annual Rpt, 1944; 187th Medical Battalion Annual Rpt, 1944, p. 2; Surg, XVIII Airborne Corps, Semiannual Rpt, January-June 1945, pp. 1–3.

casualties. Well over half of the First Army's dozen evacuation hospitals by that time had closed for movement, had lost their equipment, or—in the VIII Corps area—had become inaccessible to the majority of divisions. In addition, the displacement of the 4th Convalescent Hospital, the 618th Clearing Company exhaustion center, and the 91st Medical Gas Treatment Battalion communicable disease facility left the army unable to retain and care for short-term cases. Perforce, then, Rogers on 19 December established a total evacuation policy in place of the ten-day one hitherto in effect. Under the new policy, army hospitals evacuated all their patients as soon as they were able to travel and sent new arrivals whose conditions permitted it, without treatment, directly to COMZ facilities. Most of the bypassed patients, under an agreement between Rogers and the ADSEC surgeon, Colonel Beasley, went to the by now well-developed cluster of general hospitals around Liege. Those hospitals, according to General Hawley, "saved the First Army medical service during the counteroffensive," for without them Rogers could not have kept his remaining evacuation beds open for fresh casualties or cleared his endangered units for withdrawal.[26]

Two ADSEC units close to the combat zone temporarily served as army evacuation hospitals, receiving wounded brought from division clearing stations. One of these, the 77th Evacuation Hospital, a 750-bed unit located at Verviers, had been functioning as a holding unit and hastily reorganized to perform its original mission. Just behind the center of the new First Army front, the 77th, assisted for a time by the 9th Field Hospital, for about a week handled most of the casualties from divisions trying to stop the German advance toward the Meuse. The staff, augmented with auxiliary surgical teams and medics from nonoperating First Army hospitals, worked eighteen-hour and longer days to sort, treat, and evacuate the flood of patients. They keep eight operating and two fracture tables busy day and night. Verviers, a major road center, came under daily enemy artillery fire, V–1 bombardment, and *Luftwaffe* raids. This danger forced off-duty personnel to spend their few hours of rest in crowded, fetid underground shelters. On 20 December a shell blew off a corner of the school building that housed the 77th, wrecking a bathroom; damaging the nurses quarters, laboratory, and pharmacy, and one medical ward; and mortally wounding a Red Cross worker. The hospital staff cleaned up the wreckage and continued in operation. A week later, in addition to the regular patient influx, the 77th had to care for the 14 dead and 50 wounded from a direct bomb hit on the 9th Field Hospital. "For hours the receiving room was in a turmoil as the differentiation and treatment went on. Among the dead, decapitations and amputations made the task gruesome, even for the men who had seen many hundreds of wounded." Enemy bombardment for a time prevented hospital trains from

[26] Quotation from Ltr, Hawley to TSG, 27 Jan 45, file HD 024 ETO O/CS (Hawley-SGO Corresp). See also Surg, First U.S. Army, Annual Rpt, 1944, pp. 54, 56–57, 69–70. Some individual hospitals went to total evacuation even before the army change of policy. See 5th Evacuation Hospital Annual Rpt, 1944, p. 15, for example.

reaching Verviers. The Advance Section maintained evacuation of the 77th with ambulances, which shuttled patients back to the Liege general hospitals. The burden on the weary 77th staff eased only in the last days of the year, as First Army hospitals began opening in Verviers.[27]

The 130th General Hospital, although an ADSEC unit, lay just within the First Army area. As it turned out, this hospital, set up in a large school building at Ciney, was positioned almost exactly at the westernmost tip of the Bulge and was well placed to receive casualties from the VIII Corps. That, however, was not its function. The 130th had been reorganized before leaving England as a specialized neuropsychiatric facility. At Ciney it treated combat exhaustion casualties from the First and Ninth Armies. The hospital's mission changed abruptly on 19 December, when ambulance loads of wounded began arriving, both from retreating evacuation hospitals, such as the 107th, and directly from division clearing stations. According to the unit report, the hospital found itself "acting as a cross between a clearing company and an evacuation hospital which required revamping . . . [the] entire setup." The 130th discharged its exhaustion patients to an ADSEC replacement depot, sent its psychiatric staff to the rear, and enlarged its surgical service with people from the 12th Field Hospital and the 3d Auxiliary Surgical Group. Between the twentieth and twenty-third the hospital received and treated or bypassed over 3,000 patients. It evacuated most of them by train from a nearby siding. The unit performed surgery on about 200 casualties. The German advance rolled almost literally up to the door; fighting occurred in the hospital grounds as the 2d Armored Division and other units moved in to engage and throw back the enemy. On the twenty-third the 130th evacuated all but a skeleton staff and its nontransportables. The remaining staff and patients all left or were evacuated during the next four days, along with the most vital items of equipment. An armored combat command treatment station temporarily occupied the plant until the twenty-eighth, when an advance party of the 130th moved back in.[28]

While these ADSEC hospitals, and the few First Army ones still active, coped with the immediate flow of casualties, General Rogers tried to redeploy and reopen his evacuation hospitals. He worked within the constraints of an army G–4 order, issued on Christmas Day, to withdraw all logistical units except those absolutely essential for operations to positions north and west of the Meuse. Under this directive First Army hospitals and other medical units redeployed to a concentration area about 15 miles or so west of Liege. These included two of the three evacuation hospitals that had been working in Eupen throughout the battle, under bombardment comparable to that endured by the

[27] Quotation from Allen, ed., *Medicine Under Canvas*, pp. 142–48. See also Surg, ADSEC, COMZ, Annual Rpt, 1944, p. 20; 77th Evacuation Hospital Annual Rpt, 1944, pp. 7–8; 134th Medical Group Annual Rpt, 1944, p. 16.

[28] Quotation from 130th General Hospital Annual Rpt, 1944, pp. 4, 11, 16–17, 28–30. See also Surg, ADSEC, COMZ, Annual Rpt, 1944, p. 10.

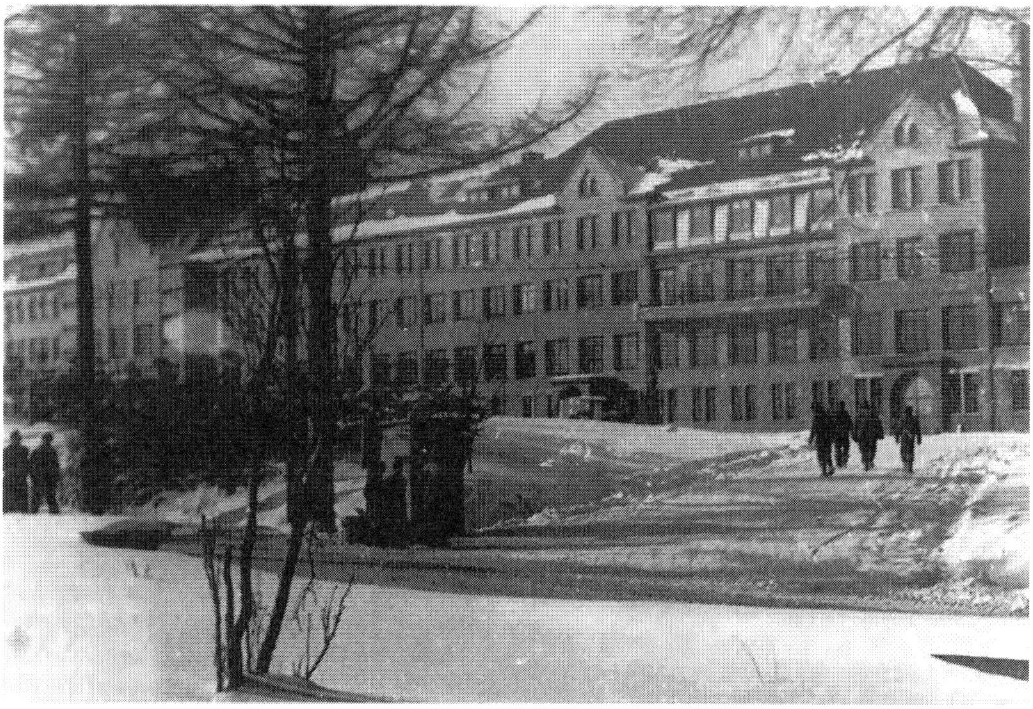

FORMER SCHOOL FACILITY HOUSING THE 130TH GENERAL HOSPITAL AT CINEY

77th at Verviers. This final withdrawal crowded First Army units back into towns already occupied by numerous ADSEC facilities. As a result, the hospitals sent there could not reopen for lack of usable buildings, tented open-field operation being out of the question in the cold wet weather. By the end of the year the First Army had a few evacuation hospitals working: the 102d and 51st (field acting as an evacuation) at Huy, the 97th and 128th at Verviers, and the 2d at Eupen. The other six evacuation hospitals then under the army, however, remained inactive, as did the convalescent hospital and most of the specialized medical facilities. General Rogers, accordingly, kept a total evacuation policy in effect until mid-January.[29]

The First Army also redeployed its medical supply installations during the last week of December and began rehabilitating those of its units that had lost equipment in the retreat. Under the 25 December withdrawal order the base depot, with most of its stock, moved by rail from Dolhain to Basse Wavre, southeast of Brussels. As later described by the army surgeon, "A series of incidents, some humorous and some serious, including

[29] Surg, First U.S. Army, Annual Rpt, 1944, p. 56; First U.S. Army Report of Operations, 1 Aug 44–22 Feb 45, bk. IV, pp. 144–45; 68th Medical Group Annual Rpt, 1944, p. 23; 134th Medical Group Annual Rpt, p. 16; 2d, 5th 45th, 97th, and 102d Evacuation Hospitals Annual Rpts, 1944; 51st Field Hospital Annual Rpt, 1944.

an international dispute as to right of tenancy, misrouted cars, and lost vehicles," prevented supply issues from this depot for the rest of the year. The two advance sections of the 1st Medical Depot Company kept most of the army supplied. The 2d Advance Section, earlier withdrawn from Malmedy, on the twenty-sixth set up a dump at Huy to support the army's right wing corps and divisions. At Dolhain the 1st Advance Section issued to the V Corps, and the army blood bank detachment, also located there, remained in operation. First Army medical units farther to the rear for a while drew directly upon COMZ depots, notably M-409 at Liege. By the end of the year the base depot was engaged in replenishing its much depleted stock. General Rogers sent liaison officers to divisions and other organizations to determine the extent of their medical equipment losses, which in many units approached 100 percent of their basic allowances. His office then worked directly with the chief surgeon's Supply Division to speed replacement items forward.[30]

Throughout the medical unit movements resulting from the Ardennes battle, the First Army Provisional Medical Department Truck Company performed indispensable service. This unit, attached to the 57th Medical Battalion, had been formed during the pursuit by pooling vehicles, primarily taken from evacuation hospitals, as a transportation reserve for moving the larger army installations. Its work, and vehicle strength, had diminished in scope during the relatively static autumn and winter battles, but in the late-December crisis the company again came into its own. Expanding quickly from 50 trucks to 100, in two weeks it transported nine evacuation and three field hospitals, the convalescent hospital with 1,400 patients, a depot company section, and a gas treatment company, as well as tons of supplies. The company significantly increased the ability of the First Army medical service to respond rapidly to the changing military situation.[31]

During the first two weeks of the German offensive, the First Army medical service redeployed most of its nondivisional units while maintaining continuous evacuation of the regrouping combat forces. Its relative success in both endeavors may be attributed to a favorable starting position, to the delays in the German advance, to an abundance of transportation, and to a high standard of unit and individual initiative and resourcefulness. By the end of December, however, the army for all practical purposes had lost its ability to hold and treat casualties; its medical service perforce had been reduced to little more than a conduit between division clearing stations and COMZ hospitals.

Bastogne: Encirclement and Relief

The battle for Bastogne began on 19 December, when the 101st Airborne Division went into action to the east of that strategic road junction.

---

[30] Quotation from Surg, First U.S. Army, Annual Rpt, 1944, p. 22. See also ibid., p. 23; First U.S. Army Report of Operations, 1 Aug 44-22 Feb 45, bk. IV, pp. 156-57; 1st Medical Depot Company Annual Rpt, 1944, p. 7.

[31] Surg, First U.S. Army, Annual Rpt, 1944, p. 61; 57th Medical Battalion Annual Rpt, 1944, pp. 22-23.

The following day the VIII Corps gave Brig. Gen. Anthony C. McAuliffe, acting division commander, overall charge of the defense, with control also of Combat Command B, 10th Armored Division; of Combat Command R, 9th Armored Division; and of an assortment of artillery, tank destroyer, and other units that had collected in Bastogne. On the twenty-first the Germans closed their ring and made their first attacks on the American perimeter. The enemy surrender demand came on the twenty-second and elicited General McAuliffe's immortal one-word rejection. For another four days the defenders fought off repeated assaults by the *Fifth Panzer Army,* making effective use of well-directed artillery fire to break up German attacks. At night they endured *Luftwaffe* bombing raids on the city. The American units within the perimeter had enough food, ammunition, and other necessities, brought in with them or foraged from abandoned First Army and VIII Corps dumps, to carry them through until 23 December, when large-scale supply airdrops began just in time to avert a critical shortage of artillery shells. At 1645 on the day after Christmas elements of the 4th Armored Division of the Third Army opened a road into Bastogne from the south. This breakthrough ended the siege, although heavy fighting continued around the city for several more weeks.[32]

American casualties during the siege amounted at least to 189 officers and men killed, 1,040 wounded, 407 sick and injured, and 412 missing—the loss reported by the 101st Division. In addition, Combat Command B of the 10th Armored Division suffered about 500 battle casualties, and there were still more among the other commands, and fragments of commands, that defended the city. The great majority of the sick and wounded were trapped in Bastogne for the duration of the encirclement.[33]

The 101st Division medical service was organized and equipped for self-sufficient operations out of contact with the normal ground chain of evacuation. Its medical detachments went into action at full strength in men and equipment and carrying along extra reserves of litters and blankets. The division's 326th Airborne Medical Company included both collecting and clearing elements and had an auxiliary surgical team attached so that it could perform the functions of a field hospital platoon (*see Map 18*).

An early stroke of misfortune deprived the division of its hospital. The 326th Company, accompanied by the division surgeon, Colonel Gold, and his staff, set up its clearing and surgical station early on 19 December at a crossroads about 8 miles west of Bastogne. Gold, in consultation with the division supply officer, placed the station there, in what he expected would be the division service area, on the assumption that the 101st would be fighting as a part of a continuous front line. Around 1030 the company deployed its collecting elements,

[32] For tactical developments, see Cole, *Ardennes,* ch. XIX.

[33] 101st Airborne Division After-Action Rpt, 17–27 Dec 44, box 14335, RG 407, NARA. Cole, *Ardennes,* pp. 480–81, provides figures on casualties in other organizations. His figures for the 101st Division differ from those in the report first cited, as do those given in Surg, 101st Airborne Division, Annual Rpt, 1944, pp. 12–13.

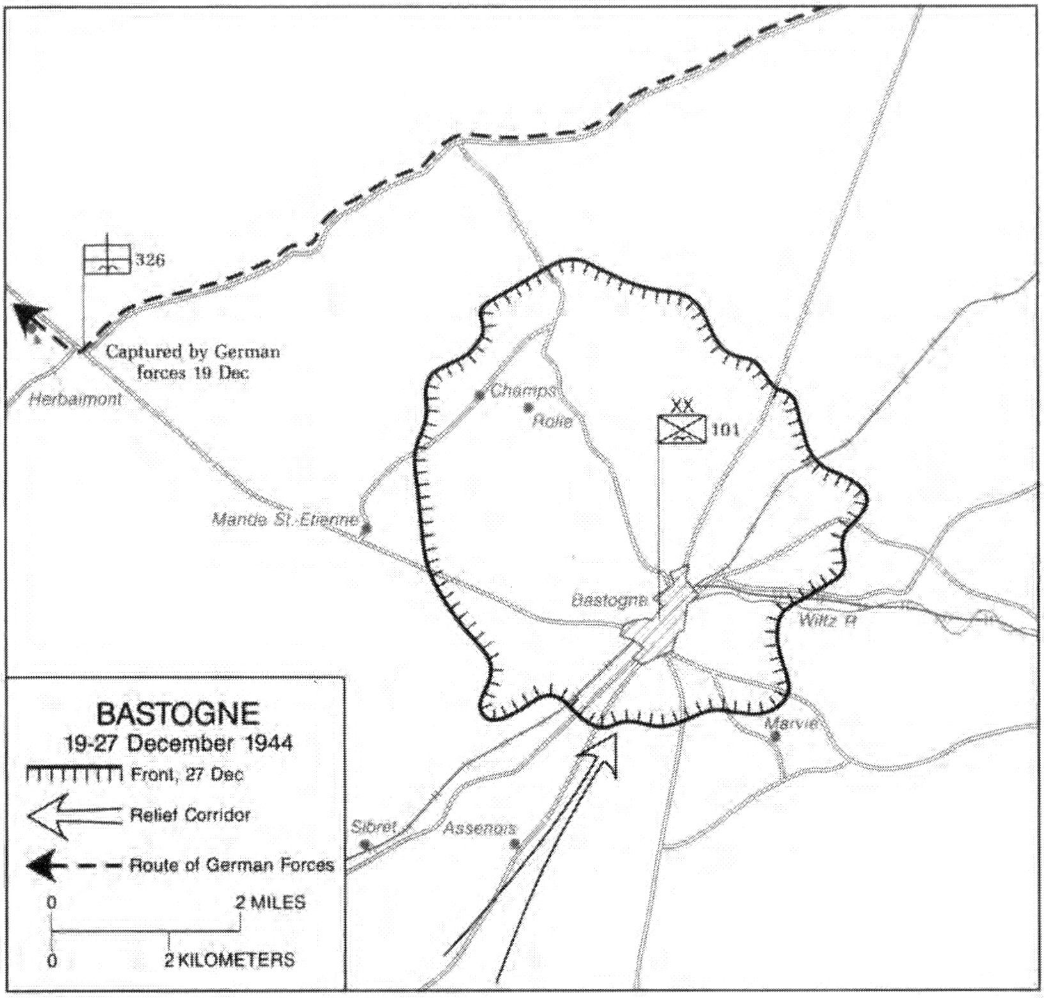

MAP 18

sending four or five ambulance jeeps and an evacuation officer to each of the four infantry regiments. The first patients arrived at about 1100. Late that afternoon the 326th Company commander, Major Barfield, left the crossroads with an ambulance convoy to take patients to the 107th Evacuation Hospital at Libin and to contact the 64th Medical Group about additional ambulances for the clearing station. On the return trip Barfield and his group found their road to Bastogne blocked by a blown bridge and columns of tanks and spent the night at the 107th.[34]

[34] Surg, 101st Airborne Division Annual Rpt, 1944, pp. 9–10; 326th Airborne Medical Company After-Action Rpt, Belgium and France, 17–28 Dec 44, p. 3; G–3 Account of Bastogne Operation, in 101st Airborne Division Combat Intervs, box 24075, RG 407, NARA; Crandall Interv, 8 Jun 45, box 222, RG 112, NARA.

At around 2200 a German force of perhaps half a dozen armored vehicles and 100 troops, some dressed in civilian clothing, attacked the 326th Company clearing station. Evidently a reconnaissance element of one of the columns beginning to encircle Bastogne, it had come down a road from the northeast and caught the medical company totally by surprise. After a few minutes of sporadic automatic weapons fire, the Germans realized that they had run into a medical installation. An enemy officer came forward and demanded the Americans' surrender. Colonel Gold, who had no alternative, complied, but a few officers and men on the west side of the company area ran off into the nearby woods. As the Germans were rounding up their prisoners, a truck column headed out of Bastogne to pick up supplies rolled unsuspectingly into the crossroads. Firing broke out again, from the Germans and from at least one of the trucks. The medics, caught in the crossfire, ducked for cover. Some were killed or wounded by stray bullets; a few managed to escape in the confusion. Soon the flames of burning American vehicles lighted the area. Americans and Germans alike made futile efforts to save the screaming wounded trapped inside the wrecks. The Germans withdrew toward the northeast, taking with them the remaining medical personnel and patients, as well as any equipment and supplies they decided not to destroy. The prisoners included Colonel Gold and his staff, an entire auxiliary surgical team, and 11 officers and 119 men of the 326th Company. With them, the 101st Airborne Division lost its hospital and its emergency surgical facility.[35]

Division headquarters learned of this misfortune shortly after midnight, from infantry patrols sent to investigate the shooting at the crossroads and from escapees of the 326th Company who made their way into Bastogne. The G–4 and the evacuation officers of the medical company in town, together with the regimental surgeons and Major Barfield, now acting division surgeon, quickly improvised a new evacuation system. They designated the regimental aid station of the 501st Parachute Infantry, centrally located within the city in a convent, as the collecting point for all division casualties. Meanwhile, the VIII Corps surgeon, at division request, deployed a collecting company and the clearing company of the corps medical battalion to move patients from Bastogne to evacuation hospitals. Some 170 men passed through this improvised evacuation chain on the twentieth. By 2330 on that day, however, the Germans had blocked the last road out of Bastogne. Completion of the encirclement left the VIII Corps collecting and clearing units outside the ring, along with Major Barfield, who had gone back to corps headquarters to report on the loss of the medical company and

[35] 101st Airborne Division After-Action Rpt, 17–27 Dec 44, box 14335, RG 407, NARA; Surg, 101st Airborne Division, Annual Rpt, 1944, pp. 10–11; 326th Airborne Medical Company After-Action Rpt, Belgium and France, 17–28 Dec 44, p. 4. For eyewitness stories, see Crandall Interv, 8 Jun 45, box 222, RG 112, NARA; Rapport and Northwood, *Rendezvous with Destiny*, pp. 467–68; Graves, *Front Line Surgeons*, p. 278; and Statement of Pfc E. E. Lucan, in 101st Airborne Division Combat Intervs, box 24075, RG 407, NARA.

bring forward additional supplies and equipment. Wounded soon began to accumulate in the regimental aid station; as early as 0630 on the twenty-first about 150 were on hand.[36]

The 101st Division now was totally cut off from evacuation. Its medical officers, to give the steadily growing number of casualties at least essential life-saving treatment until American forces broke the German siege, improvised a hospital at the convent housing the regimental aid station. Maj. Martin S. Wisely, MC, regimental surgeon of the 327th Glider Infantry, headed a pickup staff made up of doctors and aidmen from the division antiaircraft, engineer, artillery, and tank destroyer units. To obtain more space and better protection from artillery and air attack for his patients, Wisely moved the hospital from the convent to the basement garage of a Belgian Army barracks. As the hospital population increased, he placed ambulatory patients in the barracks rifle range and used still another building for trenchfoot cases. Eventually, patients were distributed among basements all over the city, with the barracks garage reserved for the most severely wounded.

These facilities were, to say the least, primitive. The main garage ward, for instance, had no latrine and only a single electric light. A field kitchen set up at one end of the large room fed both staff and patients. The wounded "were laid in rows on sawdust covered with blankets. Each row had a shift of aidmen, and an attempt was made to segregate incoming cases into specified rows depending upon the seriousness of their wounds." Those deemed unlikely to survive lay nearest the wall. "As they died they were carried out to another building where an impromptu Graves Registration Office was functioning." Wisely and his assistants worked 24-hour shifts trying to keep their patients fed, reasonably warm, and in stable condition. They attempted no major surgery. According to the participants, morale among the casualties was "extremely high." On Christmas Eve a ration of cognac and the voice of Bing Crosby singing "White Christmas" from a salvaged civilian radio provided some holiday atmosphere.[37]

Although the 101st Division hospital handled most of the casualties of the siege, it was not the only improvised medical facility in Bastogne. Combat Command B, 10th Armored Division, a Third Army unit that had entered the city from the south, improvised its own holding and treatment station after being cut off from its supporting armored medical company. On Christmas Eve the hospital took a direct hit from a German

---

[36] Surg, VIII Corps, Annual Rpt, 1944, p. 8; Surg, 101st Airborne Division, Annual Rpt, 1944, p. 11; 326th Airborne Medical Company After-Action Rpt, Belgium and France, 17–28 Dec 44, pp. 3–5; G–3 Account of Bastogne Operation and Narrative, "Medical Evacuation and Supply," both in 101st Airborne Division Combat Intervs, box 24075, RG 407, NARA; 169th Medical Battalion Annual Rpt, 1944, p. 12; 429th Collecting Company Annual Rpt, 1944, p. 3.

[37] Quotations and most details from Rapport and Northwood, *Rendezvous with Destiny*, pp. 469–71. See also Surg, 101st Airborne Division, Annual Rpt, 1944, p. 11; 326th Airborne Medical Company After-Action Rpt, Belgium and France, 17–28 Dec 44, p. 5; 501st Parachute Infantry Draft After-Action Rpt, in 101st Airborne Division Combat Intervs, box 24075, RG 407, NARA. History of the 12th Evacuation Hospital, 25 August 1942 to 25 August 1943 (hereafter cited as 12th Evac Hist), pp. 111–12, contains additional eyewitness reports.

bomb. The resulting roof cave-in and fire killed a number of patients and also a Belgian woman nurse, who had volunteered to help tend the American wounded.[38]

Around the perimeter the infantry battalions set up their aid stations in the standard manner, with the main installations well sheltered in farmhouses or other structures and forward collecting elements close to the foxhole line. Short of litterbearers, the airborne units relied heavily on their ambulance jeeps to move their casualties. Where jeeps could not go, some units used toboggans, made of sheet metal torn off roofs, to slide wounded men across the snow. Jeeps of the division's 326th Company carried patients from the battalion aid stations to the central hospital in Bastogne. One regimental surgeon, Maj. Douglas Davidson, MC, of the 502d Parachute Infantry, thought he could do as much for his wounded as the ill-equipped division facility; hence, he maintained his own holding hospital in the barn of the chateau housing the regimental command post. Davidson used horse stalls for wards and pressed the chaplains and a dentist into service as cooks. He estimated that "only about 5 men died of wounds who might have been saved had they been given medical care." On Christmas Day, when German tanks and infantry broke through the main line of resistance and momentarily threatened the command post, Davidson routed out all of his wounded men who were able to walk, gave them all rifles, and led them to join a scratch force of headquarters personnel in repelling the attack.[39]

During this week of encirclement the hospitals in Bastogne faced two major problems: medical supply and the provision of emergency surgery. Of these the supply problem proved the easier to solve. A few tons of stores and a small issuing detachment of the 1st Medical Depot Company remained in Bastogne, and paratroopers also found an abandoned VIII Corps medical supply point. From these sources the surgeons obtained necessities for the first few days. Nevertheless, by the end of the third day of the siege, the hospitals were running short of penicillin, plasma, morphine, dressings, litters, and blankets. To keep patients warm in the unheated wards, the division collected the blankets of its dead and sent parties of men to salvage quilts and bed clothing from ruined dwellings. Food also was short, although the division reserved for the hospitals the limited available quantities of sugar, coffee, Ovaltine, and ten-in-one rations. The large-scale airdrop, which began on 23 December, alleviated most medical supply deficiencies. Penicillin and other medicines, plasma, Vaseline gauze, anesthetics, morphine, distilled water, syringes, sterilizers, litters, and blankets arrived in the parachuted bundles. The parachute cloth itself, and the wrapping of the bundles, went to the hospitals to provide addi-

---

[38] Surg, 10th Armored Division, Annual Rpt, 1944, p. 15; 101st Airborne Division After-Action Rpt, 17-27 Dec 44, box 14335, RG 407, NARA; Rapport and Northwood, *Rendezvous with Destiny*, pp. 471 and 546.

[39] Rapport and Northwood, *Rendezvous with Destiny*, pp. 470-71. For Davidson, see S. L. A. Marshall, "Bastogne," pp. 197-98, and Narrative (source of quotation), 592d Parachute Infantry, both in 101st Airborne Division Combat Intervs, respectively box 24074 and box 24075, RG 407, NARA.

tional warm covering for patients. Whole blood also was among the air-delivered supplies, but the bottles broke on landing or were destroyed when a German shell blew up the room where they were stored.[40]

As the days of encirclement went by, the division surgeons realized that the number of wounded awaiting treatment was increasing and that they were going to die unless they underwent major operations immediately. Equipment for such surgery was at hand: the operating theater outfit of the 42d Field Hospital platoon that had withdrawn from Wiltz. However, the few surgeons in Bastogne either could not be spared from other tasks or lacked the qualifications to perform the work required. Seeking a way out of this dilemma, Major Wisely on 26 December obtained authority from the division to try to negotiate the passage of the most severely wounded through German lines. Wisely, assisted by a captured German medical officer, made contact with the enemy commander opposite the southwest sector of the perimeter. The German responded favorably to the evacuation proposal but postponed a final answer until the next day. By that time Third Army troops had ended the siege.[41]

Even as Wisely was trying to arrange for the wounded to come out of Bastogne, Third Army efforts to send surgeons in bore fruit. The army surgeon's office obtained six medical officers and four enlisted technicians, all volunteers, from the 4th Auxiliary Surgical Group and the 12th Evacuation Hospital to go into Bastogne and set up an emergency surgical facility. The army at first intended to drop these men into the perimeter by parachute; but, to their relief, they were able to travel by less hazardous means. One officer was flown in on Christmas Day in a light plane and the rest followed by glider during the afternoon of the twenty-sixth.

When the main body of the surgical group walked into the garage hospital, about 150 patients, all severe cases, remained, the rest having been moved elsewhere. The need for the reinforcements' services was all to apparent, as "the odor of gas gangrene permeated the room." Using the 42d Field Hospital equipment, which included an operating lamp and an autoclave, the surgeons and technicians set up a four-table theater in a small tool room adjoining the garage. They examined and sorted the patients and by nightfall had the first men on the tables. The volunteers, assisted by three Belgian women and by a 10th Armored Division battalion surgeon who was a qualified anesthetist, operated all through the night and until around noon of the twenty-seventh, trying to repair wounds that had gone from two to as many as

---

[40] Surg, First U.S. Army, Annual Rpt, 1944, p. 22; Surg, Third U.S. Army, Annual Rpt, 1944, p. 171; Surg, 101st Airborne Division, Annual Rpt, 1944, pp. 11–12; Rapport and Northwood, *Rendezvous with Destiny*, pp. 469–71; Narrative, "Medical Evacuation and Supply," and Interv, ACofS, G–4, and Others, both in 101st Airborne Division Combat Intervs, box 24075, RG 407, NARA; 101st Airborne Division After-Action Rpt, 17–27 Dec 44, box 14335, RG 407, NARA.

[41] Rapport and Northwood, *Rendezvous with Destiny*, p. 471; Narrative, "Medical Evacuation and Supply," and 327th Glider Infantry Journal, 26 Dec 44, both in 101st Airborne Division Combat Intervs, box 24075, RG 407, NARA. The Third Army's chief of staff had plans for moving surgeons into Bastogne under a white flag. See Cole, *Ardennes*, p. 609.

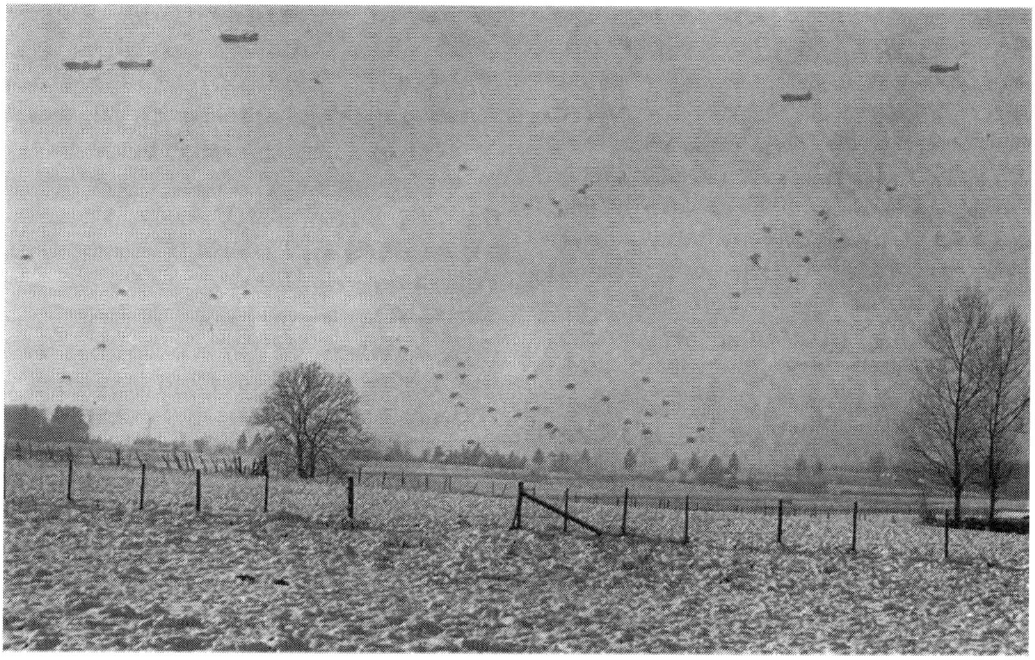

Bundles of Medical Supplies, *air-dropped from C–47s over a field near Bastogne and retrieved by 101st Airborne Division troops*

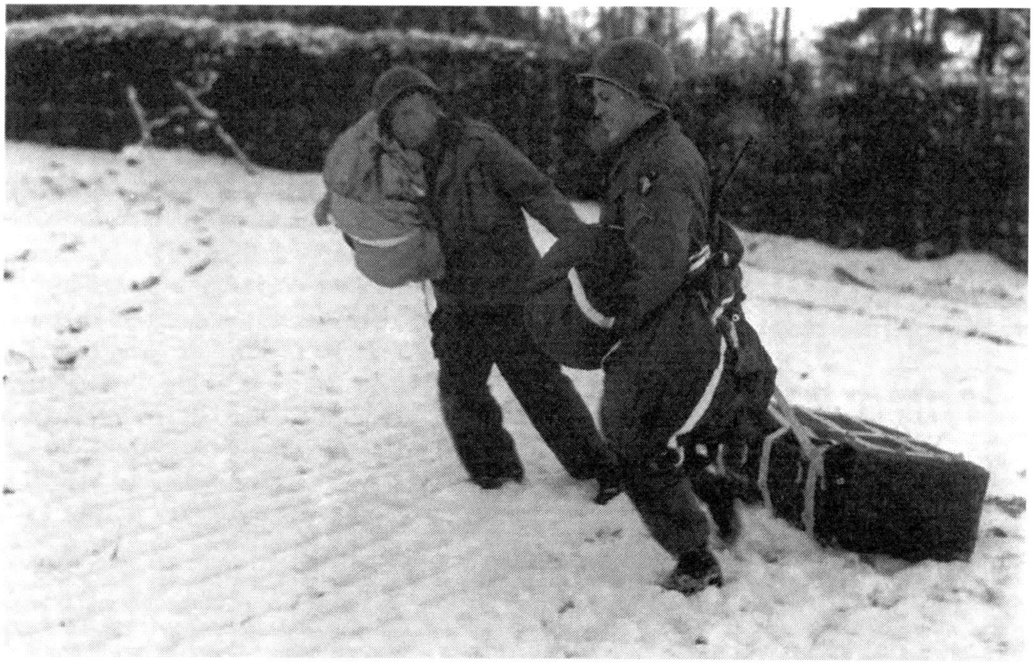

eight days without surgical attention. Of necessity, they performed many amputations. Evacuation of casualties from Bastogne began on the twenty-seventh, but the surgeons, after a rest around midday, operated for another twenty or so hours. Even after a near-miss by a German bomb blew in the operating room door and brought down part of the ceiling, they kept on, working for a time by flashlight. The volunteer group, every member of which—both officer and enlisted—received the Silver Star, completed about fifty major operations, with three postoperative deaths.[42]

As early as 21 December the surgeons of the VIII Corps and the 101st Division, together with the commander of the 64th Medical Group, had begun planning for the medical relief of Bastogne. After the Third Army took control of the VIII Corps, the army surgeon and the surgeon of the III Corps, which led the attack to break the encirclement, joined in the preparations. Besides arranging for aerial resupply and surgical reinforcement of the besieged division, the Third Army and its subordinate commands prepared to evacuate an anticipated 1,000 sick and wounded as soon as a way out of Bastogne was opened. After a couple of false starts, resulting from reports that there was to be an evacuation under flag of truce, the army set up triage and emergency treatment facilities at Attert and Villers-devant-Orval, south of Bastogne, on the most likely routes by which wounded would come out of the city. The armored medical company attached to Combat Command B, 10th Armored Division, and a platoon of the 61st Field Hospital took position at Attert. At Villers-devant-Orval the 635th Clearing Company and a collecting company, both from the VIII Corps' 169th Medical Battalion, constituted the receiving elements. In addition, the III Corps formed a provisional medical battalion for the 101st Division, consisting of a field hospital platoon, a collecting company, and a gas treatment company (to function as a clearing station). All these units were in position by the time the lead tanks of the Third Army contacted the Bastogne defenders.[43]

As it turned out, all the accumulated casualties came out through Villers-devant-Orval. Early on 27 December the first evacuation convoy of twenty-two ambulances and ten trucks rolled out of Bastogne carrying 260 patients. Men of the 635th Clearing Company unloaded the casualties, tagged them, and transferred them to 64th Medical Group ambulances for movement to evacuation hospitals. The vehicles from Bastogne then went back to the city for another load. In two days the medical units evacuated all of the 964 patients in the Bas-

[42] Quotation from 12th Evac Hist, pp. 111–12. See also ibid., pp. 63 and 110; Surg, Third U.S. Army, Rpt, December 1944, p. 31, in Third U.S. Army After-Action Rpt, 1 Aug 44–9 May 45; 4th Auxiliary Surgical Group Annual Rpt, 1944, p. 16; 101st Airborne Division After-Action Rpt, 17–27 Dec 44, box 14335, RG 407, NARA; Surg, 101st Airborne Division, Annual Rpt, 1944, p. 12; 326th Airborne Medical Company After-Action Rpt, Belgium and France, 17–28 Dec 44, p. 5; Rapport and Northwood, *Rendezvous with Destiny*, p. 471; Editorial Advisory Board, 1962, pp. 211–12.

[43] Surg, Third U.S. Army, Annual Rpt, 1944, p. 79; Surg, III Corps, Annual Rpt, 1944, an. 1; 169th Medical Battalion Annual Rpt, 1944, p. 12; 240th Medical Battalion Annual Rpt, 1944, pp. 8–9.

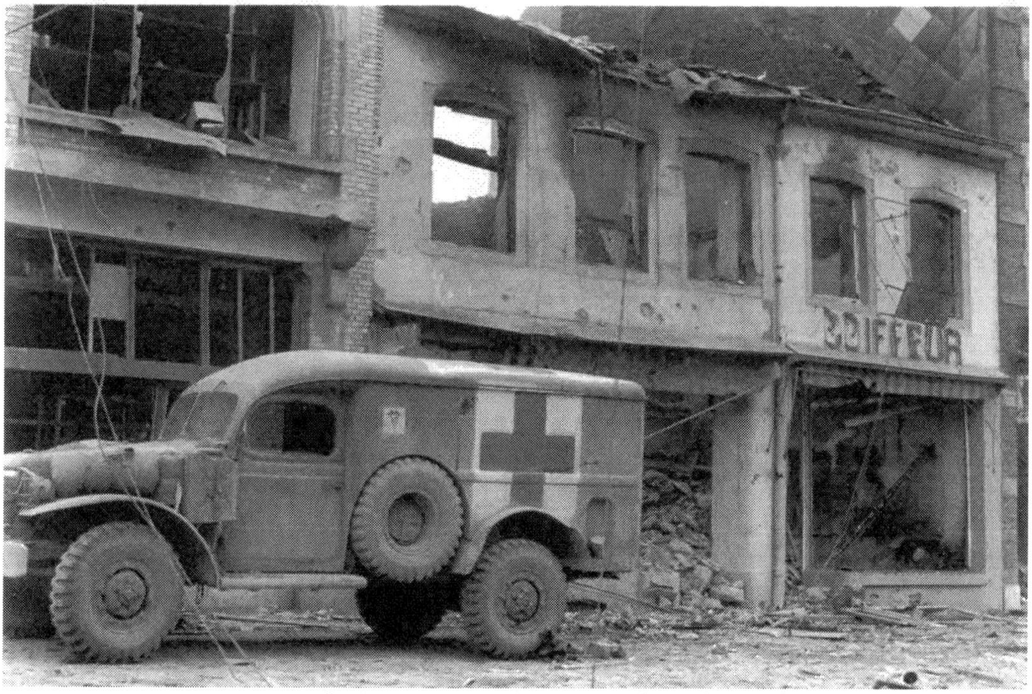

ARMY AMBULANCE IN BASTOGNE, *standing ready to load casualties of the siege*

togne hospitals.[44] At the same time, elements of the provisional medical battalion moved into the city to provide clearing station and forward surgical support for the airborne troops, who still were engaged in intense combat.[45]

In the defense and relief of Bastogne the field army, corps, and division medical services displayed a high degree of resourcefulness and adaptability. Medics inside the perimeter, after the initial disaster of the loss of the 101st Division clearing station, put together a new second-echelon facility in the midst of combat, using what human and materiel resources they had on hand. They kept most of the casualties alive until evacuation. Medics outside the ring made every effort to send in needed supplies and to reestablish forward surgical support for the besieged troops; they lost no time in evacuating the Bastogne hospitals after the relief. For the casualties, nevertheless, the siege was an ordeal. How many patients died in

[44] This figure is less than the total reported casualties of the siege. Men evacuated before the encirclement, or who returned to duty during the siege, or who died, probably account for the discrepancy.

[45] Surg, Third U.S. Army, Annual Rpt, 1944, p. 79; Surg, III Corps, Annual Rpt, 1944, an. 1; Surg, 101st Airborne Division, Annual Rpt, 1944, p. 12; 64th Medical Group Annual Rpt, 1944, pp. 8–9; 326th Airborne Medical Company After-Action Rpt, Belgium and France, 17–28 Dec 44, pp. 5–6; 169th Medical Battalion Annual Rpt, 1944, p. 12; 240th Medical Battalion Annual Rpt, 1944, pp. 9–10; Narrative, "Medical Evacuation and Supply," in 101st Airborne Division Combat Intervs, box 24075, RG 407, NARA; 16th Field Hospital Annual Hist, 1944, encl. 3; 92d Medical Gas Treatment Battalion Annual Rpt, 1944, p. 7.

Bastogne for lack of early surgery or as the result of other deficiencies of the improvised hospitals cannot be determined from the fragmentary records of those ephemeral organizations. One firm figure is the 101st Airborne Division report of 33 deaths under treatment in its facilities between 19 and 31 December. The Third Army surgical consultant, after examining the wounded brought out of Bastogne, concluded that "other than the physical discomforts, the casualties had not unduly suffered for lack of Medical Department treatment and that the mortality was extremely low." Whatever the clinical verdict, a *Stars and Stripes* correspondent who watched one of the first evacuation convoys come out of Bastogne expressed the human reality of the siege:

> The convoy of wounded came out of Bastogne in a slow trickle. The day was beautiful if you like Belgium in the winter time. The snow on the hills glistened in the sun, and the planes towed vapor trails across the big, clean sky. The wounded sat stiffly in the trucks, and they rose tautly when they came to a rut in the frozen road. The dust of the road had made their hair gray, but it did not look strange because their faces were old with suffering and fatigue.[46]

The Third Army Attack

The relief of Bastogne was one consequence of the Third Army counterattack against the southern flank of the Bulge. To launch this attack, General Patton's army performed the considerable tactical and logistical feat of disengaging from a planned offensive northeastward across the Saar River, shifting a good part of its combat strength from its right to its left wing and making a 90-degree change in the axis of its line of communications. Patton received directions for this movement from SHAEF and the 12th Army Group on 18–19 December and at the same time took over the VIII Corps from the First Army. Three days of hasty consultation, planning, and staff work ensued. On the morning of the twenty-second, the day Patton had promised Eisenhower he would attack, the III Corps,[47] with the 4th Armored and the 26th and 80th Infantry Divisions, opened its drive toward Bastogne. The XII Corps rearranged its forces and attacked on the right of the III Corps. The remaining Third Army corps, the XX, extended its line to defend what had been the main army front east of the Moselle.

With the other army staff agencies, the army medical service hastily made plans and preparations to support the new attack. The army surgeon, Colonel Hurley, with his staff section, throughout the campaign remained at Nancy with the rear echelon of Third Army headquarters. A small medical liaison group, headed by the chief surgical consultant, Colonel Odom, joined Patton's forward tactical command post at the city of Luxembourg. Hurley also dispatched liaison officers

[46] Surgical consultant quoted in Surg, 101st Airborne Division, Annual Rpt, 1944, pp. 12–13. *Stars and Stripes* quotation from Rapport and Northwood, *Rendezvous with Destiny*, pp. 596–97.

[47] The III Corps joined the Third Army just before the Ardennes battle and controlled the troops reducing the last forts around Metz until the army's turn northward.

to the III and VIII Corps, to keep him informed about the rapidly changing situation. He especially needed information about the newly acquired and badly disorganized VIII Corps. Hurley's executive officer, Lt. Col. John B. Coates, MC, who now, as he had throughout the campaign, bore the burden of directing day-to-day army medical operations, reported that at first "nobody in Third Army knew where VIII Corps was, specifically. We didn't even know where the VIII Corps headquarters was." The corps, in turn, was equally uncertain of the whereabouts of its medical units. Coates, therefore, sent two officers of his section forward to find the corps and establish communications with them, a task which took three or four days.[48]

With the VIII Corps the Third Army acquired a few nondivisional medical units in its new main area of operations, notably the 64th Medical Group and the 107th and 110th Evacuation Hospitals. To reinforce these, the army surgeon conducted a rapid large-scale redeployment of forces. As of 16 December the army's eleven evacuation hospitals and three medical groups all were located along or east of the Moselle; a number of hospitals were moving, or preparing to move, still farther to the eastward to support the projected attack across the Saar. One medical depot company, the 33d, also was shifting eastward from Toul to Chateau-Salins. Within about a week Hurley and Coates transferred six evacuation hospitals to Arlon, the city of Luxembourg, Longuyon, and Montmedy, close behind the III and VIII Corps. Two medical groups, the 65th and 69th, went to Esch, south of the Luxembourg capital and on the new main line of evacuation to the army and ADSEC holding units at Etain and Thionville. The 33d Medical Depot Company changed its destination to Longuyon.

To make these movements in so short a time, over a constricted roadnet jammed with thousands of other troops, Colonel Hurley and his subordinates dispensed with most administrative formalities. Organizations acted on verbal instructions. "The written orders," Hurley reported, "were confirmatory." Colonel Coates, who directed much of the operation, recalled that "everybody picked up as they could pick up, and started moving as quickly as possible. . . . It was first come almost first served that got on the roads." Much depended on the resourcefulness of veteran medical group, hospital, battalion, and depot commanders. These men, according to Coates, "with minimum direction . . . were able to pick up and on their own carry out a broad directive to get to some place at such and such a time the best you can." Evacuation hospitals, for instance, rushed advance parties, often recalled from scouting trips east of the Moselle, to the new locations to find usable buildings. They borrowed trucks from each other to haul people and equipment. Their personnel

[48] Quotation from Editorial Advisory Board, 1962, pp. 209–10. See also Surg, Third U.S. Army, Annual Rpt, 1944, pp. 57–58. For tactical developments, see Cole, *Ardennes*, chs. XX, XXI, and XXIV. Martin Blumenson, *The Patton Papers*, 2 vols. (Boston: Houghton Mifflin Co., 1972–74), vol. 2, *1885–1940*, pp. 595–604, recounts army headquarters conferences and planning.

worked hard and rapidly to adapt often less than suitable accommodations for hospital use.[49]

As a result of this rapid redeployment of army medical forces, the divisions attacking northward had little difficulty with evacuation, even though they suffered heavy casualties. The clearing stations of the 4th Armored Division, for example, handled 450–500 patients every twenty-four hours for five days. Early in the offensive the III Corps had to send some of its wounded by ambulance 60 miles back to Metz, for lack of facilities nearer the front. Within days, however, evacuation hosptials were pushing up close behind the corps. The 64th and 65th Medical Groups established ambulance regulating stations at Virton, Arlon, and Luxembourg City to control the flow of patients rearward from the clearing stations. Evacuation from the army to the Communications Zone continued with little change, because the Etain and Thionville rail and air holding units set up earlier in the campaign could receive patients from the north as easily as from the east.[50]

Even as the counteroffensive went on, the Third Army surgeon undertook an emergency effort to reequip the VIII Corps units that had been hit hardest in the initial German attack. These included two platoons of the 42d Field Hospital, several elements of the 28th Division, and the 326th Airborne Medical Company, all of which needed complete new outfits. Other organizations, such as the 107th Evacuation Hospital, had suffered less total but still significant losses. Colonel Hurley arranged for VIII Corps units to draw materiel directly from the COMZ medical depot at Reims, as well as from his two army depot companies. He also set up a temporary VIII Corps supply dump, stocked from the 32d Medical Depot Company at Metz, to fill emergency requisitions from the 64th Medical Group and the evacuation hospitals. For the airborne medical company Hurley had a set of equipment flown to Metz, where 101st Division trucks picked it up. As a result of these efforts all the worst-depleted organizations were in the process of reconstituting themselves by the beginning of the new year.[51]

Southern Encore: Operation NORDWIND

On the last day of 1944, as the Ardennes offensive was losing momentum, German forces in northern Alsace and along the Rhine launched *Operation NORDWIND,* a major assault on the Seventh Army. That army was spread thin along a right-angled front of over 100 miles, recently extended

[49] Hurley quotation from Surg, Third U.S. Army, Annual Rpt, 1944, p. 53; pp. 47–58 and 169–70 detail unit movements. Coates reminiscences in Editorial Advisory Board, 1962, pp. 208–10. See 64th Medical Group Annual Rpt, 1944, p. 9. For examples of evacuation hospital movements, see 101st and 104th Evacuation Hospitals Annual Rpts, 1944, and 12th Evac Hist, pp. 64–66.

[50] Surg, Third U.S. Army, Annual Rpt, 1944, pp. 79 and 90; Surg, III Corps, After-Action Rpt, December 1944, in Surg, III Corps, Annual Rpt, 1944; Surg, 4th Armored Division, Annual Rpt, 1944, p. 12 and encl. 6; Surg, 10th Armored Division, Annual Rpt, 1944, pp. 11–14; 436th Medical Battalion Annual Rpt, 1944, p. 3.

[51] Surg, Third U.S. Army, Annual Rpt, 1944, pp. 170–72; 64th Medical Group Rpt, 1944, p. 9; 326th Airborne Medical Company After-Action Rpt, Belgium and France, 17–28 Dec 44, p. 6.

to cover part of the ground formerly held by the Third Army. The Germans planned to exploit American weakness in this area by a three-pronged drive from the north, from the east across the Rhine, and from the south out of their Colmar bridgehead, aimed at destroying divisions and recapturing the politically symbolic city of Strasbourg. SHAEF, the 6th Army Group, and the Seventh Army anticipated this blow. Late in December the army developed contingency plans for withdrawing its right-flank corps, the VI from the Alsatian plain to a better defensive position on the eastern slope of the lower Vosges.

When the Germans launched their attack form the north, around midnight on 31 December, hitting the junction between the XV and VI Corps, the 6th Army Group, at SHAEF recommendation, directed the Seventh Army to execute the withdrawal. The Free French government of General Charles de Gaulle, however, objected vehemently to this maneuver, which entailed abandonment of Strasbourg. At the same time the front-line divisions of the Seventh Army contained and blunted the initial German assault while surrendering a minimum of ground. On 4 January 1945, in light of these facts, the Allies reversed their eariler decision. The Seventh Army received orders to hold its line in Alsace and defend Strasbourg. It did so in a month of bitter fighting, which ended in the complete defeat of the *NORDWIND* attack.[52]

The abortive general withdrawal resulted in much marching and countermarching of Seventh Army medical units. Under the late-December contingency plan the Seventh Army was to pull back almost all its medical installations in the Alsatian plain to towns on the western side of the Vosges. Accordingly, during the first days of January, the 2d Convalescent and 9th Evacuation Hospitals fell back from relatively exposed Sarrebourg, respectively to Epinal and Rambervillers. The 117th Evacuation Hospital at the same time retreated from its advanced position at Phalsbourg to Epinal. At that point, cancellation of the strategic withdrawal interrupted the medical redeployment, to the confusion of some units. The 95th Evacuation Hospital, for example, left Mutzig, just west of Strasbourg, on 3 January and made its way to Epinal in bitter cold, over mountain roads slippery with ice. Hardly had it reached its destination when the commanding officer received telephone orders to return to Mutzig at once, as the Seventh Army wanted forward hospitals after all. The 95th left that night for its old station and the next day was back in at least limited operation there. It continued work in Mutzig until the eighth, when it moved northwestward to Sarrebourg to help handle casualties from the main German attack on the XV and VI Corps. The 132d Evacuation Hospital, also located at Mutzig, withdrew to Epinal on the third, spent one night in bivouac there, and then

[52] Seventh U.S. Army Report of Operations 1944–1945, vol. II, chs. XXII and XXIII, and vol. III, pp. 943 and 977–78; History of the Medical Activities of VI Corps, January–June 1945 (hereafter cited as VI Corps Hist), p. 1.

moved to Sarrebourg, where it went into operation.[53]

In spite of all this backing and filling, Seventh Army medical units handled the roughly 9,000 wounded and 17,000 sick and injured of the *NORDWIND* battles with no more difficulty than was to be expected in winter combat. Several infantry regiments gave ground under the impact of the German assault; they did so gradually, evacuating their wounded and pulling back their aid stations in good order. As had been the case in the Ardennes withdrawals, the field hospital platoons attached to clearing stations had difficulty coordinating their movements with those of the divisions and complained of a shortage of transportation, but Seventh Army field hospital elements, in contrast to those in the Ardennes, suffered no equipment or personnel losses. The lot of the casualties in this winter fighting, nevertheless, was far from easy. Cold and exposure worsened the condition of many wounded men, as did the long ambulance hauls necessitated by the early retreat of some field hospital platoons and evacuation hospitals. Yet thanks to the Seventh Army's success in checking the German drive almost before it got started, the medical support problems of this southern encore to the Ardennes counterblow were minor ones and rapidly solved.[54]

Overcoming Adversity

Taken as a whole, the field army medical service suffered comparatively little damage from, and responded efficiently to, the German counteroffensive. The First Army lost significant numbers of patients, medical personnel, and equipment in the divisions initially overrun, although the great depth of the division support areas normally permitted collecting and clearing stations to extricate themselves more or less intact. As a result of unit withdrawals and redeployment, the First Army also temporarily became unable to hold and treat its sick and wounded. Nevertheless, emergency care and evacuation within the army went on throughout the battle, and, when necessary, COMZ facilities assumed some of the functions of army hospitals. The Third Army medical service speedily altered its focus of operations and took over support of those First Army elements cut off from their parent command by the enemy breakthrough. In addition, it assembled medical personnel and supplies for the relief of Bastogne. Within Bastogne 101st Airborne Division medics overcame an initial disaster, successfully improvised hospitals, and kept most of their wounded in reasonably good condition until they could be evacuated.

These achievements resulted in large part from a high order of army medical service performance, on the

[53] Surg, Seventh U.S. Army, Annual Rpt, 1944, p. 22, and the Semiannual Rpts, January–June 1945, for the following units: Seventh U.S. Army, pt. I; 95th Evacuation Hospital, encl. 1; 116th Evacuation Hospital, p. 1; 117th Evacuation Hospital, p. 1; and 132d Evacuation Hospital, p. 8 (see also pp. 1–2).

[54] Seventh U.S. Army Report of Operations, 1944–1945, vol. II, pp. 563–74, and vol. III, pp. 1,033–34; Surg, Seventh U.S. Army, Semiannual Rpt, January–June 1945, pt. I and pt. III, p. 34; Surg, 44th Infantry Division, Semiannual Rpt, January–June 1945, pp. 1–2; Surg, 45th Infantry Division, Periodic Rpt, January–June 1945, pt. 1; VI Corps Hist, p. 1; 57th Field Hospital Semiannual Rpt, January–June 1945, pp. 1–3 and 6–7.

part of both individuals and organizations, but a number of other circumstances also contributed to the outcome. One was German tactical failure. The enemy never penetrated beyond the rear boundaries of the First Army and fell entirely short of their goal of disrupting the Allies' logistics system. In addition, the Germans lacked the air power to interdict American road movements, including movement of casualties and medical units. The medical service benefited from the lavish transportation resources of the American army. The First Army alone had the use of almost 50,000 vehicles during the first week of the offensive. By regular or irregular means, enterprising medics obtained enough of these, most of the time, for themselves, their patients, and their equipment. The medical service itself had a plethora of resources at every level. At Bastogne, for instance, the 101st Airborne Division could spare enough doctors and technicians from its tactical units to staff a hospital and could equip and supply it with the residue left from earlier retreats. In this aspect of the battle as in others, "the much criticized weight of the American logistic 'tail' " enhanced the army's capacity to cope with unanticipated contingencies.[55]

The army medical service in the Ardennes possessed still another advantage: the proximity of well-developed COMZ evacuation facilities, hospitals, and supply depots. By mid-December the long effort to fill out the logistical support system attenuated by the summer pursuit largely had achieved its objective. The medical Communications Zone was in a position to relieve the armies of their casualties and replace promptly their personnel and equipment losses. The effort to do so, however, combined with the strains of supporting the earlier American offensive and building up COMZ facilities, brought to a head for the COMZ medical service a number of problems and deficiencies that had existed since the beginning of continental operations.

[55] For discussion of American transportation and logistical advantages, see Cole, *Ardennes*, pp. 665–66. Quotation on p. 666.

CHAPTER XIII

Completing COMZ

When the heavy fall and winter fighting began in November 1944, the Communications Zone still was in the process of developing intermediate and forward logistical support facilities and moving men and materiel inland from the beaches. It continued these efforts during the months of Allied attack and German counterattack, and at the same time it shifted its main logistics axis northward from Normandy to Antwerp and kept necessities flowing to the hard-pressed armies. As the First and Third Armies completed the eradication of the Bulge late in February 1945, the Communications Zone at last was coming into its full powers. Having mastered most of its major problems of supply, transportation, and evacuation, it was ready to provide the wherewithal for the coup-de-grace against Nazi Germany. This achievement, however, came at the cost of a winter of turmoil, controversy, and crisis.

The theater medical service endured and overcame its share of these troubles and contributed its share of the achievements. During the winter ETO medics completed their organization and established and confirmed command relations among their own elements and with other COMZ and field force agencies. They finished their troop buildup and coped with a variety of personnel shortages and problems. They rounded out their continental depot structure, established uniformity and efficiency in depot operations, and transferred the bulk of their supplies forward from the beaches and ports. They expanded and filled in their continental hospitalization and evacuation systems and managed, though with difficulty, to accommodate the heavy, sustained flow of casualties from the winter battles. At the same time they resolved policy controversies over evacuation, especially from the theater to the United States, which had persisted since D-Day.

The Chief Surgeon and Command Relations

Throughout the vicissitudes of the continental campaign General Hawley maintained his dominance over the increasingly widespread and organizationally compartmentalized theater medical service. By early 1945 he had under his supervision almost a quarter of a million people—in two army groups, four field armies, a fluctuating number of base sections, and hundreds of individual units. To hold onto his authority over all these forces, Hawley had to navigate through continuing crosscurrents of administrative conflict.

He had the advantage of a large, comparatively stable, and expert corps of assistants. His Paris staff consisted, in December 1944, of 102 officers, 269 enlisted men, and 26 civilians—the largest in the Medical Department outside that of the Office of the Surgeon General (*see Chart 10*). Key division chiefs, such as Gordon in Preventive Medicine, Hays in Supply, and McNinch in Medical Records, had learned their jobs during the long buildup in Great Britain and stayed in their positions throughout the campaign. The most significant high-level change came in February 1945, when Colonel Kimbrough left Professional Services to return to the United States; he was replaced by the equally experienced Colonel Cutler, who also continued as chief consultant in surgery. The staff divisions also remained stable, except for the addition, early in January, of a new Field Survey Division, created by Hawley to seek out and report deficiences in all nonclinical aspects of the medical service. This able staff, with a wealth of information and an extensive network of acquaintances and contacts throughout the American and Allied forces, decisively strengthened Hawley's hand in the persistent theater squabbling over administrative authority.[1]

Combining the ETO and COMZ headquarters early in 1944 did not end the jockeying for power between air, ground, and service commands. Indeed, the SHAEF and 12th Army Group staffs asserted their claims with increasing force. As a result, the United States high command went into operation on the Continent amid continued wrangling about the distribution, boundaries, and dimensions of authority, especially in matters of theater administration and logistics. Shortly before D-Day the American staff at Supreme Headquarters made an attempt, which General Lee blocked, to take over the theater-level functions of the Communications Zone. On D-Day itself Eisenhower, in his order formally redesignating the Services of Supply as the Communications Zone, relieved Lee of his duties as deputy ETO commander. But Lee's headquarters continued to perform most theater administrative tasks, and Lee's chiefs of technical services, such as Hawley, remained the theater chiefs of services. Nevertheless, the Americans on the SHAEF staff claimed extensive but loosely defined rights to intervene in ETO matters, especially those involving coordination or resolution of disputes between the air forces, the 12th Army Group and its component armies, and COMZ.

Resentment and distrust abounded between General Bradley's 12th Army Group headquarters and that of the Communications Zone. The tension

[1] Armfield, *Organization and Administration*, p. 341; Professional Services Division, OofCSurg, HQ, ETOUSA, Semiannual Rpt, January–June 1945, p. 2; Field Survey Division, OofCSurg, HQ, ETOUSA, Semiannual Rpt, January–June 1945, pp. 1–7 and 10–11. Administration Division, OofCSurg, HQ, ETOUSA, Annual Rpt, 1944, encl. 3, lists Hawley's principal subordinates at the end of 1944. Personnel Division, OofCSurg, HQ, ETOUSA, Annual Rpt, 1944, encl. 4(b), gives the strength of the staff. Middleton Interv, 1968–69, vol. 1, pp. 249–50, NLM, comments on Kimbrough's removal.

stemmed from the army group staff's conviction that, like its British counterpart, it should control COMZ, rather than being coordinate with the service forces under a theater headquarters that in fact was also the logistical headquarters. For a month after its activation on 1 August the 12th Army Group actually possessed authority over COMZ, but this arrangement ended when SHAEF moved to Versailles in September and took direct command of land operations. Essentially, the army group staff accused the Communications Zone of conflict of interest. They claimed that COMZ consistently favored its own requirements, and often its creature comforts, over the needs of the fighting forces and blamed this fact for the supply shortages that dogged the armies throughout late 1944. They condemned Lee's early transfer of COMZ headquarters to Paris for disrupting the supply services at a crucial point in the campaign. Similar resentment of the service command permeated the armies. The field forces tried to promote their interests by increasing SHAEF's involvement in theater affairs, especially in the allocation of supplies.[2]

Throughout the arguments over administrative authority General Hawley consistently asserted the principle that "there is no Chief Surgeon C[OM]Z. There is a Chief Surgeon, ETO, who is also Surgeon, C[OM]Z." He made his position prevail through a judicious mixture of firmness and conciliation. With General Kenner at SHAEF, Hawley had what he later characterized as "very friendly associations . . . , but not very close." On the Continent, as in Britain, Kenner and his small staff kept busy with a constant round of inspections of British and American medical installations. He conferred frequently with Hawley and Hawley's division heads on ETO problems of hospitalization, evacuation, and supply. Kenner reported regularly to Eisenhower, who considered him "one of the finest medical officers I have ever met."[3]

Nevertheless, Kenner's authority over U.S. Army medical matters remained more formal than substantive. His office transmitted policy directives to the armies; he tried to impose his views in a few instances, notably in reducing theater evacuation policy from 180 to 120 days and in changing the cross-Channel sea evacuation route. For the most part, however, his instructions and recommendations paralleled or repeated those of General Hawley, and Hawley managed to sidetrack them when they did not. Hawley, on his part, appears to have

[2] Ruppenthal, *Logistical Support*, 1:222–27, 2:26–27 and 349–51, summarizes the continuing conflicts. For an example of the 12th Army Group's view, see Memo, Brig Gen R. G. Moses to Gen Bradley, 26 Sep 44, and Paper by Moses, October 1945, both in Moses Papers, MHI. The Supreme Commander's views on how the system should work can be found in Dwight D. Eisenhower, *The Papers of Dwight David Eisenhower* (hereafter cited as *Eisenhower Papers*), eds. Alfred D. Chandler, Jr., et al. (Baltimore: Johns Hopkins Press, 1970–), vols. 1–5, *The War Years* (1970), 4:2,206. Memo, Maj Gen LeRoy Lutes to Lt Gen Somervell, 31 Dec 44, box 24, RG 160, NARA, reflects SHAEF's dissatisfaction with COMZ.

[3] First quotation from Ltr, Hawley to CofS, ETOUSA, 29 Sep 44, file HD 024 ETO CS (Hawley Chron). Second quotation from Editorial Advisory Board, 1962, p. 224. Third quotation from Ltr, Eisenhower to Gen Marshall, 28 Sep 44, in *Eisenhower Papers*, 4:2,196.

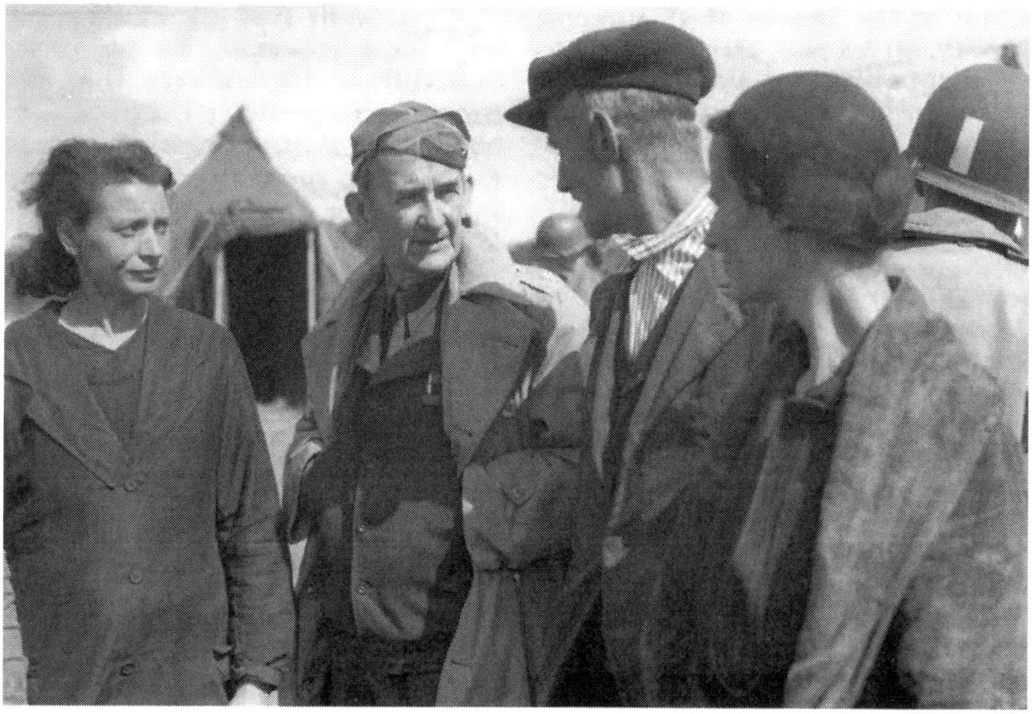

GENERAL KENNER ON ONE OF HIS MANY INSPECTION TRIPS *in northern France*

worked through Kenner, or gone around him as he thought expedient in particular situations. Yet American medical officers, in the armies and COMZ alike, generally thought of themselves as working primarily for Hawley and recalled Hawley as the dominant individual in shaping theater medical policies.[4]

[4] Kenner's activities can be followed in Medical Division, COSSAC/SHAEF, War Diary, August 1944–February 1945. For medical officer views, see Davis Interv, 19 Jun 45, box 222, RG 112, NARA, and, in file HD 000.71, CMH, the following: Interv, OSG with Maj Gen Albert W. Kenner, MC, 12 Jul 49; Gorby Interv, 1949; Interv, OSG with Brig Gen Alvin L. Gorby, MC, 22 Jun 53 (hereafter cited as Gorby Interv, 1953); Interv, OSG with Col Charles H. Beasley, 29 Sep 50; and Spruit Interv, 1949. Also in CMH, see Hartford Interv, 7–8 Oct 80, tape 1, side 1. On the theater evacuation policy, see Chapter XIV of this volume.

Hawley's success in maintaining cordial working relationships with the army groups and armies, despite the general field force mistrust of COMZ, removed what could have been the occasion for more frequent and forceful intervention by General Kenner in ETO medical affairs. Colonels Gorby and Reeder, respectively, the 12th and 6th Army Group surgeons, maintained liaison with both Kenner and Hawley, although Reeder's relations with the latter were attenuated by the connection of 6th Army Group to the separate Southern Line of Communications. In spite of the tension between the 12th Army Group and COMZ Gorby, relatively junior in rank and with a small staff, showed no disposition to assert his independence of the theater chief surgeon. Hawley, on his part, carefully respected the position of the group surgeons, such as it was, in the medical chain of command and sometimes called on them for assistance in resolving difficulties with the armies, which dealt directly with the Communications Zone on many medical as well as other logistical matters.[5]

Hawley dealt circumspectly with the army surgeons. When necessary, he emphatically reminded them that he was the theater, not merely COMZ, chief surgeon and that the entire medical service, from front to rear, had to work as a unified system. However, he preferred to rely on conciliation to secure cooperation, exploiting to the limit his range of contacts and acquaintances within and outside the Medical Department. He was willing to overlook minor infringements upon his prerogatives. He commented after the war: "I just rode out these little things and they all eventually straightened out. I thought it would do more harm in the long run than good to make an issue out of things." As often as he could, Hawley visited the army surgeons and their medical units. Several times he worked his way forward as far as the infantry battalion aid stations and came under German fire. He made these trips partly, he admitted, because "I was curious. . . . I'd gone to war. I wanted to see the fighting." He believed that when "you go forward to the battalion aid station and what's ahead of the battalion aid station, . . . you really find out what's going on." Most important, he sought to demonstrate his concern for the front-line surgeons and aidmen who bore such a disproportionate share of the hardship and danger. When at the front, Hawley emphasized helpfulness to the field army medical service, rather than criticism of it. This attitude, which the chief surgeon tried to instill throughout the COMZ medical organization, at least minimized in the theater medical service the endemic combat force distrust of the Communications Zone.[6]

Within the Communications Zone, base section boundaries changed repeatedly as the armies advanced and the Allied logistical base moved northward from Normandy toward the Channel ports and Antwerp (*Map 19*). On 1 December 1944 the Brittany Base Section absorbed the territory of the underemployed Loire Base Section, and the Normandy Base Section extended its jurisdiction toward the northeast, to include the American installations at Le Havre and Rouen, which had become major disembarkation ports for troops and supplies. The Channel Base Section, after giving up Rouen and Le Havre to Normandy, oversaw American activities in Antwerp and in a strip of Belgian territory between the British logistical area and the Advance Section. The other three base sections—ADSEC, Oise, and Seine—continued

[5] Ltr, Hawley to Gorby, 11 Aug 44, file HD 024 ETO CS (Hawley Chron); Gorby Intervs, 1949 and 1953, file HD 000.71, and 1962, pp. 7, 9–11, 13–14, 37, CMH; Hartford Interv, 7–8 Oct 80, tape 1, side 1, CMH.

[6] Quotations from Hawley Interv, 1962, pp. 68–71, 87–88, 98–102, CMH, which also contains comments from army-level medical officers. For Hawley's sterner approach, see Ltr, Hawley to Gorby, 11 Aug 44, file HD 024 ETO CS (Hawley Chron). See also Hartford Interv, 7–8 Oct 80, tape 1, side 1, CMH.

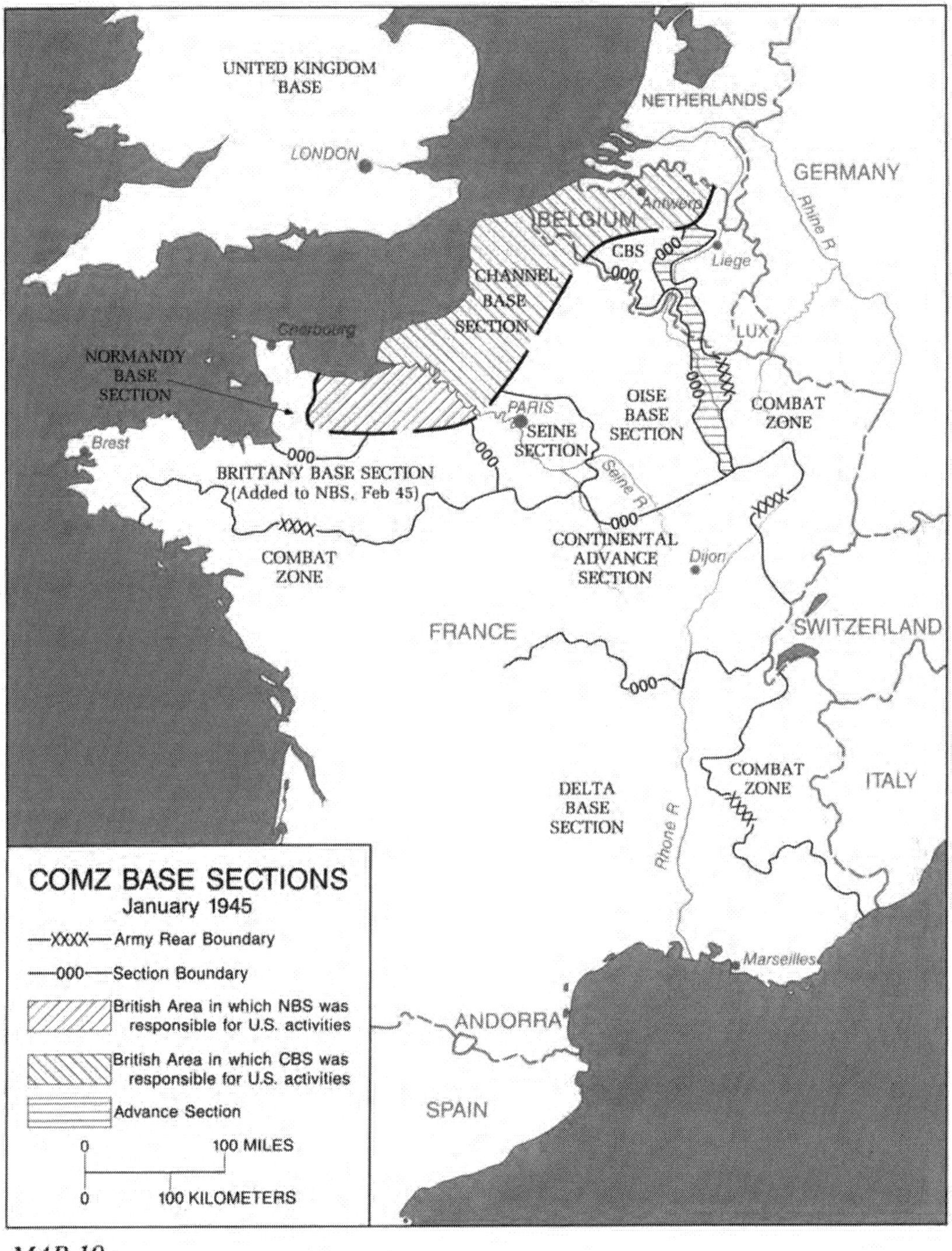
UNITED KINGDOM BASE
LONDON
NETHERLANDS
GERMANY
Rhine R
Antwerp
BELGIUM
CBS
Liege
CHANNEL BASE SECTION
LUX
Cherbourg
NORMANDY BASE SECTION
PARIS
OISE BASE SECTION
COMBAT ZONE
Brest
SEINE SECTION
BRITTANY BASE SECTION (Added to NBS, Feb 45)
Seine R
CONTINENTAL ADVANCE SECTION
COMBAT ZONE
Dijon
FRANCE
SWITZERLAND
COMBAT ZONE
ITALY
DELTA BASE SECTION
Rhone R
COMZ BASE SECTIONS
January 1945
XXXX Army Rear Boundary
000 Section Boundary
British Area in which NBS was responsible for U.S. activities
British Area in which CBS was responsible for U.S. activities
Advance Section
0 100 MILES
0 100 KILOMETERS
Marseilles
ANDORRA
SPAIN

MAP 19

their earlier functions, in some cases with slight boundary revisions.[7]

Authority over COMZ medical units and installations continued to be divided between the base section commanders, who had formal operational and administrative control over them, and General Hawley, who exercised technical supervision. In practice, Hawley, as he had in Great Britain, managed to expand technical supervision into what amounted to day-to-day direction, especially of the work of base section general hospitals. He resisted vigorously, and usually with success, occasional base section efforts to interfere in hospital command and administration. When necessary, Hawley appealed directly to the ETO-COMZ staff to overrule encroaching section commanders, but he relied more often on his ability to convince the commanders that they would serve their own interests best by doing what he wanted. He demonstrated this method in persuading the Normandy Base Section commander, Col. Theodore Wyman, to replace an inexperienced section surgeon with one better qualified and selected by him. The chief surgeon wrote to Wyman:

> I am too old a soldier not to know that the authority of a commander is practically unlimited, and that, if he so desires, he can dictate the technical operations of the services without regard to the policies of the Chiefs of Services. I also have great respect for the responsibilities and prerogatives of command.
>
> However, I have also a great responsibility to my own commander. So long as my technical policies are carried out in any echelon, and medical units are not hampered in their functions, I shall accept full responsibility for all medical failures. But, if the technical operations of the medical service are interfered with by the commander of any echelon, I have no alternative than to place squarely upon him the responsibility for any medical failure in his echelon.[8]

After moving to Paris in June 1944, Hawley enlarged upon his formal and informal techniques for keeping close watch over the medical service and enforcing high standards of professional care and compassion for the individual casualty. He continued to employ his consultants, and those of the armies and base sections, as a communication and control network, and he supplemented them in early 1945 with the new Field Survey Division. This division, Hawley told its chief, Lt. Col. Clark B. Meador, MC, one of his veteran troubleshooters, was to "act as the eyes and ears of the Chief Surgeon; and to assist Medical commanders in the field in carrying out the policies dictated by this office or higher headquarters." Hawley responded forcefully to patient complaints, from whatever source. For example, late in 1944 a number of GIs in letters to the *Stars and Stripes* made allegations of poor food, excessive inspections, and lack of amenities in general hospitals. Hawley at once directed members of his staff and the base section surgeons to survey the

[7] Troops Branch, Operations Division, OofCSurg, HQ, ETOUSA, Semiannual Rpt, January-June 1945, p. 10; Surg, Normandy Base Section, Semiannual Rpt, January-June 1945, p. 2. Ruppenthal, *Logistical Support*, 2:37-38, summarizes base section boundary changes.

[8] Quotation from Ltr, Hawley to Col Theodore Wyman, Jr., 1 Aug 44, file HD 024 ETO CS (Hawley Chron). For other examples of his methods, in same file, see Memos, Hawley to AG Personnel, ETO, 27 and 29 Jul 44, and Memo, Hawley to CofS, ETO, 30 Nov 44.

nonclinical aspects of patient care. Then he pressed section surgeons and hospital commanders to correct the minor but irritating deficiencies the surveys revealed.[9]

Hawley himself frequently inspected COMZ medical installations. When doing so, the chief surgeon, besides making ward rounds and discussing professional matters with commanders and chiefs of services, also paid attention to aspects of unit operations that many medical officers would have overlooked. At the 21st General Hospital, for instance, Hawley and his staff were invited to inspect the guard detachment.[10] To the amusement of the hospital commander, Hawley "did a good infantry officer's job of the details of seizing the rifles and upending them to squint through the barrels. Then he slammed the rifles almost viciously into the guard's hands. The guard and all the onlookers were surprised and pleased. He did not neglect to say a few words to the officer and his detail which made them feel well flattered." Hawley came down hard on the commanders of installations that fell short of his standards, on the principle that "there are no poor units; there are only poor leaders." He wrote personal letters of admonition to delinquent commanders and, if deficiencies in their units persisted, had the officers reassigned. Even minor lapses by medical personnel did not escape the chief surgeon's sharp eye. He warned the commander of the 12th Field Hospital: "A group of your nurses was seen in Paris a few days ago in improper uniform and generally untidy. I am very sorry to have heard this and I do not want to hear such a report again." [11]

During the autumn and winter of 1944–45 Hawley maneuvered to extend his authority over the medical units of the separate communications zone behind the 6th Army Group. That group, while it came under SHAEF operational control in mid-September, continued to draw its logistical support largely from the Mediterranean Theater of Operations, which had mounted the invasion of southern France. By 1 October the Mediterranean Theater had established two base sections to operate the line of communications running from Marseilles northward up to the Rhone valley. The Delta Base Section, under Brig. Gen. John P. Ratay, controlled the installations around Marseilles. The Continental Advance Section (CONAD), under Maj. Gen. Arthur R. Wilson, performed functions for the 6th Army Group similar to those of ADSEC. Both sections were part of the Mediterranean Theater Communications Zone, which established a forward headquarters at Dijon to supervise their work.

---

[9] Quotation from Field Survey Division, OofCSurg, HQ, ETOUSA, Semiannual Rpt, January–June 1945, p. 1. For hospital complaints and Hawley's response, see letters and memorandums for December 1944 in file HD 024 ETO CS (Hawley Chron).

[10] Hospital units maintained armed guard forces to protect their property and to supervise POW laborers.

[11] First and second quotations from Cady, "Notes on the 21st General Hospital (AUS)," pp. 507–09, Cady Papers, MHI. Third quotation from Ltr, Hawley to CO, 12th Field Hospital, 14 Sep 44, file HD 024 ETO CS (Hawley Chron). For examples of Hawley's dealing with delinquent commanders, see Ltrs, Hawley to CO, 90th General Hospital, 14 Sep 44, and Hawley to Col H. H. Price, 10 Nov 44, file HD 024 ETO CS (Hawley Chron).

General Lee and his staff wanted to assume command over the southern line of communications as soon as possible. They intended to enforce uniform policies and procedures throughout supply organizations that they assumed would become increasingly interdependent. The SHAEF staff, however, preferred to delay the merger in order to take maximum advantage of the surplus supplies available in the Mediterranean Theater during a period when the northern Communications Zone barely could support the 12th Army Group, not to mention the 6th. After weeks of negotiation the two theaters agreed on a compromise. They created a new organization, the Southern Line of Communications (SOLOC) around the nucleus of the Mediterranean COMZ advance headquarters at Dijon. This agency, activated on 20 November under Maj. Gen. Thomas B. Larkin, was a subdivision of the ETO Communications Zone, with Larkin designated a deputy commander COMZ under General Lee. However, SOLOC had the right to communicate directly with the Mediterranean Theater on matters of logistical support, and it was the sole channel for contact between the ETO-COMZ headquarters and CONAD, the Delta Base Section, and their subordinate units.[12]

Under the terms of this agreement, and of General Lee's letter of instructions to General Larkin, Hawley could deal with the CONAD surgeon, Col. Harry A. Bishop, MC; the Delta Base Section surgeon, Col. Vinnie H. Jeffress, MC; and the commanders of the fifteen fixed hospitals, two depots, and other medical installations in southern France only through Col. Charles F. Shook, MC, the SOLOC surgeon. Hawley's staff division chiefs could not correspond directly with their southern counterparts on any of the innumerable details of bringing SOLOC medical policies and procedures, derived from the Mediterranean Theater, into line with ETO practices. Problems resulted, for differences among the theater medical organizations were many, ranging from broad matters of supply management to questions of clinical procedure. SOLOC hospitals, for instance, treated many long-bone fractures by internal fixation (plating and pinning), whereas those in the European Theater followed the preferences of Surgeon General Kirk by relying exclusively on traction, followed by application of casts. Distressed at this and other SOLOC practices, Hawley periodically lamented the limitations on his authority in the southern area. He complained that the Southern Line of Communications "was given what amounts to complete autonomy. Believe it or not, I practically have to be invited before I can visit SOLOC." [13]

[12] Southern France, until September 1944, had been part of the North African (later Mediterranean) Theater; it reverted to the ETO on 18 September. Larkin had been commander of the Mediterranean Theater COMZ before taking over SOLOC. For details on the formation of SOLOC, see Ruppenthal, *Logistical Support*, 2:29–30 and 38–42.

[13] Quotation from Ltr, Hawley to Maj Gen J. E. Dahlquist, 11 Jan 45, box 2, Hawley Papers, MHI. See also Ruppenthal, *Logistical Support*, 2:42–45; Ltr, Lt Gen Lee to Chiefs, General and Special Staff

Continued

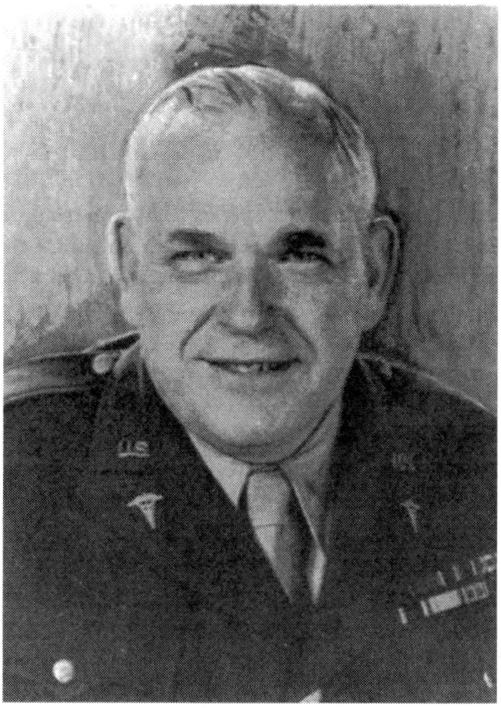

COL. CHARLES F. SHOOK

As in so many other instances, internal diplomacy within the theater medical service reduced the ill effects of divided authority. On 15–16 November Colonel Shook and his assistant visited Paris. They worked out an agreement with Colonel Cutler and other members of Hawley's staff on COMZ-SOLOC medical relations, covering general administrative principles and the details of hospitalization, evacuation, supply, records and reports, and the establishment of a consultant system for the southern base sections. The agreement reaffirmed Hawley's responsibility for "overall supervision of Medical Department technical matters" for all United States forces in the theater. It declared that Colonel Shook in SOLOC "will be guided by the technical policies and procedures that have been laid down by the Chief Surgeon, European Theater of Operations," that all ETO medical resources "will be considered as a pool of medical means, and [that] neither the Communications Zone in support of . . . [the 12th Army Group] nor that in support of the Southern Group of Armies will be considered as acting independently or as being self-sufficient." [14]

Personal and administrative relations between the two communications zones soon smoothed out. By late December Hawley was calling Shook's attitude "100 per cent" cooperative. After careful preparation, and after a delay caused by the Ardennes crisis, Hawley and Cutler made a five-day visit to the Southern Line of Communications in January. They

Secs, ETO-COMZ, 3 Nov 44, sub: Administrative Support for Southern Group of Armies and Attached Air Forces, copy in Planning Branch, Operations Division, OofCSurg, HQ, ETOUSA, Annual Rpt, 1944; Notes, Col R. E. Peyton, 17 Oct 44, sub: Visit to Dijon, DRAGOON 1944 file, CMH; Wiltse, *Mediterranean*, pp. 399–403. On internal fixation of fractures, see Ltrs, TSG to Hawley, 13 Dec 44 and 13 Jan 45, and Hawley to TSG, 29 Dec 44 and 27 Jan 45, file HD 024 ETO O/CS (Hawley-SGO Corresp).

[14] Quotation from MFR, Col D. E. Liston, 4 Dec 44, sub: Agreements Made at Conference, 15–16 November 1944, DRAGOON 1944 file, CMH. In same file, see MFR, Planning Branch, Operations Division, OofCSurg, HQ, ETOUSA, 10 Nov 44, sub: Support of DRAGOON Forces, and Memo, Lt Col J. H. Voegtly to Col Peyton, 18 Nov 44, sub: Notes Taken at Conference on Medical Service for Southern Group of Armies. See also Carter, ed., *Surgical Consultants*, 2:280–82, and Planning Branch, Operations Division, OofCSurg, HQ, ETOUSA, Annual Rpt, 1944, p. 13. Among other things, SOLOC committed itself at this time to adopt the ETO system of medical statistical reports.

conferred with Shook and his base section surgeons, and also with Colonel Rudolph, the Seventh Army surgeon, and they inspected numerous medical installations. During this trip Cutler secured SOLOC's agreement that its base section consultants could communicate directly with their ETO counterparts, integrating the southern consultants into the informal network so important in holding the theater medical service together. Hawley and Cutler at the same time gave a little ground on internal fixation of fractures, authorizing use of the procedure in certain types of cases. Through such arrangements the chief surgeon and his staff cleared the way for a full merger, and the two communications zone medical services became ever more closely integrated in supply, evacuation, and other activities. Formal merger followed on 6 February 1945, when the theater disbanded SOLOC and placed CONAD and the Delta Base Section directly under the northern Communications Zone. Colonel Shook then moved to Paris and became the ETO deputy chief surgeon.[15]

By the time the ETO-COMZ absorbed SOLOC, theater medical administrative and command relations had assumed the shape they would retain during the rest of the war in Europe. The primacy in the medical service that General Hawley had established during the buildup survived the entry into combat, the full activation of SHAEF and the 12th Army Group, and the incorporation of the forces from the Mediterranean. Throughout, the chief surgeon, while surrendering none of his prerogatives, managed to keep up smooth working relations with such potential rivals as General Kenner. Hawley's success earned the ETO medical service the praise of Surgeon General Kirk, who declared that this organization, compared to those of other theaters, was the "only [one] . . . set up and operating the way it should [be]. . . . It is so far ahead of the others there is no comparison."[16] The chief surgeon attained this favorable result despite blurred lines of authority and persistent feuds. His system, in the end, depended more on personal and professional doctor-to-doctor relationships than on sound structure. Nevertheless, it was sufficient to support the armies in their drive to final victory.

The Continuing Buildup

During the six months after D-Day the European Theater medical establishment expanded from about 130,000 officers, nurses, and enlisted men to over 212,000—an average of 5.5 doctors, 1.2 dentists, 6.3 nurses, and 68.35 medical enlisted men for each 1,000 soldiers (*Table 9*). It was, by the end of 1944, the largest single theater medical service, containing nearly 40 percent of all the Medical Department personnel in the Army.

[15] Hawley's remarks on Shook in Ltr, Hawley to Kenner, 19 Dec 44, file HD 024 ETO CS (Hawley Chron); in same file, see Ltr, Hawley to Col C. F. Shook, 23 Dec 44. Hawley's January visit is recounted in detail in Carter, ed., *Surgical Consultants*, 2:292 and 301–06. Ltrs, Hawley to TSG, 24 Jan 45, and TSG to Hawley, 17 Mar 45, file HD 024 ETO O/CS (Hawley-SGO Corresp), reflect the compromise on internal fixation. See also Ruppenthal, *Logistical Support*, 2:45.

[16] Ltr, TSG to Hawley, 18 Aug 44, file HD 024 ETO O/CS (Hawley-SGO Corresp).

TABLE 9—MEDICAL PERSONNEL STRENGTH, ETOUSA, LATE 1944

Personnel	October		November		December	
	Number	Percent	Number	Percent	Number	Percent
Officers						
Veterinary Corps	105	.06	111	.05	125	.06
Medical Corps	10,921	6.25	12,664	6.14	13,162	6.19
Sanitary Corps	378	.22	441	.21	465	.22
Dental Corps	2,633	1.51	2,960	1.43	3,175	1.49
Medical Administrative Corps	3,566	2.04	4,239	2.05	4,511	2.12
Army Nurse Corps	12,991	7.43	15,138	7.34	15,612	7.34
Other Corps	614	.36	699	.34	701	.33
Total	31,208	17.86	36,252	17.57	37,751	17.74
Warrant Officers	298	.17	370	.18	373	.18
Enlisted Men	143,266	81.97	169,687	82.25	174,653	82.08
Grand total	174,772	100.0	206,309	100.0	212,777	100.0

Source: Personnel Division, OofCSurg, HQ, ETOUSA, Annual Rpt, 1944, chart 5(d).

About 60 percent of the ETO medical personnel worked in the Communications Zone, another 35 percent served in the field armies, and the remainder were in the air forces.[17]

The composition of the medical service, in numbers and types of units, more or less conformed to the troop basis established before the invasion. However, the theater and the War Department continually added, deleted, formed, and disbanded organizations as they reconciled the projected with the actual needs of the campaign. The theater, for example, gained ten more general hospitals and almost fifty ground force medical units to support nine additional infantry divisions assigned during 1944. It broke up several station hospitals to create new T/O convalescent rehabilitation units and constantly shuffled manpower to meet the seemingly insatiable need for separate medical detachments and for casuals to staff base section and hospital center headquarters. Accounting changes brought troop basis alterations. Late in 1944 the War Department reclassified 14,400 field hospital beds as mobile instead of fixed, allowing the ETO the same number of additional beds in general or station hospitals. To absorb part of this extra allowance, the theater disbanded three newly arrived general hospitals in order to reorganize eight veteran ones as 1,500-bed hospitals and another as a 2,000-bed installation.[18]

New medical units of all types flowed into the theater during the last

[17] Personnel Division, OofCSurg, HQ, ETOUSA, Annual Rpt, 1944, app. D; McMinn and Levin, *Personnel*, p. 358.

[18] Troop Movements and Training Branch, Operations Division, OofCSurg, HQ, ETOUSA, Annual Rpt, 1944, pp. 6–10 and 38–39; Personnel Division, OofCSurg, HQ, ETOUSA, Annual Rpt, 1944, pp. 5–6 and 12–13; Troops Branch, Operations Division, OofCSurg, HQ, ETOUSA, Semiannual Rpt, January–June 1945, pp. 4, 6, 8–17, 34. Ruppenthal, *Logistical Support*, 2:289–90, describes the general changes in the service troop basis.

half of 1944 and the first few months of 1945, adhering generally to reinforcement schedules worked out before D-Day. Once these reinforcements reached Europe, General Hawley's Troop Movements and Training Branch staff, in coordination with the ETO G-4 and the base sections for COMZ units and with the 12th Army Group and later the Fifteenth Army for field force organizations, directed their movement and assignment. During the autumn of 1944 the Southern Line of Communications repeatedly demanded more field and communications zone medical units to support the additional divisions being sent to the 6th Army Group. The ETO-COMZ, in negotiations with SHAEF and SOLOC, managed to scale down these requests, on the grounds that all theater medical resources should be treated as a single pool, rather than each communications zone being set up as a self-sufficient entity. Medical reinforcements, nevertheless, did go to SOLOC, either diverted to Marseilles while at sea or sent across France after landing at Channel ports.[19]

Preinvasion plans called for new medical units, like most other reinforcements from America, to bypass the United Kingdom after about D+60 and land at ports on the Continent. Delays in opening deep-water French and Belgian harbors, however, compelled diversion of most units to Great Britain during the last half of 1944. Most medical units, therefore, entered the ETO at Scottish ports, staged in Britain for periods varying from a few hours to a couple of months, then went by train to the south coast, where they boarded landing craft or other shallow-draft vessels for the cross-Channel voyage. During the summer the reinforcements landed at Cherbourg or the Normandy beaches and bivouacked in the Cotentin until called forward to begin operations. Units arriving after the beginning of November usually disembarked at Le Havre and staged in the nearby RED HORSE cantonment area, which included a theater transient camp for medical troops at Etretat, a small seashore resort.

For the new arrivals life in the staging areas was often difficult. Frequently, units became separated from their personal baggage and TAT (to accompany troops) equipment during their journeys to France. Without cooking and mess gear, tentage, bedding, or vehicles, the unfortunate personnel set up housekeeping with what they could salvage and borrow. Officers, nurses, and enlisted men alike prepared C-rations over driftwood fires, shivered under too few blankets, and at times went for weeks without a change of clothing until their equipment finally caught up with them. Medical personnel awaiting movement orders at Etretat lived austerely in requisitioned homes, chateaus, and hotels, contending with shortages of fuel for cooking and heating and coping with insufficient latrine and bathing facilities. A few units suffered major accidents during disembarka-

[19] Troop Movements and Training Branch, Operations Division, OofCSurg, HQ, ETOUSA, Annual Rpt, 1944, pp. 13–15 and encls. 5 and 8; Troops Branch, Operations Division, OofCSurg, HQ, ETOUSA, Semiannual Rpt, January–June 1945, pp. 2–3, 12, 14, and encl. 1. For negotiations about units for SOLOC, see correspondence in DRAGOON 1944 file, CMH. For similar arguments about field units for the Seventh Army, see Chapter XI of this volume.

tion, staging, and forward movement. The 553d Medical Ambulance Company lost fifty-six men (thirty-two killed, twenty-four injured) in a train wreck near Le Havre. Staging could be prolonged, especially for general hospitals, which had to wait for sites to become available, for equipment assemblies to arrive, and for transportation to appear. The base sections tried to keep units busy during their time in staging, conducting orientation and training programs and sending personnel, particularly from hospitals, to reinforce hard-pressed organizations already in operation.[20]

The medical troop buildup substantially achieved its objectives, in terms of gross numbers of personnel and units. Strength totals, however, concealed many quantitative shortages and qualitative deficiencies. To begin with, the War Department, in order to place units in the theater on schedule, sent many of them overseas before they had completed their training. In all, 78 of the 151 general hospitals called for in the troop basis arrived "short-trained," as did 7 of the 46 400-bed evacuation hospitals, 11 of the 61 ambulance companies, and smaller proportions of other unit types. The short-trained organizations varied greatly in readiness for operations. Those that landed in Britain just before D-Day were short-trained only in the sense that a few individuals had not completed all requirements or that the unit perhaps lacked a week or so of field exercises. Such organizations could, and did, go right to work. The units that arrived later in 1944 were in worse shape. Most, activated only three–four weeks before embarkation, were random aggregations of medical officers and nurses with limited Army experience; the enlisted detachments, except for a few key men, came directly from basic Medical Department training. One such unit, the 166th General Hospital, which arrived in the Loire Base Section in November, "had never functioned as a hospital and only a small percentage of the enlisted men had ever worked in a hospital. . . . The nurses had joined the unit at the Port of Embarkation. They had never worked as a group." As these units reached the United Kingdom and France, base section and army surgeons surveyed their state of training; prescribed remedial programs of instruction; and, whenever possible, put their personnel to work in functioning installations of the same type, remedying manpower shortages while providing on-the-job training for the new arrivals. Eventually, most short-trained organizations went into satisfactory operation, though a few of the worst were broken up and their manpower used to reinforce more experienced units.[21]

[20] Operations Division, OofCSurg, HQ, ETOUSA, Annual Rpt, 1944, p. 5; Troop Movements and Training Branch, Operations Division, OofCSurg, HQ, ETOUSA, Annual Rpt, 1944, pp. 26–27; Troops Branch, Operations Division, OofCSurg, HQ, ETOUSA, Semiannual Rpt, January-June 1945, pp. 2–3, 6, 12–14; Surg, Channel Base Section, Annual Rpt, 1944, pp. 9–10 and 86–89. For examples of units in staging, see John C. Burwell, Jr., "Memoir," pp. 3–10, John C. Burwell Papers, MHI, and 170th General Hospital Annual Rpt, 1944, pp. 2–6 (this unit also was separated from its TAT equipment).

[21] Quotation from Surg, Loire Base Section, Annual Rpt, 1944, p. 3. See also ibid., p. 5; Troop Movements and Training Branch, Operations Division, OofCSurg, HQ, ETOUSA, Annual Rpt, 1944,

Continued

Most late-arriving medical units, besides being short of training, were short of people, either in absolute numbers or in important specialities. As a result of the policy forced on Surgeon General Kirk by the doctor shortage in the United States, most new hospitals arriving in Europe after D-Day lacked qualified chiefs of surgical and medical services and contained general practitioners in place of many specialists. Some general hospitals arrived in the theater with only 16 of their authorized 32 MC officers. Kirk expected the theaters—especially the ETO with its large complement of affiliated units top-heavy in professional talent—to make up these deficiencies by redistributing their own personnel. Typical of the units that this policy created, the 170th General Hospital embarked for Europe in September with "no Chief of Surgery, Medicine, Orthopedics, Neuropsychiatry, [and no] Urologist who was considered professionally qualified"; the orthopedic staff consisted of "two young officers with limited experience." [22]

The arrival of an increasing number of, in effect, undermanned organizations aggravated shortages in many categories of ETO medical personnel. MC specialists were spread ever more thinly. For instance, in early 1945, the theater had available only 63 board-certified orthopedic surgeons out of the 460 called for in the T/Os of army and COMZ hospitals and auxiliary surgical groups. They were supplemented by 95 partially trained orthopedic surgeons and by 85 others who had some background in trauma. Shortages also existed among dentists and MAC officers. The theater nurse complement had fallen 345 below authorized strength by the close of 1944, partly because the War Department, confronting a slowdown in recruiting and the probable need for a nurse draft, as a conservation measure dispatched 12 general hospitals to Europe without nurses, to be staffed from theater resources. Medical enlisted personnel also fell below strength at the end of 1944, largely as a result of heavy casualties among infantry division aidmen and litter-bearers.[23]

The ETO medical service did its best to remedy the shortages and deficiencies from its own resources. Colonels Cutler and Middleton and their assistants visited each newly landed general hospital to evaluate its professional staff. Using the Personnel Division's machine readable

pp. 9–10 and 25–26; Training Branch, Operations Division, OofCSurg, HQ, ETOUSA, Semiannual Rpt, January-June 1945, pp. 5–6. On training efforts, see Surg, Normandy Base Section, Annual Rpt, 1944, p. 3; Surg, Seine Section, Semiannual Rpt, January-June 1945, pp. 21–22; Surg, Seventh U.S. Army, Annual Rpt, 1944, p. 20.

[22] Quotation from 170th General Hospital Annual Rpt, 1944, pp. 1–2. See also Ltr, TSG to Hawley, 6 Oct 44, file HD 024 ETO O/CS (Hawley-SGO Corresp); Personnel Division, OofCSurg, HQ, ETOUSA, Annual Rpt, 1944, p. 7 and app. D; McMinn and Levin, *Personnel*, pp. 316–17. On the doctor shortage, see Chapter V of this volume.

[23] Personnel Division, OofCSurg, HQ, ETOUSA, Annual Rpt, 1944, app. D; Professional Services Division, OofCSurg, HQ, ETOUSA, Semiannual Rpt, January-June 1945, pp. 4–5; Troop Movements and Training Branch, Operations Division, OofCSurg, HQ, ETOUSA, Annual Rpt, 1944, p. 9; McMinn and Levin, *Personnel*, pp. 227–31; Ltrs, TSG to Hawley, 6 Oct 44, and Hawley to TSG, 13 Apr 45, file HD 024 ETO O/CS (Hawley-SGO Corresp); Memo, Hawley to DepTheaterCdr, 6 Jun 44, sub: Shortage of Nurses, file HD 024 ETO CS (Hawley Chron).

records of the qualifications and experience of every MC officer in Europe, the consultants arranged for transfers from veteran organizations to give the new hospitals at least adequate chiefs of surgery and medicine and as many needed specialists as possible. Army surgeons and their consultants, aided by the chief surgeon's office, similarly balanced and reinforced evacuation hospital staffs. To ensure full employment of scarce specialists, the Hospitalization Division, continuing on the Continent a practice begun in England, designated certain heavily staffed general hospitals as treatment centers for particular types of difficult cases. Staging medical units provided doctors, nurses, and enlisted men on temporary assignment to flesh out many organizations. By full exploitation of this source the theater maintained an adequate ratio of nurses to patients in its wards, in spite of the persistent numerical shortage. The ETO medical service relieved some scarcities by enhancing the skills of people it already had; the Nursing Division of General Hawley's office, for instance, established a four-week school to train hospital chief nurses. The United Kingdom Base and the Third Army both set up courses, with instructors drawn from their own hospitals, to develop additional officer and nurse anesthetists, partially remedying another perennial personnel scarcity. The 107th Evacuation Hospital, in order to take some of the burden from its one fully qualified orthopedic surgeon, trained its general surgeons in basic procedures for treating compound fractures and organized two teams of enlisted men skilled in applying plaster casts.[24]

The T/O reductions, ordered by the War Department for general and evacuation hospitals and for most other types of medical units, statistically erased many personnel shortages and actually freed people to fill vacancies. Thus a July 1944 cut in general hospital MC officer complements from 37 to 32 released over 450 ETO doctors for other assignments. To obtain nurses for the dozen general hospitals sent without them, the theater reduced all general hospital nurse complements from 83 to 73. Similar trimming of the enlisted strength of most unit types prevented, on paper at least, a shortage until late 1944. These and other reductions, however, left medical units with fewer people to do the same amount of work, and with reduced internal ability to compensate for staff casualties or to expand patient capacity in emergencies. In some instances the cuts severely hampered units in carrying out their basic missions. The commander of the 95th Evacuation Hospital complained, after a 5 percent reduction in his enlisted force:

---

[24] Personnel Division, OofCSurg, HQ, ETOUSA, Annual Rpt, 1944, pp. 7–8; Professional Services Division, OofCSurg, HQ, ETOUSA, Annual Rpt, 1944, Medical Consultation Service sec., pp. 3–4, and Chief Consultant in Orthopedic Surgery sec., pp. 4–5; Surg, United Kingdom Base, Annual Rpt, 1944, pp. 67–68, and Semiannual Rpt, January–June 1945, vol. 1, pp. 51–53; Surg, Seventh U.S. Army, Annual Rpt, 1944, p. 40. On the chief nurses, see Nursing Division, OofCSurg, HQ, ETOUSA, Annual Rpt, 1944, pp. 8 and 18, and Semiannual Rpt, January–June 1945, p. 1. On the anesthetists, see Professional Services Division, OofCSurg, HQ, ETOUSA, Annual Rpt, 1944, Chief Consultant in Anesthesia sec., pp. 1–2; Surg, Third U.S. Army, Annual Rpt, 1944, pp. 102–03; 107th Evacuation Hospital Annual Rpt, 1944, p. 22.

"It is inconceivable that anyone would think that an evacuation hospital could possibly function on a 24-hour schedule with only four men designated in the T/O as litter bearers." [25]

Such expedients enabled the ETO medical service to fill, at least partially, the ranks of its expanding number of units. Another personnel problem was more intractable: replacing over 560 officers, 400 nurses, and 4,900 enlisted men lost from various causes during 1944. Of these, about 160 officers and 3,100 men were killed, wounded, or captured in combat—the majority while serving as infantry battalion surgeons, company aidmen, and litterbearers. Attrition among these front-line medical people, who also contributed their share of non-battle casualties, was heavy and constant. In six months of fighting the 9th Infantry Division had to replace over 100 percent of its aidmen. Division medical losses approached the crisis point during the Ardennes and *NORDWIND* offensives; each of the field armies fell some 500 medical enlisted men understrength, and there was an urgent demand for over 300 replacement MC officers.[26]

The ETO medical service labored throughout the campaign under a chronic shortage of both officer and enlisted replacements. Replacements for the medical service, as for all other arms and technical services, were supposed to come from three sources: recovered sick and wounded released from the hospitals; personnel from units rendered surplus by T/O changes or transferred out for other reasons; and casuals sent from the United States in predetermined numbers, on theater requisition, specifically to replace losses. Early in 1944 the chief surgeon's Personnel Division worked up casualty projections for all categories of medical troops, based on World War I loss rates modified by World War II experience up to that point, and, on this basis, periodically requisitioned replacements from the United States. Due to the medical manpower shortage, however, the War Department never came close to filling these requisitions; throughout the campaign the replacement flow across the Atlantic was more like a trickle. Of 2,300 Medical Department officers entering the ETO replacement system between D-Day and V-E Day, only about 800 (34 percent) were casuals from the United States. The proportion of enlisted replacements from outside the theater (6,300 out of 42,000) was even smaller. Making matters worse, the officers

[25] Quotation from 95th Evacuation Hospital Annual Rpt, 1944, p. 11. See also Personnel Division, OofCSurg, HQ, ETOUSA, Annual Rpt, 1944, p. 10; Operations Division, OofCSurg, HQ, ETOUSA, Annual Rpt, 1944, p. 6; Surg, Normandy Base Section, Annual Rpt, 1944, p. 15; Training Branch, Operations Division, OofCSurg, HQ, ETOUSA, Semiannual Rpt, January-June 1945, p. 4. Hawley laments T/O reductions in Ltr, Hawley to TSG, 14 Sep 44, file HD 024 ETO O/CS (Hawley-SGO Corresp). McMinn and Levin, *Personnel*, pp. 96-97 and 301-02, discusses the general background of T/O reductions.

[26] Personnel Division, OofCSurg, HQ, ETOUSA, Annual Rpt, 1944, encl. 9, and Semiannual Rpt, January-June 1945, pp. 2-3; Surg, First U.S. Army, Annual Rpt, 1944, p. 58; Surg, 9th Infantry Division, Annual Rpt, 1944, p. 15. For examples of casualty figures for other divisions, see Surg, 1st Infantry Division, Annual Rpt, 1944, p. 30, and Surg, 4th Armored Division, Annual Rpt, 1944, p. 22. General Kenner constantly expressed concern at high front-line medical losses. See various inspection reports in Medical Division, COSSAC/SHAEF, War Diary, July-December 1944.

and men who were sent generally were unsuited for assignment to the divisions, where they were most needed. Most had received training almost exclusively for work in COMZ medical installations; they lacked knowledge of infantry tactics and battlefield survival techniques required for effectiveness as battalion surgeons or company aidmen. The 5th Infantry Division surgeon summed up a universal complaint: "As a rule, Medical Department replacements have been received not adequately trained to function under fire. . . . Many . . . had no idea of how to take care of themselves in the field in . . . darkness, rain and mud." [27]

Largely thrown back upon its own resources, the ETO medical service arranged to use its available people with maximum efficiency and to fill vacancies, especially in the armies, as expeditiously as possible. While still at Cheltenham before the invasion, the staffs of the Personnel Division and the Troop Movements and Training Branch had cultivated friendly working relations with the nearby Ground Force Reinforcement Command, which handled replacements of all services. This mutually beneficial alliance continued throughout the campaign, ensuring the medical service maximum flexibility in controlling its own personnel. The Reinforcement Command referred the names of all medical officers entering its depots to the Personnel Division for suggestions as to reassignment, thereby giving it the unique privilege of what amounted to complete assignment jurisdiction over its own officer personnel in this theater. In processing unit requisitions for medical replacements the Reinforcement Command, in the interests of speed, waived its standard procedure of waiting for the requisition to make its way up the chain of command and acted on informal certification that a vacancy existed. The medical and Reinforcement Command staffs cooperated to establish a constantly replenished replacement pool of ten nurses in each army, again reducing the time required to fill vacancies. During the Ardennes crisis they delegated to army and base section surgeons the assignment of all but a few categories of officers entering replacement depots and arranged for the automatic return of most of the recovered medical service sick and wounded to their former organizations. [28]

The chief surgeon's office and the Reinforcement Command responded jointly to field army complaints of a shortage of qualified replacement aidmen. Investigation showed that the armies themselves were creating part

[27] Quotation from Surg, 5th Infantry Division, Annual Rpt, 1944, pp. 32–33. McMinn and Levin, *Personnel,* pp. 297–300 and 303–05, describes the worldwide problem of Medical Department replacements. See also Personnel Division, OofCSurg, HQ, ETOUSA, Annual Rpt, 1944, p. 6; Study No. 88, General Board, USFET, sub: Training Status of Medical Units and Medical Department Personnel Upon Arrival in the European Theater of Operations, pp. 5–8, file 353/2.

[28] Personnel Division, OofCSurg, HQ, ETOUSA, Annual Rpt, 1944, app. B, and Semiannual Rpt, January–June 1945, pp. 2, 6–7 and encls. V–VI; Nursing Division, OofCSurg, HQ, ETOUSA, Annual Rpt, 1944, p. 10; Surg, Third U.S. Army, Annual Rpt, 1944, pp. 125 and 150; Surg, Ninth U.S. Army, Annual Rpt, 1944, p. 36; Ltrs, Hawley to Surgs, First, Third, Ninth U.S. Armies, 18 Dec 44, sub: Medical Department Replacements, and Hawley to Col C. F. Shook, 24 Dec 44, file HD 024 ETO CS (Hawley Chron).

of the shortage by requisitioning medical and surgical technicians for inappropriate slots, such as drivers and cooks, and that great confusion existed throughout the replacement system in matching actual tasks with military occupational specialty numbers. Early in 1945 Hawley's people and the Reinforcement Command issued new enlisted replacement and requisitioning rules to prevent misassignment of highly trained medics, and they arranged conferences to teach army medical personnel officers to use the revised system.[29]

These measures promoted efficient use of what medical replacements were available in the theater, but they did not themselves produce any more people. Especially to replace combat losses, the theater continually robbed Peter to pay Paul, Peter in this instance being rear-area medical units. The process began within the armies. Corps medical battalions and medical groups routinely loaned officers and enlisted men to the divisions to replace casualties until regularly requisitioned replacements arrived from the depots. COMZ units also loaned doctors, nurses, and enlisted men to the armies, and they gave up people permanently for reassignment forward. During the Ardennes battle COMZ hospitals and other installations furnished over 300 officers and 3,100 enlisted men to fill the gaps left by army casualties. Such replacements, however, were less than satisfactory to the divisions. The officers often were overage or physically unfit for the strenuous life of infantry battalion surgeons; both they and the enlisted men, like replacements from the United States, lacked training as front-line medics. Of 21 medical officer replacements in the 2d Armored Division during 1944, for example, 8 had to be evacuated or kept in the division rear because they were unsuited to combat. The arrival during the summer of significant numbers of MAC assistant battalion surgeons created a large pool of medical officers available to serve as battalion surgeons, but the pool was emptied almost immediately to cover the losses of the first two months of fighting. By late 1944 a MAC officer shortage had developed in turn, in spite of army efforts to commission qualified Medical Department NCOs in this corps.

To meet the constant need for more aidmen, the Troop Movements and Training Branch and the Ground Force Reinforcement Command early in 1945 established a school at the 19th Reinforcement Depot to retrain Medical Department cooks, clerks, and drivers, who were in oversupply, as medical and surgical technicians. Within the armies several corps and divisions set up similar courses of their own, to make aidmen out of selected infantry replacements and less skilled medical soldiers. The willingness of combat units to divert riflemen, who also were scarce, for this purpose indicated the value they placed upon their aidmen.[30]

---

[29] Troop Movements and Training Branch, Operations Division, OofCSurg, HQ, ETOUSA, Annual Rpt, 1944, pp. 30-31; Training Branch, Operations Division, OofCSurg, HQ, ETOUSA, Semiannual Rpt, January-June 1945, pp. 1-2 and encl. 1; First U.S. Army Report of Operations, 1 Aug 44-22 Feb 45, bk. IV, p. 194.

[30] McMinn and Levin, *Personnel*, pp. 302-03; Personnel Division, OofCSurg, HQ, ETOUSA, Annual

Continued

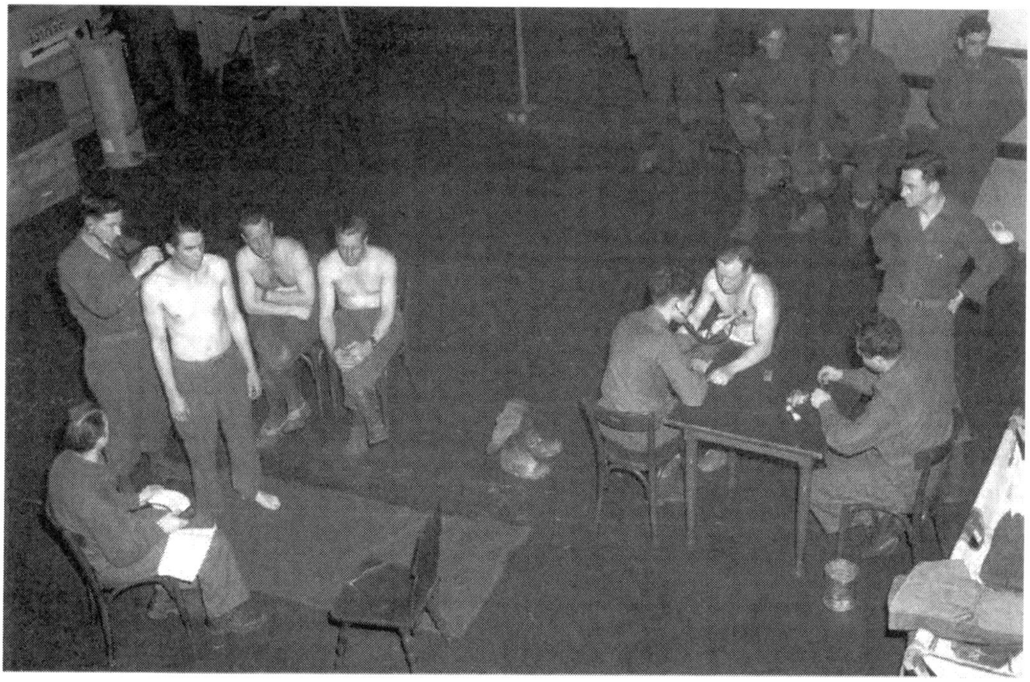

TROOPS UNDERGOING A PHYSICAL EXAMINATION *to determine their fitness for reassignment to combat duty*

Some of the riflemen so retrained may well have been former medical soldiers. The medical service, even while straining to replace its own casualties, also had to help fill the ranks of the infantry, dangerously depleted by the autumn offensive and the German counterattacks. Since the hedgerow battles, the European Theater had conducted a running argument with the War Department over its requisitions for infantry replacements, which the department considered excessive. The theater finally acceded to demands from Washington that it make infantrymen out of some of the tens of thousands of General Assignment soldiers (those physically and mentally qualified for combat) in its Communications Zone and that it replace them in rear-area installations with Limited Assignment men (unfit for front-line duty). Accordingly, in January 1945, the theater began combing General Assignment men out of all the technical ser-

Rpt, 1944, pp. 8-10, and Semiannual Rpt, January-June 1945, pp. 2-3; Training Branch, Operations Division, OofCSurg, HQ, ETOUSA, Semiannual Rpt, January-June 1945, pp. 2-3; Surg, ADSEC, COMZ, Semiannual Rpt, January-June 1945, p. 8; First U.S. Army Reports of Operations, 20 Oct 43-1 Aug 44, bk. VII, p. 107, and 1 Aug 44-22 Feb 45, bk. IV, p. 194; Surg, Third U.S. Army, Annual Rpt, 1944, pp. 148-52; Surg, Seventh U.S. Army, Annual Rpt, 1944, pp. 39-42. For an example of the intra-army borrowing system, see Surg, V Corps, Annual Rpt, 1944, p. 8. For examples of corps and division medics training, see Surg, XII Corps, Annual Rpt, 1944, p. 10; Surg, 2d Armored Division, Annual Rpt, 1944, pp. 2-3 and encl. 4; Surg, 4th Armored Division, Annual Rpt, 1944, p. 10; and Surg, 80th Infantry Division, Annual Rpt, 1944, p. 9.

vices for retraining as riflemen. It tapped the Medical Department for 12,000 enlisted men, a quota which the chief surgeon's office divided among the base sections. General Hawley and his staff managed to soften this blow to their already burdened personnel system through informal arrangements with the Ground Force Reinforcement Command and the newly created Theater Manpower Section, under which a majority of the men taken, especially the technicians, in fact went to the divisions as aidmen and litterbearer replacements instead of ordinary infantry.

COMZ medical installations still suffered substantial quantitative and qualitative manpower losses as a result of the theater policy. The ADSEC medical service between January and March gave up over 1,300 men, 540 of them enlisted specialists, and received only 260 Limited Assignment men in return. The United Kingdom Base in the same period lost over 2,300 medical soldiers to the infantry and 1,200 more as Medical Department replacements, with only 1,000 Limited Assignment personnel arriving in exchange. Individual general hospitals surrendered up to 15 percent of their technicians; some fell as many as 50 or 60 men below their already barely adequate T/O enlisted strength of 450. The Limited Assignment men who arrived as replacements usually had no previous Medical Department service. Many were former infantrymen, reclassified after being wounded. They often were less than enthusiastic at becoming medics; many held noncommissioned ratings inappropriate to unskilled hospital assignments. ADSEC units received large numbers of combat exhaustion convalescents, who broke down again under the shelling and bombing to which many forward holding units and hospitals were subjected and who had to be returned to the replacement depots. Hospitals and other units trained their new men as best they could, on the job whenever possible, and many eventually developed into first-rate medical soldiers. The training effort, however, further taxed already overworked and undermanned organizations.[31]

With their total work force steadily being reduced and their skilled people spread ever more thinly, army and COMZ medical units, especially hospitals and supply depots, got through the winter by making extensive use of civilian and prisoner-of-war (POW) labor. In France and Belgium evacuation hospitals regularly employed 80–100 local people, general hospitals hired as many as 500–1,000, and some depots used up to 200. These men and women, usually selected by their national government's labor agencies and paid by their governments under reverse lend-lease, took over much of the menial work in wards, kitchens, and

[31] McMinn and Levin, *Personnel*, pp. 240–41; Personnel Division, OofCSurg, HQ, ETOUSA, Semiannual Rpt, January–June 1945, p. 3; Training Branch, Operations Division, OofCSurg, HQ, ETOUSA, Semiannual Rpt, January–June 1945, pp. 3–4; Surg, ADSEC, COMZ, Annual Rpt, 1944, pp. 64–65, and Semiannual Rpt, January–June 1945, pp. 16–17 and 41; Surg, United Kingdom Base, Semiannual Rpt, January–June 1945, vol. 1, pp. 106–08 and 112. For general background on the infantry replacement issue, see Ruppenthal, *Logistical Support*, 1:458–63 and 2:304–32. For typical effects of the manpower drain, see Surg, Seine Section, Semiannual Rpt, January–June 1945, pp. 36 and 45–47; 5th General Hospital Annual Rpt, 1945, pp. 3–4; 298th General Hospital Annual Rpt, 1945, p. 237; and 15th Medical Depot Company Annual Rpt, 1945, p. 2.

warehouses. They also maintained hospital buildings, provided clerical help, and operated telephone switchboards. Some general hospitals employed French or Belgian nurses; but, because of the language barrier and limits of their training, the Americans generally confined these women to only the most elementary nursing chores. Not all civilian helpers were paid. In Holland the 111th Evacuation Hospital drew volunteer nurse's aides from the Dutch Red Cross. These women, who came from the "leading families" of their community, provided "invaluable" assistance on the wards and also in central supply and the laboratory. In recognition of their social status, they were allowed to eat in the officers mess.[32]

Working with civilians had its difficulties. Units had to hire interpreters or conduct English classes in order to maintain effective communication with their local help. Some reported instances of theft, absenteeism, and security violations, not to mention demands, in one instance instigated by the Resistance, for higher wages and more days off. Efforts to train civilians had mixed results. At Depot M-402 in Normandy, "when an officer or enlisted man endeavors to explain errors, the civilians apparently interpret explanations as reprimands and in several cases the officer has found himself with crying civilians on his hand[s]." On balance, nevertheless, these employees proved indispensable in supplementing theater medical manpower.[33]

POW laborers, exclusively Germans in the 12th Army Group and the northern Communications Zone and both Germans and Italians in SOLOC, proved as useful as civilians and better disciplined. First Army evacuation hospitals in Normandy began using POWs during June and July as litterbearers and for other unskilled tasks. The experiment worked so well that in August the Advance Section began attaching prisoners to its general hospitals and arranged for construction of a POW enclosure at each new hospital plant. By late 1944 most evacuation and general hospitals and depots on the Continent employed POWs, in numbers ranging from 40 or so in the evacuation hospitals to as many as 500 in the general hospitals.

Each facility obtained prisoners from its army or base section provost marshal, housed them in a barbed wire enclosure on its grounds, and guarded them with medical enlisted men, who bore arms for this duty but not their brassards or their Geneva Convention identification cards. The Germans, in keeping with general theater policy, lived in tents or huts

[32] 111th Evacuation Hospital Annual Rpt, 1944, p. 10.

[33] Quotation from Memo, 1st Lt J. E. Holimeyer, MAC, to OofCSurg, HQ, ETOUSA, 5 Feb 45, sub: Depot Personnel, in 26th Medical Depot Company Hist File, 1945. See also McMinn and Levin, *Personnel*, pp. 255 and 260-62; Nursing Division, OofCSurg, HQ, ETOUSA, Annual Rpt, 1944, p. 6, and Semiannual Rpt, January-June 1945, pp. 5-6; Surg, ADSEC, COMZ, Annual Rpt, 1944, p. 39; Surg, Seine Section, Annual Rpt, 1944, p. 24, and Semiannual Rpt, January-June 1945, pp. 45-46 and 87; Surg, CONAD, Semiannual Rpt, January-June 1945, p. 11. For a sampling of unit experience, see 9th Evacuation Hospital Annual Rpt, 1944, pp. 10-11; 59th Evacuation Hospital Annual Rpt, 1944, sec. XIII; 111th Evacuation Hospital Annual Rpt, 1944, p. 10; 5th General Hospital Annual Rpt, 1945, p. 4; 99th General Hospital Annual Rpt, 1944, p. 7; 127th General Hospital Annual Rpt, 1944, p. 5; and 298th General Hospital Annual Rpt, 1945, pp. 231-32.

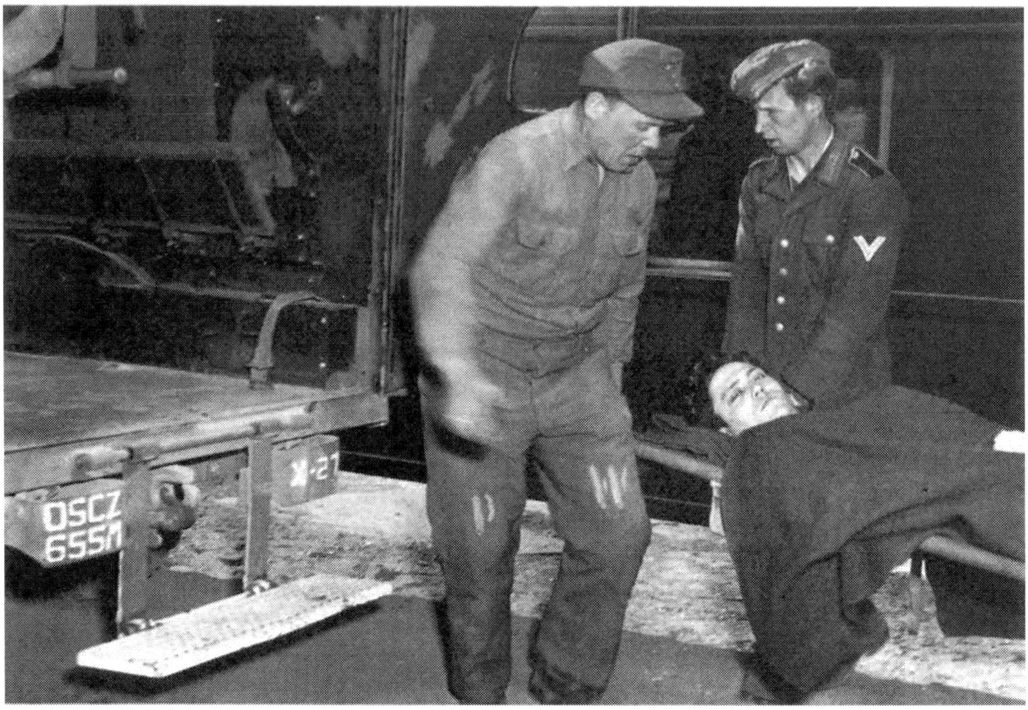

GERMAN POWs UNLOADING CASUALTIES FROM A HOSPITAL TRAIN AT REIMS

under austere conditions; hospitals tried to provide medical care and limited amenities, such as weekly hot showers and sports equipment, to maintain their health and morale. On and off the job, the prisoners were supervised by their own noncommissioned officers and, in the case of the Italians, were organized into sanitary companies and engineer platoons. While the great majority did manual labor, prisoners with special skills—for example, former members of their army medical services—worked in almost all departments of hospitals and depots, although they never administered treatment to Allied patients. Innovative hospital commanders put their prisoners' talents to good use. Col. Lee Cady, MC, of the 21st General Hospital found enough musicians among his contingent for a small orchestra, which played for the enjoyment of staff and patients. Most hospitals preferred POW laborers to civilians. The Germans, in particular, were orderly, obedient, harshly punished any of their own who stole or misbehaved, and uncomplainingly worked long hours. Although rumors of uprisings and escape plots circulated during the Battle of the Bulge, the POWs displayed no defiance of American authority. As later recalled by Colonel Cady, "The 21st could have won the rest of their war with POWS." [34]

[34]Quotation from Cady, "Notes on the 21st General Hospital (AUS), p. 485, Cady Papers, MHI. See

Continued

Morale Problems

For ETO medical personnel, whether in the armies or in the Communications Zone, the demands of active operations left little time for the training and professional activities that had been so prominent a part of their pre-D-Day life in Great Britain. The Medical Field Service and Army Nurse Corps Schools at Shrivenham graduated their last classes in October. Efforts to move them, and the rest of the school center, to France were frustrated by the theater's inability to secure a suitable site. Within individual units, except for those that arrived "short-trained" and went through accelerated catch-up cycles, regular refresher and professional enhancement courses were a casualty of the campaign. Some base sections attempted to enforce minimal training requirements, and both the armies and COMZ conducted conferences and courses for especially vital categories of personnel, for example, hospital chief nurses. When they could, theater medics tried to continue professional meetings and conferences with each other and foreign colleagues. Thus the staff of the 15th General Hospital at Liege held meetings with the medical faculty of the local university, who were eager to catch up on the latest development in their fields after the long intellectual drought of the Nazi occupation. At theater level the Inter-Allied Conference on War Medicine resumed its London sessions in October. Later that same month, in Paris, American and British consultants held the first of what they hoped would be periodic Allied conferences.[35]

While most medical units coalesced into smoothly functioning teams, human nature and the circumstances of war occasionally strained personal and professional relationships and organizational cohesion. Rank and promotion were a cause of much bitter feeling among MC specialists, who resented the fact that unit T/Os did not always allocate officer grades in conformity to the professional heirarchies of medicine and surgery. Factionalism, based on clashing personalities or differences of professional opinion, divided some unit staffs. In one evacuation hospital, according to its commander, the chief of the operating section "does not understand the handling of officers and men," causing "widespread resentment" and "considerable discord," and had

also ibid., pp. 437–38, 494, 506, 587–88; McMinn and Levin, *Personnel*, pp. 326–28; Troop Movements and Training Branch, Operations Branch, OofCSurg, HQ ETOUSA, Annual Rpt, 1944, p. 40; Surg, United Kingdom Base, Semiannual Rpt, January-June 1945, vol. 1, p. 112; Surg, CONAD, Annual Rpt, 1944, pp. 12–13; Surg, ADSEC, Daily Activities Rpts, 5–7 Aug 44, and Hospitalization Division, OofSurg, ADSEC, Weekly Activities Rpts, weeks ending 12 and 19 Aug 44, Beasley Papers, MHI; Surg, ADSEC, COMZ, Annual Rpt, 1944, p. 68. For an example of use of POWs, see 298th General Hospital Annual Rpts, 1944, pp. 270–71, and 1945, pp. 232–36.

[35] Troop Movements and Training Branch, Operations Division, OofCSurg, HQ ETOUSA, Annual Rpt, 1944, p. 17; Troops Branch, Operations Division, OofCSurg, HQ ETOUSA, Semiannual Rpt, January-June 1945, pp. 4–5; Nursing Division, OofCSurg, HQ ETOUSA, Semiannual Rpt, January-June 1945, p. 1; Training Memo No. 1, Surg, Seine Section, 29 Jan 45, in Surg, Seine Section, Semiannual Rpt, January-June 1945, pp. 81–92; Surg, ADSEC, COMZ, Annual Rpt, 1944, pp. 49–50; First U.S. Army Report of Operations, 1 Aug 44–22 Feb 45, bk. IV, p. 193; 15th General Hospital Annual Report, 1944, pp. 19–20; Professional Services Division, OofCSurg, HQ ETOUSA, Annual Report, 1944, Medical Consultation Service sec., pp. 4–5; Carter, ed., *Surgical Consultants*, 2:256–57.

failed to enforce orders against "drinking of liquor during operations." The chief nurse, while "efficient above reproach," had "a poor understanding of human nature" and did not "possess satisfactory qualities of tact and leadership." Over and above promotions and personalities the oppressive realities of war loomed strong. In a Third Army field hospital the ward nurses, "in a period of heavy operation, do little but work and catch sleep as they can." They "see so much death, have so many problems regarding proper care of patients and so many patients to care for . . . that they tend to grow depressed. . . . Very excellent nurses become short tempered and difficult. . . ."[36]

By late 1944 the morale problems of front-line medical officers and enlisted men, especially those in infantry battalion and regimental detachments, had become a matter of concern to the army surgeons and General Hawley. Many of these combat medics had been under fire in North Africa, Sicily, and Italy before D-Day and in nearly constant action since then. They were approaching the limits of emotional and physical endurance. In addition, the medical officers, who had little opportunity to practice their professional specialties, feared that they were falling behind their hospital colleagues, with whom they would have to compete when they returned to civilian life.

Division, corps, and army surgeons tried to transfer their oldest, tiredest officers and men to less arduous duty, with medical detachments of artillery and support units in divisions and corps and in evacuation or other hospitals in the armies. In October General Hawley instituted a theater-wide system for rotating commissioned and enlisted medical personnel between the ground forces and COMZ, both to replace veterans of prolonged front-line service with fresh men from the rear and to give specialists from general and station hospitals three-month tours of duty with evacuation and field hospitals and auxiliary surgical groups. This program got off to a promising start, although commanders inevitably took advantage of it to discard their least desirable men, including in one draft from the First Army a cocaine addict and a chronic alcoholic. However, the midwinter manpower crisis soon submerged the rotation program, forcing its replacement by a one-way flow of people from COMZ to the armies. As the tactical and personnel situations stabilized in early 1945, General Hawley revived rotation, setting a monthly transfer quota from each army of ten officers and twenty-five enlisted men, but hostilities ended before the system could make its beneficial effects felt on any significant scale.[37]

[36] Comments on evacuation hospital from Memo, Col C. D. Goodiel to Surg, Ninth U.S. Army, 7 Sep 44, Shambora Papers, MHI. Comments on field hospital from 60th Field Hospital Annual Rpt, 1944, pp. 6–7. For other unit morale problems, see Cady, "Notes on the 21st General Hospital (AUS), pp. 463–64, Cady Papers, MHI, and Gosman, "War without Blood," passim. In fixed hospitals neurosurgeons complained that the highest-ranking slots open to them were captaincies while chief dentists were lieutenant colonels. See Professional Services Division, OofCSurg, HQ, ETOUSA, Annual Rpt, 1944, Chief Consultant in Surgery sec., p. 19, Chief Consultant in Orthopedic Surgery sec., p. 7, and Chief Consultant in Anesthesia sec., p. 15.

[37] On forward area morale, see Surg, Seventh U.S. Army, Annual Rpt, 1944, pp. 40–42; Surg, XII

Continued

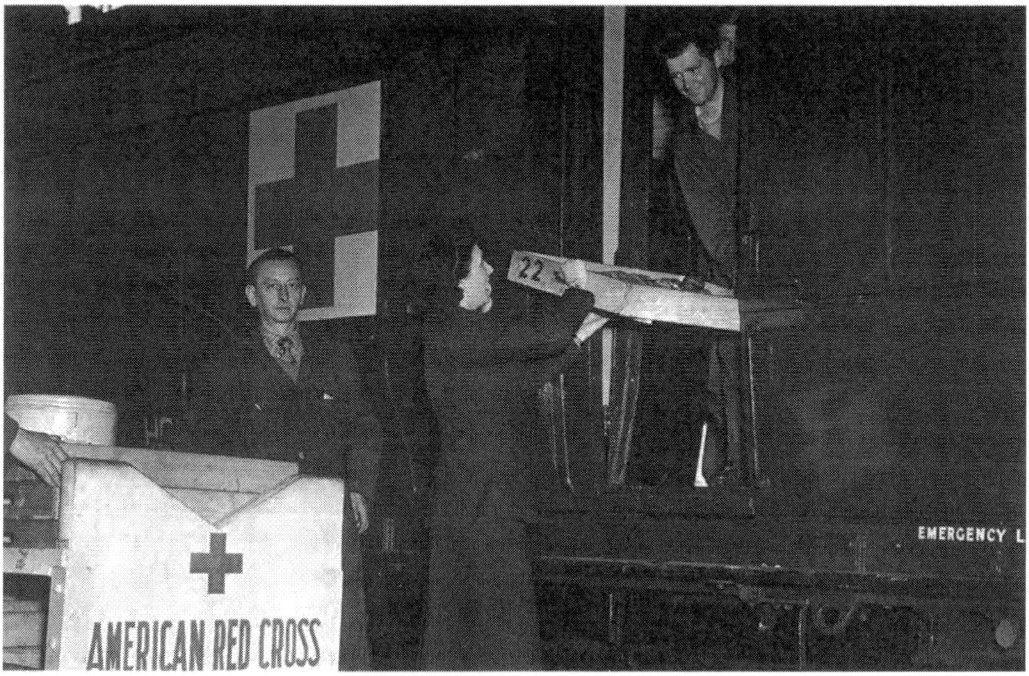

AMERICAN RED CROSS WORKERS SUPPLYING DOUGHNUTS FOR CASUALTIES *to improve morale while traveling on a hospital train*

Whether in the armies or the Communications Zone, medical units employed every resource provided by the theater and of their own devising to give staff and patients some respite from the often grim daily routine. They sent officers, nurses, and enlisted men on pass to nearby towns, when such were not off limits to American personnel. Other medical people received much-coveted 48-hour passes to Paris, and a few extremely fortunate individuals went home to the United States on thirty-day leaves. Within units, Special Service detachments scheduled films and an occasional traveling USO show for staff and patients. Radios and record-players, both government issued and "liberated," were precious possessions. Clubs, for officers, nurses, and enlisted men, ranged from austerely furnished recreation tents to com-

Corps, Annual Rpt, 1944, p. 11; Surg, 1st Infantry Division, Annual Rpt, 1944, p. 34; Surg, 5th Infantry Division, Annual Rpt, 1944, p. 39. On rotation within the armies, see First U.S. Army Report of Operations, 1 Aug 44–22 Feb 45, bk. IV, p. 194; Surg, V Corps, Annual Rpt, 1944, pp. 16–17; Surg, 2d Armored Division, Annual Rpt, 1944, p. 49; Surg, 3d Infantry Division, Annual Rpt, 1944, p. 10. On theater rotation, see McMinn and Levin, *Personnel*, pp. 332–36; Personnel Division, OofCSurg, HQ, ETOUSA, Annual Rpt, 1944, p. 13; Professional Services Division, OofCSurg, HQ, ETOUSA, Annual Rpt, 1944, Chief Consultant in Surgery sec., ex. L, Medical Consultation Service sec., p. 14, and Chief Consultant in Anesthesia sec., pp. 2–3; Middleton Interv, 1968–69, vol. 1, pp. 205–06; Surg, 1st Infantry Division, Annual Rpt, 1944, pp. 24 and 34–35; Editorial Advisory Board, 1962, pp. 215–17. On cases of addiction and alcoholism, see Ltr, Hawley to Col J. A. Rogers, 20 Nov 44, file HD 024 ETO CS (Hawley Chron).

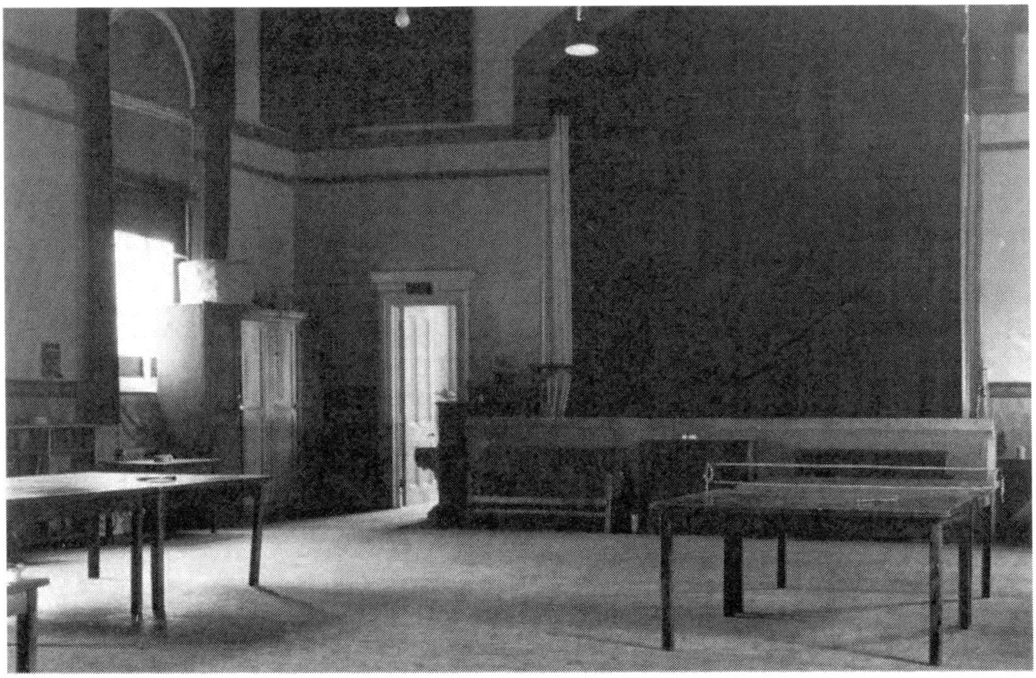

STATION HOSPITAL DAYROOM, *used by staff and patients for recreational purposes*

paratively well-appointed barrooms and lounges, depending on the type of unit, how long it had been in one place, and the foraging skill of the staff. When time and weather permitted, sports teams and leagues made their appearance. Amateur theatricals provided a showcase for homegrown talent. In the hospitals Red Cross workers supplied the patients with reading material, small toilet articles and luxuries; wrote letters for them; organized games and parties; and acted as counselors and sympathetic listeners. Holiday celebrations, especially at Thanksgiving and Christmas, brought out the best of everyone's ingenuity. In the 93d Evacuation Hospital, a Seventh Army unit,

trees were decorated in every ward. Sprigs of pine were hung from doors, windows, and light fixtures. In the chapel a manger scene was set up behind the altar, and a large unit tree was decorated with colored paper and 'balls' made by inflating the fingers of old rubber operating room gloves, and then dipping them in paint. There were candle light services, singing of carols, Red Cross stockings for the patients, and a couple of turkey dinners. [At a Christmas night dance] there was an orchestra, and a 'snack bar' contributed from boxes from home.[38]

[38] Quotation from 93d Evacuation Hospital Unit Hist, 1944, p. 51. For other examples of unit recreation and morale building, see Surg, Ninth U.S. Army, Annual Rpt, 1944, p. 37; Surg, Seventh U.S. Army, Annual Rpt, 1944, p. 46; Surg, Third U.S. Army, Annual Rpt, 1944, p. 125; Surg, ADSEC, COMZ, Annual Rpt, 1944, p. 51; 32d Medical Depot Company Annual Rpt, 1944; 66th, 67th, and 68th Medical Groups Annual Rpts, 1944; 12th, 41st, and 91st Evacuation Hospitals Annual Rpts, 1944; 99th, 101st, 130th, and 298th General Hospitals Annual

Continued

Medical Supply

While key medical personnel became scarcer during the winter of 1944–45, supplies in the theater grew more abundant, and the Communications Zone placed more of them where most needed. The medical service, like the other supply services, benefited from the November opening of Le Havre, Rouen, and Antwerp, deep-water ports much nearer the front than Cherbourg and the no longer usable invasion beaches. The Communications Zone, with an enlarged port capacity and a steadily expanding railroad network, brought more tonnage ashore and pushed more of it forward, ending the supply famine that had stalled the armies in September. On 9 December, when SHAEF discontinued its tonnage allocation system, ADSEC and 12th Army Group supply reserves each were approaching a quarter of a million tons. The Southern Line of Communications, meanwhile, increased the flow of goods through Marseilles so that by mid-December the Continental Advance Section had stockpiled over 50,000 tons and the Seventh Army about 80,000 tons.

Yet the theater supply system continued to work only with friction, inefficiency, and disagreement among commands. Delays in discharging the huge backlog of ships that had built up in European waters during the summer caused shortages of particular items throughout the fall and winter. COMZ stocks still were geographically ill-distributed, with too large a proportion concentrated at the ports or—as the result of a late-year forward movement—in advanced depots that were congested by too-rapid, indiscriminate deliveries. When the German Ardennes breakthrough jeopardized these depots, the Communications Zone reacted by temporarily stopping shipments to forward installations. This action, in turn, caused renewed backups at the ports. As these events indicated, supply movement planning was not a COMZ strongpoint. Neither were documentation and control of shipments on the still ramshackle, overburdened continental railroads. Commands complained constantly of delayed, misdirected, and lost cargoes. The armies, as ever distrustful of the Communications Zone, padded their requisitions to accumulate excessive reserves; sent their own vehicles to collect supplies; and dealt unilaterally and disruptively with the various technical services. COMZ supply accounting left much to be desired. Its depots were little more than huge dumps, lacking systems and facilities for classifying and keeping track of the goods they received, stored, and issued. The theater had not imposed any uniform systems for stock control and the calculation of requisitioning requirements. Working with the resulting unreliable information, the European Theater and the War Department could not agree on how much of such key items as artillery ammunition the theater had on hand and how much it

Rpts, 1944. See also Cady, "Notes on the 21st General Hospital (AUS)," pp. 454 and 491, Cady Papers, MHI; Brown Interv, 1979, CMH; Gosman Interv, 24 Mar 82, CMH; and Lee Interv, 1981, CMH. On Red Cross work, see Surg, Third U.S. Army, Annual Rpt, 1944, pp. 175–77; 60th Field Hospital Annual Rpt, 1944, p. 7; 91st Evacuation Hospital Annual Rpt, 1944, pp. 34–35.

needed. The theater insisted that the War Department was not sending enough; the Washington authorities replied that they were furnishing sufficient supplies and demanded that the theater put its own administrative house in order so that it could find them.

In December General Somervell, at Eisenhower's request, sent the Army Service Forces director of operations, Maj. Gen. LeRoy R. Lutes, to survey the ETO supply situation. Lutes and his delegation spent several weeks in the theater. They documented the logistical deficiencies and recommended remedies that the Communications Zone, under constant pressure from SHAEF and the War Department, gradually implemented. By the time the armies prepared to cross the Rhine, the supply system behind them was functioning in relatively good order.[39]

By contrast with the general situation in the theater, the ETO medical service had already gone through its own experience of mismanagement and reform. Thanks to the work of the Voorhees mission early in 1944, and to the subsequent efforts of Colonel Hays and his assistants, the medical service had solved before D-Day many of the supply problems that still plagued the other technical services and the theater as a whole six months after the invasion. It possessed, for instance, an efficient system of depot management and stock control. General Hawley, as agent of the theater commander, directed the disposition of all medical stores in continental depots, treating them as a single pool of goods rather than as the property of the individual base sections. He also exercised technical supervision over depot operations. This amounted in practice very nearly to full operational control, as neither the base section commanders nor their surgeons had the staff or the expertise to manage the details of depot work. Closely overseen by the chief surgeon's Supply Division, COMZ depots, including eventually those of SOLOC, all followed uniform operating procedures prescribed in the Medical Department Depot Manual, which the Supply Division revised late in 1944 to incorporate the lessons of continental experience. These procedures included a simple, accurate method for determining and reporting regularly the amount of stock on hand, due in, and issued. In Paris the Stock Control Branch of the Supply Division consolidated reports from the depots on automatic data processing machines to produce timely statistics for a variety of purposes. Among other things, this information helped Supply Division transfer stock between depots, maintaining adequate working levels computed on the basis of the number of troops and the type of installations the depot served.[40]

Because the Supply Division could furnish stock information that all con-

[39] Discussion based on Ruppenthal, *Logistical Support*, 2:96, 103–16, 126–33, 176–86, 348–63. Lutes report and supporting documents in Maj Gen LeRoy R. Lutes, Official Report: Mission to European Theater of Operations, 4 December 1944–13 January 1945 (hereafter cited as ETO Rpt, 1944–45), box 44, RG 200, NARA.

[40] Supply Division, OofCSurg, HQ, ETOUSA, Semiannual Rpt, January–June 1945, sec. II, pp. 5–7, sec. III, pp. 4–6, sec. IV, pp. 5–6; Wiltse, ed., *Medical Supply*, pp. 314–17; Kelley Interv, 27 Jan 45, box 221, RG 112, NARA.

cerned judged reliable, the requisitioning and shipment of medical supplies from the United States involved little confusion or conflict between Washington and the theater. For its initial continental buildup the Supply Division, before D-Day, ordered large prescheduled shipments of goods for delivery to French ports beginning about 1 September 1944. Thereafter, the division issued biweekly maintenance and replacement requisitions to keep up a 60-day reserve of all items as well as a 120-day reserve to cover ordering and shipping time. During late autumn Colonel Hays' office integrated the Southern Line of Communications into this system. Under a provision of the mid-November agreements SOLOC computed its requirements on the same basis as its northern counterpart and submitted its requisitions through the theater Communications Zone, which partially filled them from its own surpluses before passing the reduced, or "edited," requisitions on to the New York Port of Embarkation. After the February 1945 merger of COMZ and SOLOC, the Supply Division developed requirements for the entire theater and arranged for deliveries to Marseilles and the Channel ports in proportion to the respective troop strengths of the 6th and 12th Army Groups and their supporting base sections. This procedure kept supplies flowing across the Atlantic with a minimum of delay, duplication, and dispute. In December the Lutes mission had reported that an average of 45 days elapsed between the requisitioning of medical supplies from America and the first deliveries to COMZ depots; the corresponding time for Quartermaster stores was 145 days. The mission had also found only three minor medical items in short supply in the theater. Separate from the rest of the supply system, transatlantic blood flights also went without a hitch, reaching a delivery rate of over 8,000 pints per week during January.[41]

The distribution network kept pace. By late October 1944 a chain of depots stretched from Normandy and the Riviera to Belgium and northeastern France (*see Map 20*). Depot M–402, at Chef-du-Pont and Carentan, besides supporting the Normandy Base Section, received supplies landed at Cherbourg and shipped them forward to other depots. Depot M–405 at Le Mans distributed supplies to the Loire and Brittany Base Sections. At the center of the supply network Depot M–407 at Paris, in addition to serving the many Seine Section medical installations, received materiel sent forward by rail from M–402, by barge up the Seine from Rouen and Le Havre, and by air from Great Britain and the United States. This depot, largest in the system, forwarded supplies to the Advance Section and the armies by

[41] Supply Division, OofCSurg, HQ, ETOUSA, Annual Rpt, 1944, sec. II, ex. III (Memo, Col S. B. Hays to Hawley, 24 Dec 44, sub: Difficulties in Moving Medical Supplies and Equipment), and Semiannual Rpt, January–June 1945, sec. II, pp. 1–3; Wiltse, ed., *Medical Supply*, pp. 315–16. For SOLOC arrangements, see correspondence in DRAGOON 1944 file, CMH. On Lutes report and shortages, see Ruppenthal, *Logistical Support*, 2:353; Lutes, ETO Rpt, 1944–45, box 44, RG 200, NARA; and Memo, Lutes to CG, SHAEF, via CG, COMZ, 25 Dec 44, sub: Report on Supply Situation—Northern France, tab 2E, box 44, RG 200, NARA. On blood flights, see Ltr, Hawley to TSG, 27 Jan 45, file HD 024 ETO O/CS (Hawley-SGO Corresp).

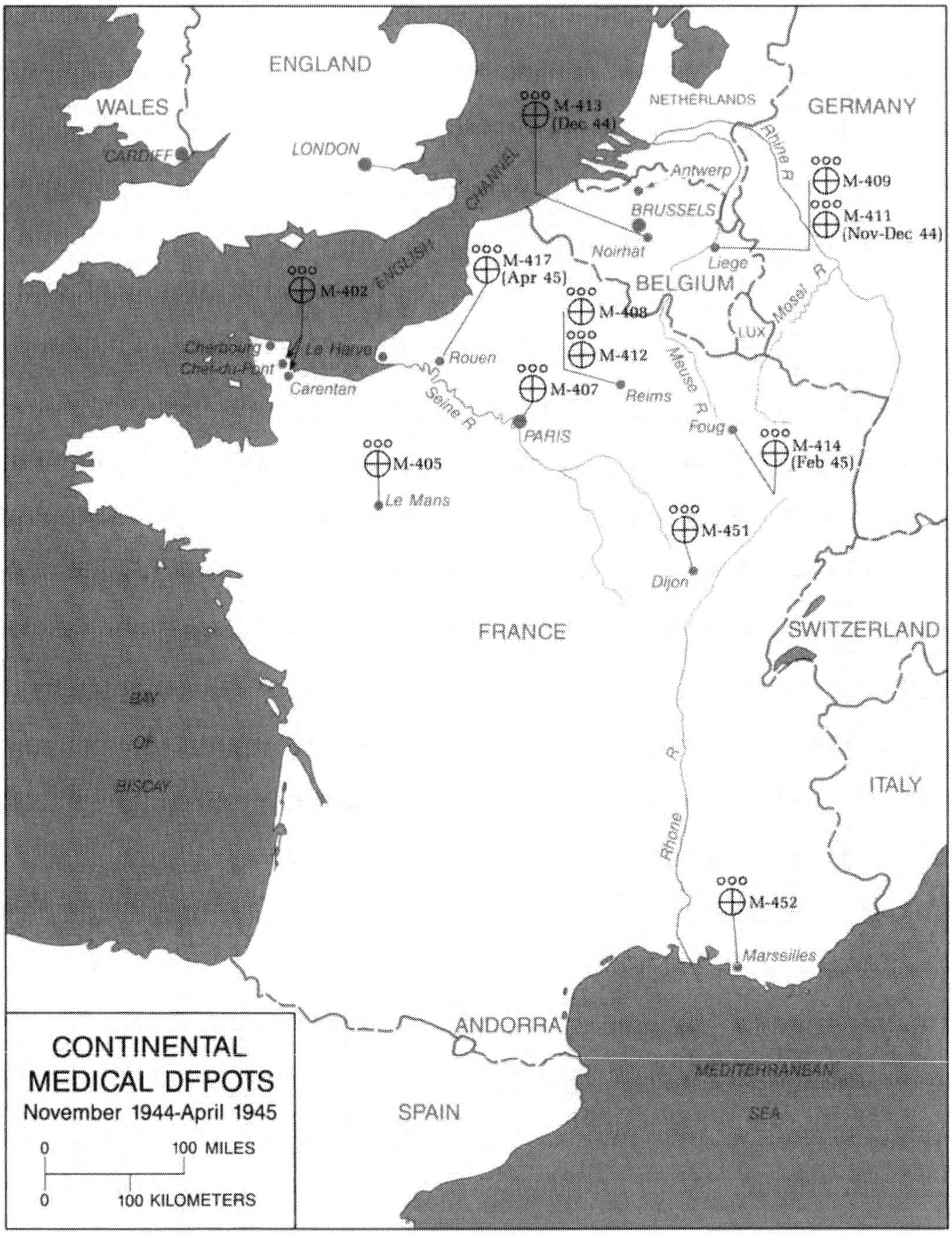
ENGLAND
WALES
CARDIFF
LONDON
ENGLISH CHANNEL
NETHERLANDS
GERMANY
M-413 (Dec 44)
Antwerp
BRUSSELS
Rhine R
M-409
M-411 (Nov-Dec 44)
Noirhat
Liege
M-417 (Apr 45)
BELGIUM
Mosel R
M-402
M-408
LUX
M-412
Cherbourg
Le Harve
Chef-du-Pont
Carentan
Rouen
M-407
Reims
Meuse R
Seine R
PARIS
Foug
M-414 (Feb 45)
M-405
Le Mans
M-451
Dijon
FRANCE
SWITZERLAND
BAY OF BISCAY
ITALY
Rhone R
M-452
Marsseilles
ANDORRA
MEDITERRANEAN SEA
SPAIN
CONTINENTAL MEDICAL DFPOTS
November 1944-April 1945
0 100 MILES
0 100 KILOMETERS

MAP 20

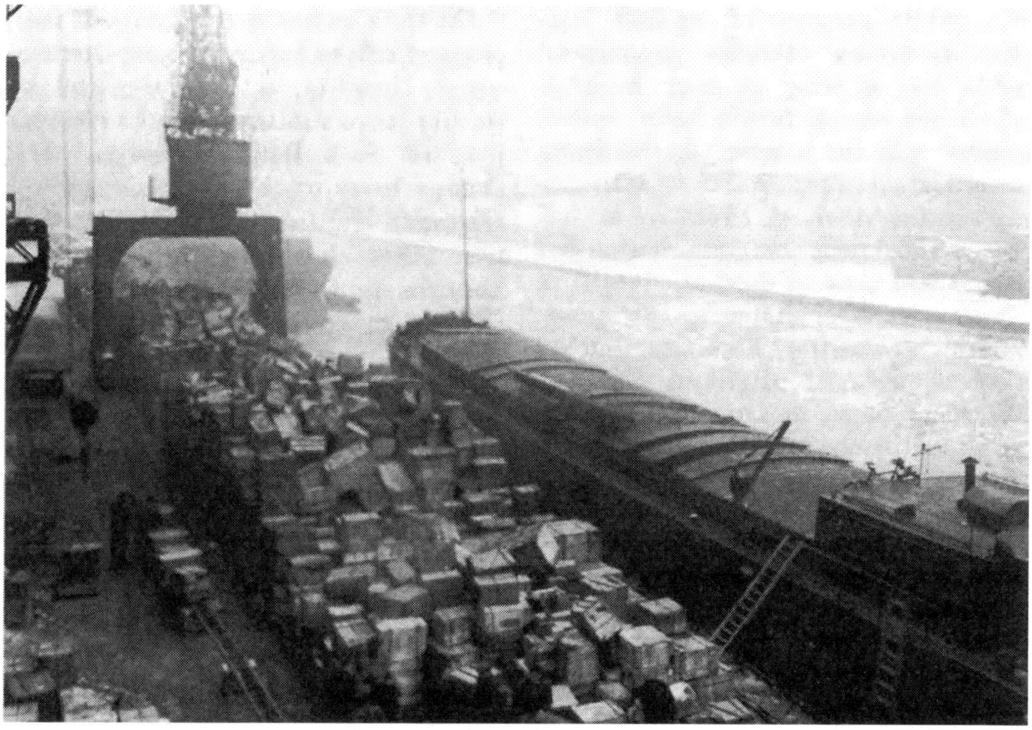

MEDICAL SUPPLIES AT MEDICAL DEPOT M-407, *the largest facility of this type on the Continent served by barges as well as railroads*

air, road, and rail; it was the central continental issuing point for Medical Department forms, spare parts, and items in short supply; and it repaired major pieces of hospital equipment. Two advance depots—M-409 at Liege, which went into operation early in November, and M-408 at Reims—directly supported ADSEC and the First, Third, and Ninth Armies. Depot M-412, also at Reims, continued its specialized work of collecting, processing, and issuing captured German medical supplies. With SOLOC the theater acquired two additional depots: M-352 (later redesignated M-452) at Marseilles, with functions similar to those of M-402, and M-351 (later M-451) at Dijon, which supported CONAD and the U.S. Seventh and French First Armies.[42]

The theater medical service possessed both sufficient supplies and well-located depots for their storage and issue. What was lacking during the autumn and winter was reliable transportation. Difficulties began at the overworked continental ports, where the theater gave unloading priority to ammunition, rations, and

[42] Fenton Interv, 7 Jun 45, box 222, RG 112, NARA. Locations and functions of depots summarized in Supply Division, OofCSurg, HQ, ETOUSA, Annual Rpt, 1944, sec. II, pp. 10-17 and ex. VIII. The SOLOC depots were redesignated in February 1945 to conform to the ETO numbering system. See Supply Division, OofCSurg, HQ, ETOUSA, Semiannual Rpt, January-June 1945, sec. III, p. 16, and Wiltse, *Mediterranean*, pp. 406-08.

POL while cargoes of medical supplies remained offshore in vessels' holds for as long as four months. When this logjam finally broke in November with the opening of the Seine ports and Antwerp, it did so with disruptive suddenness. Within a few days a dozen ships discharged over 9,000 tons of medical freight at Cherbourg, overwhelming the Chef-du-Pont receiving facilities. Other medical materiel destined for the Continent went to Great Britain instead, as the theater diverted ships to reduce its backlog. The United Kingdom Base, with its limited allotment of cross-Channel shipping already committed to prescheduled transfers of supplies from its own depots to the Continent, could not readily transship the diverted cargo. The base also had little warehouse room available, for it was reducing the number and capacity of its depots as part of a general scaling down of American installations in Britain. Base medical supply officers sent as much tonnage as they could to France by air, or by expedients, such as loading goods on trucks and hospital trains being ferried across the Channel. They perforce stacked the rest of the overflow in open fields. Fortunately, the New York Port of Embarkation packed ETO-bound medical supplies to withstand at least 90 days of outdoor storage. In both the United Kingdom and France large quantities survived exposure to the elements for much longer than that.[43]

On the Continent the railroads supplanted trucks for most long-distance supply hauling, a shift signaled by theater discontinuance, on 14 November, of Red Ball operations. The change from trucks to trains did not eliminate difficulties with transportation. After the end of the Red Ball Express the COMZ G–4 daily authorized the medical service to send a certain number of tons of supplies from Normandy to the front by train. Days went by, but no rail cars appeared at Depot M–402 and no supplies moved. Finally, late in November, Colonel Hays discovered the reason: The daily medical tonnage was not enough to fill an entire train, and "because of rail operating difficulties" the transportation authorities moved from Normandy only fully loaded trains bound for a single destination. "In other words," Hays stressed in his report to General Hawley, "although G–4 was setting up tonnage allocations and forwarding them to Normandy Base, no provision was made to move these supplies." The Supply Division chief negotiated with the G–4 a rearrangement of his allocation, under which, every few days, the Normandy Base Section could send a full trainload to Paris, where Depot M–407 then would reconsign individual cars to the armies and ADSEC. Such small shipments, however, were prone to loss and delay. One group of eight cars dispatched from M–407 took three to fourteen days, depending on the individual car, just to get through the Paris switching yards. On another occasion, only fourteen cars of a special forty-car train from Chef-du-Pont

---

[43] Supply Division, OofCSurg, HQ, ETOUSA, Annual Rpt, 1944, sec. II, p. 11 and ex. III, pp. 2–4; Wiltse, ed., *Medical Supply*, p. 321; Kelley Interv, 27 Jan 45, box 221, RG 112, NARA.

actually reached their destination at Reims.[44]

To keep tonnage moving forward, the Supply Division, the base sections, and the armies continued to employ the expedients of the summer pursuit. The Supply Division late in 1944 borrowed 150 trucks from the Ninth Air Force to haul 300 tons of badly needed items from Chef-du-Pont to Reims. The armies, as they had earlier, sent their own vehicles long distances back to the Communications Zone to collect what they needed. Between 1 and 15 December Third Army trucks picked up 50 tons of medical supplies in Paris and about 100 in Reims. Hospital trains evacuating casualties from Liege to Paris carried emergency supplies for the First and Ninth armies, and for Depot M–409 and the Liege general hospitals on their northbound runs. At times, also, the Paris depot coupled regular freight cars to these trains for the trip to Liege. Aircraft—C–47s across the Channel to Le Bourget field and the UC–64s of the 320th Air Transport Squadron from Paris to the front—hauled millions of pounds of blood, biologicals, and high-priority cargo. All these expedients, however, contributed little to the heavy-duty job of filling the forward depots. Because of lack of transportation, at the end of November the great bulk of reserve medical supplies still were concentrated at Chef-du-Pont and Paris, with only comparatively small stock accumulated in the COMZ depots nearest the front.[45]

During the last weeks of 1944 and the early months of the new year the ETO medical service, assisted by a general improvement in the theater logistical situation, largely resolved its supply movement and distribution problems. The port of Antwerp went into full operation, in spite of harassing bombardment by German V-weapons, and the shipping backlog rapidly diminished, as did the frequency of cargo diversions to Great Britain. The United Kingdom Base managed to move across the Channel much of the excess stock it had accumulated. On the Continent the end of the SHAEF tonnage allocation system freed more of the available transportation for the movement of reserve supplies. To expedite medical shipments and reduce losses in transit, the Supply Division in December established a Movement Control Section. Officers of this section, stationed at strategic road and rail junctions, followed each truck convoy or rail car carrying medical supplies from originating depot to final destination. Colonel Hays admitted that these efforts duplicated "to a large extent the work of the Transportation Corps but

[44] Quotations from Supply Division, OofCSurg, HQ, ETOUSA, Annual Rpt, 1944, sec. II, ex. III, pp. 9–10 and 12–13. See also ADSEC Hist, p. 76; Wiltse, ed., *Medical Supply*, pp. 339–40.

[45] Supply Division, OofCSurg, HQ, ETOUSA, Annual Rpt, 1944, sec. II, pp. 19–22 and ex. III, pp. 13–15, and Semiannual Rpt, January–June 1945, sec. II, p. 11 and exs. X and XI; Surg, Seine Section, Annual Rpt, 1944, pp. 39–41, and Semiannual Rpt, January–June 1945, p. 40. Hawley thanks the Air Force for its support in Ltr, Hawley to Lt Gen Carl T. Spaatz, 14 Nov 44, file HD 024 ETO CS (Hawley Chron). For continental reserve distribution, see Memo, Col S. B. Hays to Operations Division, OofCSurg, HQ, ETOUSA, 25 Nov 44, sub: Tonnage Reports at Depots, box 63, RG 112, NARA.

it has been found to be necessary, and . . . it has paid dividends." [46]

The efficiency and reliability of railroad freight service improved steadily, partly because of continuing physical rehabilitation of the French and Belgian lines and partly because of better medical service and Transportation Corps documentation of shipments. Under a new cargo identification system, for instance, each carload of medical supplies had a distinctive exterior label—the familiar Red Cross on a white field—placed on it. With more efficient transportation available, and greater freedom to use it, the medical service within a couple of months evened out the distribution of its reserves. Of the about 40,700 tons of medical stores on the Continent, only 6,000 or so remained at Chef-du-Pont and Marseilles by the end of February. The rest of the supplies were at Paris, the largest single concentration, and in intermediate and advance depots.[47]

As had been the case since the beginning of BOLERO in 1942, movement of equipment assemblies for the many new medical units arriving in the theater, especially the 4,000-piece outfits of the general hospitals, continued to be plagued with difficulties. Equipment became separated from units during transshipment in Britain or split between depots there and on the Continent when port congestion forced diversion of vessels. Rail and road movement in France and Belgium suffered from the vicissitudes of the overloaded transportation systems, including the usual losses and diversions. Medical units newly arrived on the Continent often waited weeks for Communications Zone to locate and deliver their assemblies. Without equipment, General Hawley complained, these organizations constituted "merely . . . more mouths to feed and bodies to shelter, without any return in service," an exaggeration since many of them reinforced operating units. Nevertheless, when the theater during November and December was racing desperately to set up more continental beds to take care of ever-increasing casualties, it helped little to have nineteen general hospitals sitting idle for lack of equipment. During the Ardennes emergency the Paris supply depot built two general hospital outfits from its own stock, to hasten activation of units. Such expedients used up replacement equipment reserves and could not begin to compensate for nondelivery of the original assemblies.[48]

Even the persistent assembly problem, however, gradually yielded to

[46] Quotation from Supply Division, OofCSurg, HQ, ETOUSA, Annual Rpt, 1944, sec. II, ex. III, p. 16. See also ibid., sec. I, p. 2, sec. II, p. 22 and ex. III, pp. 11 and 13, and Semiannual Rpt, 1945, sec. II, p. 5.

[47] Supply Division, OofCSurg, HQ, ETOUSA, Semiannual Rpt, January-June 1945, sec. III, p. 20; Surg, United Kingdom Base, Semiannual Rpt, January-June 1945, vol. 1, p. 127. The movement of stocks can be followed in Memos, Col S. B. Hays to Operations Division, OofCSurg, HQ, ETOUSA, 9 and 30 Oct, 27 Nov, 5 Dec 44 and 28 Jan, 26 Feb 45, sub: Tonnage Balances at Depots, box 63, RG 112, NARA.

[48] Quotation from Ltr, Hawley to G-4, ETOUSA, 14 Nov 44, sub: Delays in Movement of Medical Units and Unit Equipment, in Supply Division, OofCSurg, HQ, ETOUSA, Annual Rpt, 1944, sec. V, ex. VI. See also ibid., sec. II, ex. III, pp. 5-7 and 11, sec. IV, pp. 6-7 and ex. VII, sec. V, pp. 2-6 and exs. IV(a), VI, and XI; Surg, Normandy Base Section, Annual Rpt, p. 20; Surg, Seine Section, Annual Rpt, 1944, p. 41; Wiltse, ed., *Medical Supply*, pp. 337-39; Ltr, Hawley to Maj Gen W. M. Goodman, 14 Nov 44, file HD 024 ETO CS (Hawley Chron).

theater remedial efforts and improving transportation facilities. Under new staging procedures, adopted on 1 November, units that disembarked in Britain remained there until both their TAT equipment and their assemblies were on hand and ready to accompany them across the Channel. The New York and Boston port authorities, after a barrage of letters, telegrams, and teletype messages from Hawley, on the twenty-ninth agreed to a plan that at least ended the practice of splitting general hospital outfits among several ships and ensured delivery of "functionally complete" assemblies. Diversion of assemblies to Great Britain ended early in 1945, and they received higher unloading priority at continental ports. The Supply Division established procedures for following each assembly from its departure from the United States to an operating site. It also secured permission from the Transportation chief to send escort officers from the owning unit with each assembly during both cross-Channel and continental movement. This practice, long informally followed by veteran units, greatly increased the chances that an assembly would arrive at its destination complete and on time.[49]

Meanwhile, the major medical depots improved their operating efficiency and solved a variety of practical problems, sometimes by sheer hard work. At Depot M–402 the 11th Medical Depot Company used bulldozer-drawn mud sleds and 750 POW laborers to sort out and ship forward the mass of supplies suddenly unloaded at Cherbourg during November. In mid-January 1945 the same company took over Depot M–407 at Paris. Here its men, reinforced by a second company and by more than 260 French civilians, in six weeks unloaded a backlog of 120 freight cars and 7 barges. Working in cold and snow, they filled over 850 accumulated requisitions and thereafter more or less kept abreast of the new ones, which arrived at a rate of about 100 a day. They acquired additional buildings for the equipment repair shop and for storage of slow-moving items, and they rearranged the shipping and receiving sections for more efficient operation in less space. At Depot M–452 in Marseilles the 46th Medical Depot Company, an ETO unit, early in January reinforced the 231st Composite Medical Battalion, a veteran Mediterranean Theater organization. The new company, besides providing badly needed additional manpower for this busy port depot, introduced the European Theater stock control system. With the 231st Battalion it developed M–452 into the most completely mechanized depot in the theater, with stock stored on pallets for movement by forklift trucks and with over 3,000 feet of roller conveyor.[50]

[49] Supply Division, OofCSurg, HQ, ETOUSA, Annual Rpt, 1944, sec. II, ex. III, pp. 16–17, sec. IV, p. 7, sec. V, pp. 5–6 and exs. VI and VII, and Semiannual Rpt, January–June 1945, sec. IV, pp. 2–3 and 6–8; Surg, Normandy Base Section, Annual Rpt, p. 20. For an example of the practice of escorting assemblies, see 28th Field Hospital Annual Rpt, 1944, pp. 15–16.

[50] Supply Division, OofCSurg, HQ, ETOUSA, Annual Rpt, 1944, sec. II, p. 12, and Semiannual Rpt, January–June 1945, sec. III, pp. 9–11 and 16; Surg, Delta Base Section, Annual Rpts, 1944, p. 1, and 1945, p. 4; Surg, Normandy Base Section, Annual Rpt, 1944, encl. 8; Surg, Seine Section, Annual Rpt, 1944, p. 41, and Semiannual Rpt, Janu-

Continued

Two COMZ depots, M-409 at Liege and M-408 at Reims, felt the direct impact of the Ardennes counteroffensive. For the better part of a month the 66th Medical Depot Company at M-409 worked under constant V-1 and V-2 bombardment and nightly air raids. Near-misses damaged the depot buildings and destroyed some supplies, but the company and its reinforcing detachment of the 165th Medical Battalion suffered no casualties and never had to cease operations. Besides its regular work of supplying the Liege hospitals and the First and Ninth Army depots, M-409 for a couple of weeks acted as base depot for the First Army. At Reims, amidst air attacks, Depot M-408, reinforced by 45 POW laborers (double guarded to prevent breakout or mutiny), worked under blackout conditions in subfreezing weather to supply the divisions holding the southern flank of the Bulge. M-408 provided medical supplies and equipment for the 82d and 101st Airborne Divisions before they entered the battle, and later helped to replace their combat losses. It also outfitted six provisional collecting companies and established two advance supply points for COMZ units preparing a last-ditch defense line along the Meuse, as well as making contingency plans for its own withdrawal.[51]

To take advantage of the northern ports and to facilitate supply of the armies, the medical service established three additional depots. Depot M-409 on 29 November 1944 opened a satellite facility (M-411) at Liege to handle the expected large volume of incoming stores from Antwerp, which lacked space for extensive supply dumps. However, German bombardment of Liege forced closing of this subdepot after less than a month of operation and its replacement by a new depot, M-413, in a less exposed position at Noirhat, near Brussels. Another depot, eventually designated M-417, went into operation near Rouen in January 1945, to hold general hospital assemblies landed at the Seine ports. The third new depot, M-414, opened in mid-February in an unused foundry at Foug, just west of Toul, after a prolonged COMZ effort to obtain from Third Army a usable site closer to that army's rear than M-408 at Reims. When finally opened, M-414, in Continental Advance Section territory, issued to both the Third and Seventh Armies, and also to the general hospitals clustered around Nancy, Commercy, and Bar-le-Duc. Through it the Seventh Army and CONAD began drawing the bulk of their medical supplies from the Channel ports and Antwerp instead of from Marseilles.[52]

ary-June 1945, pp. 39–40; 11th Medical Depot Company Hist, January-June 1945, pp. 1-3; 46th Medical Depot Company Semiannual Rpt, January-June 1945, pp. 1-4.

[51] Surg, ADSEC, COMZ, Semiannual Rpt, January-June 1945, p. 37; 66th Medical Depot Company Annual Rpt, 1944, p. 4; 165th Medical Battalion Annual Rpt, 1944, pp. 2-3, and Semiannual Rpt, January-June 1945, p. 2; 13th Medical Depot Company Annual Rpts, 1944, p. 13, and 1945, pp. 4 and 33-34.

[52] Wiltse, ed., *Medical Supply*, pp. 328-29; Supply Division, OofCSurg, HQ, ETOUSA, Annual Rpt, 1944, sec. II, pp. 15-17, and Semiannual Rpt, January-June 1945, sec. III, pp. 6 and 13-15; Surg, ADSEC, COMZ, Annual Rpt, 1944, pp. 29-30; Surg, CONAD, Semiannual Rpt, January-June 1945, pp. 12-13; 13th Medical Depot Company Annual Rpt, 1944, p. 12; 30th Medical Depot Company Annual Rpt, 1944, p. 7; 66th Medical Depot Company Annual Rpt, 1944, p. 4.

With its depot network in place and with reserve stocks well forward, the ETO medical service early in 1945 at last could implement the system for supplying the armies long envisioned in plans and SOPs. Every ten days each army dispatched a requisition, covering anticipated maintenance and replacement requirements, to a single designated COMZ advance depot through the appropriate regulating station; it could also make emergency requisitions as necessary. The supporting depot filled orders from its own stock and was automatically replenished in turn by the Communications Zone. Emergency shipments and supplies from rear COMZ depots normally went forward by air. Advance depots usually dispatched goods to the armies by truck, for road transport took less time than rail over short distances. Forward depots responded rapidly to army demands, sometimes within seventy-two hours. The Supply Division, through a set of simple reports from the issuing depots, monitored service to the armies.[53]

[53] Supply Division, OofCSurg, HQ, ETOUSA, Semiannual Rpt, January-June 1945, sec. II, pp. 8-9, sec. III, p. 6, sec. IV, pp. 4-5; Surg, ADSEC, COMZ, Semiannual Rpt, January-June 1945, pp. 36-37.

By the beginning of 1945 the medical service possessed a fully functioning continental supply system. It had established advance, intermediate, and rear depots, efficiently and uniformly administered, and with reliable stock accounting and control. Supplies from the United States flowed steadily and in ample quantities into this depot system and, to an increasing extent, smoothly through it to the armies. After a January visit to the theater by General Somervell, Hawley noted with gratification that the Army Service Forces commander and his entourage "had no criticism of medical supply" and that one officer, "after inspecting Medical Depot No. 409, said that he had never seen a finer depot."[54] Hawley, unfortunately, could not report such optimistic comments, from visitors and from within the theater, on the most important functions of the medical service, for which organization, personnel, and supply were simply the foundations. The chief surgeon's hospitalization and evacuation systems and policies came under increasing strain and mounting criticism as the Communications Zone struggled to cope with the flood of casualties from the fall and winter battles.

[54] Ltr, Hawley to TSG, 27 Jan 45, file HD 024 ETO O/CS (Hawley-SGO Corresp).

CHAPTER XIV

Hospitalization and Evacuation Crisis

By late 1944 the hospitalization and evacuation system had become a complex, dynamic chain of many links. Closest to the front were the Advance Section air and rail holding units. Those at Verviers and Liege served the First and Ninth Armies, and those at Nancy, Etain, and Thionville supported the Third. Behind the holding units were two forward clusters of general hospitals at Liege and Bar-le-Duc, astride the principal lines of communication north and south of the Ardennes. Backing up these hospital centers, the medical complex at Paris, hub of the entire system, consisted of seven general hospitals, extensive rail and air evacuation facilities, and a large convalescent camp. To the rear of Paris the Normandy and Brittany Base Sections contained additional general hospitals, the majority located in the Cotentin Peninsula and on the old battlefields inland from OMAHA beach. The Normandy Section also maintained a holding unit and casualty embarkation facilities at Cherbourg, the only cross-Channel evacuation port used by the American forces. Across the water, in the United Kingdom Base, a medical battalion and transit hospital at Southampton and field hospital platoon holding units at nearby Membury and Ramsbury airfields received casualties from France and transferred them to the final links of the chain: the dozens of general hospitals spread over the countryside of southern and western England.

From his Paris office, Colonel Mowrey, General Hawley's chief of evacuation, and his small, usually overworked staff regulated patient flow through these facilities in accord with a 30-day policy for the Continent and a 180-day policy (reduced in October to 120) for the theater as a whole. The system at each stage featured much sorting and many alternate movement paths. Forward holding units first divided incoming casualties into two groups: those requiring less then 30 days of hospitalization, and those needing longer-term care or evacuation to the United States. They dispatched the latter directly to Britain by air whenever planes were available. Of the under-30-day patients, those requiring less than two weeks of hospitalization went by rail and road to the Liege and Bar-le-Duc general hospitals. The rest, and longer-term cases for whom aircraft space was not available, were loaded on trains for the run to Paris, where Seine Section medics detrained

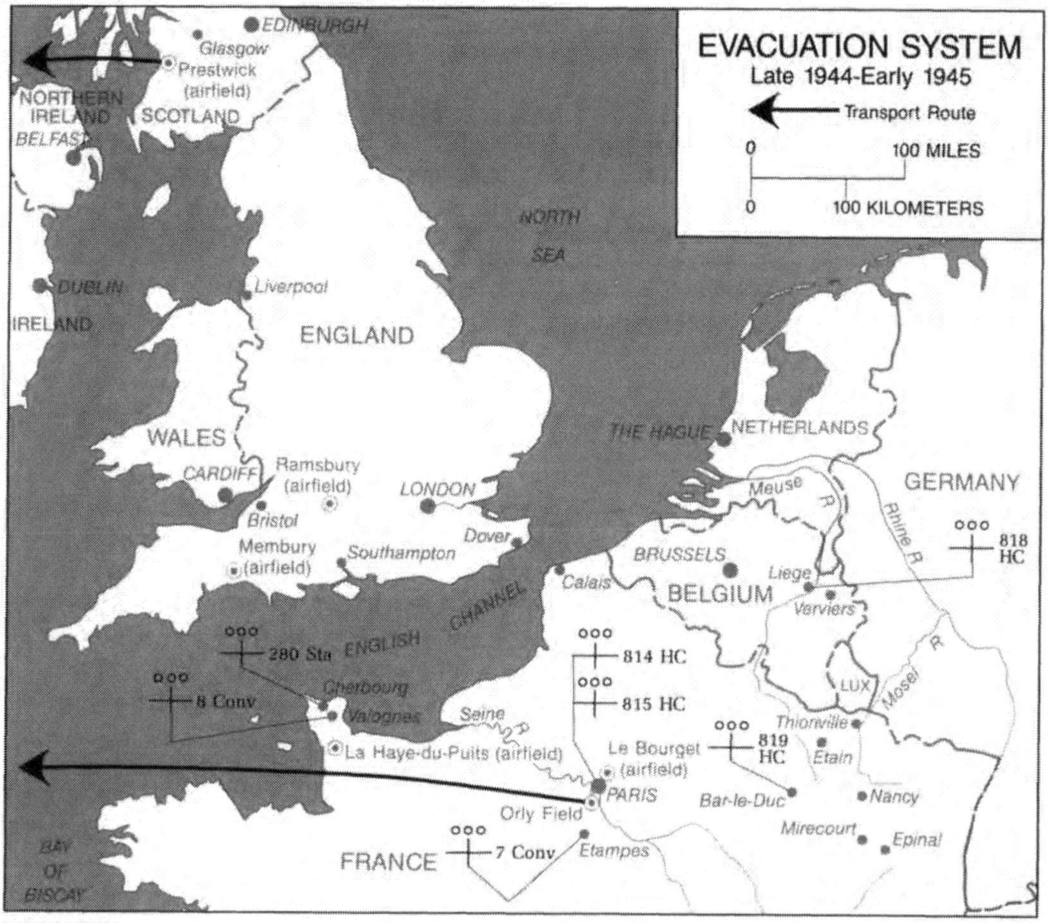

MAP 21

and sorted them. Continental patients, if not retained in the Paris general hospitals, traveled by rail to hospitals in the Normandy and Brittany Base Sections. Patients destined for the United Kingdom and the United States went directly to Britain by air from Le Bourget field or to Normandy by train for embarkation at Cherbourg.

The entire system was highly flexible and opportunistic. It gave preference to air evacuation whenever craft could be obtained and weather permitted, but it also could move a large volume of casualties by surface means alone. By varying the evacuation policies of the general hospitals in Paris, Liege, and Bar-le-Duc Colonel Mowrey could open up reserves of beds for sudden surges of casualties from the armies, while in quieter times he could keep many short-term patients near the front for rapid return to duty (*Map 21*).[1]

[1] Memo, Hawley to G–4, ETO, 19 Jan 45, file 705:Admission to and Operations in Hospitals; Evacuation Branch, Operations Division, OofCSurg, HQ, ETOUSA, Annual Rpt, 1944, pp. 5 and 10;

Continued

Behind the 6th Army Group, the Southern Line of Communications maintained a separate but similar evacuation system. From air and rail holding units in the Continental Advance Section, patients, depending on their expected length of time in the hospital, went to forward general hospitals around Epinal, Besancon, and Dijon or to rear installations at Marseilles, which was also the evacuation port for SOLOC patients bound for the United States. SOLOC initially did not send casualties to Great Britain or to the northern Communications Zone, but this practice changed under the November agreement between the two logistical commands. From then on, SOLOC, while retaining its separate line of evacuation, accepted the principle that all its facilities were part of a single theater pool. In return, it received assurance that COMZ would evacuate and hospitalize a portion of its patients if the limited facilities in southern France became overloaded. When this occurred, aircraft and hospital trains from Paris collected the overflow directly from forward CONAD installations.[2]

At each link in the evacuation chain, medical units, as they gained experience, steadily improved and refined their techniques for maximum efficiency and patient comfort and safety. Holding units learned to place in different wards their "COMZ short," "COMZ long," and "UK" cases. They took hourly patient censuses to facilitate the rapid makeup of train- and planeloads. By various expedients they mastered the always difficult problem of keeping each man and his records together through reception, sorting, and evacuation. Through channels both official and unofficial, evacuation officers secured the earliest possible notice of the arrival of planes and trains. This information was necessary to prepare for air evacuation, because flights of C–47s often landed on a few minutes' warning and could stay on the ground for only a short time. Also important were such details as the number of incoming "strap" and "bracket" craft, for the method of on-board litter suspension was critical in load planning—the two types had different patient capacities. Once the transportation was at hand, quick transfer of patients from wards to airstrips and platforms and then to airplanes and rail cars became the main consideration. Ambulance crews and litter detachments, their every movement precisely choreographed, became expert at combining speed and gentleness in this process.[3]

In Paris Colonel Mowrey's Evacuation Branch, after some initial confusion, delegated most of the day-to-day conduct of evacuation to Colonel Rich, the Seine Section surgeon, and

Surg, Seine Section, Annual Rpt, 1944, pp. 18–19; Surg, Normandy Base Section, Annual Rpt, 1944, pp. 5, 8–9 and encl. 3; 819th Hospital Center Annual Rpt, 1944, pp. 5–6; 15th General Hospital Annual Rpt, 1944, pp. 4–5; 94th Medical Gas Treatment Battalion Annual Rpt, 1944, p. 34; 186th Medical Battalion Annual Rpt, 1944, pp. 14–16; 552d Ambulance Company Annual Rpt, 1944, pp. 6–7.

[2] Evacuation Branch, Operations Division, OofCSurg, HQ, ETOUSA, Annual Rpt, 1944, p. 14; Wiltse, *Mediterranean*, pp. 401–04; MFR, Col D. E. Liston, 4 Dec 44, sub: Agreements Made at Conference, 15–16 November 1944, DRAGOON 1944 file, CMH.

[3] 94th Medical Gas Treatment Battalion Annual Rpt, 1944; 28th Field Hospital Annual Rpt, 1944, p. 21.

his staff. The two offices jointly established an evacuation priority for each class of patients so that the Seine Section, by loading low- as well as high-priority cases when large numbers of casualties were due in from the front, could fill all available outgoing transportation and quickly clear hospital beds. Late in the year the Seine Section placed the headquarters of the 343d Medical Battalion in administrative and operational control of its hospital train units, ambulance companies, litter detachments, and air holding units. This action relieved the overburdened section surgeon's staff of most details of evacuation management, and it permitted more efficient use of resources. The battalion organized a centrally dispatched pool of more than 100 ambulances, drawn from units throughout the section, for mass movement of patients between medical installations, airfields, and railway stations. The Seine Section made the most efficient use possible of its general hospitals. Those closest to the stations were assigned to casualty reception and triage, while others performed specialized surgical work, reducing the waste of professional talent that resulted when the big hospitals were used as holding and transit facilities.[4]

Means of casualty transportation were in steadily increasing supply. Air evacuation, the first choice of surgeons for moving the seriously ill and injured, continued on a large scale throughout the late autumn and winter, in spite of worsening weather and persistent administrative uncertainties. C-47s of the IX Troop Carrier Command and the 302d Air Transport Wing during the last three months of 1944 carried the majority of patients who crossed the Channel. On one peak day in November they evacuated more than 3,000 casualties from France to Great Britain. By late 1944 the air forces and the chief surgeon's office had established workable procedures for timely transmission of aircraft requests from forward holding units to SHAEF's Combined Air Transport Operations Room. Air Force authorities were increasingly generous in allocating planes for evacuation, and the basing of a C-47 wing at Le Mans made more craft regularly available.

By formal or informal means, medics and cooperative air liaison officers almost always managed to produce planes where and when they were needed. Late in the year the 302d Wing converted the theater's only designated aeromedical transport squadron, the Paris-based 320th, from single-engine UC-64s, which had proved less than totally suitable for evacuation and resupply, to the larger C-47s, further increasing medical service airlift capacity. SHAEF periodically reiterated that air evacuation should be considered only a

[4] Evacuation Branch, Operations Division, OofCSurg, HQ, ETOUSA, Daily Diary, 16 and 25-26 Oct 44, file HD 024 ETO; Surg, Seine Section, Annual Rpt, 1944, pp. 21-22, 28-29, 49-50; 40th General Hospital Annual Rpt, 1944, pp. 55 and 81; 48th General Hospital Annual Rpt, 1944, pp. 35-36; 425th Ambulance Company Annual Rpt, 1944, pp. 2-3, and Hist, January-June 1945, pp. 3-4. See also, in file HD:ETO:370.05:Evacuation, Sep-Dec 44, MFR, Col Mowrey, n.d.; Memo, Col Cutler to Chief, Professional Services Division, OofCSurg, 26 Oct 44, sub: Meeting of Surgical Chiefs, Paris Hospitals . . . ; Memo, Maj D. J. Twohig to Chief, Evacuation Branch, Operations Division, OofCSurg, 31 Oct 44, sub: Evacuation of Patients From Paris General Hospitals to Cherbourg.

bonus, but by the end of the year its transportation agencies were treating medical evacuation flights as a permanent and indispensable element in their planning.[5]

The ETO medical service acquired more hospital trains during the fall and winter and operated them with increasing efficiency. Between 30 September and the end of the year the northern Communications Zone doubled its medical rolling stock from 17 trains to 34. Most of the additional trains were brought over from Great Britain; others were built on the Continent, to medical service specifications, by the reconstituted French railway authorities. The Southern Line of Communications in the same period acquired six trains of its own, four shipped directly from the United States and two constructed by the French. The trains of both zones had an aggregate capacity of over 8,000 litter and 3,700 ambulatory patients and well exceeded in numbers the theater's planned ratio of trains to divisions. Except for a chronic lack of heat in the cars, the equipment was adequate for the task, especially when improved by the ingenuity of the medical crews, who added furniture and enlarged kitchens and water storage facilities.

Train running times remained irregular and usually slow. The French railroads were battle-damaged and congested, and subject to interruption by accidents and occasional enemy air attacks. Nevertheless, General Hawley, by constant pressure on the Transportation Corps, gradually secured higher scheduling priority for his trains. In late December the average round trip between Paris and Cherbourg took about 47 hours, compared to 96 to 120 earlier in the campaign. Hospital train units and dispatching and receiving hospitals and holding units, as they acquired greater proficiency in their work, steadily reduced turnaround times in the forward areas and at Paris. The Seine Section, which provided stabling and servicing for the entire COMZ train complement, during October acquired trackage at a second station, the Gare de l'Est, as the terminal for trains shuttling between the capital and the Third Army area. The section thus reduced congestion at the Gare St.-Lazare, which continued to handle all trains from the First and Ninth Armies and also those running between Paris and Cherbourg. To speed the turnaround of trains, the section set up a medical supply point for them at the Gare St.-Lazare, as well as rest and bathing facilities at both terminals for the hard-worked staffs. Even with these improvements, the combination of slow runs and increasing casualty flow kept every train in

[5] Admin Memo No. 147, OofCSurg, HQ, ETOUSA, 2 Nov 44, AirEvacCorresp, file HD 580 ETO; Evacuation Branch, Operations Division, OofCSurg, HQ, ETOUSA, Daily Diary, 30 Dec 44, file HD 024 ETO, and Annual Rpt, 1944, pp. 12-14 and encl. 10; Robert F. Futrell, *Development of Aeromedical Evacuation in the USAF, 1909-1960*, USAF Historical Study no. 23 (Maxwell Air Force Base, Ala.: USAF Historical Division, Research Studies Institute, Air University, 1960), pp. 238, 240, 242-43. On SHAEF acknowledgement, see Extract from Thirtieth Weekly Military Shipments Priority Meeting, 16 Dec 44, EvacCorresp, 1944-45, file HD 370.05 ETO, and Memo, HQ, COMZ, to SHAEF, 26 Dec 44, file 370.05 Evacuation (Planning).

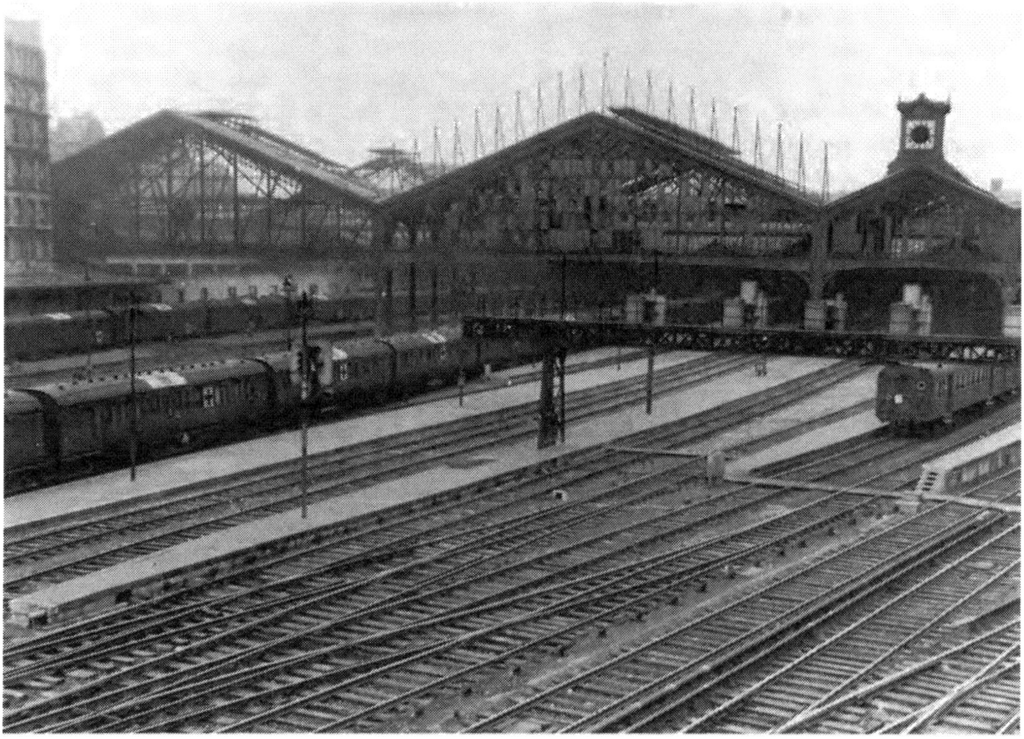

GARE ST.-LAZARE, PARIS

almost constant service, with little time between trips for maintenance of the equipment or leave for the medical personnel.[6]

Persistent Problems

Despite much progress, three persistent problems hampered—and, on occasion, almost paralyzed—the theater hospitalization and evacuation system during the winter battles of 1944–45. The theater faced a shortage of fixed hospital beds, largely resulting from delays in setting up enough general hospitals on the Continent. At the same time a lack of cross-Channel shipping, combined with the long, inefficient line of evacuation through Cherbourg, jeopardized the smooth flow of patients to the more numerous hospital beds in England. Finally, the United Kingdom

[6] Evacuation Branch, Operations Division, OofCSurg, HQ, ETOUSA, Daily Diary, 6, 9, 10, 23 Oct 44, file HD 024 ETO, and Annual Rpt, 1944, pp. 10–11 and encl. 4, and Semiannual Rpt, January–June 1945, encl. 2, pp. 2–3; Surg, ADSEC, COMZ, Annual Rpt, 1944, pp. 17–18; Surg, Seine Section, Annual Rpt, 1944, pp. 39–40; Memo, Kenner to G–4, SHAEF, 11 Nov 44, Medical Division, COSSAC/SHAEF, War Diary, November 1944; Memo, HQ, COMZ, to SHAEF, 26 Dec 44, file 370.05:Evacuation (Planning). For details of train operations, see 14th, 16th, 18th, 43d, and 45th Hospital Trains Annual Rpts, 1944; 99th General Hospital Annual Rpt, 1944, p. 17; and 552d Ambulance Company Annual Rpt, 1944, p. 10.

hospitals themselves were becoming overloaded, due to a combination of General Hawley's 180-day evacuation policy, a shortage of transatlantic shipping for casualties, and disputes within the theater and between the theater and the War Department over the proper method of using what shipping there was. Throughout the autumn Generals Kenner and Hawley and their superiors in Paris, London, and Washington argued and worried about these problems. By mid-December they were beginning to hammer out solutions to some of them. The solutions, however, were only partially in effect when winter and war imposed on the medical service the most severe challenge yet to confront it.

Establishing hospitals on the Continent as close as possible behind the advancing armies had been a major concern of General Hawley since before D-Day. During the last three months of 1944 alone the Hospitalization Division put twenty-two new continental plants in operation, the majority in the advanced clusters around Liege and Bar-le-Duc. Other general hospitals opened in Paris, Le Mans, Rouen, and Antwerp. The Southern Line of Communications effectively doubled its fixed bed capacity during the same period, with most of the new beds in general hospitals close behind the Seventh Army. Late in the year the two communications zones between them had about 50,000 general, station, and convalescent hospital beds in operation, roughly two-thirds of them in the northern COMZ. The United Kingdom Base, with the BOLERO hospital construction program fully completed, contained over 96,000 T/O and about 35,000 emergency expansion beds. On the Continent two hospital centers went into operation in December, the 818th at Liege and the 819th at Bar-le-Duc. In the United Kingdom Base seven centers were at work, coordinating the activities of dozens of general hospitals. At each center the headquarters, by consolidating administration, supply, and evacuation and redistributing professional staff when necessary, greatly increased the efficiency of its attached units.[7]

Yet the continental hospitalization program, progress notwithstanding, had fallen considerably short of its objectives. Before D-Day the Hospitalization Division had set the goal of having twenty-five general hospitals open in France by 31 August; it did not reach that objective until late October. By the end of December the division was less than halfway to its new target of seventy-nine continental plants in operation by 30 April 1945. Not all the units opened during the autumn were of direct use in handling battle casualties. In the Channel Base Section, for example, new general hospitals served primarily COMZ units in Antwerp and other ports, or received sick and injured from the tens of thousands of incoming troops

[7] Hospitalization Division, OofCSurg, HQ, ETOUSA, Annual Rpt, 1944, pp. 11–12 and 15–20, and Semiannual Rpt, January–June 1945, encl. 34; Surg, CONAD, Annual Rpt, 1944, pp. 4–7; Memo, HQ, COMZ, to SHAEF, 26 Dec 44, file 370.05:Evacuation (Planning); Surg, Normandy Base Section, Semiannual Rpt, January–June 1945, p. 13. On hospital centers, see James B. Mason, "The Surgeon of the Higher Echelon and the Hospital Center," *The Military Surgeon* 3 (November 1952): 321, and 819th Hospital Center Annual Rpt, 1944, pp. 1–2.

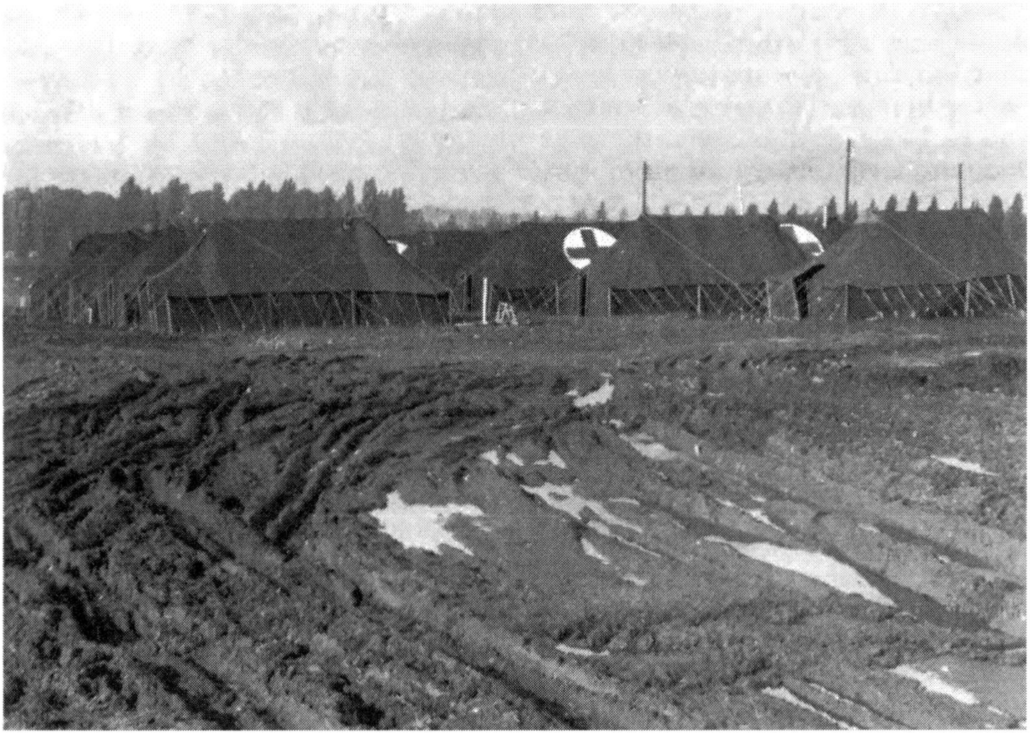

TENTS OF THE 76TH GENERAL HOSPITAL *near Liege*

who passed through the vast RED HORSE staging area around Rouen.[8]

The delay in setting up more hospitals was not due to a lack of operating units. At most times during the autumn and winter between twelve and twenty general hospitals were idle on the Continent and in Britain, awaiting equipment and plants. The latter proved increasingly difficult to secure. The Hospitalization Division reconnoitered and requested more than enough sites, almost all with suitable standing buildings, at locations as far forward as Aachen, Verdun, and Luxembourg. However, as winter descended, the medics had to compete for space under roofs with other Army elements and with French and Belgian civilian agencies. Elaborate negotiations, conducted through SHAEF, were often needed before the civilian authorities grudgingly gave way. The field armies, needing shelter for their own medical and other units, also resisted handing over facilities, and the slowed pace of the advance in late autumn further delayed medical service occupation of forward sites. Hospitals that did get into their plants then had to cope with the effects of battle damage and German sabotage; the difficulty of obtaining engineer construction support; the

[8] Hospitalization Division, OofCSurg, HQ, ETOUSA, Semiannual Rpt, January-June 1945, encl. 4; Surg, Channel Base Section, Annual Rpt, 1944, pp. 7-9 and enclosures.

shortage of building materials; and the vagaries of scarce, unreliable civilian labor. For units setting up or operating in tents, like some in Normandy and Liege, cold winds, rain, snow, and mud compounded all other difficulties.[9]

In early December General Kenner opined that the hospital bed shortage was approaching crisis proportions. He pointed out that the fixed hospitals of COMZ, SOLOC, and the United Kingdom Base were already treating 7,000 patients more than their operating capacity. In addition, a large backlog of casualties awaited evacuation across the Channel and to the United States. The SHAEF chief surgeon recommended that the theater give highest priority to establishing 100,000 fixed beds on the Continent. He pressed Hawley both to find a way of speeding cross-Channel transportation and to reduce his evacuation policy, clearing more patients out of the United Kingdom. While Hawley fully concurred with Kenner's call for more beds on the Continent, he insisted that the situation was not as critical as it seemed, because Kenner counted only the T/O bed capacities of hospitals, which could accommodate larger emergency patient loads if necessary. By COMZ's reckoning, which included over 35,000 emergency expansion beds in Great Britain and 20,000 on the Continent, the theater still had a thin but viable cushion of unused capacity. Inconsistent counting methods obscured the entire issue. Both Kenner and Hawley ignored COMZ's thousands of holding and transit beds, nor did they consider the fact that many patients in the continental fixed hospitals were actually short-term cases, rather than true general hospital patients requiring prolonged and elaborate treatment. Nevertheless, it was clear that the system was operating somewhere near the upper limit of its capacity.[10]

Over and above the question of whether the hospitals could accommodate all the American Army's casualties was another issue: that of caring for the sick and wounded among the nearly 300,000 German troops taken prisoner since D-Day. During the summer and fall the United Kingdom Base designated a steadily lengthening list of station hospitals to provide minimal treatment for these patients, before they were evacuated to the United States under a 30-day theater policy for POWs. Many Germans eventually wound up in hospitals in such exotic places as Tennessee and Arizona. The European Theater already was having difficulty finding

[9] Memo, Hawley to CofS, COMZ, 14 Dec 44, file HD:ETO:370.05:Evacuation, Sep–Dec 44; Memo, HQ, COMZ, to SHAEF, 26 Dec 44, file 370.05:Evacuation (Planning); Surg, ADSEC, COMZ, Annual Rpt, 1944, p. 11; Surg, Seine Section, Annual Rpt, 1944, pp. 17–21; Surg, Normandy Base Section, Annual Rpt, 1944, p. 8; Darnall, "Sidelights," p. 27, and "Breakthrough to Paris, " pp. 271–72. For examples of general hospital difficulties, see 167th General Hospital Annual Rpt, 1944, p. 6; 170th General Hospital Annual Rpt, 1944, pp. 4–8; and Cady, "Notes on the 21st General Hospital (AUS)," pp. 437–38, 446, 466, 484, 487–89, Cady Papers, MHI.

[10] Quotation from Memo, Kenner to CofS, SHAEF, 7 Dec 44, file HD:ETO:370.05:Evacuation, Sep–Dec 44. In same file, see Ltr, AG, SHAEF, to CG, COMZ, ETO, 9 Dec 44, sub: Status of US Hospitalization and Evacuation. . . . See also MFR, Kenner and Hawley, 2 Dec 44, sub: US Hospital Bed Situation, Casualty Evacuation and Other Medical Matters, in Medical Division, COSSAC/SHAEF, War Diary, December 1944; Memo, HQ, COMZ, to SHAEF, 26 Dec 44, file 370.05:Evacuation (Planning).

beds for its POW patients, and personnel to attend them, when the War Department in mid-November compounded its troubles. Anticipating an early collapse of the Reich, the department ordered a halt to movement of almost all prisoners, including patients, across the Atlantic. As a result, by late December United Kingdom Base hospitals contained over 14,000 Germans. General Hawley's planners, looking ahead to another Allied breakthrough, produced astronomical estimates of the number of captured enemy to be cared for and warned that a high proportion would likely be severely ill or suffering from untreated, infected wounds. The stabilization of the front and the German counterattacks made this a future rather than a present problem. Nevertheless, the need to make decisions and take measures on POW hospitalization hung ominously over all discussions of the theater bed shortage.[11]

Whether for POWs or American casualties, additional hospital beds on the Continent obviously were needed. But no quick way could be found to put more plants in operation. General Kenner, through SHAEF, pressed the 12th Army Group to give up some sites in its possession and expedited negotiations with the Allies to obtain others. He and Hawley both worked through every possible channel to win the hospitals higher priority in the allocation of engineer support and transportation. Hawley's Supply Division improved the handling of hospital assemblies. Nevertheless, command attention and directives could not at once overcome manpower and materiel shortages, ice and snow, and tactical setbacks.[12]

Inefficiencies in cross-Channel sea evacuation also concerned General Kenner. Under army-navy arrangements made soon after D-Day, all casualty movement over the Normandy beaches and most transportation of patients on LSTs ended in late autumn. At the same time the United Kingdom Base discontinued casualty reception at Portland-Weymouth. From then on, all American patients not sent to Great Britain by air traveled on British hospital carriers shuttling between Cherbourg and Southampton. The Normandy Base Section surgeon, who had charge of embarkation, established the 280th Station Hospital at Cherbourg to hold trainloads of patients from Paris until a carrier came in; he employed ambulance and sanitary companies to move evacuees to the docks. Late in the autumn he acquired hospital train stabling facilities at the dockside Gare Maritime, which in peacetime served passengers on the French transatlantic liners. This arrangement permitted direct transfer of patients from rail cars to ships when schedules dovetailed. When they did not, the station hospital in Cherbourg, and in emergencies the Normandy general hospi-

[11] Smith, *Hospitalization and Evacuation*, pp. 234–35; Surg, United Kingdom Base, Annual Rpt, 1944, p. 15; MFR, Planning Branch, Operations Division, OofCSurg, ETO, 29 Nov 44, file HD 383.6 (Hospitalization and Medical Services for Prisoners of War, 1942–45).

[12] For examples of efforts to speed up the establishment of new hospitals, see MFR, Kenner and Hawley Conference, 22 Dec 44, sub: Evacuation and Medical Problems, in Medical Division, COSSAC/SHAEF, War Diary, December 1944; Memo, HQ, COMZ, to SHAEF, 26 Dec 44, file 370.05:Evacuation (Planning).

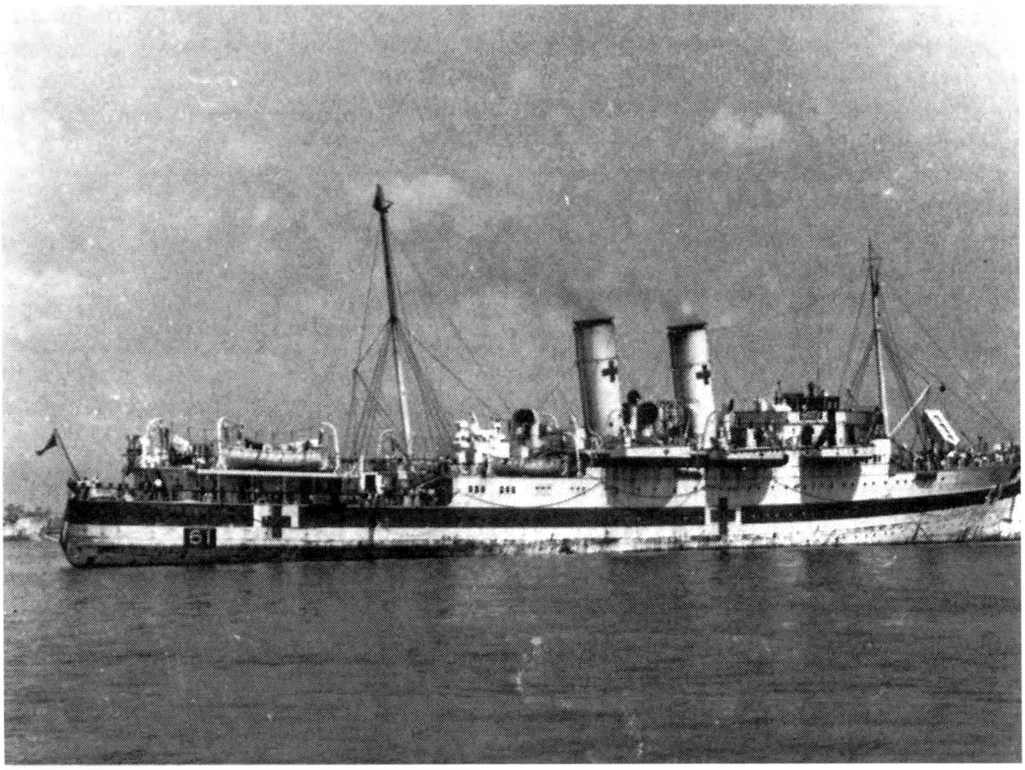

CROSS-CHANNEL EVACUATION ON HOSPITAL CARRIER *PRAGUE*

tals, temporarily housed and cared for the evacuees. During the last three months of 1944 the Normandy Base Section embarked over 50,000 sick and wounded GIs; the section sent off another 3,500 by air from a field near La Haye-du-Puits in the Cotentin.[13]

Casualty embarkation at Cherbourg was about as efficient as port congestion and increasingly treacherous Channel weather allowed. However, there simply were not enough ships to carry all the evacuees, especially if the Communications Zone took literally the periodic SHAEF injunctions to plan for evacuation entirely by surface means. After much negotiation, General Hawley by late autumn had secured from the British seven of their hospital carriers and two small hospital ships for the cross-Channel run. These vessels, on the rare occasions when all were in service at the same time, could carry about 1,000 patients per day, roughly half the rate

[13] Memos, Cdr, U.S. Naval Forces, Europe, to CG, ETOUSA, 18 Jul 44, sub: Inter-Theater Evacuation of Casualties, and Lt Col E. C. Andreassen to G–4, United Kingdom Base, 15 Sep 44, sub: Responsibility of Surgeon, UK Base, for . . . Evacuation . . . thru . . . Portland-Weymouth, EvacCorresp, 1944–45, file HD 370.05 ETO; Evacuation Branch, Operations Division, OofCSurg, HQ, ETOUSA, Daily Diary, 5 Oct 44, file HD 024 ETO, and Annual Rpt, 1944, p. 11; Surg, Normandy Base Section, Annual Rpt, 1944, pp. 4–6; 298th General Hospital Annual Rpt, 1944, p. 108 (the 298th preceded the 280th as the holding unit at Cherbourg).

required if COMZ were to function without air evacuation. The theater could increase the ships' effective capacity by opening a shorter cross-Channel route than the three-day, 350-mile round trip between Cherbourg and Southampton. Accordingly, at General Kenner's direction, various Allied committees and agencies explored alternative routes, such as that between Calais and Dover. All involved a shorter sea passage, and in some cases a shorter rail haul from Paris as well, but each possessed difficulties of its own. Docking and bunkerage for vessels and holding unit space for patients were limited on both sides of the Channel. On the British side, rail movement from east coast ports inland to the general hospitals would be longer and more complicated than from Southampton. Hospital trains from Dover would have to pass through the congested London metropolitan complex, a prospect that dismayed the British railway authorities. In addition, as long as numerous general hospitals were in operation in Normandy, some sea evacuation from Cherbourg would have to continue, regardless of what other routes were opened. Taking all these considerations into account, Allied evacuation and transportation officers, among them Colonel Mowrey, concluded at a mid-December London conference that they would have to make do for the time being with the Cherbourg-Southampton route, supplemented by continued maximum use of aircraft.[14]

Moving patients more efficiently within the system, even when it was possible, threatened to transfer the overload from the continental COMZ hospitals to those in Great Britain. If the medical service could not set up more beds, preferably in France, it could relieve the pressure only by getting patients out of the system more rapidly. Aside from death (so rare outside the forward emergency surgical units as to be statistically insignificant), a patient could leave the system in only two ways: by return to duty or by being evacuated to the United States.

Many patients leaving COMZ hospitals by the first route passed through the convalescent camps and centers administered by Colonel Diveley's Rehabilitation Division. By the time Colonel Diveley moved his office from London to Paris in January 1945, the program he had been instrumental in instituting had grown into a formidable complex. Its installations in Great Britain, after much exchanging of sites with other agencies, consisted of five rehabilitation and reconditioning centers with a total capacity of more than 12,000 men, staffed by medical personnel and nonmedical Limited Assignment officers and men from the Ground Force Reinforcement Command

[14] Evacuation Branch, Operations Division, OofCSurg, HQ, ETOUSA, Daily Diary, 2 Oct, 17 and 29 Nov, and 1, 10, 11, 16 Dec 44, file HD 024 ETO, and Annual Rpt, 1944, pp. 11–12; Memo, HQ, COMZ, to SHAEF, 26 Dec 44, file 370.05:Evacuation (Planning); and, in file EvacCorresp, 1944–45, file HD 370.05 ETO, Memo, CSurg, ETO, to CofTrans, ETO, 13 Dec 44, sub: Cross-Channel Sea Evacuation; Memo, Hawley to CMedOff, SHAEF, 12 Dec 44, sub: Cross-Channel Sea Evacuation; Extract from Thirtieth Weekly Military Shipments Priority Meeting, 16 Dec 44. All the shorter routes would have involved moving American casualties into or across the lines of communications of the 21 Army Group, something Allied logistical planners had tried to avoid throughout the campaign.

(GFRC). Late in 1944, after the War Department adopted a T/O for convalescent center units, the medical service organized five to operate the United Kingdom facilities, using personnel from four disbanded station hospitals. Besides the centers, the Rehabilitation Division in Great Britain oversaw reconditioning activities in thirteen station hospitals assigned to relieve general hospitals of nearly recovered patients, as well as programs in many of the general hospitals themselves. On the Continent the 7th and 8th Convalescent Hospitals, field army units under COMZ control, located respectively at Etampes near Paris and at Valognes in the Cotentin, prepared recovered soldiers from two of the largest general hospital clusters for return to the front. The facilities in the United Kingdom Base and on the Continent could accommodate in all about 31,500 trainees. About 85 percent of their graduates returned to some form of duty.[15]

But moving patients out of convalescent centers and hospitals into GFRC depots did not always go smoothly. General hospital commanders at times were less than prompt in clearing their wards, either out of professional desire to follow through on particularly interesting cases or because able-bodied convalescents helped to solve their perpetual shortage of labor. The chief surgeon, through his consultants, made constant efforts to suppress such practices. Some delays were not the hospitals' fault. General hospitals in the Normandy Base Section, for example, had difficulty obtaining clothing and equipment for soldiers ready for discharge; at times they had to hold fit men for as long as a week for lack of small but indispensable items, such as canteen cups. Making matters still more difficult for the Normandy hospitals and convalescent camp, the Ground Force Reinforcement Command closed its Cotentin depot during the autumn. The medics then had to secure rail transportation for the returnees to the Paris reinforcement depot, and also find them rations and mess gear for the trip.[16]

When discharged patients entered the reinforcement system, the medical service still had some responsibility for them. The close relationship between the Reinforcement Command and General Hawley has already been noted.[17] In England the command's headquarters and Hawley's office had occupied adjacent buildings in Cheltenham and were only a block apart in Paris. Physical proximity made easier the informal cooperation that, here as elsewhere in the European Theater, took up the slack caused by organizational confusion. Each GFRC depot centralized and controlled the flow of replacements—former hospital patients and also new arrivals from the States and returning AWOLs—and each had a depot surgeon and a small complement of enlisted corpsmen, themselves often Limited Assignment men retained by the depot

[15] Rehabilitation Division, OofCSurg, HQ ETOUSA, Annual Rpt, 1944, pp. 10-21, 23-24, and Semiannual Rpt, January-June 1945, p. 1.

[16] For use of convalescent labor, see Cady, "Notes on the 21st General Hospital (AUS)," p. 449, Cady Papers, MHI, and Ltr, Hawley to Consultants, 10 Dec 44, box 3, Hawley Papers, MHI. On Normandy difficulties, see Surg, Normandy Base Section, Annual Rpt, 1944, p. 9, and 298th General Hospital Annual Rpt, 1944, pp. 108-09.

[17] See Chapter XIII of this volume.

to free able-bodied medics for frontline duty. The surgeons, under technical direction from both the base sections and the GFRC surgeon, Col. George G. Durst, MC, were the only medical men in daily contact with the stream of replacements.[18]

Depot surgeons spent much of their time on preventive medicine, because the pooling of men from many different sources raised the specter of communicable disease and demanded constant vigilance. "Repo depot" transients were particularly apt to catch and spread venereal disease, to which depot surgeons responded with the customary devices of propaganda, physical inspection, and treatment as necessary.

More fundamental was the depot surgeons' task of examining each replacement, making a medical profile of the man, and rating him as either General or Limited Assignment, if screening revealed a more permanent defect. In many instances, it did. According to the GFRC commander, Brig. Gen. Walter G. Layman, about 18 percent of hospital returnees had "some physical or emotional condition," usually directly related to the injuries that had caused their evacuation, and required "special consideration in reassignment." Limited Assignment men piled up in the depots because many jobs were closed to them and because commanders preferred to take General Assignment men, if possible. For a time in mid-1944 the theater brought chaos to the depots by allowing combat exhaustion centers to dump on the replacement system thousands of men recently released from narcosis therapy but unable to control their tremors long enough to stand inspection—and still far from able to resume combat. General Layman insisted that such cases not be sent to his facilities until they had "completed their full period of convalescence in suitable Medical Department installations," and he won his point. The General Assignment men sent forward to the divisions were again checked by unit surgeons and dentists, and complaints came back to the depots if any were found unfit for duty. In spite of difficulties the system moved men in large numbers. During November, December, and January about 207,000 U.S. Army patients returned to duty through COMZ hospitals, about half of them in the United Kingdom and half on the Continent.[19]

Compared to the flow back to duty via the Reinforcement Command, the number of patients evacuated from the theater to the United States, a little over 78,000 during all of 1944, was small. General Hawley, in adopting his 180-day evacuation policy, had intended it to be, for he wanted to

[18] Depot surgeons received technical direction on routine matters from the base section surgeons and special guidance on physical standards and other such questions from Colonel Durst. This somewhat anomalous dual responsibility worked out well in practice and, at Durst's recommendation, survived the July 1944 redesignation of the Reinforcement Command as a major command of ETOUSA.

[19] Quotations from Medical History of the Ground Force Reinforcement Command, ETO, 23 October 1943–30 June 1945, pp. 4, 13, 16, 18, 32–34, file 319.1-2 (GFRC). For an example of division processing, see 76th Infantry Division SOP (Medical Processing of Division Reinforcements), in Surg, 76th Infantry Division, Semiannual Rpt, January–June 1945. See also Memo, Anon. to Col Doan, 22 Feb 45, sub: Status of Hospitalization and Evacuation, file 705:Admission to and Operations in Hospitals.

retain in Europe as many salvageable veteran soldiers as possible. His policy, however, required a very large hospital system in the theater, and for that and other reasons it came under serious attack by late 1944. Beginning soon after D-Day, General Kenner repeatedly urged Hawley to reduce the policy to 120 days. The SHAEF chief medical officer wanted to lighten the load of patients he saw building up in the hospitals, especially those of the United Kingdom Base. Also, anticipating an early German collapse and a large post-surrender demand for beds for POWs and recovered Allied prisoners, Kenner wanted to clear out as many American patients as possible before the end of hostilities, when the European Theater was certain to lose its high priority for shipping. Hawley, throughout the summer, stuck by his position. He reiterated the desirability of conserving experienced manpower, and also argued that medical sea- and airlifts were only barely adequate for the number of men to be moved under the 180-day policy; hence, a shorter policy would do nothing but enlarge the backlog of patients awaiting transatlantic evacuation.[20]

Hawley's resistance prevailed because Kenner was unwilling to seek a SHAEF directive forcing a change. In the end, therefore, the decisive action came from the Office of the Surgeon General and the Army Service Forces in Washington. Surgeon General Kirk from the beginning had preferred a 120-day policy and had enforced it in all overseas theaters except the European Theater, where he had deferred to Hawley's wishes. By midsummer of 1944, however, Kirk had problems of his own. He possessed in the United States an embarrassing surplus of thousands of empty general hospital beds and was under pressure to close excess facilities to ease the nationwide doctor shortage. At the same time Kirk was having difficulty staffing all the hospital units requested by the theaters. Because overseas hospital bed requirements would decrease with a shorter evacuation policy and because the number of patients returning to fill zone-of-interior beds would correspondingly increase, a cut in the theater's evacuation policy was an obvious way to solve both problems. Accordingly, in August General Kirk recommended a reduction of the ETO policy from 180 to 120 days. Army Service Forces headquarters, to which Kirk was subordinate, after its own study of the problem, concurred in the recommendation. On 5 October the War Department instructed the theater to make the change.[21]

General Hawley considered the new evacuation policy "a fine example of an order that cannot be carried out" for lack of transportation. In the case of transatlantic air movement of patients, he clearly was correct. Evacuation by long-range four-engine C–54s of the Air Transport Command, initially promising, proved dis-

[20] Figures from Evacuation Branch, Operations Divison, OofCSurg, HQ, ETOUSA, Annual Rpt, 1944, encl. 11. On Kenner's views, see Notes of Kenner-Hawley Conference, SHAEF Main, 14 Aug 44, and MFR, Kenner, 4 Sep 44, sub: Evacuation Policy . . . , in Medical Divison, COSSAC/SHAEF, War Diary, August–September 1944. On Hawley's views, see Memo, Hawley to Inspector General, WD, 10 Oct 44, and Ltr, Hawley to TSG, 13 Oct 44, file HD 024 ETO O/CS (Hawley-SGO Corresp).

[21] For background to this decision, see Smith, *Hospitalization and Evacuation*, pp. 228–30, and Ltr, TSG to Hawley, 4 Sep 44, file HD 024 ETO O/CS (Hawley-SGO Corresp).

appointing after D-Day. Before the invasion the Transport Command assured the medical service of space on its planes for 6,000–10,000 patients per month; at its best, it delivered only about one-third of that. Making matters worse, the command, for lack of medical attendance on board and at stopovers, would take litter patients—those most needing air evacuation—up to only 30 percent of the average planeload. The medical service, too, encountered difficulty in moving patients from hospitals to the remote transatlantic air terminal at Prestwick.[22]

Most important, the theater Air Transport Board gave relatively low priority for space to casualties as opposed, for example, to air crews rotating back to the United States after completing their required number of combat missions. During autumn the board actually cut medical evacuation space allocations to a little over 1,000 a month. In partial compensation the Air Transport Command in October committed itself to move 2,000 patients per month directly from France to the United States via its new transatlantic terminal at Orly Field, just south of Paris. While the Air Force restored the heavily sabotaged airport, the Seine Section established a 400-bed holding unit for United States–bound casualties at a nearby general hospital. The new airlift began on 7 December when a C–54 took off, carrying 16 patients. Other flights soon followed, but inclement weather during the rest of the month restricted the total number of men lifted to 351. As 1944 ended, transatlantic air evacuation remained more promise than reality.[23]

With airlift negligible, most evacuees to the United States had to travel by ship. Sea transportation, especially of bed patients and of ambulatory cases who still required considerable medical attention (respectively Classes II and III in the War Department classification system) long had been a matter of contention between General Hawley and his Washington and ETO superiors. The chief surgeon from the earliest days of the theater had insisted, on grounds of patient welfare and safety, that bed-confined men should be sent to sea only on specially outfitted hospital ships, marked and protected as required by the Geneva Convention. During 1943 the War Department had adopted Hawley's position as its own and had undertaken an ambitious hospital ship procurement program. The effort, however, fell far short of its goals during 1944, and most of the vessels that were obtained were sent to the Pacific. With too few hospital ships to move even the nonambulatory fraction of its over-180-day patients, the European Theater obviously had to rely for further evacuation on westbound troop transports. These were in ample supply due to the continuing flow of reinforcements to Europe. Following standard War Department

[22] Quotation from Ltr, Hawley to TSG, 13 Oct 44, file HD 024 ETO O/CS (Hawley-SGO Corresp). In same file, see also Memo, Hawley to Inspector General, WD, 10 Oct 44.

[23] Memo, Col. F. H. Mowrey to Chief, Hospitalization Division, OofCSurg, 26 Sep 44, sub: Air Evacuation to the U.S., AirEvacCorresp, file HD 580 ETO; Evacuation Branch, Operations Division, OofCSurg, HQ, ETOUSA, Annual Rpt, 1944, pp. 15–16; Surg, Seine Section, Annual Rpt, 1944, p. 28; Futrell, *Aeromedical Evacuation*, pp. 379–82; Darnall, "Sidelights," p. 26.

procedures, surgeons at the ports of embarkation surveyed each of these vessels to determine its carrying capacity for each of the four classes of patients. The ports then furnished hospital equipment and supplies to each transport, as well as assigning on-board medical personnel.[24]

Until very late in 1944 the theater consistently made use only of a fraction of the sealift thus provided. There were practical reasons for this. Glasgow, Liverpool, and Bristol, the ports at which most troopships from the United States unloaded, were a considerable train ride from the United Kingdom Base hospital centers and provided no space for holding units of any size. The base surgeon was obliged to collect patients from the widely dispersed hospitals and to move them to the ports just in time to meet the vessels; yet, he rarely received sufficient notice of convoy arrivals for patients to be moved before the rigidly scheduled return sailing dates. The hospital ship platoons that provided on-board care often were short of professional personnel—nurses, for example—whom the theater had to furnish from its own limited reserves. A similar lack of advance sailing notice, remoteness of home ports from Army hospitals, and inadequate shipboard medical attendance restricted American use of British transports, notably the huge liners *Queen Elizabeth* and *Queen Mary,* each of which could carry 1,000 or more patients on every rapid, unescorted crossing. In addition, the big ships, which loaded from lighters in the Firth of Clyde, required prohibitively time-consuming efforts to embark litter patients, who had to be manhandled through side ports and up elevators and stairways not designed to accommodate them.

Policy questions also entered in. General Hawley's staff and the port surgeons frequently disagreed about the patient-carrying capacity of particular ships, with the European Theater generally producing the lower estimates, and loading vessels accordingly. Patient classification also was an issue. Hawley persistently designated patients as Class IIs or IIIs, requiring care and assistance, whom the port authorities and General Kenner thought could be considered Class IVs, able to travel as ordinary troops. The chief surgeon had grounds for his position. He pointed out that an amputee with one leg, who might be ambulatory on crutches in a hospital ward, became a bed patient on a ship, where he could not negotiate ladders or manage a tray in a mess line on a rolling deck. Hawley refused to place men whom he considered helpless in troop accommodations even if the result was a vessel that sailed half-empty.

Authorities in the United States and Great Britain tried manfully and, in the main, successfully to eliminate the practical obstacles to full use of the transports and also to reach a meeting of minds with Hawley and his staff on vessel capacities and patient classification. Nevertheless, Hawley dragged his feet throughout the autumn, and transport space continued to go unused while patients accu-

[24] The four classes (see Chapter IV) were: I (mental patient); II (hospital bed patient); III (ambulatory hospital patient); and IV (troop class patient, that is, able to travel in ordinary troop accommodations and take care of himself).

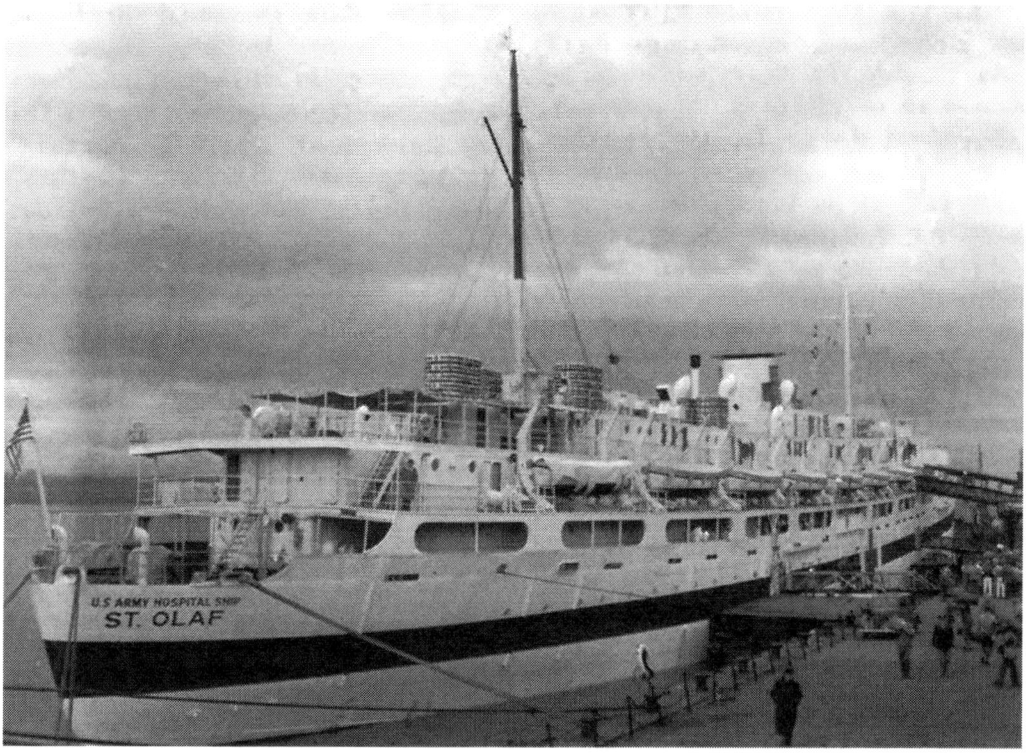

SEA EVACUATION ON U.S. ARMY HOSPITAL *ST. OLAF*

mulated in Britain. Behind the near-deadlock, reported an inspecting officer sent by the surgeon general, was a fundamental difference in outlook. Washington saw transoceanic evacuation as "basically an ambulance ride" on a grand scale, while Hawley viewed it as a continuation of the "definitive general hospitalization" that had begun in the United Kingdom Base or the big continental hospitals. A tenacious fighter on what he considered matters of principle, Hawley was also a shrewd administrator who kept a close eye on public relations. Very likely he held out in order to force the higher authorities to take unequivocal (and documented) responsibility for sending sick and wounded men to sea under conditions that he deemed to be substandard and unsafe.[25]

---

[25] Quotations from Rpt (to TSG), Lt Col John S. Poe, 12 Nov 44, sub: Visit to ETOUSA, box 256, RG 112, NARA. See also Memo, Chief, Passenger Branch, ETO, to ACofTrans (Movements), ETO, 2 Mar 44, sub: Evacuation of Sick and Wounded From the Continent . . . , EvacCorresp, 1942–44, file HD 024 ETO; Notes of Kenner–Col Davis–Col Mowrey Conference, 20 Oct 44, and Memo, Kenner to CofS, SHAEF, 26 Oct 44, sub: ZI Evacuation Problem, in Medical Division, COSSAC/SHAEF, War Diary, October 1944; Ltr, Hawley to TSG, 25 Oct 44, file HD 024 ETO O/CS (Hawley-SGO Corresp); Memo, Col F. H. Mowrey to CSurg, ETO, 2 Oct 44, sub: Utilization of the Queens, EvacCorresp, 1944–45, file HD 370.05 ETO; Evacuation Branch, Operations Division, OofCSurg, HQ, ETOUSA, Annual Rpt, 1944, pp. 14–15. For background on the shipping problem, see Joseph Bykofsky and Harold Larson,

Continued

The War Department, after weeks of inconclusive exchanges, finally gave Hawley the direct order he appeared to want. On 3 December the Army chief of staff, General Marshall, instructed the European Theater to make full use of United States transports for evacuation, filling them to their capacities as defined by the War Department. The theater was to do the same with the *Queen Elizabeth* and *Queen Mary*, as soon as it could make satisfactory arrangements with the British. If necessary to fill transport space, the theater was to reduce its evacuation policy temporarily to 90 days.[26]

Marshall's order had immediate effects. General Hawley on 10 December instructed United Kingdom Base and SOLOC surgeons to use 100 percent of the available evacuation lift and to include patients who needed 90 days of hospitalization, or even less, if necessary. He directed his consultants to scrutinize hospital disposition procedures, to make certain that commanders sent off promptly all evacuable patients. Even before the Marshall directive arrived, Hawley and the ETO Transportation chief, Maj. Gen. Frank S. Ross, completed arrangements with the British to augment the medical staffs of the *Queens* and to improve their hospital facilities so that each liner could accommodate about 1,700 Class II and III patients. To speed movement of evacuees to the embarkation ports, the United Kingdom Base borrowed six British hospital trains to supplement the eight already in its possession. Evacuation from the European Theater visibly accelerated. Under Washington's prodding, even before Marshall's order, the theater, which had evacuated a little over 8,200 men in September, shipped out over 12,500 in October and 11,300 in November. After the chief of staff's directive, the outward flow during December increased to 20,800.[27]

At the end of 1944 the theater and the War Department also made basic policy decisions on POW hospitalization. General Hawley late in the year sent a request to the War Department for 100,000 additional general hospital beds to accommodate POWs and the large number of displaced persons expected after the surrender of Germany. However, realizing that the chances of obtaining such a medical reinforcement were slim, he and his staff also explored the only remaining alternative: use of the over 350 captive German medical officers, 390 nurses, and 7,200 medical enlisted men in the theater to care for their own countrymen, either in separate wards of American hospitals or in all-prisoner facilities. Theater hospitals already had begun using limited numbers of Germans for this purpose. One SOLOC general hospital, the 21st, in November organized an entire prisoner section with a German

The Transportation Corps: Operations Overseas, United States Army in World War II (Washington, D.C.: Office of the Chief of Military History, Department of the Army, 1957), pp. 365–66.

[26] Msg, Marshall to ETOUSA, 3 Dec 44, copy in file HD:ETO:370.05:Evacuation, Sep–Dec 44. See also Smith, *Hospitalization and Evacuation,* p. 236.

[27] Ltr, Hawley to Surgs, SOLOC and United Kingdom Base, 10 Dec 44, sub: Evacuation to the ZI, file HD:ETO:370.05:Evacuation, Sep–Dec 44; Ltr, Hawley to Consultants, 10 Dec 44, box 3, Hawley Papers, MHI; Bykofsky and Larson, *Transportation Corps,* pp. 366–67; Memo, HQ, COMZ, to SHAEF, 26 Dec 44, file 370.05:Evacuation (Planning).

professional staff. Hawley approached this solution with caution, as did most other medical officers. Early reports on the performance of German medics were mixed; some proved insubordinate and poorly trained. Further, this policy would entail retention of German POW medical personnel for the duration of hostilities, in technical violation of the Geneva Convention requirement for the earliest possible repatriation. No belligerent power in this war had honored that provision of the Convention, but deliberate large-scale disregard of it by the United States might afford the Germans a pretext for violating other provisions, to the detriment of wounded Allied prisoners and those who cared for them. Necessity, however, left no alternative. Early in December Hawley approved a study by his Operations Division calling for broader, more systematic use of captured talent. Three weeks later, he endorsed the idea of hospitals staffed entirely by Germans, with only a small American supervisory cadre. The United Kingdom Base late in December reorganized the 327th Station Hospital as the first such all-POW facility.[28]

General Marshall, even more aware than Hawley that the bottom of the American medical manpower barrel had been reached, came to the same conclusion as the ETO chief surgeon. Just before Christmas, he and Secretary of War Henry L. Stimson decided, in spite of misgivings about the Geneva Convention, that the European Theater must use German medical personnel and entirely POW-staffed hospitals to care for prisoners. The Army simply could not provide staffing for Hawley's requested 100,000 beds. To confirm the feasibility of prisoner hospitals, and to investigate other aspects of the theater medical service, Marshall dispatched to Europe a medical officer then serving in the War Department G-4, Lt. Col. Crawford F. Sams.

Sams flew to Paris in a snowstorm, visited SHAEF, and embarked on a grand tour. He trekked through forward areas where the Ardennes battle was raging, he visited the POW camps of COMZ and SOLOC, and he saw the hospitals of both the northern and southern lines of communications. (In a curious coincidence, he was able to tell a German nurse working in SOLOC that her doctor husband was alive and well, working in another American hospital in northern France.) Everywhere, Sams found among the prisoners an abundance of medical talent. Some of the doctors had not been well trained by current American standards, for the once excellent German medical education system had suffered under the Nazis. But prisoners preferred to be cared

[28] Memo, Col Cutler to CSurg, ETO, 17 Nov 44, sub: Care of POWs by German Medical Officers; Memo, Professional Services Division, OofCSurg, to Operations Division, OofCSurg, 30 Nov 44; Staff Study No. 1, OofCSurg, HQ, ETOUSA, 1 Dec 44, sub: Medical Service for Enemy Prisoners of War (and related memo for Hawley, with his concurrence, 2 Dec 44); Ltr, Hawley to Surg, United Kingdom Base, 27 Dec 44; Memo, Hawley to ACofS, G-4, ETO, 20 Dec 44, sub: Medical Means Required for Prisoners of War. All in file HD 383.6 (Hospitalization and Medical Services for Prisoners of War, 1942-45). See also Surg, United Kingdom Base, Annual Rpt, 1944, p. 15; Cady, "Notes on the 21st General Hospital (AUS)," pp. 455-56 and 470-71, Cady Papers, MHI. For discussion of the Geneva Convention issue, see Crawford F. Sams, "Medic," pp. 295-96, CMH.

for by their own people. Sams concluded, confirming what Marshall already had decided, that equipment for the 100,000 additional beds should be sent to Europe, but no staff. As the new equipment arrived, it should be issued to the rearmost American hospitals that would be sent forward to support the armies. The equipment and plants left behind should be turned over to the POW medics, who would work under no more than general American supervision.[29]

On 28 December, even before Sams returned and reported, the War Department directed the European Theater to implement essentially the policy he recommended. General Hawley, with a new flood of prisoners in prospect from the cleanup of the Bulge and the resumption of the Allied offensive, lost no time in doing so. The United Kingdom Base converted half a dozen more station hospitals into POW facilities. On the Continent the Normandy Base Section in January 1945 began reorganizing its general hospitals in the Cotentin and near OMAHA beach into prisoner hospitals. Except for one unit, which remained to supervise the Germans, the American hospitals that had occupied these sites moved to new plants nearer the front, leaving behind their tentage and equipment and receiving new outfits as they went forward.[30]

By breaking the transatlantic evacuation deadlock and deciding to establish German-staffed POW hospitals, the War Department assured the eventual solution of two major ETO medical logistical problems. These actions, however, had only a marginal impact on the medical service's ability to respond to the German attack in the Ardennes. Indeed, setting up POW hospitals depended upon the ability of American general hospitals to occupy new sites farther forward. The delay in securing such sites was a principal component of the winter crisis. Theater medical personnel had to rely on resources and facilities already on hand, as they coped not only with battle casualties but also with victims of a pernicious combination of severe weather, poor supply planning, and inadequate health precautions.

Trenchfoot: The Other Enemy

The winter of 1944–45 was the coldest and wettest that Europe had seen in many years. To plague the already miserable American front-line infantry, winter brought an undramatic but crippling ailment: trenchfoot. Cases began to appear in October, and rapidly increased thereafter. In December, when the systems of evacuation and hospitalization were straining under the weight of wounded, the casualties of cold injury resulting from the Ardennes battle arrived in numbers that exceeded all expectations.

[29] Sams, "Medic," pp. 293–322, CMH.

[30] MFR, Planning Branch, Operations Division, OofCSurg, ETO, 10 Feb 45, sub: Prisoners of War Held by U.S. Forces in ETO; Memo, Planning Branch, Operations Division, OofCSurg, to Chief, Operations Division, OofCSurg, 13 Jan 45; Ltr, Col D. E. Liston to G-1, ETO, 13 Jan 45. All in file HD 383.6 (Hospitalization and Medical Services for Prisoners of War, 1942–45). See also Smith, *Hospitalization and Evacuation*, p. 236; Surg, Normandy Base Section, Semiannual Rpt, January–June 1945, pp. 2–4.

Cold injury took various forms depending on the depth of the chill and the length of exposure. Severe cold, notably at high altitudes where some bomber crewmen were subject to the direct blast of freezing winds, could cause quick tissue death. Milder frostbite occurred among the infantry as well. Slower and subtler was the ground type of cold injury, which did not even require especially low temperatures. In chilled feet the small blood vessels initially contracted, reducing the oxygen supply to the tissues; in serious cases the arterioles and the nerve endings were "irreversibly damaged" so that the effect of the injury persisted. Wetness increased the speed and severity of injury by conducting heat away from the body. Anything, such as tight shoelaces, that obstructed the flow of blood likewise hastened the onset of trenchfoot's unpleasant symptoms—numbness followed by swelling; then by intense pain; and, in some cases, by tissue death, with gangrene. Once injury occurred, the victim could look forward to a long course of treatment, and possible recurrence of the condition caused by the inability of damaged tissue to resist cold. Trenchfoot proved to be most dangerous to the front-line troops, who lived for long periods without shelter or dry clothing and who were often immobilized under enemy fire. No one died of trenchfoot, but its impact was heavy, both upon fighting regiments that lost their riflemen and upon the hospitals that cared for them.[31]

Americans met cold injury in three areas during the war—the Aleutians, Italy, and the European Theater. Little information moved from one theater to another and the lessons learned in one region had to be relearned elsewhere. Troops in Italy underwent their most severe trial in the winter of 1943–44, when more than 5,700 cases occurred. By the time of D-Day the Mediterranean Theater had worked out methods of control that reduced the number of cases in the following winter by almost three-fourths: Cases fell to 1,572, and admission rates tumbled from 54 per 1,000 troops per annum to 20. Better equipment and more rigorous discipline were the primary factors. Commanders ensured that boots were not laced too tight, that socks were changed as frequently as possible, that feet were massaged daily, and that warm tents were available where forward troops could gain a few hours' rest, whenever possible. The Mediterranean Theater's official report on trenchfoot was in the hands of its chief surgeon in January 1944 but failed to reach the European Theater until a year later, and then only in response to a direct request. The ETO chief consultant in surgery, Colonel Cutler, visited the Mediterranean and returned to urge timely preparations for meeting cold injury. But ETO medical officers were too preoccupied to heed his warning.

Cold injury approached the European Theater as a silent crisis, its possibility dimly foreseen but its poten-

[31] Unless otherwise noted, this section, to include statistics, is based on Tom F. Whayne and Michael E. DeBakey, *Cold Injury, Ground Type*, Medical Department, United States Army in World War II (Washington, D.C.: Office of the Surgeon General, Department of the Army, 1958), pp. 127–210. Quotation from Whayne Comments, 4 Dec 86, p. 17, CMH.

tial for havoc unappreciated. The problem became lost in the vast complexity of the planning and buildup for invasion, when medical planners were occupied with more pressing needs. The medical annex to OVERLORD did not mention cold injury; COMZ's NEPTUNE plan remarked only that "the cold, wet weather prevailing during the winter season in the area will predispose combat troops to this affection" and that "supplying seasonal changes of clothing opportunely, giving particular attention to the furnishing of proper footwear" was important in preventing trenchfoot.[32] Several ETO publications recommended that shoes be laced tightly. The 1944 *Manual of Therapy*, issued over Hawley's signature, summed up its contribution to the prevention of cold injury in a single sentence: "The importance of a footbath with soap and water cleansing, vigorous massage (20 minutes), dry socks, and a change of shoes in the prophylaxis of foot disability resulting from exposure to cold and moisture, cannot be overemphasized." [33] A comprehensive command directive on care of the feet, prepared by Colonel Gordon, the Preventive Medicine Division chief was disapproved for publication by the Adjutant General, ETOUSA, on the ground that existing manuals covered the subject and that, in any case, cold injury prevention was the responsibility of subordinate commands. By the time publication of a circular letter took place on 24 November, massive losses from cold injury had already been sustained.

Conceptual problems helped to confuse the issue. To many doctors "injury" seemed a different category from "disease." Forms used to report cold injury were ambiguous and nomenclature varied; at one time or another trenchfoot and immersion foot were reported as nonbattle injuries or as disease, and frostbite as battle or nonbattle injury, all depending on the outlook of the individual unit or command. In consequence, the dimensions of the problem were not at first perceived.[34]

While commanders and surgeons alike thought of other things, American soldiers in the European Theater entered the winter fighting inadequately clothed. Disagreements in the hierarchy, errors fostered by the course of battle, and inadequacies in the footgear on hand contributed to the situation. The theater Quartermaster chief, Maj. Gen. Robert M. Littlejohn, disagreed with the quartermaster general in Washington over the composition of the winter uniform. This circumstance, combined with optimistic midsummer expectations of an early end of hostilities—the First Army commander asked a medical officer in mid-September, "Don't you know that this war is going to be over in a few weeks?"—led to delayed and insufficient winter clothing requisitions by the theater. Making matters worse, the armies during the pursuit gave low priority to the shipment forward of what cold

[32] An. 9—Medical, p. 23, to FECOMZ Plan, 14 May 44, file HD 370 ETO.

[33] ETO, *Manual of Therapy*, 5 May 44, file Manual of Therapy, ETO, box 405, RG 112, NARA.

[34] Above paragraphs based on Cir No. 108, HQ, ETOUSA, 24 Nov 44, reproduced in Whayne and DeBakey, *Cold Injury*, pp. 525–28.

weather clothing was available. General Bradley of the 12th Army Group later candidly described the calculated risk he took in pressing the foe:

> When the rains first came in November with a blast of wintry air, our troops were ill-prepared for winter-time campaigning. This was traceable in part to the September crisis in supply for, during our race to the Rhine, I had deliberately by-passed shipments of winter clothing in favor of ammunition and gasoline. As a consequence, we now found ourselves caught short, particularly in bad-weather footgear. We had gambled in our choice and now were paying for the bad guess.[35]

Winter footgear was especially inadequate, in both quantity and type. Later investigators concluded that feet could be kept in condition by heavy socks or foot wrappings to wick away moisture, worn inside water-repellent shoes or boots that were loose enough not to constrict the blood flow. During his European inspection tour Colonel Sams kept his boots loosely laced and had no problem, despite the fact that he spent much time in the field and, for experimental purposes, never changed his socks. American field shoes and combat boots were not waterproof, though a substance called dubbin was supplied to make them so. (Hawley emphatically declared that dubbin was useless.) Both forms of footwear could be laced tightly, as could a winterized rubber-soled boot called the shoepac. Supply problems multiplied difficulties. The theater Quartermaster chief did not have sufficient galoshes, and troops who received them often discarded them during good weather as an encumbrance. In December the theater cabled for 500,000 additional pairs of shoepacs over and above the 446,000 pairs already shipped and the 90,000 pairs that had been issued to Seventh Army. Production and transport problems, however, ensured that none arrived until mid-January 1945. Distribution foul-ups then imposed new delays. The emergency order of shoepacs did not reach the troops in great numbers until the problem of cold injury had ended.

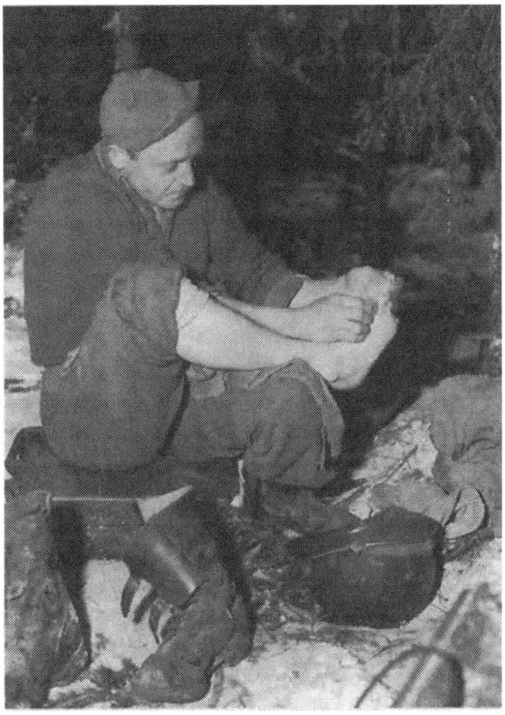

CARE OF THE FEET

Even men who received shoepacs, the most sophisticated form of winter footgear available to American forces, had difficulty using them. The tops were permeable to water; the rubber

[35] First quotation from Whayne Comments, p. 18, CMH. Second quotation from Omar N. Bradley, *A Soldier's Story* (New York: Henry Holt and Co., 1951), p. 445. For a general account of the clothing controversy, see Ruppenthal, *Logistical Support*, 2:218–35.

soles wore out quickly in field use; most were too large; and the need to wear multiple socks and felt insoles made them unsuitable for men in battle. Inside the shoepacs the soldier's feet were not ventilated and excessive sweating soaked the skin as thoroughly as if the wet had come from the outside. In time, a form of injury—shoepac foot—was named for the footgear; surgeons complained that sweating and maceration of the skin produced "a foot which is as bad as any seen thus far," often bringing hospitalization for ten to fifteen days. When the victim returned to duty, the cycle then repeated itself. In February the perspiration problem caused the 8th Infantry Division to order its troops to turn in shoepacs previously issued. In other units, surgeons rendered more favorable verdicts on the shoepac; unquestionably, it was the best footwear that the American Army then possessed for wet and cold weather. But there was also much to be said for Hawley's blunt assessment: "The plain truth is that the footwear furnished U.S. troops is, in general, lousy." [36]

In late November and early December 1944 many factors, large and small, combined to produce a crisis. Startled officers—in the medical service, the supply chain, and the line—learned first-hand how General Winter could disable an army. Then the Germans launched their counteroffensive, and troops pinned down in the snow and mud suffered the equivalent of a major epidemic. Soon the Army faced the loss of what amounted to several divisions of front-line soldiers.

Reports in November painted a picture of radical discomfort for the riflemen. Heavy rains ran off over saturated ground, streams and marshes flooded, and the first frosts struck at men who were almost never dry or warm. In the Third Army, men waded rather than marched, fought in deep mud, and rested in water-filled foxholes. As the month advanced, night frosts became commoner. Vehicles churned roads into sloughs. The 5th Infantry Division ordered 11,000 pairs of galoshes that were badly needed. In the 90th Infantry Division all trenchfoot victims were evacuated as litter cases. In the Seventh Army's 3d Infantry Division the surgeon wrote a sharp criticism of the shoepac: With the issue of the winterized boots he had anticipated that trenchfoot would decrease; instead, ill-fitted water-soaked shoepacs were themselves injuring feet. All along the line dry socks became a critical item and units struggled to obtain supplies and to provide some means of drying and cleaning wet socks. Unit reports often spoke reassuringly of corrective measures; men were instructed to remove their shoes or boots daily, massage their feet, and so forth. But the 79th Infantry Division of the Seventh Army had 1,400 battle casualties and 210 cases of trenchfoot for the month. In the Third Army six men were evacuated for cold injury for every ten evacuated as battle casualties. Losses of 10 to 15 percent of unit strength became common.

[36] First quotation from Essential Technical Medical Data Rpt, HQ, ETOUSA, December 1944, p. 9. Second quotation from Ltr, Hawley to TSG, 29 Dec 44, file HD 024 ETO O/CS (Hawley-SGO Corresp). See also Surg, 8th Infantry Division, Annual Rpt, 1945, p. 10.

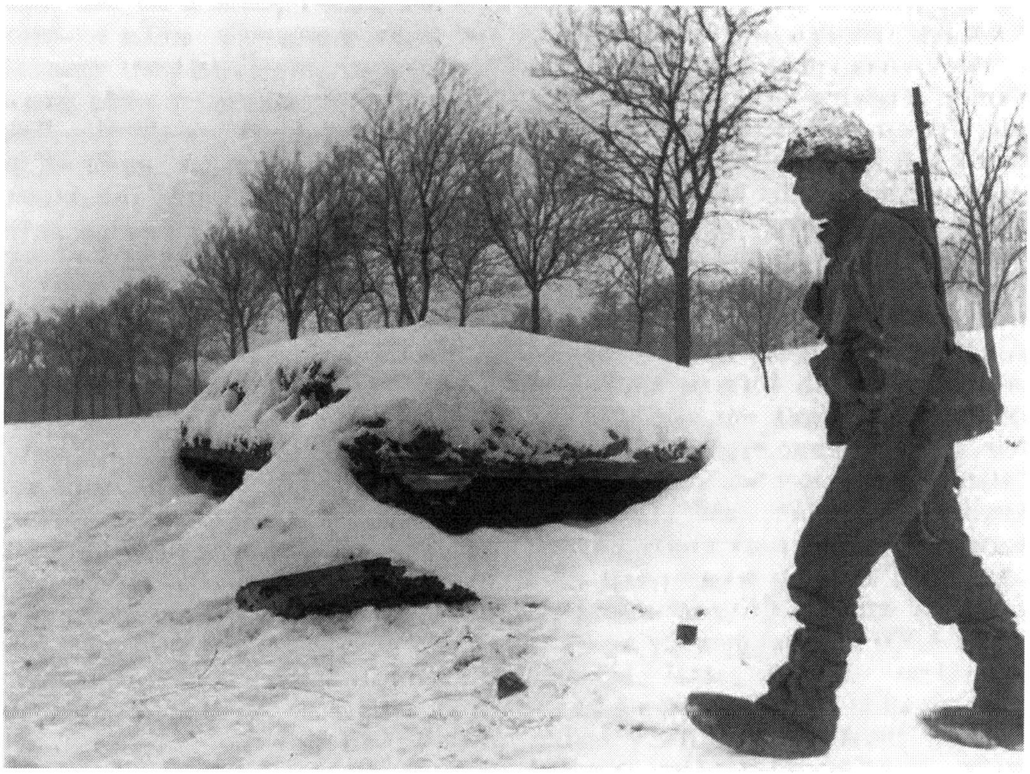

SENTRY WEARING IMPROVISED BOOTS OF STRAW-FILLED BLANKETS

Too often men on the line were obliged to improvise their own protective gear while the battle raged. In the Third Army, officers of the 35th Infantry Division had been unable to get shoepacs for their men. Combat boots and overshoes proved inadequate protection for front-line soldiers pinned down by hostile fire. Men tried putting paper between two pairs of socks, but found it insufficient; besides, their boots were not large enough to permit wearing more than two pairs of socks without constricting the feet, reducing the blood supply, and causing cold injury. Overshoes were so unsatisfactory when worn over combat boots that 60 percent of the cold injury victims in the division were found to have become disabled while wearing them. The best protection resulted from discarding the combat boots altogether and wearing six or eight pairs of wool socks or a kind of homemade boot made out of two thicknesses of a GI blanket, inside the overshoes, which were waterproof and large enough to hold such a mass of material. But the clumsy multilayered wrappings reduced the soldier's mobility, and the overshoes were noisy and unsuitable for stealthy movements in close combat. From the end of December to mid-January the division lost 479 front-line riflemen to cold injury.[37]

Many units could have told similar stories. Fighting in Lorraine during the German offensive, the 328th Infantry lost 500 men to trenchfoot and exposure during the first days of the battle. One company of the 11th Infantry had only 14 men available for duty, and the chief cause of ineffectiveness was trenchfoot. Cold injury combined with heavy battle losses to render the 358th Infantry unable to continue an attack on the German line. For the same reason the 357th Infantry had to be pulled back. During November and December losses to cold numbered 23,000, almost all combat infantrymen. Because an infantry division contained about 4,000 such soldiers the loss was equivalent to the total infantry strength of at least five and a half divisions. Striking selectively, cold injury, said General Bradley, "sapped assault strength and thus weakened the offensive." [38]

In this respect Americans seemingly fared worse than both their Allies and their enemies. The British record, among the few units engaged in the winter fighting, was far better and resulted, at least in part, from their practice of rotating units on the line to rest areas. The enemy's situation was less clear. German regular units apparently prevented cold injury more successfully than Americans because their veterans, at least, had longer experience of winter warfare. Yet the many replacements who filled the ranks appeared to suffer severely. Some enemy front-line units reported 10 to 15 percent losses to cold injury. The German Army possessed a field boot without laces, but most of its men who fell prisoner to the Americans were found to be wearing laced leather field shoes. German surgeons understood, as did their American counterparts, the importance of not constricting the blood flow and placed some faith in an ointment called Pernionin. The salve was simply oil of wintergreen and aromatics in a lanolin base, but its smell and feel may well have encouraged more frequent massage. Nevertheless, 12th Army Group medical officers who surveyed four POW enclosures concluded that, in most enemy units, foot discipline was poor and the "preventive program . . . similar to our own." [39]

The impact of cold injury losses upon American hospitals and the evacuation system was heavy. During October and November more than 11,000 trenchfoot casualties were admitted to the Paris general hospitals from the four American field armies. Cold injury accounted progressively for 1.3, 4, 20, and 24 percent of weekly admissions during November. The nature of the injury worsened its effects upon the patients, the hospital staffs, and the capabilities of the field

[37] Surg, 35th Infantry Division, Semiannual Rpt, January–June 1945, p. 1.

[38] Quotation from Bradley, *Soldier's Story*, p. 445. See also Essential Technical Medical Data Rpt, HQ, ETOUSA, December 1944.

[39] Quotation from "Frostbite Problems in the German Army During World War II," OCMH Ms P–602, pp. 25–27, MHI. See also Surg, 303d Medical Battalion, After-Action Rpt, February 1945, pp. 5–7, encl. to History of the Medical Units of the 78th Infantry Division for the Year 1945; Surg, 12th Army Group, Hist, January–June 1945, an. 16, p. 7; Army Service Forces Monthly Progress Rpt, 31 Mar 45, sec. 7 (Health), p. 6, file HD 700 (Health).

armies alike. Victims, unable to walk upon exquisitely painful feet, required litter carry at the front and bed care in the hospitals. As already noted, the disability was long-term, and apt to recur upon exposure—nature's most ingenious contrivance for the embarrassment of the foot soldier and those who cared for him.

As early as September and October the medical service attempted to make up for earlier omissions by distributing War Department publications that gave concise instructions to troops and commanders for avoiding injury. Various command directives and memoranda followed, drawing attention to the problem, repeating official policies, and underlining the fact that (as a Third Army circular dated 9 November phrased it) "excessive development of trenchfoot in an organization will be considered as indicative of inadequate [command] supervision and control." [40] Unfortunately, such action came late in the day for an army in which large numbers of officers, NCOs, and enlisted men were ignorant of the nature and potential seriousness of the threat.[41]

November found General Bradley taking action at the urging of his surgeon, Colonel Gorby. Bradley followed up a command directive with personal letters to the commanders of his field armies. In turn, the commanders ordered immediate action to control the epidemic. General Patton's memorandum to the Third Army's corps and division commanders declared with characteristic vigor that "the most serious menace confronting us today is not the German Army, which we have practically destroyed, but the weather which, if we do not exert ouselves, may well destroy us through the incidence of trench foot." [42]

By December, admission of past errors and assumption of responsibility by commanders was general. To Gorby, Hawley admitted, "I am not sure that the Medical Department has been aggressive enough. . . . We have published long dissertations on the prevention of trench foot which are too long for anyone to read." In January General Eisenhower emphasized the need for commanders to pay "unremitting attention" to the problem, and officers of lesser rank followed their chief's lead. A barrage of publicity began, with articles and editorials in the *Stars and Stripes* and other publications widely read by theater soldiers. Radio broadcasts carried the message to front-line troops. The theater prepared and circulated millions of copies of a brochure and initiated efforts to indoctrinate replacements. The armies set up trenchfoot control teams.[43]

Yet all of these measures, necessary and helpful as they were, came too late to modify the impact of cold injury upon the winter fighting. Instead, after reaching a new high in January, the cold injury casualty rate

[40] As quoted in Whayne and DeBakey, *Cold Injury*, p. 167.

[41] Polls of the overseas army, wrote Assistant Secretary of War John J. McCloy to the surgeon general on 16 August, showed that 85 percent of those questioned felt that they had received little training in avoiding or treating trenchfoot. The only other training failure equally marked was in the handling of land mines. See ibid., pp. 66, 166–67, 509–15.

[42] Quotation from the memorandum (21 Nov 44) reproduced in ibid., p. 529. See also Gorby Interv, 1962, p. 20, CMH.

[43] Whayne and DeBakey, *Cold Injury*, p. 169.

fell in response to the reduced level of combat, perhaps aided by a thaw that arrived providentially during the second week of February. (Because the weather remained chilly and the thaw increased wetness, its effects are difficult to assess.) By that time the European Theater had suffered a medical misfortune that cost the ground forces a total of 45,283 casualties at a most critical period. In searching for the causes of that extraordinary failure, no simple assignment of blame is possible. Errors, mainly of omission by medical, quartermaster, staff, and line, gave a new meaning to the old formula for disaster of too little and too late. Now the medical service could only try to deal with the results.[44]

Coping With the Crisis

During the autumn and winter discussions of hospitalization and evacuation policy, none of the participants expected a major enemy counterattack. Their concern rather was with the implications for the ETO medical service of the imminent German collapse that all anticipated. The Ardennes attack caught senior theater medical officers, like everyone else, off guard. General Hawley recalled his own complete surprise. "All I can remember," he said, "is the chaos. . . . Nobody knew anything. We were pretty much in the dark." Hawley hastily issued instructions for evacuation of hospitals in danger of being overrun, and the ADSEC surgeon, Colonel Beasley, made plans for withdrawing his people and equipment. But neither had to be implemented. As a result of the stout defense put up by the First Army, the German attack columns barely penetrated the fringes of COMZ territory. Some disorder followed; the 130th General Hospital at Ciney was temporarily displaced, and another field hospital holding unit closed and moved because of bomb damage. But all other COMZ medical units remained in place, and continued working.[45]

Yet the impact of the offensive spread far and wide. Some units, hospitals and holding units in and around Liege, suffered casualties and plant damage from enemy V-weapons, conventional bombing, and long-range artillery fire. Hardest hit was the 76th General Hospital, struck on 8 January 1945 by a V-1 that killed 24 patients and staff, injured 20, and heavily damaged buildings and equipment. This unit, and most others that were struck, cared for their own casualties, cleared away rubble, and kept on working. These same Liege hospitals, because of the closing and movement of most First Army medical units, in effect assumed the functions of that army's evacuation hospitals and holding units. Occasionally re-

[44] Ltr, HQ, ETOUSA, to CGs, 30 Jan 45, sub: Trenchfoot Control Officers, reproduced in 12th Army Group Report of Operations, vol. XIII (Medical Section), pp. 204–05. The rate per 1,000 troops per year was 127.7 in November, 135.2 in December, 139.8 in January, and 84.9 in February, after which it rapidly declines. See Preventive Medicine Division, OofCSurg, HQ, ETOUSA, Semiannual Rpt, January–June 1945, pp. 43–44.

[45] Quotation from Hawley Interv, 1962, pp. 106–07, CMH. See also Memos, Hawley to CofS, ETO, 22 Dec 44, sub: Destruction of Medical Supplies To Prevent Capture by the Enemy, and Hawley to Surg, ADSEC, 24 Dec 44, sub: Abandonment of Fixed Hospitals, file HD 024 ETO CS (Hawley Chron); Surg, ADSEC, COMZ, Semiannual Rpt, January–June 1945, p. 8.

ceiving wounded directly from the battlefield without any preliminary treatment except first aid, the general hospitals and the controlling 818th Hospital Center, which had been in operation for only two days when the offensive began, hastily reorganized for quick triage, rapid-fire stabilizing surgery, and mass evacuation. The Battle of the Bulge also affected medical communications, especially the Advance Section, where telephone contact with the armies became sporadic due to bad weather as well as enemy action. To keep in touch with the army surgeons, Colonel Beasley had to send liaison officers on frequent dangerous journeys over the snow and ice-clogged roads, often under fire.[46]

Throughout the weeks of bitter fighting, all COMZ medical elements had one overriding task: keeping the field armies cleared of casualties and free to maneuver. Conditions as the battle began were relatively favorable: a temporary pileup of casualties in the armies during late November, caused mainly by a shortage of transportation, had soon been alleviated and the flow of patients from the front went relatively smoothly until 16 December. By that time enough hospital trains were in service to permit idling some for crew rest and equipment maintenance; cross-Channel air and sea evacuation were proceeding with only minor delays and mishaps; the Paris general hospitals had 3,600–5,600 empty beds each day; and the Liege and Bar-le-Duc hospitals were far from full. Farther to the rear, the situation was less favorable. The Normandy Base Section reported few empty beds, except in the Cherbourg holding unit, and United Kingdom Base hospitals contained almost 117,000 patients.[47]

On 17–18 December large numbers of casualties, including about 2,000 patients hastily unloaded by First Army installations, began flowing toward Paris from the Ardennes battlefields. On the nineteenth the Evacuation Branch reported that the situation was "becoming tense." The Liege hospitals were filling; thirteen trains were on the Liege-Paris shuttle; and the weather was curtailing both air and sea evacuation. Colonel Mowrey, trying to minimize the patient load in endangered First Army hospitals and in the ADSEC holding units immediately behind them, gave those facilities priority for evacuation, further increasing the pressure on transportation and on installations farther to the rear.[48]

For the rest of the month the Evacuation Branch and the Seine Section lived from hand to mouth. As trainload after trainload of wounded from Liege rolled into the Gare St.-Lazare and a lesser but increasing flow from the Third Army arrived at the Gare de l'Est, the reserve of empty beds in the capital dwindled to 2,600 or fewer

[46] Surg, ADSEC, COMZ, Semiannual Rpt, January–June 1945, p. 8; Evacuation Branch, Operations Division, OofCSurg, HQ, ETOUSA, Annual Rpt, 1944, p. 12; 818th Hospital Center Semiannual Rpt, January–June 1945, p. 9; 298th General Hospital Annual Rpt, 1945, pp. 8, 11, 137; 32d General Hospital Semiannual Rpt, January–June 1945, pp. 1–6. Liege, a major target because of its key logistics role, was hit by over 1,000 V-bombs between mid-September 1944 and early 1945. See MacDonald, *Siegfried Line*, pp. 229–30.

[47] Evacuation Branch, Operations Division, OofCSurg, HQ, ETOUSA, Daily Diary, 16–30 Nov and 1–16 Dec 44, file HD 024 ETO.

[48] Ibid., 16–19 Dec 44, file HD 024 ETO.

per day. To keep the Paris regulating tank from overflowing, the Seine Section rushed patients to Le Bourget field whenever the skies cleared and C–47s came in; it sent daily trainloads to Cherbourg, where patients at times waited twenty-four hours or more in the ward cars for the arrival of fog or storm-bound hospital carriers. Enemy action compounded the section's difficulties. On the night of 26 December German bombs destroyed a hospital train at the Gare St.-Lazare and put the station out of service for forty-eight hours. With all medical rail operations shifted to the Gare de l'Est, the loading of trains for Cherbourg temporarily stopped due to yard and station tieups. By the twenty-eighth the Seine Section, with 14,000 patients in its wards, effectively was out of empty beds. Then, as was to happen repeatedly during the crisis, the jam broke. Planes began flying again from Le Bourget and the forward airstrips; trains for Cherbourg began moving; and carriers pulled into the harbor. The Seine Section hastily opened two more general hospitals, one a temporary convalescent facility in a commandeered Paris hotel formerly used as a SHAEF officers club. By the thirty-first, with 1,200 empty beds reported in Liege and 3,600 in Paris, evacuation officers could breathe a little easier.[49]

During January 1945 evacuation continued at a hectic pace. "Hospital trains were overworked," the Evacuation Branch reported, "all available planes were utilized; Paris was a hub of activity; and the port of Cherbourg was busy day and night outloading patients. . . ." The Communications Zone routinely transferred 2,000 patients per day from forward areas to its continental and United Kingdom hospitals. On a record day, the twenty-first, over 4,800 casualties crossed the Channel, 2,200 of them by air. These patients included a growing number from the 6th Army Group, diverted to the northern COMZ from SOLOC, where casualties of the *NORDWIND* offensive had swamped the available medical facilities. To keep the ADSEC holding units clear and to maintain empty beds in Liege, Bar-le-Duc, and Paris, the Evacuation Branch tried to crowd the system toward the rear, filling the Normandy and Brittany Base Section general hospitals and deliberately overloading the United Kingdom Base. This policy worked, but at the cost of evacuating many less serious casualties too far back for convenient return to duty. Inclement weather, which hampered both air and sea transportation, periodically blocked the rearward flow of patients, causing the Paris bed reserve to shrink alarmingly. On two occasions during the month, when the Continent had more beds open than the United Kingdom, General Hawley temporarily halted cross-Channel evacuation. At the end of the first of these embargoes, deteriorating weather prevented an immediate resumption of air and sea movement, giving the Evacuation Branch its worst days of a bad month. After each natural or man-made stoppage, however, the patient flow resumed and evacuation conditions returned to normal—if a constant high volume of casualties, interminable hard work for all hands, and the need to stretch human and material resources to and

[49] Ibid., 20–31 Dec 44, file HD 024 ETO.

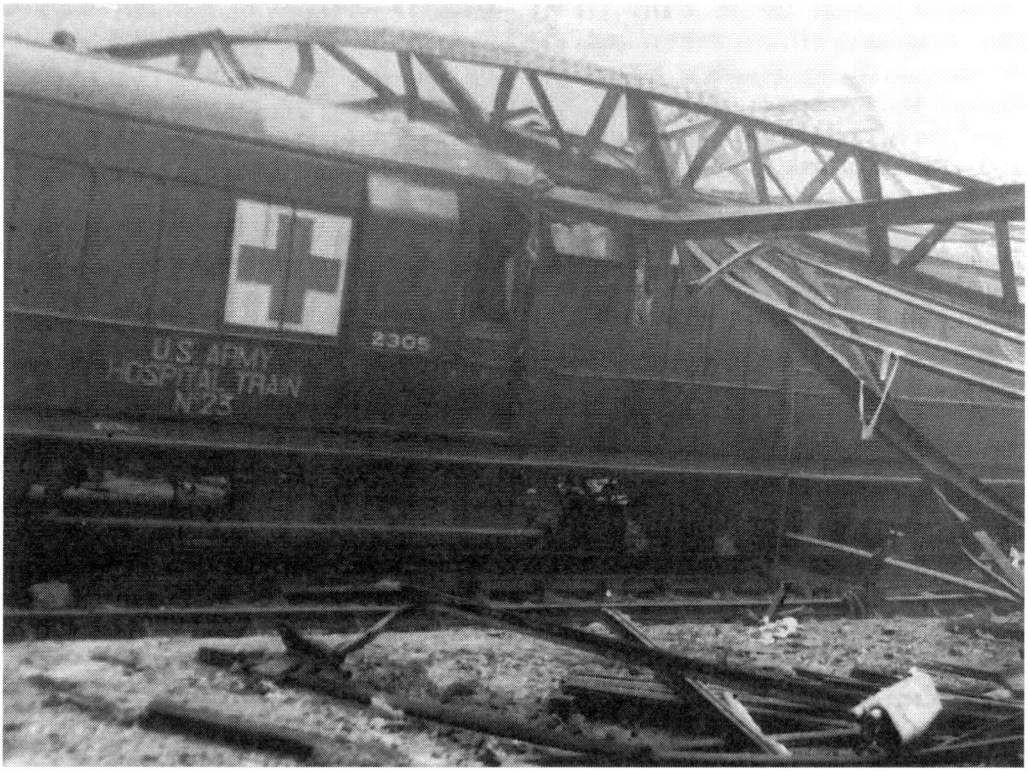

WRECKAGE OF HOSPITAL TRAIN AFTER GARE ST.-LAZARE BOMBING

beyond the limit could be so characterized.[50]

The Ardennes crisis put the medical service's rail transportation facilities to the severest test they yet had faced. Hospital train personnel and equipment operated at full capacity day after day, week after week. They did so in spite of cold and snow that froze steam lines and switches and exposed the inadequacies of car heating systems, in spite of equipment breakdowns from overuse and lack of maintenance and in spite of damage and casualties from air raids and accidents. (On 11 January, for example, an ammunition dump explosion in Normandy temporarily put three trains out of action and caused 70 casualties.) The Evacuation Branch tried to shorten running times on the most important routes, but an effort in January to establish regular schedules governing the Paris-Cherbourg and Paris-Nancy runs brought little improvement. Only in late February, after the shift of cargo shipments to

[50] Quotation from Evacuation Branch, Operations Division, OofCSurg, HQ, ETOUSA, Semiannual Rpt, January–June 1945, pp. 3–4. See also ibid., pp. 1–2, and Daily Diary, 1–31 Jan 45, file HD 024 ETO; Surg, Seine Section, Annual Rpt, 1944, p. 28; Surg, CONAD, Annual Rpt, 1944, pp. 9–10, and Semiannual Rpt, January–June 1945, p. 7. On the triage problem see Ltr, Brig Gen T. J. Davis, AG, SHAEF, to CG, COMZ, 13 Jan 45, file 705:Admission to and Operations in Hospitals.

Antwerp reduced freight traffic on the lines radiating from Paris, did the Evacuation Branch notice any major change for the better. The Seine Section, meanwhile, further streamlined and decentralized train loading and unloading procedures. In mid-February, for greater efficiency, the section moved all reception of incoming hospital trains to the Gare de l'Est and used the Gare St.-Lazare only for loading outgoing trains bound for Cherbourg. During January General Hawley requested still more trains than the forty he had in operation, both to compensate for slow running times and to allow sidetracking of the older rolling stock for now urgently needed repairs. Three trains previously ordered from the French came into service early in the new year. In addition, the theater Transportation chief agreed to provide a dozen more for delivery during the next several months; the first three became available in February. To staff them, and the others to be delivered, the Seine Section had to comb doctors, nurses, and enlisted men out of its general hospitals to form provisional hospital train units.[51]

Fog and clouds grounded most transport planes during the first week of the Battle of the Bulge. But when clear skies returned on 23 December, so did the C-47s, to drop supplies to beleaguered American troops and to pick up casualties at Le Bourget and the forward airstrips. Throughout the battle, aircraft, often flying in marginal weather, moved large numbers of patients—14,000 in the last days of December and about 17,000 in each of the ensuing months. In spite of hazardous flying conditions, they accomplished this feat with only one major mishap. On 30 December a plane on a night evacuation flight, lost in the fog and out of fuel, crash landed near Le Havre. Thanks to "heroic action" on the part of the flight nurse, Lt. Ann M. Krueger of the 817th Medical Air Evacuation Squadron, the 27 patients on board were extricated before the wreck burst into flames.[52]

In spite of storms and fog, hospital ships and carriers—all that SHAEF and the European Theater could obtain—maintained the sea shuttle between Cherbourg and Southampton, moving almost 85,000 patients during December, January, and February. Though General Kenner continued to press the search for a shorter cross-Channel evacuation route, his efforts led to no real improvements. Early in February, after weeks of deliberation, a SHAEF committee of medical, engineer, and transportation officers recommended opening a line between Boulogne and Dover. Colonel Mowrey, Hawley's Evacuation Branch chief, objected to this proposal. He pointed out that Boulogne could accommodate only two of the smallest carriers at a time, that the train run from Liege would take fifteen hours, and that a large holding

[51] Evacuation Branch, Operations Division, OofCSurg, HQ, ETOUSA, Semiannual Rpt, January-June 1945, pp. 3-5 and encl. 2, pp. 1-2; Surg, Seine Section, Semiannual Rpt, January-June 1945, pp. 12-13 and 46-47.

[52] Evacuation Branch, Operations Division, OofCSurg, HQ, ETOUSA, Semiannual Rpt, January-June 1945, encl. 6; Futrell, *Aeromedical Evacuation*, pp. 241-42 and 244-45. Quoted words from Memo, Maj Wesley C. Oliver, HQ, IX Troop Carrier Command, to CO, 9th History Unit, U.S. Army, 31 Jan 45, box 407, RG 112, NARA. Krueger was recommended for the Soldier's Medal.

unit would have to be set up at the port—all to move no more than 450 additional patients a day. American and British transportation officers also were unenthusiastic about the new route. Nevertheless, Kenner in mid-February directed the theater to initiate the service. Due to delays in preparing the facilities, and probably to some medical service foot-dragging, it took another month to begin operations. By that time the need for an additional cross-Channel sea route long had passed.[53]

Throughout the midwinter battles, Generals Kenner and Hawley anxiously watched the fixed hospital patient census inexorably rise. Yet the Communications Zone always managed to have a bed for every casualty and maintained a surplus, razor-thin at times, of beds over patients. Hospitals in the United Kingdom Base and on the Continent expanded their capacities by a variety of expedients. The United Kingdom Base made permanent and fitted for winter use most of the 30,000 supposedly temporary tented expansion beds it had set up at its general and station hospitals before D-Day. The base also reassigned to regular patient care a number of station hospitals previously

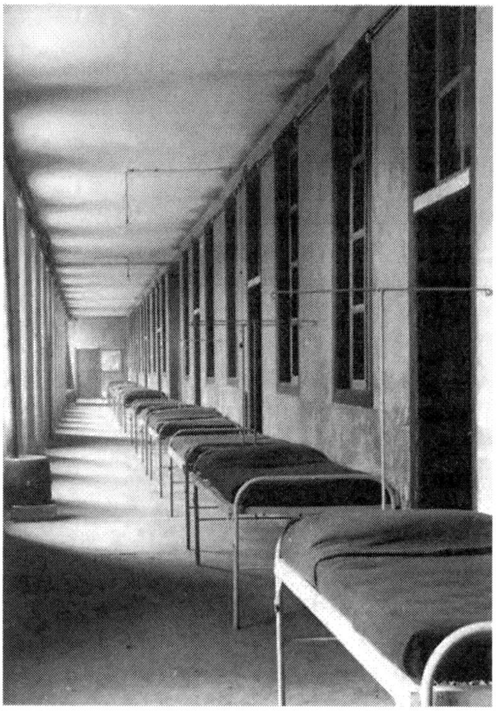

HOSPITAL EMERGENCY BEDS

employed to hold convalescents. To add still more beds, each hospital, both in Britain and on the Continent, packed more patients into its existing space, first by filling its wards to their actual rather than T/O capacity, then by reducing the floor space per bed in the wards, and finally by placing still more emergency beds in laboratories, barracks, offices, and hallways. By such means most theater general hospitals operated at 50 percent or more above their rated capacity.[54]

[53] Evacuation Branch, Operations Division, OofCSurg, HQ, ETOUSA, Daily Diary, 2 Jan, 3 and 16–17 Feb, 1 Mar 45, file HD 024 ETO, and Annual Rpt, 1944, encl. 10, and Semiannual Rpt, January–June 1945, p. 6 and encl. 6; Surg, Normandy Base Section, Semiannual Rpt, January–June 1945, pp. 10–11; Ltr, Brig Gen T. J. Davis, AG, SHAEF, to CG, COMZ, 13 Jan 45, file 705:Admission to and Operations in Hospitals; Memos, Lt Col I. A. Marshall, MC, to Chief, Operations Division, OofCSurg, 6 Feb 45, sub: Cross-Channel Evacuation, and Col F. H. Mowrey to Chief, Operations Division, OofCSurg, 7 Feb 45, sub: Cross-Channel Evacuation, Boulogne-Dover, file HD:ETO:370.05:Evacuation, Jan–Oct 45.

[54] Rehabilitation Division, OofCSurg, HQ, ETOUSA, Semiannual Rpt, 1945, pp. 2–3; Surg, United Kingdom Base, Annual Rpt, 1944, pp. 11–13 and app. 9; Surg, Normandy Base Section, Semiannual Rpt, January–June 1945, pp. 13–14; Surg, Seine Section, Annual Rpt, 1944, pp. 24 and 27, and Semiannual Rpt, January–June 1945, pp. 30–31

Continued

Throughout the theater, extra patients overcrowded recreational and Red Cross facilities in many hospitals and overtaxed water and sewage disposal systems. They also placed a strain on hospital personnel who, after the various T/O reductions, were barely adequate to handle even their regular patient loads. To staff additional beds, hospitals drew heavily upon civilian and POW labor and obtained additional people from hospital units not yet in operation. The 21st General Hospital at Mirecourt, operating 3,500 beds despite its T/O strength of 2,000, for a while had the personnel of an entire newly arrived 1,000-bed unit attached to it as reinforcements and for on-the-job training. Some augmentations became permanent. The War Department late in December allowed the theater to add 14,400 general and station hospital beds, provided it could find within its boundaries the required plants and personnel. Due to a lack of both, the theater made only limited use of this authority. However, it did expand nine veteran 1,000-bed general hospitals, the majority in Paris, which already were working above rated capacity, into T/O 1,500- and 2,000-bed units. To increase their personnel, the theater disbanded three inadequately trained general hospitals not yet in operation.[55]

Besides enlarging existing hospitals, General Hawley and his Hospitalization Division chief, Colonel Darnall, struggled to place more units and plants in operation. They received considerable assistance from General Kenner and his staff, especially in prevailing upon the armies and Allied governments to turn over sites. As a result of these efforts, during January and February, the Communications Zone opened twenty-six new continental general hospitals at locations selected in late fall, around Verdun, Nancy, Toul, Evreux, and Soissons. Between mid-December and mid-February the total number of T/O fixed beds in COMZ and SOLOC, exclusive of emergency beds, rose from about 50,000 to over 76,000. Planning for still further expansion of the hospital system to support the eventual push across the Rhine, Hawley's staff picked out additional locations along the lines of communication radiating from Paris and made plans with the theater G–4 and Engineer chief for their phased development. These sites, clustered around Aachen, Luxembourg, Mourmelon, and Chalons, would accommodate all the remaining general hospi-

and 84; Surg, CONAD, Annual Rpt, 1944, pp. 7–8; Cady, "Notes on the 21st General Hospital (AUS)," p. 492, Cady Papers, MHI. For policy on use of emergency expansion beds, see, Ltr, HQ, SHAEF, to CG, COMZ, 6 Feb 45, and MFR, Col D. E. Liston, DepCSurg, ETO, 12 Feb 45, both in file 705:Admission to and Operations in Hospitals. Day-to-day figures on beds and patients may be found in Status of Hospitalization, UK-Continent, March 1944–February 1945.

[55] For plant problems of expansion, see Surg, United Kingdom Base, Annual Rpt, 1944, pp. 11–13; Cady, "Notes on the 21st General Hospital (AUS)," pp. 477–78, 495, 501, Cady Papers, MHI. On hospital reorganization, see Smith, *Hospitalization and Evacuation*, pp. 236–37; Troops Branch, Operations Division, OofCSurg, HQ, ETOUSA, Semiannual Rpt, January–June 1945, p. 34; Surg, Seine Section, Semiannual Rpt, January–June 1945, p. 10. Enlarged units were the 1st, 48th, 50th, 62d, 108th, 178th, 191st, 217th (1,500 beds), and 203d (2,000 beds). Disbanded units were the 190th, 252d, and 253d.

tals in the ETO troop basis scheduled to arrive through mid-April, as well as some veteran organizations brought forward from Normandy and the United Kingdom. When all these plants were occupied, the Communications Zone would have over 118,000 fixed beds in operation on the Continent, well in excess of the number declared necessary by General Kenner back in December.[56]

Additional hospital centers went into operation during the crisis. The 811th and 812th, activated in January, took control of hospitals and other medical installations in the Normandy Base Section. The Seine Section by late February also contained two centers. The 814th coordinated hospital activities north of the Seine, while the 815th did the same south of the river. Other center headquarters were projected to oversee the new hospital clusters forming north and east of Paris.[57]

Providing limited relief to the crowded theater hospitals, transatlantic evacuation increased during the winter. General Kenner especially concerned himself with this problem. He repeatedly pressed Hawley to designate more Class II and III patients as Class IVs so that fuller use could be made of the ordinary troop accommodations on returning transports. Hawley, successfully in the main, resisted these pressures. More productive were efforts to obtain additional hospital-type accommodations. Early in 1945 the British, at American urging, further enlarged the capacity of the *Queens* to accommodate 2,500 Class IIs and IVs and 1,000 Class IIIs on the *Elizabeth* and a slightly smaller number on the *Mary*. The Joint Chiefs of Staff, meanwhile, authorized the conversion of six troopships into ambulance vessels, less completely staffed and equipped medically than hospital ships but better able to care for patients than regular transports. These ships, however, were not available until March.

Of more immediate help was air evacuation, which finally came into its own. Beginning in February the Air Transport Command, dispatching C–54s from both its Orly and Prestwick terminals, finally achieved its long-promised evacuation rate of over 2,000 patients a month. The airborne flow of casualties from Europe became so rapid that it overloaded Air Force medical reception facilities at New York, compelling diversion of flights to other East Coast points. In March, at the request of SHAEF, the Transport Command more than doubled even this rate, moving nearly 4,700 patients across the ocean. By plane and ship 24,666 evacuees crossed the Atlantic in January, 29,743 in February, and 30,410 in March. Yet, despite continuation of the 90-day theater evacuation policy, the United Kingdom Base patient

[56] Status of Hospitalization, UK-Continent, March 1944–February 1945; Memo, Hawley to G–4, ETO, 19 Jan 45, file 705:Admission to and Operations in Hospitals; Evacuation Branch, Operations Division, OofCSurg, HQ, ETOUSA, Daily Diary, 5 and 12 Feb 45, file HD 024 ETO; Surg, CONAD, Semiannual Rpt, January–June 1945, p. 5; 819th Hospital Center Semiannual Rpt, January–June 1945, pp. 1–2; Staff Study, OofCSurg, HQ, ETOUSA, 20 Feb 45, sub: Medical Service in the Operation to, and East of, the Rhine, pp. 8–10.

[57] Surg, Normandy Base Section, Semiannual Rpt, January–June 1945, p. 3; Surg, Seine Section, Semiannual Rpt, January–June 1945, pp. 32–33; Staff Study, OofCSurg, HQ, ETOUSA, 20 Feb 45, sub: Medical Service in the Operation to, and East of, the Rhine, pp. 9–10.

census declined only slowly, apparently because the accelerated outflow during December and January served mainly to remove a backlog of men awaiting evacuation under the old 120-day policy. Only the figures for February and subsequent months represented a real increase attributable to the December War Department mandate (*Chart 11*).[58]

Throughout late December and January Colonel Sams, General Marshall's representative on the POW hospitalization question, circulated around the theater on his other larger mission: examining the overall workings of the medical service. Hawley viewed Sams' activities with considerable suspicion. He feared that Sams represented an effort within the War Department to undermine and possibly unseat both himself and Surgeon General Kirk. Hawley's assessment contained a grain of truth. Marshall's sending of Sams to Europe did reflect the chief of staff's distrust of Kirk, as well as his dissatisfaction with the Army Service Forces in general. These internal War Department political machinations, however, in the end had little effect on the ETO medical service. Sams expressed the highest regard for both Kenner and Hawley. At the end of his trip he reported to General Marshall that Medical Department deficiencies in the European Theater were the result, not of personal failures by either man, but rather of the absence of a true theater headquarters able to control both the armies and the Communications Zone. He emphasized that Kenner and Hawley were working together effectively to overcome their problems. Indeed, Sams could find few things in the medical service to criticize. His major recommendations, that general hospitals be set up closer behind the armies and that the intermediate medical COMZ between ADSEC and the United Kingdom Base be strengthened, were simply reiterations of what Kenner and Hawley had been recommending, and working to accomplish, since the breakout from Normandy.[59]

The anticlimactic outcome of Sams' mission was only one indication of a fundamental reality: By early February the ETO hospitalization and evacuation crisis was over. Lighter battle casualties, a declining number of trenchfoot cases, and the opening of more continental general hospitals produced a steadily growing bed sur-

[58] Evacuation Branch, Operations Division, OofCSurg, HQ, ETOUSA, Semiannual Rpt, January–June 1945, encl. 8; Memos, Kenner to CofS, SHAEF, 31 Jan 45, sub: Evacuation of Casualties to ZI, and Hawley to CG, COMZ, 24 Mar 45, sub: Casualty Evacuation to ZI and Conservation of Theater Manpower, EvacCorresp, 1944–45, file 370.05 ETO; Memo, Col R. E. Peyton to DepCSurg, ETO, n.d. [ca. February 1945], file 705:Admission to and Operations in Hospitals; Bykofsky and Larson, *Transportation Corps*, pp. 367–68; Futrell, *Aeromedical Evacuation*, pp. 383–84; Theater Service Forces, ETO, Progress Rpt, July 1945, sec. 1, p. 35.

[59] Marshall's distrust of Kirk stemmed from the political battle in 1943 over the replacement of Surgeon General Magee, in which Marshall and his candidate, Kenner, had been outmaneuvered by the civilian and medical profession, which backed Kirk. See Chapter III of this volume and Interv, OSG with Brig Gen Crawford F. Sams, USA (Ret.), 18 Jan 50, CMH. For Sams' mission and recommendations, see Sams, "Medic," pp. 293–324, CMH. For Hawley's suspicions, see Ltr, Hawley to TSG, 27 Jan 45, with postscript, 2 Feb 45, file HD 024 ETO O/CS (Hawley-SGO Corresp). Kirk, ironically, welcomed Marshall's intervention in Army Service Forces affairs, on the grounds that the Medical Department had "pretty near lost our pants to ASF." See Ltr, TSG to Hawley, 7 Mar 45, file HD 024 ETO O/CS (Hawley-SGO Corresp).

CHART 11—EVACUATION TO THE ZONE OF INTERIOR, OCTOBER 1944–JULY 1945

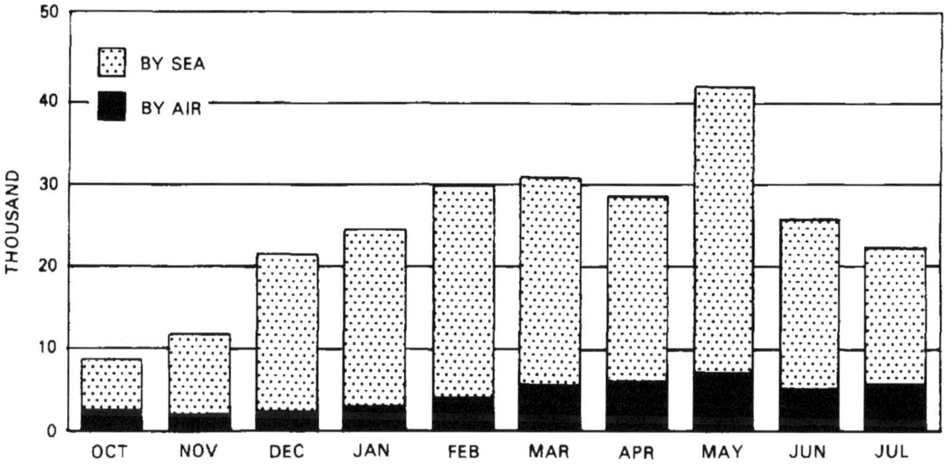

Source: HQ, TSFET, Progress Rpt, July 1945, sec. 1, p. 35.

plus, even though SOLOC continued to evacuate large numbers of its patients to the main Communications Zone. With little strain on continental hospitals, General Hawley again stopped cross-Channel evacuation for a couple of days in order to relieve the United Kingdom Base, whose patient census had at last begun to decline. By mid-February, as the railheads advanced behind the armies, hospital trains began picking up wounded as far to the east as Aachen. A surplus of medical rolling stock now was available; the Evacuation Branch stabled the majority of its trains for long-needed repairs and welcome rest for crews and medical staff. Late in the month, with over 30,000 T/O and expansion beds empty in France and Belgium, Hawley and his staff adopted a sixty-day evacuation policy for the Continent, to go into effect on 1 March. Even though new First and Ninth Army attacks during the last week of February again increased the flow of casualties, the new evacuation policy went into effect on schedule.[60]

Throughout the winter battles the COMZ medical service accomplished its principal task of keeping casualties moving steadily rearward from the armies. General Rogers, the First Army surgeon, attested: "Evacuation to the rear of First U.S. Army kept pace with all demands placed upon it."[61] The medical service overcame in this process the effects of bad weather, delays in completing its continental hospitals, an unplanned-for volume of cold injury victims, and the shutdown of most of one field army's hospital system. The favorable result stemmed in good measure from the basic soundness of the hospitalization and evacuation structure that General Hawley and his associates had built

[60] Evacuation Branch, Operations Division, OofCSurg, HQ, ETOUSA, Semiannual Rpt, January–June 1945, pp. 5–7, and Daily Diary, 1–28 Feb 45, file HD 024 ETO. See the 19 Feb 45 diary entry for the decision on the sixty-day policy.

[61] Surg, First U.S. Army, Annual Rpt, 1944, p. 58.

since the St.-Lo breakout. It also stemmed from the fact that those portions of the structure in place when the crisis erupted had been substantially overbuilt, thanks to Hawley's consistent practice of setting the highest attainable quality standards and making the largest possible demands for personnel, units, and materiel. As a result, the medical service by late 1944 had enough extra at so many points that it could ride out temporary setbacks and overloads with minimal loss in efficiency or quality of patient care. Then, too, throughout the winter, Hawley, strongly supported at SHAEF by General Kenner, was able to continue building his medical infrastructure; he set up new hospitals and supply depots, obtained additional hospital trains, and further improved air and sea evacuation. War Department decisions and interventions also helped. This was especially true of General Marshall's breaking of the transatlantic evacuation deadlock, which increased the flow of patients out of the United Kingdom at just the right time.

Finally, as at every stage of the campaign, credit belonged to the ETO medics of all ranks and in all jobs. They willingly endured weeks of overwork, discomfort, and occasional personal danger in order to provide their wounded comrades with an improved chance for life. Their days of adversity now were ending. With ample resources at last on hand, they began planning and preparing to support the final offensive against the exhausted and depleted German armies.

CHAPTER XV

The Last Campaign

Allied campaign plans for the spring of 1945 looked to simultaneous pressure against Germany from east and west. General Eisenhower planned and Field Marshal Montgomery's 21 Army Group would make the first push into Germany, and the British commander, after overrunning part of the Rhineland, embarked on elaborate preparations for his grand assault. But the actual course of the last campaign featured opportunism and bold exploitation. German forces were so depleted that the American field armies were able to win quick gains. Once across the Rhine, a near-blitzkrieg developed that tested to the full the ability of medical units to keep up with the rapidly advancing armies.

The U.S. First Army, having borne the brunt of the enemy's offensive in the Ardennes in February, prepared for a renewed attack. Its surgeon, General Rogers, routinely attended G–2 and G–3 briefings, and map overlays of interest to his personnel were posted in the medical section. His veteran units made their own preparations with a high degree of professionalism. Basic organization had not changed markedly since the early days of the fighting. Each corps was supported by a medical battalion, under the corps surgeon, and by a medical group, which controlled evacuation and a variety of miscellaneous units, under the army surgeon. Hospitals too were under the operational control of the army surgeon. While organizing medical evacuation from the divisions back, the medical groups kept Rogers informed of a variety of operational details—the state of the roads, planned hospital sites, division casualty rates, and a wealth of information gathered by divisional medics. Evacuation hospitals were alerted and their commanders given a rundown on their future locations and duties; buildings behind enemy lines that might prove suitable as hospitals were identified via aerial photography for subsequent medical use.

Intelligence on enemy troop concentrations and defensive works indicated the areas where the greatest number of wounded might be encountered. Plans were laid for evacuation, and arrangements for delivering additional supplies to forward elements. Air evacuation required much coordination, for SHAEF provided the planes, and First Army holding units had to be alerted to take up their posts as new airstrips were cleared for use. Reinforcements ranging from medical officers to litterbearers were called up for the divisions that were expected to bear the brunt of the fighting. The commander of the auxiliary surgical group planned the most effective disposition of his teams to provide support for the field hospitals. The engineers were alerted to medical needs for hospital construction, road building, and repair. Ambulance control posts were established to ensure an even flow of casualties to the various hospitals, and medical truck companies readied their vehicles to move the evacuation hospitals forward as ground was gained and as new sites were selected. In armored divisions special arrangements were necessary, because these units normally did their fighting divided into three combat commands, one of which remained in reserve. Medical support followed suit, one company supporting each command, while the division psychiatrist served with the reserve in order to care for combat exhaustion cases.[1]

Encouraging were the weather and the state of enemy morale. The end of the deep snow and bitter frosts meant much reduced danger of cold injury. Among the German troops, a spreading fatalistic acceptance of defeat likewise brought hopes for less bitter fighting and fewer wounded. "Noncommissioned officers and men had reached a state of indifference," and even battalion and regimental commanders increasingly faced up to the inevitability of losing the war. Almost the only exceptions to the general rule were young junior officers, some of whom still believed Nazi promises of ultimate victory. Civilians in the Rhineland were "totally passive" and content to have their villages taken with as little fuss as possible. While some enemy troops continued desperate rearguard actions, most lacked spirit and the *Volkssturm* militiamen were "of no military value and reverted to civilian life at our approach." Americans would still be wounded and would die in the last battles, but the outcome was not really in doubt, even to the enemy.[2]

Medics in the Attack

First Army Units

Under these conditions the First Army struck at Cologne. Early attacks over clogged roads and through sometimes waist-deep snow brought the forward units toward the Roer River with its seven flood-control dams. *Volkssturm* battalions, replacements, and other makeshift forces only partly manned the West Wall defenses in the army's path, and many pillboxes and bunkers were captured empty. Yet stiff resistance developed in some areas. In the first week of February 1945 the VII, XVIII Airborne, and V Corps led the way. The last, under Maj. Gen. A. Ralph Huebner, struck at the dams. Here early good fortune quickly faded in the face of a dogged defense. Advancing troops fought in gloomy forests of wintry fir trees, slowed by mines hidden by the snow. Nevertheless, by

[1] Combat Operations Data, First U.S. Army, sub: Europe, 1944–1945, file 319.1-2 (12th Army Group).

[2] First U.S. Army Report of Operations, 23 Feb–8 May 45, p. 11.

10 February the dams had fallen to the American advance.

Evacuation problems met varied responses. The West Wall proved to be "a mass of dragon's teeth, pill boxes, barbed wire, and mine fields." The First Army's 2d Infantry Division, attacking toward the Schwammenauel Dam, had sleds especially made to pull the wounded over the snow. Mounted on broad runners to reduce friction, and fitted with litter stirrups, the devices were a marked improvement over the simple toboggans furnished by the medical supply depots. The weasels again put in an appearance, winning praise especially for their performance in deep snow. Moving forward to the battle line, the "strange looking contraptions" carried blankets, litters, drugs, bandages, plasma, food and water. Returning, they brought two patients on litters and pulled one or more on sleds over landscape so rough and snowy that hours would have been required for a litter carry. Broad treads, spreading their weight, enabled the weasels to move over minefields without setting off a blast. They were, to be sure, cranky vehicles, and the rule in the 78th Infantry Division was 2 running to 1 undergoing repairs. But for supporting the advance against the dams they proved indispensable. Working together, weasels and sleds were judged by the 2d Division surgeon "a 'must' in deep over-snow operations." The First Army also experimented with light planes—cub liaison craft—to evacuate the seriously wounded. But the attempt encountered great difficulties: Dispatching the planes when and where needed was a problem and casualties had to endure lengthy trips by road to the landing strips.[3]

On 1 March the First Army won new crossings over the Roer River and followed the enemy as he withdrew toward the Rhine. Resistance varied from none to bitter house-to-house fighting that left some villages in ruins. As American forces invested Cologne during early March—the city, except for its ancient cathedral, was all but leveled by bombing and artillery fire—the importance of the remaining Rhine bridges increased. Four still stood, at Cologne itself and at Bonn, Engers, and Remagen.[4] Then, on the seventh, quick-moving First Army forces seized intact a planked railway bridge at Remagen. Fortunately, two elements of the 51st Field Hospital were moving by chance in the direction of Remagen, and within a week of the capture, hospital personnel were at work east of the Rhine (*see Map 22*).

American troops poured across, reinforcing the first foothold the invaders had won. Typical of many were the adventures of division medics in Maj. Gen. Walter E. Lauer's 99th Infantry Division. Elements of the 99th began crossing the Rhine on 10 March, using the newly captured Ludendorff Bridge. Applying steady pressure, they reached the Wied River twelve days later, assaulted the defenders' line, and established a beach-

[3]First quotation from History of Medical Units of the 78th Infantry Division for the Year 1945, p. 2. Second quotation from Surg, 303d Medical Battalion, After-Action Rpt, February 1945, pp. 2-3, encl. to ibid. Third quotation from Surg, 2d Infantry Division, Annual Rpt, 1945, pp. 4-5.

[4]The Hohenzollern Bridge at Cologne and the spans at Engers and Bonn were destroyed by German engineers.

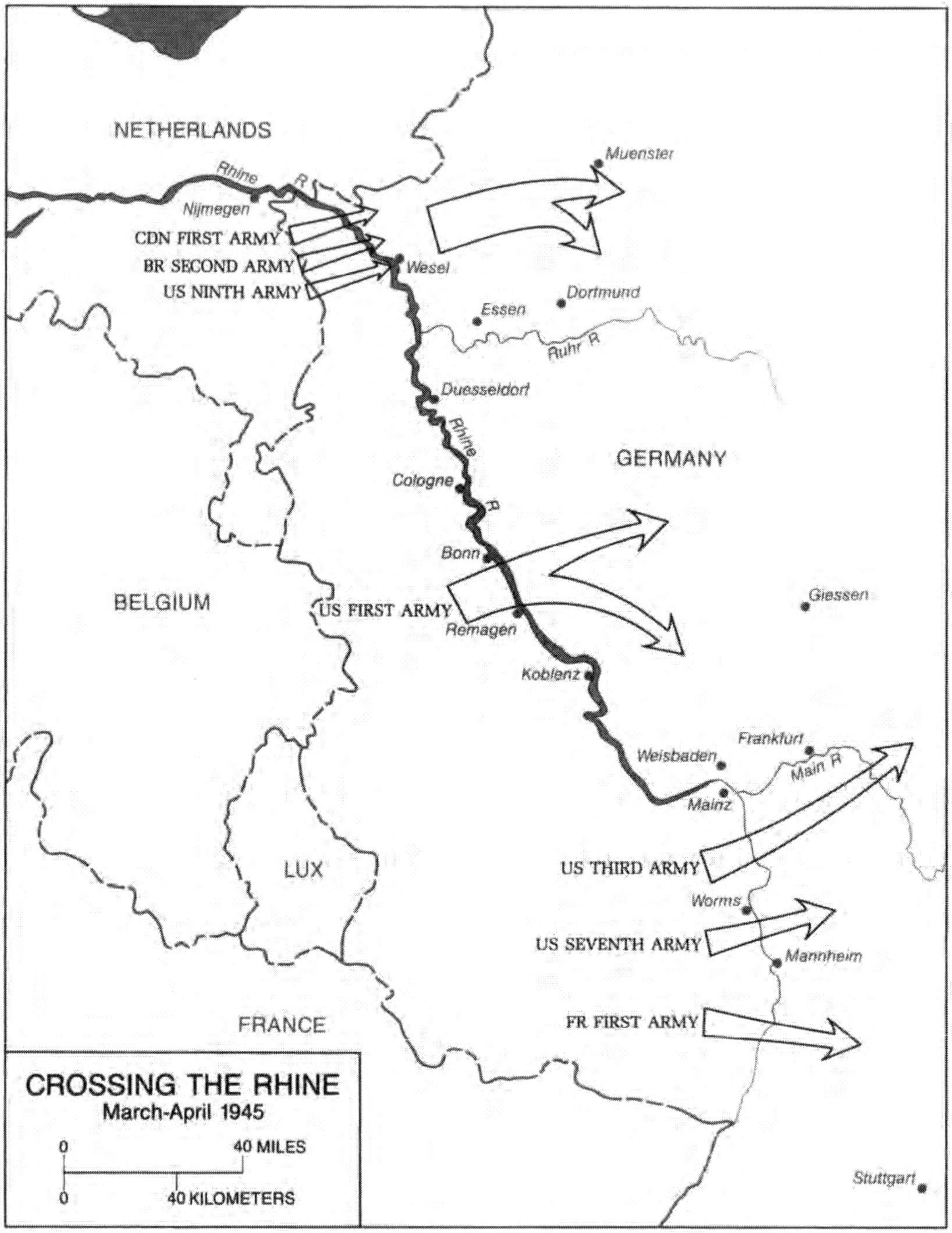
NETHERLANDS
Muenster
Rhine R
Nijmegen
CDN FIRST ARMY
BR SECOND ARMY
US NINTH ARMY
Wesel
Essen
Dortmund
Ruhr R
Duesseldorf
Rhine R
Cologne
GERMANY
Bonn
BELGIUM
US FIRST ARMY
Remagen
Giessen
Koblenz
Frankfurt
Weisbaden
Main R
Mainz
LUX
US THIRD ARMY
Worms
US SEVENTH ARMY
Mannheim
FRANCE
FR FIRST ARMY
CROSSING THE RHINE
March-April 1945
0
40 MILES
0
40 KILOMETERS
Stuttgart

MAP 22

head beyond it. Medics quickly found that the light casualties typical of the new campaign could suddenly become concentrated around surviving enemy strongpoints and especially at the rivers, all of which had to be crossed under fire. Thus enemy planes and artillery zeroed in on the Ludendorff Bridge, and many wounded had to be carried back. At the crossing of the Wied litterbearers splashed through fords, hand-carrying the injured until ponton bridges could be thrown across to facilitate ambulance evacuation. Meanwhile, field hospital units set up in villages near Remagen to receive casualties from the expanding front.[5]

The growth of the bridgehead brought the 45th Evacuation Hospital across the Rhinc to Honnef, where it opened on 25 March. Four more evacuation hospitals followed, while five clustered near the west bank to receive casualties from both sides of the river. The First Army had evacuated all its casualties to the Communications Zone during the height of the Ardennes offensive but, faced with personnel losses and inadequate replacements, had been quick to reestablish a convalescent capability as the level of fighting dropped. For a time, when the advance left the 4th Convalescent Hospital far to the rear, two evacuation hospitals, a clearing company, and the 91st Medical Gas Treatment Battalion inherited the task of holding the lightly injured through brief periods of recovery within the army area. On 22 March, however, the convalescent facility reopened in the Rhineland at Euskirchen, and the other units moved forward to resume their primary functions.[6]

As the hospitals moved up, a powerful three-corps attack broke out of the Remagen bridgehead and shattered the thin crust of defending units. The first days of April found the First Army fighting in two directions: Two corps sought to make contact with the Russians to the east, while the other two cooperated with the Ninth Army in the encirclement of enemy forces caught in the Ruhr pocket. Five evacuation hospitals, the 51st Field Hospital, and the 64th Medical Group supported the action in the Ruhr, while the 68th and 134th Medical Groups and the remaining field hospitals backed up the eastward line of advance. In either case, the evacuation hospitals encountered the usual difficulties of semimobile organizations operating in a blitzkrieg. Leapfrogging in two echelons was the best method that had been found to compensate for insufficient organic transport; only half the hospital had to be moved at a time, and in theory half was always in service. Despite this expedient, the speed of the advance and the lack of adequate Transportation Corps support often left the evacuation hospitals out of contact with the fighting units. Hence, throughout the campaign, the autonomous units into which the field hospitals had been split served as evacuation hospitals, while the latter some-

[5] Surg, 99th Infantry Division, Hist, January–August 1945, pp. 28–29; Francis P. Kintz and John Edgar, "Medical Group . . . of First U.S. Army in European Campaign: Siegfried Line, Ardennes, Rhine River, and German Collapse," *The Military Surgeon* 106 (February 1950): 139–47.

[6] Surg, First U.S. Army, Annual Rpt, 1945, pp. 23–24.

times lost all mobility, becoming holding units at airstrips or station hospitals for the care of noncombatants.

The problem posed by such patients appeared early and swiftly grew larger. Already in March hospitals were being diverted from the support of operations to care for recovered Allied military personnel (RAMPs). The 99th Division began to liberate Allied prisoners while still in the Remagen bridgehead, where its troops overran a train with 227 sick and wounded Americans aboard, freed a POW enclosure, and overtook a column of some 1,200 American and British airmen on the road near Giessen, scattering the guards. More discoveries followed as the advance to the east began. Conditions in camps where Allied prisoners had been held ranged from acceptable to indescribable; quick action was demanded to delouse, clean, immunize, and treat the inmates. At Nordhausen the VII Corps liberated a concentration camp, where personnel of the medical groups viewed—for the first but not the last time—scenes that they found "very difficult to describe"; [7] some 2,500 emaciated bodies were strewn over the camp or piled like firewood for disposal in the crematory. But the liberated formed only part of the burden. New throngs of POWs were also swept up from the beginning of the advance, growing to an inundation as the Ruhr pocket collapsed. German soldiers began to surrender en masse—"in some cases straglers [*sic*] trying to reach their own lines and in other cases . . . deserters or individuals who were content to let the war roll by them." [8] Some 300,000 POWs, many ill or wounded, swamped the two victorious armies as they attempted to finish the war.

Three evacuation hospitals took on the rapidly increasing burden of supervising German military hospitals that had been overrun by the advance. The quality of these enemy facilities varied greatly. The 110th Evacuation Hospital moved into a plant that was "splendidly equipped," [9] and the ingenuity of German surgeons in using nails to fix fractures of the long bones won praise from American doctors. But other captured hospitals were small, housed in schools or in the cellars of public buildings, and suffered from vermin, deficient supplies, and unskilled staffs whose doctors had received preferment on political not medical grounds. Patients had to be sorted and moved, and dumps of enemy medical supplies had to be taken over, inventoried, moved and reissued for the care of prisoners and displaced persons (DPs). After a high-ranking German medical officer, Maj. Gen. Walter Scherf, surgeon of the enemy's *Army Group B,* was captured, he was placed in a central headquarters at Weimar and given charge, under American oversight, of civilian and military patients from his own nation. While Scherf's group struggled to organize itself, and to find personnel and transport to carry out its duties, First Army medical groups increasingly took on the responsibilities it was unable to assume. By the

[7] First U.S. Army Report of Operations, 23 Feb–8 May 45, p. 28.

[8] Ibid., an. 11, p. 104.

[9] 110th Evacuation Hospital Semiannual Rpt, January–June 1945, p. 4

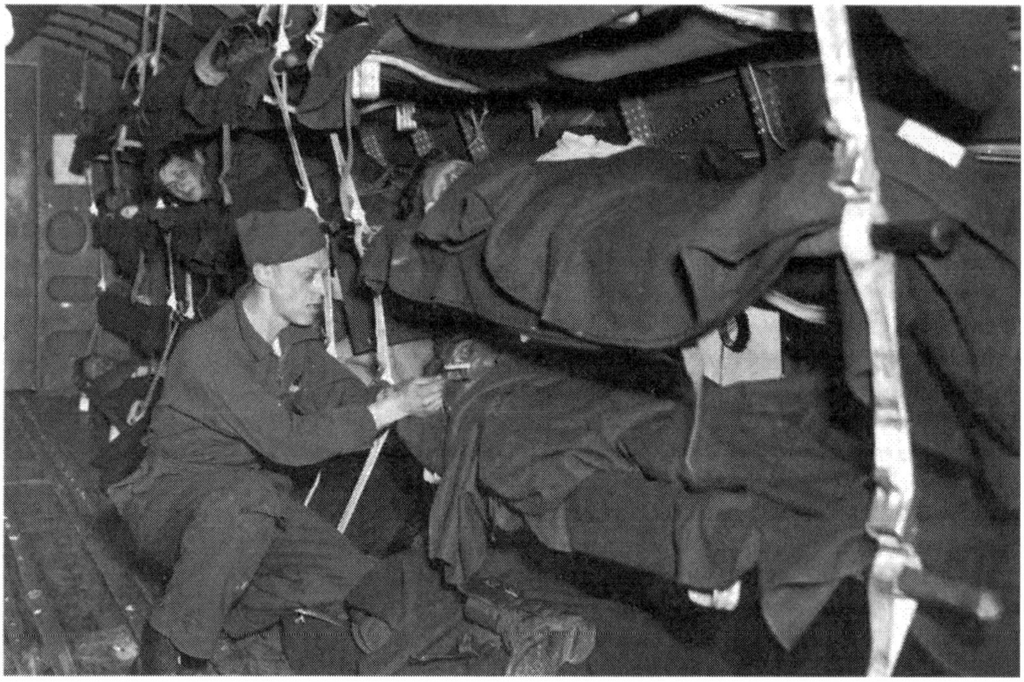

AIR EVACUATION OF WOUNDED IN A C–47, *en route from a holding unit in Germany to a general hospital in France*

end of April First Army groups controlled 216 German military hospitals, 4 POW camps, 22 DP centers, and 3 RAMP hospitals—in all, about 90,000 patients. Several evacuation hospitals—notably the 5th, 45th, 67th, 96th, 118th, and 127th—served both the combat forces and the noncombatants, the changeover from direct support to the care of noncombatants and prisoners coming for most about 1 May. Thereafter, the 5th aided transient RAMPs at Gotha; the 45th became a station hospital for the Buchenwald Concentration Camp near Weimar; and the others saw similar service.[10]

The fighting of March and April and the changeover to occupation duties in early May demanded utmost flexibility in evacuation as well. All cases requiring 10 or less days of treatment were retained in the army area while the fighting continued. For more seriously wounded soldiers the first reliance was now upon air evacuation. Even west of the Rhine poor road conditions gave new importance to air, and the First Army arranged with the IX Troop Carrier Command to make C–47s available to carry wounded. East of the Rhine the rail

[10] Surg, First U.S. Army, Annual Rpt, 1945, pp. 26–27; First U.S. Army Report of Operations, 23 Feb–8 May 45, pp. 43–84 and 105–07; Surg, V Corps, Annual Rpt, 1945; Kintz and Edgar, "Medical Groups," p. 142. The typhus threat and the treatment of liberated prisoners and DPs are recounted in some detail in Chapter XVI.

system, due to the bombing of its tracks and bridges, could no longer support the armies. Motor transport could not entirely compensate. Bridges over the Rhine were few, with priorities given to the eastward flow of men and supplies in support of the attack; and roads were poor, with distances to the front ever increasing because of the rapid advance.

Various expedients were tried. In a few cases L-5 reconnaissance aircraft were exploited as light litter planes to concentrate casualties at the airfields. In an experiment on 22 March a C-47 picked up two gliders, each holding twelve litter patients, from a small airstrip on the east bank near the 51st Field Hospital and successfully delivered them to an airfield on the west. But the main reliance was upon the "big birds," and upon their now proven ability to take over the routine movement of patients hitherto entrusted to railways. New airfields at Eudenbach and Giessen became casualty shipment points, each with its holding unit—the 618th Clearing Company and Company A, 91st Medical Gas Treatment Battalion, respectively—and hard-driven ambulances brought in the wounded from the rapidly moving front.

Medical supplies proved adequate to the needs of the army. February was a time devoted largely to restocking after the Ardennes. When the First Army moved into the Roer region, supply operations were handicapped by the miserable roads, the winter weather, the ruin of the rail lines, and the destruction of buildings that left few protected places to store medical materiel, whose packaging was not waterproof. Nevertheless, the 1st Medical Depot Company moved its advance section across the Roer, from Malmedy to the German town of Zuelpich, with 50 tons of supplies. On 16 March the section crossed the Rhine, to provide close support to the units in the newly created Remagen perimeter. As other depot advance sections moved deeper into Germany they encountered damaged and congested rail lines and widespread bomb and shell damage to potential warehouses. Clearances at the crowded bridgeheads were hard to get, but toward the end of the month trucks were able to move two sections forward to Dollendorf and Honnef. Though low-priority items were often stranded along the railways to the rear, essential supplies were kept moving from the ADSEC depots into the fighting zone. Air evacuation, a blessing to the wounded, brought a new version of one familiar problem for medical supply: Casualties were put aboard on litters covered with blankets, essential items which thereupon vanished into the COMZ, depleting supplies needed for the fighting men. Hence, special supply points had to be set up in conjunction with holding units at the airstrips.

Despite every effort, during April the front moved too rapidly for medical supply to keep pace. Supply officers would select a site for a forward depot; clear their choice with division, corps, and army headquarters, and with the military government; get transport; pack their goods; and move—only to find that the new location had become obsolete before issue could begin. The main depot chose a site at Giessen, but on opening for business found itself too far to the rear to supply the forces adequately. It moved again to Korbach, leaving behind some 20 long tons of excess and slow-moving items to be taken over by the Advance Section. In this case air transport came to the rescue in supporting the fight for the Ruhr pocket. Forty-eight tons of medical materiel—enough to stock a complete depot advance section—were flown in from the United Kingdom, enabling the 47th Medical Depot Company's first advance section to open at Siegen in support of the XVIII Airborne Corps. One big German dump became an American base, where captured supplies were concentrated. During April alone, more than 100 tons were issued for the care of POWs and DPs. German supplies were all-important to the care of noncombatants. Without them, the First Army surgeon reported, meeting the needs of such unfortunates "would have been impossible." Another massive enemy depot was turned over to the Third Army, and the stock transported by ADSEC vehicles and labor to the American forces then engaged in liberating the newly discovered concentration camps in Bavaria and Austria.[11]

Overall, the final campaign experience of the First Army was one of great difficulties overcome by a medical service that had reached its highpoint of clinical and military competence. The need to fight in two directions at once, with half the army engaged in a headlong advance, stretched to the limit medical capacities for communication and evacuation. Yet, though stressed, the medics contrived to meet their commitments, aided by the declining needs of a victorious and largely healthy army. Ironically, triumph was followed almost immediately by dissolution. On 15 May the First Army's role in the European fighting came to an end, as all assigned and attached medical units were transferred to the Ninth Army. The army surgeon and his office departed with the rest of the headquarters for the United States, and then Manila, there to command a new First Army in the planned invasion of Japan.

Ninth Army Units

To the north of the First Army zone, medics of the U.S. Ninth Army, after spending the Ardennes battle in defensive positions with Montgomery's 21 Army Group, experienced a spectacular final campaign. Preparations began in January as the Bulge disappeared. The Ninth Army shifted to the American-led 12th Army Group, and units that had been sent south to aid the First Army's stand returned. Medical organization in the Ninth Army had not changed significantly from earlier campaigns. Seven evacuation hospitals supported the army, and field hospital platoons attached to clearing stations provided direct support to its five divisions spread along the west bank of the Roer River from Wuerm to Monschau. Three medical groups controlled a variety of separate battalions, companies, and small cellular units, such as laboratories and dental prosthetic units. Divisional units managed evacuation up to the clearing

[11] Quoted words from Surg, First U.S. Army, Annual Rpt, 1945, p. 70. See also ibid., pp. 62 and 78; First U.S. Army Reprt of Operations, 23 Feb–8 May 45, pp. 111–13.

station level; above, the groups were in charge. Delayed by floods on the Roer (the Germans had expertly damaged the dams before yielding them, to ensure high water), the army moved from its positions on 23 February, at 0330, as elements began to cross in a three-corps front.

Initially, tough enemy resistance cost 6,000 casualties. While medics evacuated the injured and some 4,300 cases of disease, German resistance faded and the army swung north to meet Canadian forces that had broken out of their own bridgehead. Moenchen-Gladbach fell on 1 March, and the Ninth Army reached the Rhine the next day. By midmonth the bank from Neuss to Wesel was under its control. The medical section moved with the forward echelon of the army command post to Moenchen-Gladbach, where planning for the invasion of the inner Reich began. Among other plans, Colonel Shambora, the army surgeon, projected the use of provisional holding detachments on the east bank to allow divisional units to remain mobile, once the invasion had begun (*Diagram 5*). However, early success and the role of air evacuation soon ended all problems except those of supporting a rapid advance.[12]

After a thunderous artillery barrage, Ninth Army forces crossed the Rhine on 24 March and poured into the Westphalian plain. An airborne drop had been planned to support the movement by seizing a strategic area on the east bank near Wesel. Maj. Gen. Matthew B. Ridgway's XVIII Airborne Corps was to carry out the action; its chief American component was the 17th Airborne Division, blooded in the Ardennes. Division medics began their preparations during March in rest billets near Chalons in France. Two surgical teams were attached to the division; their six surgeons and four enlisted corpsmen were to accompany the medical company into combat by glider, to perform stabilizing surgery on the wounded who would necessarily be cut off for a time behind enemy lines. Gliders were equipped with blankets and litters, and every officer and man in the division received additional first aid packets and bandages. Medics laid in ample plasma supplies, and on D−1 the ETO blood bank delivered whole blood in thermos containers. Between 0700 and 0800 on 24 March the first combat elements took off, accompanied by their own medical detachments and liaison men from the medical company, who would jump or glide in with them. Ground troops, then engaged in forcing their way across the Rhine, raised their eyes to see an awesome sight—a "vast air armada" that required two and a half hours to pass overhead.[13]

Across the Rhine the medical company, surgical teams, and the division surgeon in their gliders encountered intense fire from small arms, machine guns, and 20-mm. and 88-mm. antiaircraft guns. Some medical gliders burst into flame. The surviving medics landed in their designated

[12] Surg, Ninth U.S. Army, Semiannual Rpt, January–June 1945, pp. 1–2, 14 and sec. III, p. 4; ibid., Daily Journal, 1 Feb 45, p. 3, Shambora Papers, MHI.

[13] Charles B. MacDonald, *The Last Offensive*, United States Army in World War II (Washington, D.C.: Office of the Chief of Military History, Department of the Army, 1973), p. 309.

DIAGRAM 5—TYPICAL DIVISIONAL EVACUATION AND MEDICAL SUPPLY PLAN FOR RHINE CROSSING

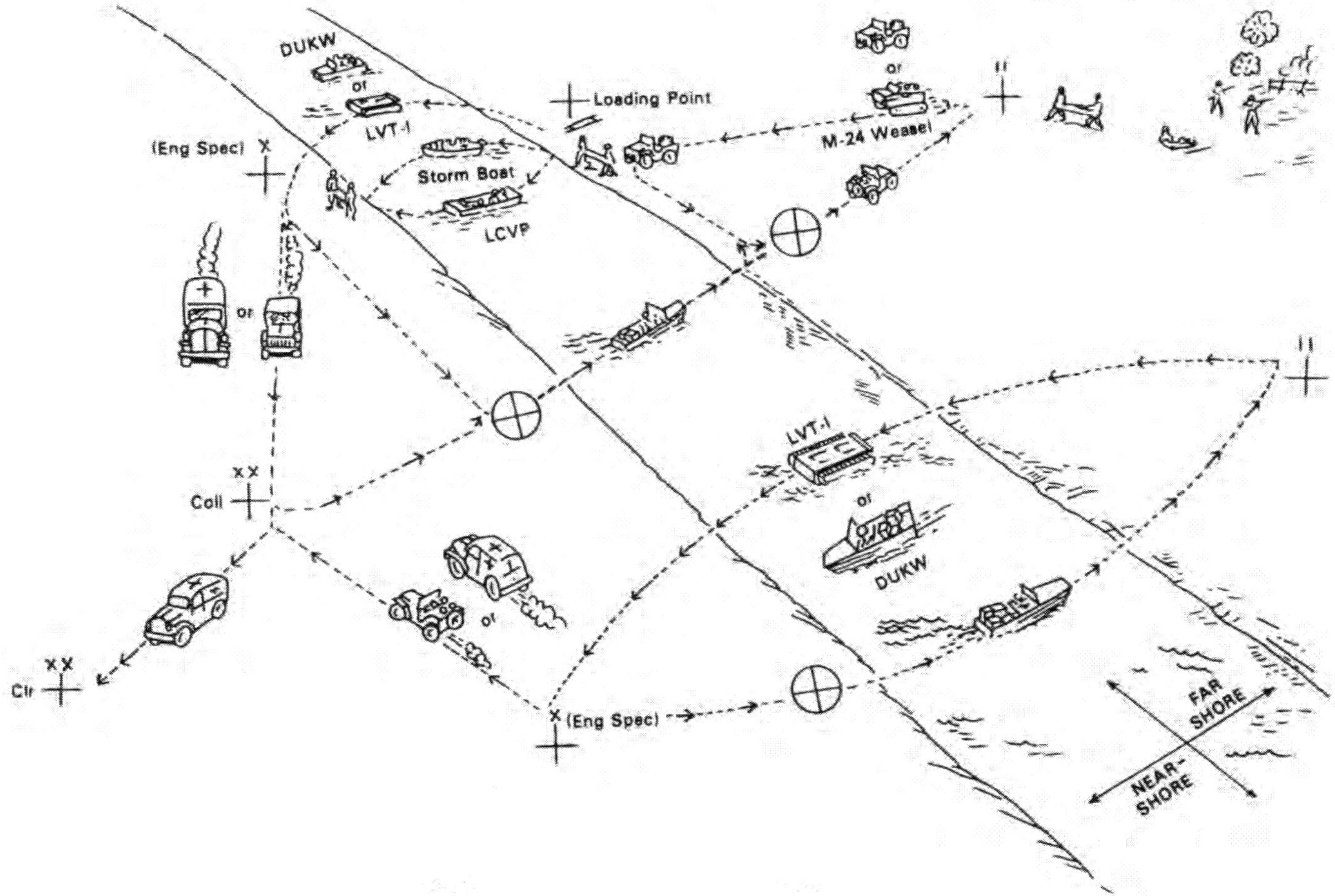

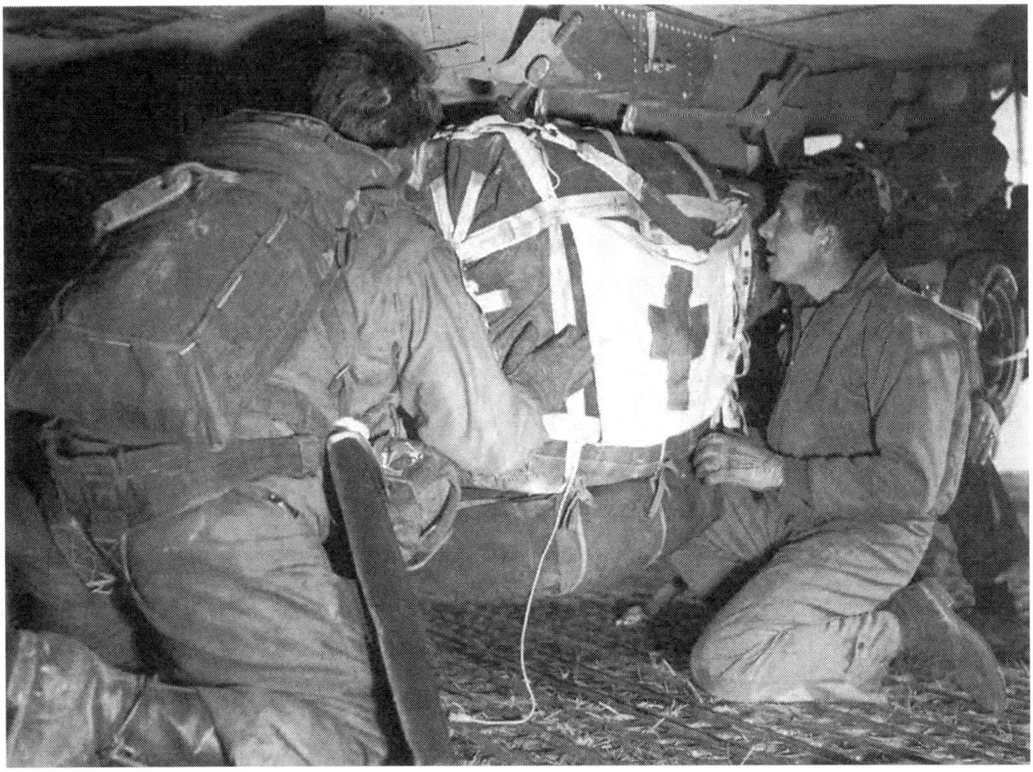

AIRBORNE MEDICS LOADING MEDICAL EQUIPMENT FOR ASSAULT DROP

drop zone only to find that combat troops had not yet cleared it of the enemy, and they took heavy casualties until the zone was secured. Small groups of medics, which grew in size as isolated personnel found one another, made their way across 2 miles of enemy-held fields and woods to set up a clearing station at a predetermined site. Within an hour of landing the station was functioning under canvas; within two, major surgery was under way. Meanwhile, combat forces had contacted British paratroopers to the north, and by 1800 had linked up with ground troops in the Rhine bridgehead. Throughout the night a platoon of infantry guarded the clearing station, while enemy patrols blundered past in the darkness. Firefights erupted, and enemy artillery blocked a truck and ambulance convoy trying to reach the embattled division from the west bank of the Rhine to evacuate its wounded. Despite the alarms, the hours of darkness passed without further injury or death among the wounded, though the ground was covered with helpless patients. By 0800, 25 March, the convoy was rolling, and by 1000 hours the wounded were being loaded into ambulances, some American issue, some captured German machines; into jeep ambulances; and into enemy trucks that now displayed the Red Cross. In the

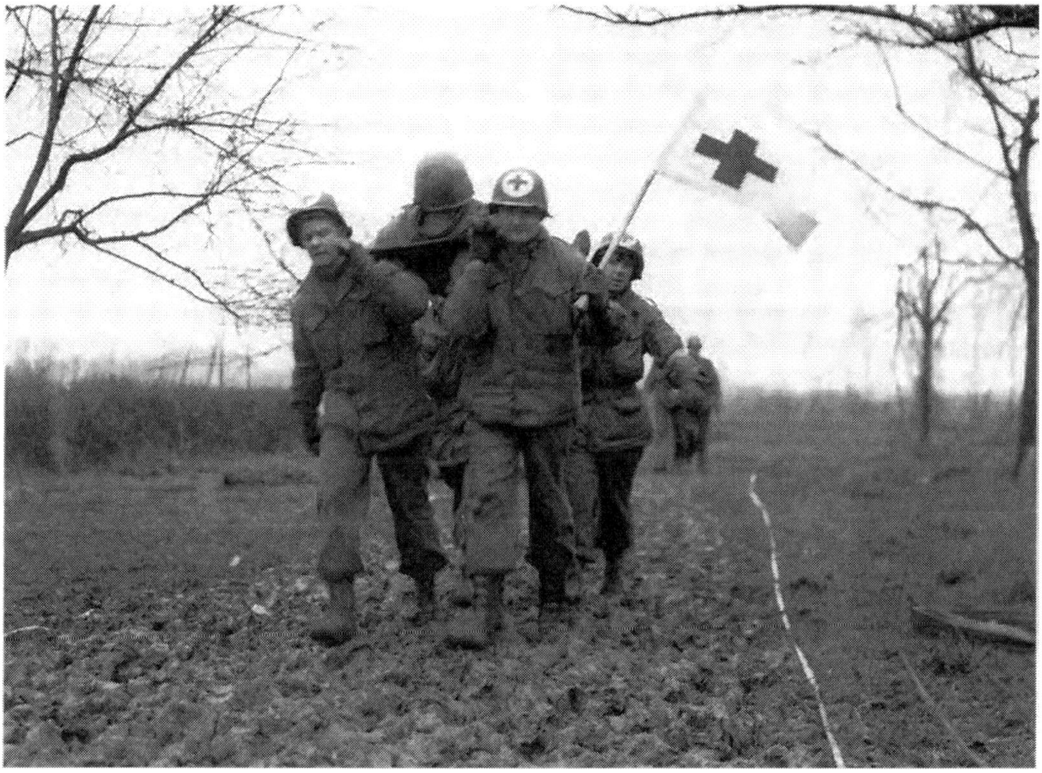

LITTERBEARERS CARRYING A CASUALTY BACK THROUGH A MINEFIELD

convoy rode German as well as American wounded, for all prisoners had received treatment either by their own captive doctors and aidmen or by clearing station personnel.

Now armored units swept through the bridgehead into the roadnet around captured Wesel, and the race to the east began. The airborne troopers did more walking than flying, and the chief task of their medical support was the usual one of trying to keep up. The initial drop had exhibited bravery and skill, but the cost was high—392 casualties the first day, with many more to follow—and the necessity for the bravura show would later be seriously questioned. The medics themselves suffered heavily, but were able to save many lives nevertheless. Able execution of a doubtful tactical plan marked the last hurrah of airborne medics in the European war.[14]

Henceforth the course of the invasion was an itinerary of sites famous in German history—Muenster, the Teutoburg Forest (on whose ridge line the 2d Armored Division met stiff resistance), Magdeburg, the Elbe River—as the Americans gained 225 miles in nineteen days. The problems encountered by the medics were the technical ones of supporting two corps advancing through a third that

[14] Surg, 17th Airborne Division, Final Rpt, 1 Jan–6 Sep 45.

was engaging the enemy; then of supporting a divided army as two corps attacked eastward against little opposition, while a third struck south into the Ruhr, against stiff resistance; and finally and always of keeping contact with line units that felt victory in their grasp. Evacuation distances stretched out despite the common practice of splitting the divisional medical battalions into forward and rear elements. In the 2d Armored Division average ambulance hauls in early April reached 93 miles, and in the 15th Armored Division medical companies reported ambulance roundtrips of 200 miles. Linking up to the First Army in the south, Ninth Army forces helped to complete the liquidation of the Ruhr pocket. During ten days, 4–14 April, its hundreds of thousands of defenders were killed or captured. At 1330 on 30 April troops of the XIX Corps encountered Russian forces, halted, and began to scoop up thousands of Germans who were in flight from the Red Army. By this time the enemy forces had virtually dissolved, and ceasefire orders came a little after sunrise on 7 May.

Few innovations marked the campaign. Instead, practice in 1945 represented the matured employment of methods earlier developed. The Ninth Army's three medical groups, besides coordinating the activities of their component units, provided Shambora's medical section a means of maintaining liaison with the medical service at all echelons. Each group headquarters ran a courier system, enabling the army surgeon to keep abreast of the changing tactical situation when signal communications became overloaded or failed. The chief problems noted with the groups' many cellular units were in personnel administration, vehicle maintenance, and messing; for these flexible units, despite their fitness for operations, the lack of a settled home in the command structure still created unresolved difficulties.

The theater-directed practice of rotating Medical Department officers and enlisted men, initiated in November 1944, continued to demonstrate its value. Each month the Ninth Army transferred five Medical Corps officers, five other Medical Department officers, and twenty-five enlisted men to the Communications Zone, attempting to select those who had endured the "most prolonged and trying combat experiences." In turn, COMZ supplied replacements whose quality drew praise from Colonel Shambora. The need for physically fit replacements meant that professional skills alone could not exempt a physician from forward service, if he was otherwise qualified. This produced some problems in utilizing specialists in forward units. Overall, however, the program's main difficulty was that many more officers and men applied for transfer to COMZ than could be accommodated.[15]

Evacuation took many forms. As in the other field armies, evacuation hospitals proved in practice to be somewhat less than semimobile, and field hospitals augmented by auxiliary surgical group personnel took over

[15] Surg, Ninth U.S. Army, Semiannual Rpt, January–June 1945, sec. II, p. 1. Similar limited rotation policies were adopted by the Third Army, extending in some cases to the level of corpsmen, who were rotated to service companies out of artillery range of the enemy for a few days of rest.

many of their normal duties. For the most seriously wounded, the bomb-battered but still functioning general hospitals of Liege were the usual destination, with ADSEC ambulances providing transport. For the Ninth Army air evacuation from Germany began in March 1945. The army surgeon selected airstrips near field and evacuation hospitals, and SHAEF dispatched a flight surgeon to each to supervise the loading of wounded. Holding units capable of handling 300 to 600 patients were set up and staffed by the medical gas treatment battalions and the field hospitals. For reasons that are unclear, communications presented a difficulty. The holding units requisitioned aircraft from the army, which in turn forwarded requests to SHAEF's air evacuation section. Because radio communication between forward units and the army surgeon failed, TWX (teletype) messages had to be used to dispatch planes. Movement of wounded continued, however, and by mid-May RAMPs and some western European DPs were also being flown out of Germany. Except during a brief gas warfare alert, the medical gas treatment battalions performed their usual variety of tasks—mainly setting up and staffing provisional centers for treatment of venereal and communicable diseases, self-inflicted wounds, neuropsychiatric cases, or convalescents. Aided by elements of the army's 3,000-bed convalescent hospitals, such centers absorbed casualties who might otherwise have been evacuated out of its control.[16]

From the hard-fought opening of the campaign, losses declined rapidly. In the first half of March the army recorded about 5,600 casualties from wounds, injuries, and stress. Despite the Rhine crossing, the number fell in the second half of the month to 5,200. Sometimes, desperate last-ditch resistance raised the total for early April to about 6,600, but it fell to 4,300 in the second half of the month and in early May to 1,900, of whom only 284 were wounded. Instead, POWs, DPs, and RAMPs burdened the evacuation system. Occupation duties began to replace the problems of speed, changing front, communications breakdowns, and long ambulance hauls that had bedeviled the invasion. Medical supply kept up with the rapidly moving front by the well-tried device of leapfrogging depot sections. As supply lines lengthened and railroads became unusable, the inadequacy of the depot companies' organic transport became increasingly evident and compelled them to depend upon the Quartermaster truck companies. But, though spot shortages developed in all classes of supplies, no critical failures occurred to impede operations.[17]

As in the other armies, the changeover to occupation duties in the Ninth Army began even as the attack proceeded. By V–E Day army units had taken on aspects of area commands and were carrying out many duties of military government. In June the ex-

[16] Surg, 2d Armored Division, Semiannual Rpt, January–June 1945, pp. 6 and 30; Surg, 5th Armored Division, Semiannual Rpt, January–June 1945, p. 39; Surg, Ninth U.S. Army, Semiannual Rpt, January–June 1945, sec. II, p. 45.

[17] Surg, Ninth U.S. Army, Semiannual Rpt, January–June 1945, sec. III, pp. 18, 22, 26, 31, 33, 37 and sec. IX, p. 1.

istence of the Ninth Army as a separate force ended, much of its area passing to the British Zone of Occupation, and the remainder to the Seventh Army, along with its soldiers.

Third Army Units

Meanwhile, General Patton's Third Army had written its own epic. Following the reduction of the Bulge, many of its units were shifted north to support the planned main attack. Those that remained were assigned a limited defensive mission. The VIII, III, and XII Corps confronted the flood-swollen Our River, beyond which lay the rugged snowy uplands of the Eifel. Here the fixed fortifications of the West Wall were anchored in the towns of Pruem to the north and Bitburg to the south. The country was "studded with steep broken hills and ravines," roads were poor, and the "cold, wet, muddy February weather" lowered over all. Seldom had a roof and walls been more desirable for the wounded, but buildings for hospital use were few. Fierce fighting had reduced most to rubble, and "ventilated [the others] to such an extent that they were unusable." Under these conditions the advance into Germany began, an aggressive defense aimed at preventing the enemy from consolidating and moving his own forces to meet the northern threat.[18]

While the VIII Corps pushed forward into the West Wall east of St.-Vith, aiming at Pruem, the XII Corps moved against Bitburg. By 5 February the 4th Infantry Division had breached the main line of resistance. On the twelfth Pruem fell, while in the XII Corps sector the 5th and 80th Infantry Divisions, crossing the Our, consolidated a wide beachhead whose depth of more than 2 miles promised a durable lodgement. Meanwhile, the XX Corps assaulted an enemy salient called the Saar-Moselle Triangle, gaining the high ground overlooking the Saar River by the twentieth. So far the campaign featured a grinding advance in dreadful weather against prepared defenses, and the Third Army was fortunate that the foe was already more than half beaten. Mines and booby traps were a continuing danger, for the defenders wired explosives to corpses, both German and American. The army counted nearly 16,000 evacuees, of whom more than 10,000 had to be moved out by road. Weather and war combined in familiar fashion to harass the troops; cold injury remained common; and the shoepacs issued in January caused the usual difficulties.

The problems of evacuation mirrored those of the fighting. Road conditions were wretched. Heavy traffic during the Ardennes battle had churned the roadbeds, and in the second week of February a sudden thaw turned them into channels of mud and slush. Carrying wounded over the soft, slippery surfaces became one of the major difficulties of the advance. Ambulances labored hub-deep toward evacuation hospitals that, impeded by the same conditions, were until midmonth located too far to the rear. Hence, division medical officers experimented with weasels and made use of litter sleds or tobog-

[18] Surg, Third U.S. Army, Semiannual Rpt, January-June 1945, pp. 13 and 20.

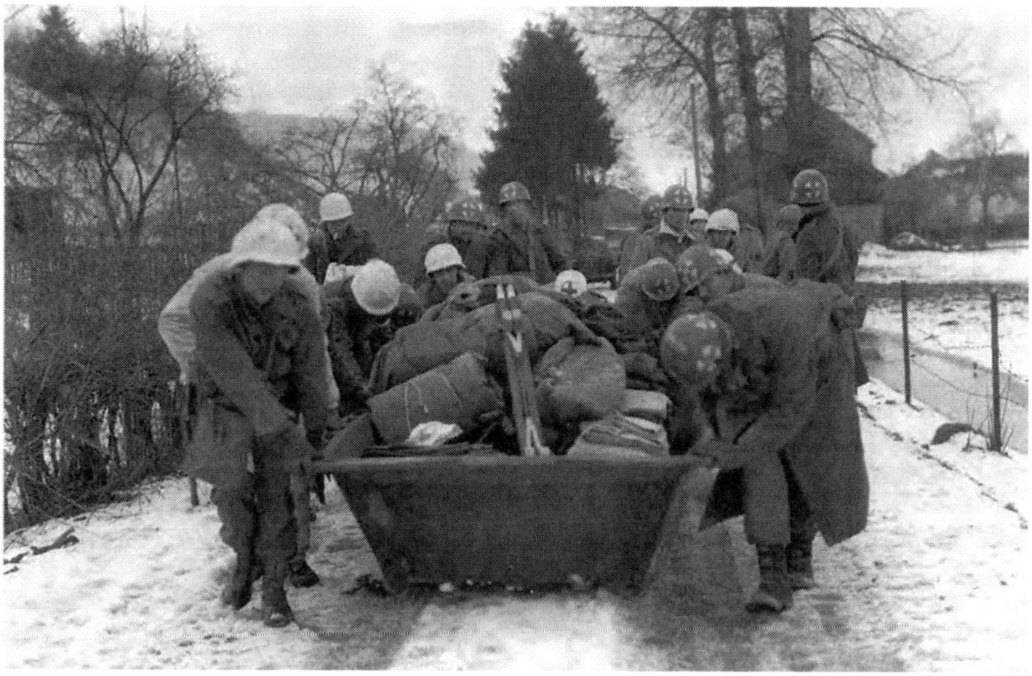

MEDICS PULLING AN ASSAULT BOAT FILLED WITH MEDICAL SUPPLIES *for wounded troops on the other side of a nearby stream*

gans. In the 90th Infantry Division it was "necessary to relieve litterbearers at frequent intervals because of physical exhaustion brought on by travelling in the deep snow." The Third Army ordered thirteen dog teams from the Air Rescue Squadron in Labrador, but by the time the contingent of 130 dogs, 14 enlisted men, and 13 officers arrived at Thionville, on 13 February, the weather had broken, the snow was melting under the thaw, and the teams were never employed.[19]

Typical of the campaign were the experiences of medics in the 80th Division. Serving with the XII Corps, the division on 7 February attacked across the Our River and its tributary, the Sauer, into prepared defenses. In the 318th Infantry's sector only one passable road led down to the river, and it was under heavy fire. While litterbearers manhandled the wounded up the banks of a steep ravine to avoid the road, medics pulled back the aid station as enemy artillery zeroed in. From the head of the ravine, over ground too muddy to support a jeep, a weasel carried the patients back to an advance ambulance loading point. Not until the second day of the attack were the Germans pushed back far enough to allow a collecting point to be established on the riverbank. The road

[19] Quotation from Surg, 90th Infantry Division, Periodic Rpt, January–June 1945, p. 6. See also Surg, Third U.S. Army Semiannual Rpt, January–June 1945, pp. 16–22.

became fairly secure, and litter jeeps took over the task of hauling casualties from the collecting to the loading point.

Meanwhile, the troops had passed east of the Sauer, fighting in harsh mountainous terrain. Here evacuation was entirely by litter, an exhausting hand-carry that ultimately stretched out to 4 miles. At its end, while shells crashed into the woods, the wounded were loaded on rafts for passage of the swift flood-swollen waters. Even at the assembly point on the west bank danger continued; here "a battalion surgeon who attempted to provide medical care for the casualties . . . soon became a casualty himself." Still more difficult were conditions where the ground was less broken and enemy observation better. In some areas the wounded could be moved only under cover of darkness; surgical technicians, accompanying assault troops across the river, turned captured pillboxes into daytime refuges for the wounded until nightfall allowed litterbearers to resume their labor. In these most difficult circumstances the advance continued: On 22 February a platoon of the clearing company opened its station on German soil. Shortly thereafter the enemy's fierce resistance came to an end as his weakened forces withdrew to the east.[20]

March brought spring and a taste of victory. The sorely tried infantry and armor won a series of rapid break-throughs. In the central XII Corps area a tank-led column sent back reports that "read like a bus or railroad timetable—0845: Orsfeld; 1135: Steinborn. . . ."[21] Confused and disheartened Germans surrendered in thousands, so many that at one point a German general fell into American hands because he thought a large crowd of prisoners was a Wehrmacht unit still in being. In two and a half days the 4th Armored Division, leaving the nearest evacuation hospital far to the rear, drove 44 airline miles and halted on high ground overlooking the Rhine. Meanwhile, the Third Army's XII and XX Corps pushed south into the Saar. Fighting on the high ground overlooking the river, Third Army forces captured Saarburg on 20 February and Trier in early March. The last German industrial area west of the river that was still under the Reich's control rapidly passed into Allied hands as the Saar-Moselle Triangle ceased to exist. On the Rhine, Koblenz fell on 19 March. With support from the Supreme Commander, the Third Army now moved to exploit its successes, embarking with his blessing on a plan to invade the Reich with ten divisions.

At 2200 on 22 March, as a bright spring moon illuminated the famous river and the broad open fields beyond, XII Corps troops, supported by four evacuation hospitals at Bad Kreuznach and Alzey, crossed the Rhine at Nierstein, without serious opposition. The surgeon of the 5th Division, the assault force, established a collecting point on the east bank to gather the light casualties and an unloading point on the west bank; both were operated by the collecting com-

[20] Surg, 80th Infantry Division, Semiannual Rpt, January–June 1945, pp 2–4. Quotation on p. 2.

[21] MacDonald, *Last Offensive*, p. 201. See also pp. 202, 205, 259.

panies of the first medical battalion to cross. The first wounded were evacuated by assault boats; later, when the bridgehead had been firmly established, by DUKWs and LVT-1s. Ferrying operations continued for four days, because engineer-built ponton bridges were filled with eastbound traffic.[22]

A swift advance followed, through Bavaria into Austria and Czechoslovakia—one which, as far as the medics were concerned, created a repetition of the difficulties they had faced in the sweep across France in August 1944. Yet the thrill of approaching victory compensated for many problems. "It was France all over again," recalled Col. James C. Van Valin, MC, commander of the 110th Evacuation Hospital, "save that this time the end was in sight, once and for all." Trucks loaded with medics and hospital gear thundered down "the fabulous autobahns, which brought back the sight and smell of the Jersey plains" to homesick soldiers who had undergone their first military training at Fort Dix nearly two years before.[23]

Three days after the Rhine crossing, Patton's armor bridged the river Main. The 80th Division crossed at Mainz in darkness, in an operation bearing little resemblance to its epic struggles at the small rivers of the Eifel a month before. Resistance faded quickly, and the aid stations crossed and set up in buildings near the water's edge. Each had a litter jeep, ferried by an LCVP across the Rhine to speed evacuation to the collecting stations on the west bank. When the aid stations moved east, following the troops, a collecting point at the site of the original landing received casualties by ambulance. Meanwhile, the engineers constructed a treadway bridge, and in due course the collecting stations shifted to the far shore. With fewer casualties and excellent roads opening out before it, the Third Army evacuated about 75 percent of its 23,192 patients by road, about 5,700 by air, and only 2,000 by rail.[24]

Patton's forces slashed across southern Germany (*see Map 23*). Behind armored spearheads the motorized or marching infantry followed (the 80th Division, for example, covered 125 miles in six days). In general, casualties were few, the problems of field medicine reduced to a matter of logistics—keeping up with the advance, moving supplies, hauling evacuees over long distances. Three medical groups supported the advance: The 65th evacuated casualties of the VIII and XII Corps; the 66th supported the XX Corps; and the 69th, strengthened by ambulances from ADSEC, evacuated wounded from Third Army hospitals. On 1 April, however, the 65th, strengthened by an additional battalion headquarters, undertook to provide evacuation for all tactical units of the army. By this time casualties were low but liaison difficult, because of the fluidity of the front. With one battalion headquar-

[22] Surg, Third U.S. Army, Semiannual Rpt, January-June 1945, pp. 28-30 and 32; Surg, 4th Armored Division, Semiannual Rpt, January-June 1945, p. 4: Surg, 5th Infantry Division, Semiannual Rpt, January-June 1945, pp. 3-4.

[23] 110th Evacuation Hospital Semiannual Rpt, January-June 1945, p. 5.

[24] Surg, 80th Infantry Division, Semiannual Rpt, January-June 1945, p. 5.

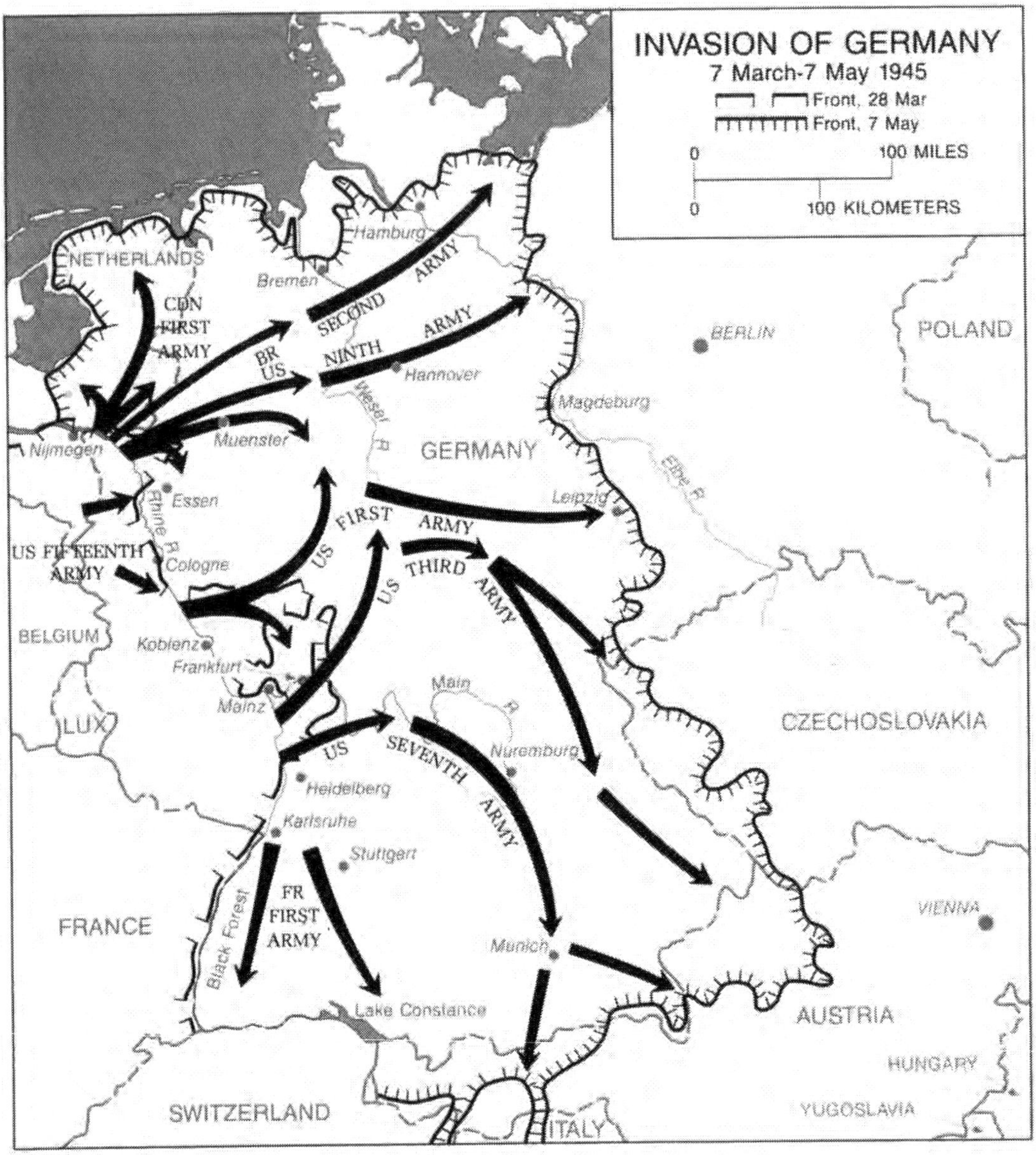
INVASION OF GERMANY
7 March-7 May 1945
Front, 28 Mar
Front, 7 May
0
100 MILES
0
100 KILOMETERS
NETHERLANDS
CDN FIRST ARMY
BR
US
SECOND ARMY
NINTH ARMY
Hamburg
Bremen
Hannover
BERLIN
POLAND
Magdeburg
Nijmegen
Muenster
Weser R.
GERMANY
Elbe R.
Essen
Rhine R.
Leipzig
US FIFTEENTH ARMY
Cologne
US FIRST ARMY
US THIRD ARMY
BELGIUM
Koblenz
Frankfurt
Mainz
Main R.
LUX
CZECHOSLOVAKIA
US SEVENTH ARMY
Nuremburg
Heidelberg
Karlsruhe
Stuttgart
FR FIRST ARMY
FRANCE
Black Forest
VIENNA
Munich
Lake Constance
AUSTRIA
HUNGARY
SWITZERLAND
YUGOSLAVIA
ITALY

MAP 23

ters for each corps, the group commander, Col. Carl G. Griesecke, felt that "the ideal utilization of a Medical Group was at last being carried out," enabling him to exercise maximum flexibility in shifting vehicles and subordinate units as needed. Internally, the group, having no fixed makeup, needed firm control as well, if its array of separate medical units was to function as a team. Unified evacuation had come late to the Third Army in response to the problems of the rapid advance and the reassignment of medical personnel to the care of prisoners and DPs. Under the special conditions of the campaign, it succeeded well.[25]

Despite the organizational simplicity, the speed of the advance created unorthodox situations. Evacuation was more than ordinarily confused. In some divisions, clearing stations got ahead of aid and collecting stations so that casualties were evacuated forward. In others, ambulances absent for a few hours found on their return only empty fields where their units had been. At one point six Third Army evacuation hospitals found themselves in what had newly been defined as the First Army zone, and the closing, moving, and reopening that resulted put all out of operation for a time, leaving only three to support all of General Patton's forces. Struggling to stay mobile, medical units pressed into service every available vehicle; they set up as seldom as possible, under the least amount of canvas that would protect them and their patients. Only the weather aided them, for as the season warmed they were freed of the necessity to search out suitable buildings to house the wounded.[26]

Fighting continued. Despite light casualties the ratio of serious wounds was high, with many puncture wounds of the chest and abdomen caused by small arms. Bloody little actions developed to mar the general picture of minor resistance and few losses. The last gestures of the *Luftwaffe* were random strafing attacks by Hitler's new jet planes. On the ground, resistance took many forms—from absurd wooden barricades to sharp skirmishes with determined fighters. Disorganized groups of enemy, cut off by the advancing armor, lingered in the woods and mountains between Wiesbaden and Bad Nauheim. On 1 April SS troops ambushed a platoon of the 16th Field Hospital, supporting the 4th Armored Division. The Germans killed the chief of surgery and captured the unit, only to see it liberated the following day by American forces.

Despite such alarms, the Third Army found itself changing willy-nilly into an occupation force as it conquered German cities, liberated prison camps, and entered Hitler's homeland, Austria. The confused last days of the war overlapped the coming postwar period; both had urgent problems demanding the same scarce resources, and neither could be ignored. "The scope of governmental problems, including much needed treatment of those suffering from illnesses, both Allied and

[25] Quotation from 65th Medical Group Semiannual Rpt, January–June 1945, p. 3. See also ibid., pp. 12–13; 94th Medical Gas Treatment Battalion Semiannual Rpt, January–June 1945.

[26] Surg, Third U.S. Army, Semiannual Rpt, January–June 1945, p. 42.

enemy, were the most complex that have been faced, perhaps, in all history," recalled the Third Army surgeon. "[Yet] the operational end of the war was a dire necessity. Each problem was huge in itself." [27]

In clearing casualties from the army area, air evacuation played a larger role during April. Nearly four-fifths of the 15,000 patients rode by ambulance to five airfields, where ADSEC or army holding units waited to receive and send them on. As usual, such units were frequently drawn from medical gas treatment battalions. The 94th had served in this way before crossing the Rhine, and might have continued to do so until the end of the war. But in March, alarms over possible use of gas by the Nazis caused the Third Army to order the unit and its counterpart, the 92d Medical Gas Treatment Battalion, to resume close support of the divisions. Failure of the Germans to resort to chemical weapons then sent the 94th back to its former occupation, and it established a holding unit at Rothenbergen beside an airfield designated Y-67. Here almost 6,000 recovered American and British prisoners were processed along with 3,000 U.S. Army patients.

As elsewhere east of the Rhine, arrival of the "big birds" signaled quick evacuation for many a wounded man. The workhorse cargo-carriers were equipped either with roll-down straps or with brackets to hold litters in place. A flight nurse and a medical technician waited aboard. Each plane could hold either 24 litter cases or 27 "walkers" (ambulatory patients). In loading, litterbearers arranged patients under the flight nurse's direction for the most convenient care during the trip; men with bulky casts, for example, were placed in the lowest litter row, at floor level. When all was secure, the plane returned to the United Kingdom or to COMZ airfields.[28]

Seventh Army Units

Among the 6th Army Group forces to the south, the Seventh Army began to prepare for its advance in the lull that followed clearance of the Colmar pocket. For a time its units operated in a sea of mud caused by the February thaw, for many rivers were swelling and water rose in low-lying areas and swampy bottoms. Drainage became a medical problem; sanitation was difficult in unit areas, and constant vigilance by the trenchfoot control teams was needed. Though cold injury fell off rapidly in consequence of the thaw, the teams were obliged to remain active throughout March.[29]

Meanwhile, the medical units readied themselves. Three 750-bed evacuation hospitals moved forward as far as possible in the XV and XXI Corps areas, where the advance was to begin, and a supply buildup brought all stocks to the maximum operating levels. The medical section acquired

---

[27] Surg, Third U.S. Army, Semiannual Rpt, January–June 1945, pp. 26 and 35 (source of quotation); Surg, 10th Armored Division, Semiannual Rpt, January–June 1945, p. 16; Surg, 76th Infantry Division, Semiannual Rpt, January–June 1945, tab April, p. 1.

[28] On air evacuation, see 94th Medical Gas Treatment Battalion Semiannual Rpt, January–June 1945, Evacuation app.

[29] Surg, Seventh U.S. Army, Semiannual Rpt, January–June 1945, p. 1, and Preventive Medicine sec., pp. 1 and 3–5.

two pilots for air evacuation missions and two boats to move the wounded by water. Resuming its attack in mid-March, the Seventh Army rapidly advanced to the Rhine's left bank. On the twenty-sixth the XV Corps crossed the river near Worms, and soon a blitzkrieg advance like that of the First, Third, and Ninth Armies was under way. As with those forces, the basic medical problem was soon reduced to one of keeping up. In the 4th Division, where combat elements were making 20 miles a day, "the Clearing Station moved almost every day and the Field Hospital about once in five days." With each advance, hospitals faced the chores of packing, loading, unpacking, and setting up again. Nurses found their hours "long and busy . . . under great strain," for new casualties often arrived while the unpacking was under way, and there was no break between the labor of movement and the care of patients.[30]

Fresh wounded continued to arrive. The 10th Armored and 44th Infantry Divisions rolled through Ulm, across the Danube and into the Tyrolean Alps, only to encounter dynamited roads and machine-gun nests, where diehard Germans offered "fanatic hostile resistance." Infantry outflanked the defenders on steep slopes and in defiles, where no vehicle could follow them. Litterbearers accompanied the assault forces, and unit medics packed in supplies on their backs. When the wounded had been manhandled to an open section of road, ambulances shuttled them back to the next roadblock, where they were unloaded, carried to other vehicles waiting beyond, and reloaded again for the trip to the clearing station. The bitter skirmishes were brief. On the following day the remnants of the German *Nineteenth* and *Twenty-fourth Armies* surrendered, and the Americans resumed their march.[31]

Evacuation hospitals apparently moved every ten to fourteen days during the campaign, aided by the Seventh Army surgeon who obtained more than a hundred trucks. With adequate transport, the hospitals frequently moved as units, rather than leapfrogging by echelons. Medical groups played a role like that in the northern armies, evacuating corps and division casualties to Seventh Army installations, strengthening the evacuation hospitals with additional personnel as needed, and performing a variety of other duties, including venereal disease control through prophylactic stations that they staffed and operated. Combat had not ended when other duties crowded in. The 31st Medical Group took on the added mission of setting up hospitals for POWs, RAMPs, and DPs, to include a 10,000-bed hospital at Goslar to serve the German wounded. The Seventh Army's line of advance through southern Germany enabled its forces to liberate (or uncover, as the records usually say) many concentration camps and to occupy and administer others after initial liberation by Third Army spearheads. Here doctors, nurses, and corpsmen worked

[30] First quotation from Surg, 4th Infantry Division, Semiannual Rpt, January–June 1945, p. 2. Second quotation from Surg, Seventh U.S. Army, Semiannual Rpt, January–June 1945, ANC sec., p. 1.

[31] Surg, 44th Infantry Division, Medical Hist, 1945, p. 2.

fourteen-hour days over patients more dead than alive, in a cresendo of fatigue made more difficult to bear by emotions of anger, revulsion, and horror. To administer hospitals, evacuate western Europeans, run the camps, fight disease, establish quarantines, and prevent epidemics were formidable problems that overlapped the purely military ones in the chaos of April 1945.[32]

Air evacuation again played an important role in the attack. During the approach to the Rhine an air holding station was set up at Goellheim. After the crossing, another opened at Darmstadt, where Seventh Army air evacuation thenceforth originated. Inside Germany, only airplanes were available to carry out American casualties, for no railroad bridge was constructed over the upper Rhine. Though spells of bad weather occasionally interrupted the airlift of wounded, no serious problems were encountered until heavy rains in early May, and by that time the German railroad system was again in operation.[33]

Fifteenth Army Units

Supporting the field armies during the spring campaign was a new organization, the U.S. Fifteenth Army. Last of the Allied armies to enter the conflict, the Fifteenth, under Lt. Gen. Leonard T. Gerow, took on a variety of tactical and logistical duties. Following the army's arrival on the Continent in December 1944, it was ordered to contain two surviving German enclaves on the western coast of France; to receive, train, and equip units arriving from the United States and the United Kingdom; and to provide operational control for the SHAEF reserve.

During the March 1945 assaults the Fifteenth Army took over a section of the Rhineland between the First and Ninth Armies, which included the cities of Aachen and Cologne, and began to restore order by performing, amid the confusion of a newly conquered region, the tasks of military government. Its forces occupied and defended the western bank of the Rhine from Bonn northward almost to the Wesel, preventing the escape of the German forces trapped in the Ruhr pocket. However, its surgeon, Col. L. Holmes Ginn, Jr., MC, was concerned primarily with support for the troops in the Rhine Province Military District—the area occupied by the army—which grew during March and April to include areas abandoned by the First, Third, Seventh, and Ninth Armies stretching from the Saar in the south to the Maas in the north. Though Fifteenth Army hospitals received almost 15,000 patients, who were evacuated to the Communications Zone, the army's most distinctive work consisted in providing a transition to peace in what would later become the British and French Zones of Occupation.[34]

[32] Surg, Seventh U.S. Army, Semiannual Rpt, January-June 1945, p. 2, and ANC sec., p. 3; Surg, 94th Infantry Division, Semiannual Rpt, January–June 1945, pp. 12–14; 31st Medical Group Annual Rpt, 1 Jan–31 May 45. For further information on these topics, see Chapter XVI of this volume.

[33] Surg, Seventh U.S. Army, Semiannual Rpt, January-June 1945, Evacuation sec. and Medical Supply sec., p. 8.

[34] History of the Fifteenth United States Army, 21 August 1944 to 11 July 1945, especially pp. 18–19;

Continued

Lessons Learned

Despite the overall picture of competence and success, the last campaign turned up some medical problems that related to command and others that concerned mobility. At the divisional level the separation between the division surgeon and the commander of the medical battalion caused difficulties, and brought proposals from many medical officers to combine the two. During action, some division surgeons solved the problem ad hoc by staying with the battalion throughout the advance. The practice of dividing field hospitals into three hospitalization units continued to work well; even in the fast-moving armored columns, nontransportables continued to receive treatment well forward. The surgical teams were furnished with two 2½-ton trucks and with sufficient tentage, instruments, and supplies for their needs. Team members rode the same trucks and set up their own tents beside those of the clearing station they supported. The third element in the combination, the field hospital unit, arrived last and took over the job of holding and caring for the wounded as the surgical team finished with them. When time came for the whole divisional support system to move forward again, a group from the collecting company remained behind with the patients who were still not able to travel. Some surgeons in the Third Army were so satisfied with this method of treating nontransportables that they declared: "The problem of handling the casualties of armored divisions was solved." Others, however, wondered whether a new unit might not perform the job better than an improvisation using portions of three.[35]

The Third Army surgeon made some suggestions that have, in retrospect, a prophetic ring. "A completely mobile surgical hospital," he wrote, "was a necessity for the support of a division." The T/O of such a unit should provide a "two-platoon arrangement which would permit leapfrog movement of the platoons or forward displacement of one while the second retain[s] the post-operative cases until they become transportable." In such proposals the duties and typical movement of the future MASH (mobile army surgical hospital) seem to be foreshadowed.[36]

Underlining the emphasis on mobility was the continued realization that in practice "the 400-bed evacuation hospital is not semi-mobile." With only its organic vehicles, the unit proved unable to move itself even in two echelons. Because about half the evacuation hospitals were closed and in motion at any given time, their patients were thrown upon the others, which handled the load by expanding their bed capacity and augmenting their equipment—and so reducing their own ability to move when the time came. Though the hospitals shuffled transport back and forth among themselves, there was seldom enough to permit them to op-

Fifteenth U.S. Army in Germany, 16 April–10 July 1945, pp. 37–38. On the Occupation, see Chapter XVII of this volume.

[35] Surg, Third U.S. Army, Semiannual Rpt, January–June 1945, p. 92.

[36] Ibid., p. 83.

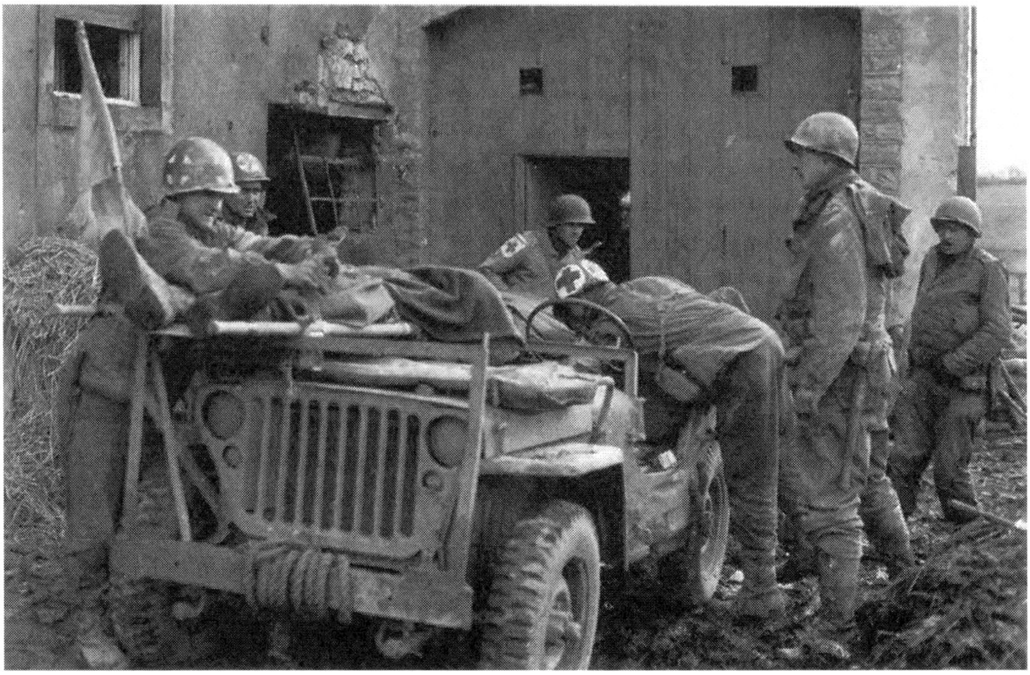

JEEP AMBULANCE EVACUATION

erate as theory demanded. The hospitals also lacked surgeons to handle peak loads so that surgical teams had to be added to their complements to cope with the demands of heavy fighting. Inadequate holding capacity during forward displacement also meant adding a clearing company platoon as a holding unit. The tendency of the "semi-mobile" evacuation hospital to grow in size and decrease in mobility apparently was not solved, for ambulance hauls increased whenever the army was in rapid motion, and only the fact that casualties usually decreased at the same time kept serious problems from developing.[37]

For evident reasons, army surgeons judged that the even larger 750-bed evacuation hospital had "little or no place in a field campaign in a war of movement." On the other hand, the convalescent hospital, "large and immobile though it may be," was an important unit when well-trained replacements for the wounded were not available. It sopped up patients who would have been lost to field army control and returned them to their units with a minimum of fuss. Here too venereal disease cases often were concentrated and treated, relieving the evacuation hospitals of a burden while preventing patients from being evacuated to the COMZ.[38]

[37] Ibid., pp. 82–83 (quoted words on p. 82); Surg, 10th Armored Division, Semiannual Rpt, January–June 1945, p. 37; Surg, 5th Infantry Division, Semiannual Rpt, January-June 1945, p. 5.

[38] Surg, Third U.S. Army, Semiannual Rpt, January–June 1945, p. 85.

Ambulance evacuation required special attention in warfare like that of the spring of 1945. The durable, ubiquitous jeep again proved its worth as an impromptu ambulance. But methods changed as the initiative for evacuation shifted forward. The notion that the higher echelon in each case could evacuate the lower on request proved to be nonsense when the front was in such rapid motion. Instead, each echelon had to consign its vehicles to the next lower one so that evacuation could be constant and instantly responsive to need. The Third Army surgeon reported:

> This same concept of constant evacuation carried down to the first and second echelon medical service. Collecting company ambulances were kept or near battalion aid stations where possible or the one-quarter-ton truck ambulance was used. Litter bearers of the medical detachments were kept available near company CP's and aid stations, rather than waiting for someone to locate the aid stations prior to sending up litter bearers.

Overall, however, the lessons of medical mobility had proved hard to learn, easy to forget, and difficult to implement when a whole army cried simultaneously for transport in a lightning campaign.[39]

Supporting the Front

Behind the Fifteenth Army the Communications Zone reached its final form. The Advance Section, which supported the 12th Army Group, had been little affected by the Ardennes fighting. In thinly populated, hilly regions of the front there were few depots or supply lines to be disrupted. The German advance had been halted short of the Meuse River, and thus of the main logistical network. What losses did occur were easily replaced: some forward dumps, a few rail lines and trains damaged by strafing or bombing, lost equipment in a few truck companies. At the rear the most serious damage to ADSEC generally and to the medics in particular was caused by V–1 "buzz bombs," for almost 2,500 beds suffered some degree of injury, especially in and around Liege. Yet the Advance Section was able to begin its planning for the new campaign without the need of a period of recovery and without replacing extensive losses.[40]

Certain installations were regrouped to provide backup for the anticipated Allied offensive. Thus the 12th Field Hospital moved to Namur, where it opened a railhead holding unit to serve the evacuation hospitals of the First Army. The 77th Evacuation Hospital relocated to La Louviere to speed the return of the lightly wounded to replacement centers. The hard-pressed 130th General Hospital, driven out of Ciney by the German attack, resumed operation in mid-January. But the primary change was a shift in the character of ADSEC itself. Recognizing the need for mobility to support the invasion of Germany, the Communications Zone began to restructure its Advance Section, transferring to the rear base sections the chain of general hospitals

[39] Ibid., p. 86. See also Surg, 10th Armored Division, Semiannual Rpt, January–June 1945, p. 36.

[40] ADSEC Hist, p. 111.

running south from Liege to Nancy. Between January and May ADSEC lost 82 percent of its general hospitals but almost doubled its number of field hospitals, and also increased its ambulance companies, sanitary companies, and its medical and dental detachments. This was a lesson the Ardennes fighting had taught. The effort to support a rapid advance with fixed facilities had ended.[41]

Transport, despite the battle and the winter weather, promised to be adequate for the advance to the Rhine. The area of the Bulge itself was devastated by Allied bombing and by demolitions carried out systematically by both sides. The rail bridges were mostly gone, the lines out of commission. However, repair got under way quickly. The lines had been pushed as close to the front as ADSEC engineers could manage, often within medium artillery range. Maintenance crews had kept roads and tracks fairly clear even during the deep snows, and the only real obstacle to resupply by rail had been caused by frozen switches. The coming of warmer weather both aided and slowed the buildup. The Meuse thawed in February, and thereafter dropping flood stages permitted the gradual resumption of barge traffic that moved heavy bulk supplies south from Antwerp. However, heavy vehicles had to be barred from roads made impassable by the thaw. Meanwhile, express supply trains—called "Toot Sweet Express"—rolled into Liege daily at 1000 hours. From Liege and Verdun in turn came virtually all the supplies that fueled Bradley's 12th Army Group.[42]

Under General Lee's orders, planning began in the latter part of February. The medical plan went to G–4 a few days later. The assumption at the time was that the main attack would be launched north of the Ruhr, with a secondary thrust south of the Moselle. The opportunistic character of the actual Rhine crossings could not be foreseen, but many of the problems presented by the river were. The medics asked for 125 C–47s a day for air evacuation. Colonel Beasley, the ADSEC surgeon, planned to establish holding units both east and west of the Rhine. Those to the east would receive the wounded by jeeps or, if necessary, by returning supply vehicles, such as the weasel. West of the river the holding units were to be set up at railheads. As the Rhine bridges were repaired and trains began to run again, the need for the western units would gradually cease.[43]

The events of March demonstrated that the end of the war was rapidly approaching. In April the Advance Section prepared its ECLIPSE plan, following SHAEF's more general plan for dealing with the final collapse of Germany. Rapid occupation of the Reich, followed by redeployment to the borders of the American Zone, formed the two phases of the plan. At the collapse or capitulation of the major German forces—or the surrender of the government or high command—the Supreme Commander

---

[41] Surg, ADSEC, COMZ, Semiannual Rpt, January-June 1945, pp. 1 and 9–10.

[42] ADSEC Hist, p. 115. The name was a pun on the French phrase *toute de suite* (quickly).

[43] Directive, COMZ, ETO, 19 Feb 45, sub: Emergency Plan for Support of Rapid Advance, with encls., file HD:ETO:320.

would announce "A-Day," when the plan would go into effect. By that time ADSEC expected the First, Third, and Ninth Armies to be completely east of the Rhine; the Fifteenth to be performing occupation duties west of the river; and its own sphere of action to be entirely inside Germany.[44]

The actual course of operations allowed the Advance Section to turn over its former territory and responsibilities to other base sections, to enter Germany, and to establish its headquarters at Bonn during April. Here it was no longer an area command—territorial control was swiftly vested in the armies—but it continued to be a logistical command. In consequence, control of road and rail traffic also passed largely to the armies. ADSEC found that its supply responsibilities were least burdensome in the north, where the reduction of the Ruhr pocket slowed the invaders; in the south, where American armor pressed deep into central Europe, supply was far more difficult. The major technical problem, however, came from the capture of vast quantities of German materiel. As already noted, such supplies were crucial to meeting the needs of sick and injured noncombatants of all types, but the job of inventorying and controlling the vast stocks proved too much for ADSEC's medical supply officers. Completing the work would be a task for the occupation authorities to come.

Evacuation mirrored the experience of the field forces. Two 1,000-bed holding units at Aachen represented the effective limit of rail transport. During the advance to the Rhine ever-lengthening ambulance hauls, improving weather, and the conquest of enemy airfields brought increased evacuation by plane. Near Moenchen-Gladbach both rail and air holding units were established. When the armies crossed the Rhine, forward airfields were used whenever weather permitted, and as soon as the engineer-built bridges spanning the river were operational, casualties were carried by ambulance to the railheads on the west bank. Even when trains began to cross the Rhine, however, priorities denied passage to hospital trains. Not until late April, when the armies were deep in Germany and the war nearly ended, did the first hospital train cross into the inner Reich.

Beasley's medics found themselves facing few surprises in hospitalization. Plans for new construction went ahead as long as the fighting continued. ADSEC officers sought out hospital sites in the wake of the advancing armies, and construction or rehabilitation got under way with the aid of the engineers. But such problems belonged essentially to the period of occupation. The complex and very rapid changes in ADSEC's status brought on by the last campaign gave way to the general transformation brought by peace and civil governance of a conquered people.[45]

The Continental Advance Section provided immediate support to the Seventh Army—fixed hospitalization,

---

[44] ADSEC, COMZ, Operation Plan "ECLIPSE," in ADSEC Hist.

[45] Ibid., pp. 131 and 149. For the problems presented by POWs, RAMPs, and DPs, as well as an account of the military government, see Chapter XVI of this volume.

evacuation, and medical supply—and to the French First Army after it entered Germany. Like ADSEC, it underwent a process of lightening in preparation for the advance. As its surgeon remarked, the section began the year adhering to the established policy of locating fixed hospitals as far forward as possible. Indeed, toward the end of January it acquired six general hospitals in the Nancy-Toul area, giving it briefly the luxury, which it had not enjoyed before, of accepting casualties without first evacuating a similar number to empty the necessary beds. But by March the spring offensive had made the policy impractical. When CONAD moved into Germany in early April, it turned its fixed installations over to the Oise Base Section. Unlike ADSEC, its hospitalization henceforward was limited to the care of its own troops and that of increasing numbers of displaced persons and prisoners of war.

Its experience with rail and air evacuation resembled closely that of the northern section, intensified, perhaps, by geography: Southern Germany is mountainous, the north an extensive plain. A hospital train base was moved to the west bank of the Rhine, but rail evacuation "lagged far behind" the need, and the rail holding units were converted to air holding units, which were then leapfrogged as necessary to keep up with the movement of the Seventh Army. Flying weather was excellent, and the lack of functioning rail facilities east of the Rhine merely underlined the advantages of the new system.[46]

Both ADSEC and CONAD drew their support from the Oise Base Section, which expanded rapidly by gathering in areas and installations as the advance sections left them behind. Fixed hospitals were established no further forward, and air transport increasingly was used to return casualties to the west bank of the Rhine. Hence, the Oise medical section, which controlled one general hospital in January, operated forty-three of the latter plus three station hospitals in April, with a concurrent expansion in depots and dispensaries. At its highpoint that month medical personnel in the base section numbered 2,700 male officers, 3,900 nurses, and 26,000 enlisted men. Its general hospitals were organized into two hospital centers, and its medical facilities all told employed some 30,000 DPs and 300,000 POWs. To the rear the Seine Section remained the key to the medical logistics system, for it contained the city of Paris, COMZ headquarters, a system of general hospitals also organized by two hospital centers north and south of the Seine, and the elaborate transport hub centered in and around the French capital. Here conditions did not change essentially during the last offensive; as before, base section medical personnel were occupied primarily with triage and evacuation. Each center had a holding hospital, where arriving patients were assigned to one of three basic categories: COMZ (less than 30 days hospitalization until 1 March, then less than 60), United Kingdom (60–90 days), and zone of interior (over 90 days). By mid-March few patients were being received by rail, marking not only the transit of the Rhine by

[46] Surg, CONAD, Semiannual Rpt, January-June 1945, pp. 4 and 8. Quoted words on p. 5.

the fighting forces but the fact that air transport often returned casualties direct to the Paris airfields, skipping the system of railheads and hospital trains entirely. COMZ patients went to the hospital appropriate for their injury within the center where they were triaged; United Kingdom patients were usually evacuated by air; and zone-of-interior patients were sent to the air holding unit of the 1st General Hospital, at Le Bourget airport, for loading on planes bound for the United States. Like ADSEC and the other base sections closer to Germany, the Seine Section also handled an increasing burden of sick and injured Allied nationals, though here mainly civilian DPs. Russians had to be sent to Germany for transfer to their own medical services, while hospital trains bore Belgians to Liege and Italians to Marseilles, while airplanes returned recovered British and Canadian prisoners to the United Kingdom.[47]

The Normandy Base Section, like Oise, grew rapidly in 1945, absorbing the Brittany Base Section, taking over the ports of Le Havre and Rouen from the Channel Base Section, and providing support to Fifteenth Army troops whose mission was to contain the holdout German garrisons in the coastal enclaves of Lorient and St.-Nazaire, on the Bay of Biscay. In March an influx of German battle casualties compelled the conversion of hospitals serving Americans to POW facilities and in April the liberation of large numbers of Allied prisoners caused the section to redesignate Camp Lucky Strike, heretofore used by replacements entering the Continent, as RAMP Camp No. 1. Meanwhile, the Channel Base Section advanced into Belgium, taking over areas formerly controlled by the Advance Section. Its surgeon was responsible for American medical needs in the area of British control along the Channel coast that included Antwerp. Indeed, by the end of the war a good third of the section's medical installations lay in British areas. Its RED HORSE expansion staging area mushroomed, becoming for a time the key debarkation point for reinforcements arriving from the United States; DP camps were established, using civil affairs medical supplies, and staffed by Belgian nurses and doctors; and section doctors and nurses, working at Camp Lucky Strike, treated liberated Americans whose condition they found to be worse than anticipated. At COMZ's request the section sent six teams—each consisting of three doctors, a medical administrative officer, and twelve enlisted technicians—to ADSEC in Germany to aid in providing immediate medical care for RAMPs. Thus the burden of aiding noncombatants stretched from the most forward areas back to the rear sections. Even in the Delta Base Section, around Marseilles, whose small medical establishment served primarily its own forces, the number of POWs rapidly increased, and German prisoners built a model 1,000-bed general hospital adjacent to their en-

[47] Surg, Oise Intermediate Section, Semiannual Rpt, January-June 1945, pp. 2-3 and 10-11; Surg, Delta Base Section, Annual Rpt, 1945, p. 1. See also Surg, Seine Section, Semiannual Rpt, January-June 1945, pp. 16-17.

closure, where their own medical personnel cared for their needs.[48]

No aspect of the medical system saw more striking changes than evacuation during the last offensive. The transformation from the crisis conditions of midwinter was extraordinary. Even when casualties began to rise in late February as a result of action along the West Wall, Paris still counted 11,000 empty beds and the hospitals of the United Kingdon recorded a falling census. With ample bed strength, the temptation for forward surgeons was to evacuate too many patients, rather than too few. Complaints registered at Colonel Mowrey's Evacuation Branch indicated that triage decisions were also being distorted by an overabundance of transport—a remarkable fact, given the conditions of the months just past. Air evacuation was, with few and brief exceptions, consistently good throughout the system. Poor weather in late April did impose some delays, but the first week of May found hospital trains at last across the Rhine, while improving weather enabled C–47s to join in clearing out the choked forward holding units, evacuating nearly 5,000 patients on the third of the month. Air evacuation to Great Britain became ever more important, not because alternatives were unavailable but because it was better for the wounded. In an effort to fill its empty beds on the Continent, ETOUSA raised the evacuation policy. The planes flying out of Liege, Paris, and Thionville were able to handle all the severely wounded who still required treatment in the United Kingdom, and whole weeks passed in which no casualty had to endure the delays and frequent rough water of the Channel crossing.

By 8 May, when Mowrey noted in his diary that "La Guerre est finis," he and Hawley had formulated and set in motion a new policy for the immediate postwar period. Patients on the Continent were to be held there, until their cases could be reviewed by medical boards. Those tagged for quick return home were then to be taken to the 1st General Hospital at Paris, airlifted to the embarkation hospitals at Cherbourg and Marseilles, and returned to the United States by sea. The status of some DP patients and the disposition of POW patients remained to be decided, and some shuffling of cases among the various hospitals in Germany would become necessary as soon as occupation authorities determined the fate of various categories. But these were little more than details. The systems of evacuation and hospitalization, overbuilt in the planning phase and stretched to their limits during the winter, provided a surplus of everything for the casualties of the last campaign.[49]

Triumph of Preventive Medicine

Despite appearances to the contrary, the same good fortune accompanied the Army in regard to sickness. By comparison with the

[48] Surg, Normandy Base Section, Semiannual Rpt, January-June 1945, p. 4; Surg, Channel Base Section, Hist, January-June 1945, pp. 2 and 5–6; Surg, Delta Base Section, Annual Rpt, 1945, p. 2.

[49] Above paragraphs based on Evacuation Branch, Operations Division, OofCSurg, HQ, ETOUSA, Daily Diary, May 1944–May 1945, file HD 024 ETO.

Mediterranean, Pacific, and Asiatic theaters, the European Theater was the healthiest in which Americans served. It was true that a year of fighting, a hard winter, and the collapse of Germany set the stage in 1945 for unusually high numbers of casualties from disease. Of the 1,950,812 admissions for disease recorded in the theater from January 1942 to December 1945, 1,027,500 (or 58 percent) occurred in 1945 alone. During the months of fighting—January through April—the number of fixed beds occupied by disease and nonbattle-injury victims consistently ran ahead of those occupied by battle casualties, while the reverse had been true in 1944. By comparison with 1944, half of which had also been devoted to fighting, syphilis increased among American soldiers in the theater from 9,190 to 25,520; gonococcal infections from 36,850 to 162,785; chancroid, from 2,500 to 12,550—a VD epidemic unleashed by the conditions of devastated Europe and the release of many troops from front-line duty. But most other diseases increased as well (malaria and certain types of pneumonia were exceptions). Diarrheal diseases increased from 33,125 to 46,585; skin afflictions from 43,840 to 73,170; infectious hepatitis from 4,310 to 20,530. Diphtheria, by reason of its virulence, brought concern to Army physicians despite its comparatively low incidence.

However, comparison of admission rates—the number of admissions for disease per 1,000 average strength per year—indicates that the impressive absolute increase resulted largely from the growth in the number of troops in the theater. Admission rates that had increased in 1943 declined sharply in 1944 and rose only slightly in 1945, never regaining the levels of the two years spent largely in training in the United Kingdom. In sum, the effects of acclimatization and the influenza outbreak of 1943 were more severe than those of combat. On the Continent the health problems with greatest impact on operations were psychoneurosis, or combat fatigue, and cold injury. Americans, well fed and cared for, formed probably the healthiest population in devastated Europe; their death rate from all diseases in 1944 was only .52 and in 1945 only .59 per 1,000 average strength per year. Typhus epidemics, worst in eastern Europe, flared also in occupied Germany, but only five Americans caught the disease, and none died. Many factors contributed to this picture of success in the control of disease, which contrasted so strongly with the failure to prevent widespread cold injury. Fundamental were the European environment, with its temperate climate and freedom from most exotic diseases; the generally adequate diet and equipment of the American soldier; and the program of preventive medicine that guarded his health.[50]

Successfully controlling disease on a continent torn by war presented complex problems to Colonel Gordon and the Preventive Medicine Division. None were more difficult than those surrounding venereal disease, a traditional plague of soldiers and a persistent outrider of war. The work done in

[50] Statistics for above paragraphs from Reister, ed., *Medical Statistics*, pp. 608, 804, 826.

England during the buildup provided few useful guides on the Continent, where, even apart from the prevailing disorder, cultural norms differed widely from those of the British Isles. On the Continent prostitution was a recognized endeavor, legally protected and regulated, and brothels formed a normal part of the urban scene. Medical officers, looking primarily to the health of the troops, tried to control disease by suppressing the brothels. Commanders, on the other hand, often viewed sex as a recreation needed and deserved by fighting men, and some attempted to provide it through regulated prostitution. On 6 July 1944 Colonel Gordon, visiting France, found in Cherbourg "houses of prostitution being run for, and indirectly by, U.S. troops." One establishment had been designated for black soldiers, the others for whites, and "military police [were] stationed at the doors to keep order in the queues which formed." The next day Cherbourg passed to ADSEC's control, and the new commander, on advice of his surgeon, Colonel Beasley, closed the houses.[51]

During the summer campaigns, policy continued to depend largely upon the attitudes of local commanders. War Department and ETO policy requiring that prostitution be suppressed was not always enforced. In the medical view, inspection of prostitutes formed no real protection against the spread of venereal disease, for a woman could harbor the disease with no apparent symptoms. The stubborn belief in licensed brothels, protested some medical officers, "is based on the sort of faith that leads a small boy to believe that if he places a horsehair in a bottle of water it will turn into a snake." [52] But the existence of an official policy merely inhibited open and rational debate, without securing compliance. It was fortunate, then, that many factors conspired to keep continental sick rates from venereal disease low—indeed, lower than those of the British Isles. Many women of the type who would normally have served the needs of the Army had compromised themselves with the Germans and fled to escape the wrath of the Resistance. Friendly, noncommercial sex was inhibited by the language barrier, which made the early stages of acquaintanceship difficult, especially for GIs on the move. Americans who did succeed in finding partners had seemingly been sufficiently impressed by the perils graphically presented to them during training to make use of excellent prophylactic stations, which the Germans had built and equipped for their own forces and which now fell to the Allies as prizes of war.

Behind the lines, however, the potential for future trouble was easy to see. Some commanders remained adamant in favor of military brothels. Civil affairs officers held varied opinions and seemingly had no consensus on which policy was best. French civil officials, while anxious to please their liberators, viewed efforts to suppress prostitution as "mildly mad" and in any case tended to follow the norms of their own country. Often the men

[51] Information on venereal disease, except as otherwise noted, from Hoff, ed., *Diseases Transmitted Through Contact,* pp. 242–66. Quoted words on p. 243.

[52] Ibid., p. 245.

themselves could give little practical help in tracing their sexual contacts.

In a foreign country where the soldier is contacting a girl who speaks a different language, lives on a dark street, has a name which the soldier cannot spell or pronounce, it is difficult for him to have her name and address. The towns are all blacked out, the streets are not laid out in squares but in a circular fashion and it is not unusual for a street to have six unpronounceable and unspellable names in six blocks.[53]

The liberation of Paris in August 1944 brought within Allied lines a world metropolis that quickly became SHAEF headquarters and a gigantic magnet for every soldier on furlough. Medical officers told of entire convoys that "got lost" on their way to this or that objective and wound up in Paris. Traditionally an easygoing city, the French capital in 1944 was particularly attractive to Americans in search of sex, for food was in short supply and even the lowliest GI found himself in "an unbeatable bargaining position." Wartime psychology was a factor: "The soldier cannot possibly worry about venereal disease when he has to worry about getting shot," remarked the Ninth Army surgeon. GIs on leave sought a last fling before possible wounding or death.[54]

When the fighting man who had undergone a lengthy period of enforced continence found himself presented with the opportunities of Paris, some remarkable performances resulted. A private from a Quartermaster company picked up, according to his VD contact form, nine different women in the vicinity of the same corner, took them to six different hotels, and actually managed seven sexual exposures. Total time elapsed: eight hours. The VD rate in the European Theater doubled during the year, and studies showed that more than two-thirds of all venereal infections acquired in France originated in Paris. The Seine Section officers were less than sympathetic to medical alarms. One medic recalled that in September 1944 the provost marshal of the section made a tour of Paris brothels to select some for officers, others for white, and still others for black enlisted men. Despite their reputation for sexual puritanism, Americans showed a marked preference for the other national faith of pragmatism, tempered by racial taboos.[55]

However, VD control officers succeeded in setting up additional prophylactic stations, often in Red Cross hostels, and programs of education and propaganda got under way with an assist from *Stars and Stripes.* The French government was cooperative and helpful, and its aid proved to be essential, not only for reasons of language but because familiarity with French cultural norms was necessary in overcoming the reluctance of women to admit the problem and seek treatment. In fact, the police and the theater medical service were closely tied together despite the ef-

[53] Quotation from Surg, Ninth U.S. Army, Daily Journal, 30 Jan 45, p. 7, Shambora Papers, MHI. See also Ltr, Hawley to CG, ETOUSA, 9 Jan 45, sub: Official Recognition of House of Prostitution, file HD 024 ETO CS (Hawley Chron). Further information on civil affairs will be found in Chapter XVI of this volume.

[54] Hoff, ed., *Diseases Transmitted Through Contact,* p. 246.

[55] Surg, Ninth U.S. Army, Daily Journal, 30 Jan 45, p. 7, Shambora Papers, MHI.

forts of the latter to claim otherwise. Medics did not as a rule supply information directly to the police, but they turned their information on venereal contacts over to French health agencies, knowing that they would do so. Belgian authorities were similarly helpful in prevention and treatment, especially in the road and rail hub of Liege. Throughout the war, rates remained highest among base section troops, replacement commands, and in the Air Force units that continued to operate from the British Isles.[56]

But the most important developments in VD control during the war were in the area of treatment, not of prevention. Even as late as 1943 an uncomplicated case of gonorrhea could occupy a hospital bed for 30 days, while the treatment of syphilis remained a tedious six-month ordeal. While sulfa drugs improved the picture, sulfathiazole rapidly lost its effectiveness as resistant strains of the gonococcus developed. Then the surgeon general's Preventive Medicine Service learned that the new antibiotic, penicillin, had proved useful against sulfa-resistant gonorrhea. A large-scale study led to the adoption of penicillin treatment throughout the Army. The results were startling: The number of days needed to treat the average case of gonorrhea was reduced from 20 to 5, and many cases could be treated while the patient remained on duty status. Penicillin treatment of syphilis began in 1944. In the Ninth Army a VD center operated by the 95th Medical Gas Treatment Battalion returned 99.9 percent of its patients to duty within the army area, underlining the fact that reduced treatment time enabled line units to exploit forward holding facilities to prevent manpower loss.

The revolution in treatment gained in significance as the end of the war approached in the spring of 1945. Command support for VD control continued to vary from one organization tc another, with the First and Ninth Armies providing strong support for the control efforts of the 12th Army Group surgeon, while the Third Army manifested little interest in the problem. The impending end of the conflict meant that soldiers of the field forces would soon enjoy the same opportunities to find sex as the support troops and could be expected to take advantage of them in the same manner. But even as the postwar VD epidemic impended, the significance of the venereal diseases had been radically transformed by improved therapy to the point that gonorrhea, at least, had become an insignificant cause of ineffectiveness among the men of the European Theater.[57]

Apart from venereal disease, few illness afflicted the troops. Influenza failed to reappear in epidemic form; the incidence of primary atypical pneumonia remained low; meningococcal infections did not become widespread; and even the fatalities

[56] Medical History of the Ground Force Reinforcement Command, ETO, 23 October 1943–30 June 1945, file 319.1-2 (GFRC); Ltr, Hawley to Le Ministre, Ministere de la Sante Publique, 3 Mar 45, file HD 024 ETO CS (Hawley Chron).

[57] VD Control Branch, Preventive Medicine Service, OSG, WD, Annual Rpt, 1943, pp. 135–57; Memo, sub: Penicillin Treatment of VD, in Preventive Medicine Service, OSG, WD, Annual Rpt, 1945. Both in box 24, RG 112, NARA. See also Technical Bulletin MED 106, 11 Oct 44, sub: Penicillin Treatment of Syphilis, CMH.

among American troops caused by diphtheria apparently resulted mainly from the fact that the younger American doctors had never encountered the disease and, awaiting positive laboratory diagnosis, delayed too long before administering antitoxin. Careful screening of American soldiers helped to keep tuberculosis from becoming a significant problem, though liberated American POWs were an exception, their susceptibility apparently caused by exposure to the disease and by malnutrition while in the enemy's hands. Soldiers from the Mediterranean Theater brought not only malaria but also infectious hepatitis to the European Theater, spreading the disease to units new from the States and causing 12,509 cases between October 1944 and early May 1945. A few cases of typhoid and paratyphoid occurred, and units suffered occasional outbreaks of food poisoning. Diarrheal diseases, after reaching epidemic peaks in December 1944 and February 1945, were sharply reduced among the troops, perhaps by tighter water discipline in the forward zones. Frequently of obscure origin, this class of ailments caused about 45,000 hospital admissions in the European Theater throughout the war, but only about 5 deaths.

Overall, this was an extraordinary record for a combat zone. Undergirding the health of the troops was good nutrition. A new C-ration proved more palatable than the old; hot B-rations became commoner in the field; and fresh fruits and vegetables were often available, especially for hospital patients. Well fed, inoculated, fighting in the heartland of their civilization, American soldiers faced no significant peril of disease for which medical science lacked an answer.[58]

The last campaign was a showpiece for the ETO medical service, rather than a test. The innovations that appeared—the abandonment of fixed hospitals in forward areas; and the heavy, in some areas exclusive, dependence on air evacuation—indicated a willingness to learn and to improvise. But no severe test of the service occurred in the handling of American sick and wounded. The true test of the system came rather in the care of noncombatants of every type, and it was here that Army medics found their most poignant experiences, their worst failures, and some of their finest hours during the memorable spring of 1945.

[58] Larkey "Hist," ch. XVI, pp. 1–6; Army Service Forces Monthly Progress Rpt, sec. 7 (Health), 30 Apr 45, p. 12, file HD 700 (Health). See also Preventive Medicine Division, OofCSurg, HQ, ETOUSA, Semiannual Rpt, January-June 1945, Nutrition Branch sec., p. 2; Grodon "Hist", vol. 1, pt. 3, pp. 10 and 32; Surg, Ninth U.S. Army, Semiannual Rpt, sec. IV, p. 3, and sec. VI, p. 3. On the Third Army and venereal disease, see Surg, 12th Army Group, Hist, January-June 1945, p. 16. On hepatitis, see also Surg, Seventh U.S. Army, Semiannual Rpt, January-June 1945, Preventive Medicine sec., p. 1.

CHAPTER XVI

Victims of War

How were noncombatants to be cared for once the tide of battle had passed them by? Facing the prospect of fighting in many populated regions around the world, American policymakers from the early days of World War II were aware that some provision must be made for the governance of liberated peoples (civil affairs) and ultimately for that of conquered nations (military government). Yet Americans traditionally viewed civil rule by the military almost as a contradiction in terms, limited to extraordinary times—the aftermath of natural disaster or civil war. At first opposed, President Roosevelt, because he could see no other way, committed himself to a period of military rule in order to avoid having both a military commander and a civil governor at work in the same territory at the same time. "It is quite apparent," he remarked in 1943, "that if prompt results are to be obtained the Army will have to assume the initial burden." [1]

So much had long been clear to military planners. The Army embodied its basic policy in *Military Government,* Field Manual 27-5, and in early 1942 it established a school of military government at the University of Virginia, with public health experts as part of its faculty. Army policy made the commanding general of a theater of operations the "military governor of the occupied territory," his "supreme authority . . . limited only by the laws and customs of war." He was to select personnel to be charged with establishing a government that was "just, humane, and as mild as practicable." Their work included many medical responsibilities: to oversee sanitation; to control communicable diseases; to protect food, milk, and the water supply from contamination; to manage the hospital system; and to organize the health care professions. Under Army guidance the civilian health officers of states, provinces, counties, and cities were to continue their duties. Anyone who failed to obey the laws and regulations promulgated by the military government faced punishment by a military tribunal. [2]

Yet civil affairs and military government remained a concept, rather than a functioning part of the Army

[1] As quoted in Earl F. Ziemke, *The U.S. Army in the Occupation of Germany, 1944–1946,* Army Historical Series (Washington, D.C.: U.S. Army Center of Military History, 1975), p. 22.

[2] Basic Field Manual 27-5, *Military Government,* 30 Jul 40, pp. 4, 8, 44–45. The first class at the Charlottesville school met on 1 May 1942.

system. In any combat area military imperatives were likely to conflict with the care of civilians. The idea of a separate civil affairs organization was new to American military doctrine and formed no part of Army training, either in staff exercises or maneuvers. If it was to become a functioning aspect of the Army's activities, its practice had to be worked out in the field.

Civil Affairs

Civil affairs, in General Eisenhower's view, was critical "not merely from a humanitarian viewpoint, but to the success of our armies." [3] For most of the ETO's existence the American field armies operated within the borders of Allied nations. The civil affairs structure, weak in resources yet complex in organization, carried out its mission at all levels of command—from the division to the Supreme Headquarters. By 1944 SHAEF had a fully functioning Civil Affairs (G–5) Section. The latter's Public Health Branch bore responsibility for advising the Supreme Commander on the dangers to civilian health, for establishing theater-wide standards for remedial action, and for providing technical supervision to civil affairs units. Subordinate commands also had similar G–5 sections.

The umbrella organization for civil affairs field workers of all types was ETOUSA's European Civil Affairs Division (ECAD). The division was organized into four component regiments, and each of these units had its own surgeon. In September 1944 all ECAD medical personnel were gathered into the European Civil Affairs Medical Group. At this time the ECAD surgeon, Lt. Col. James P. Pappas, MC, a meticulous organizer who demanded superior work ("I shall not tolerate lackadaisical nor satisfactory nor even very satisfactory performance on anyone's part," he warned) also assumed command of the group.[4]

Civil affairs detachments were formed from the European Civil Affairs Division at the request of field force commanders. Their makeup depended on local needs, and many had public health responsibilities. While in the field, they served under the local commander, with policy guidance from his G–5 section. Small groups of experts, they worked as advisers to the liberated civilians, provided liaison with the military authorities, sought out medical supplies to aid local recovery, and did all in their power to reestablish sanitation and normal health discipline after the disruption of battle.[5]

Regulations and common sense both required civil affairs personnel to cooperate closely with the field force medics. In turn, many unit surgeons were sympathetic to the con-

[3] Dwight D. Eisenhower, *Crusade in Europe* (Garden City, N.Y.: Doubleday, 1948), p. 192.

[4] Pappas was a Regular Army medical officer whose work with the European Civil Affairs Division led to a diversified career in preventive medicine. Ultimately, he became the inspector general in the Office of the Surgeon General. Quoted words from Memo, Pappas to All Officers and EM, ECA Medical Group, 13 Mar 45, sub: ECA Medical Group Efficiency—Discipline—Morale, Corresp fldr, file 816541, box 59, RG 338/332, NARA.

[5] Ebbe Curtis Hoff, ed., *Civil Affairs/Military Government Public Health Activities,* Medical Department, United States Army in World War II (Washington, D.C.: Office of the Surgeon General, Department of the Army, 1976), p. 405–29.

cept of civil affairs, if only because the health of troops was closely linked to that of the people among whom they lived and fought. But sources of friction also existed. The theater chief surgeon did not set civil affairs policy, and yet unit surgeons, controlling most manpower and transport, were often called upon to aid at least the emergency care of civilians. Confusion, if not conflict, was systemic because civil affairs units had the mission but not the means to meet civilian needs and the field forces had the means but not the mission.

Despite a situation prolific of minor irritants, civil affairs personnel made many positive contributions to the Allied cause, from the beaches of Normandy to the borders of the Reich. The first physician with a civil affairs detachment came ashore on 14 June 1944 and, shortly afterward, began work in newly liberated Cherbourg. Here the detachment made contact with the French authorities and assisted in the repair of the water system. Finding medical supplies was an important duty. Civil affairs personnel broke down medical maintenance units, obtained captured supplies from German dumps, and made French stocks that had survived the Occupation available to the towns and refugee camps of Normandy. They also tracked down reports of communicable disease outbreaks and served as middlemen between the civil authorities and the military commanders.[6]

Problems were varied. Many civilians felt more than a little bitterness over the destruction of lives and property—beyond the demands of military necessity, many inhabitants of Normandy believed—and over the loss of often profitable arrangements by which local farmers had supplied German occupiers with food. Nonetheless, cooperation developed out of necessity. Within a few days after a town's liberation, refugees began to filter back. With homes wrecked, and often with heavy rains falling (the summer of 1944 was wet), French authorities and civil affairs personnel found shelter for the returnees in ruined buildings, which were often dangerous as well as cheerless lodgings because of German booby traps. Only limited quantities of Army food were needed because Normandy, a farming region, possessed resources of its own, even in the aftermath of battle. The end of fighting brought better health conditions. Venereal disease declined as the troops moved out, and outbreaks of diarrhea among the refugees ended as sanitation improved.[7]

As they worked, civil affairs officers came to appreciate their own good fortune in finding a farming region, rather than a populous industrial area, as the first place to put their classroom lessons into practice. The region produced much of its own food, and the people were sturdy and self-reliant. "Stolid, almost impossible to panic," the tough, durable Norman

[6] Thomas B. Turner and Glen W. McDonald, "Civil Health in Theaters of Operations," *The Military Surgeon* 96 (January 1945): 131–34.

[7] Rpt, G–5, SHAEF, 1 Jul 44, sub: Summary of CA Field Operations for Period Ending 30 Jun 44, file HD 014 (CA/Public Health, ETO-CA Branch, May 44–Mar 45); Study No. 35, G–5, USFET, sub: Report of General Board, USFET, on Displaced Persons, Refugees, and Recovered Allied Military Personnel, pp. 4–5, file HD 319.4

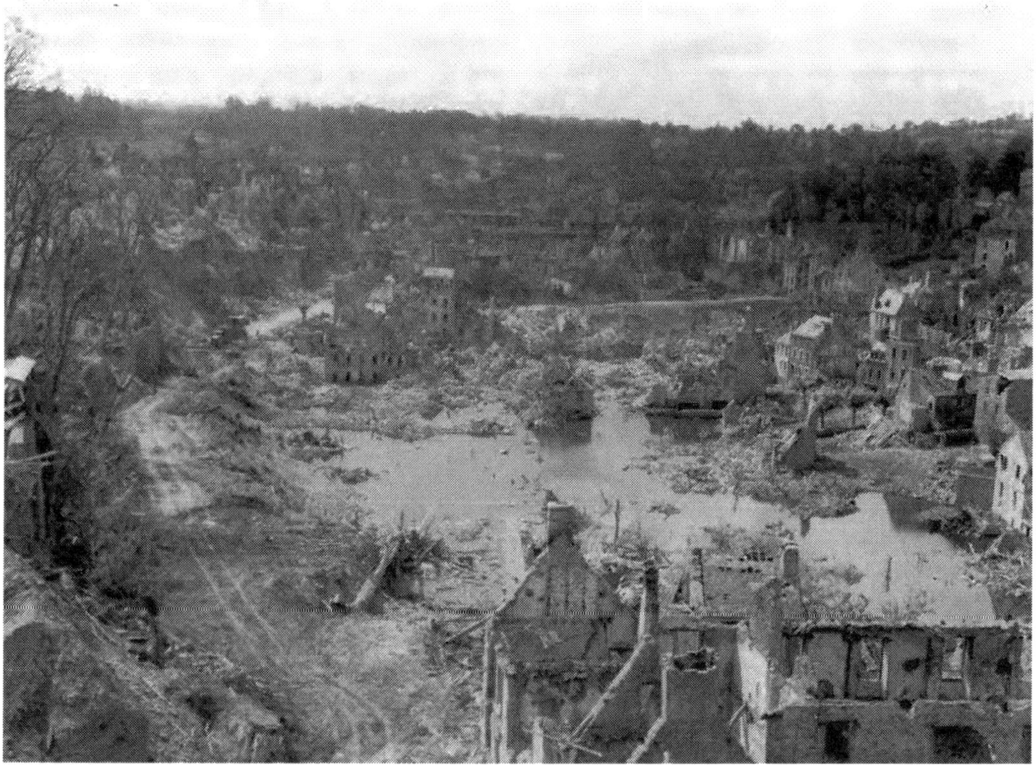

A JOB FOR CIVIL AFFAIRS: ST.-LO

peasants—even with their large proportion of children, women, and the aged—proved to be thoroughly "imbued with the will to live despite the catastrophe that [had] swept down upon them." [8]

Difficulties were greater in towns, where heavy bomb damage and the organizational confusion caused by the presence of multiple occupying units plagued efforts at reconstruction. In Le Havre an ECA detachment's public health officer was at work. But so were many others. An ECA regimental surgeon reported that not only the public health officer but his French counterpart, a military port surgeon, and the surgeon of the Channel Base Section were all attempting to do related and overlapping tasks and that none were talking to the others. Yet there was work in plenty for all of them. One section of the town had been totally demolished; thirty of the fifty-two local doctors had been bombed out of their offices, and three had been killed; a third of the water supply was nonpotable. The problem was coordination, and for this no comprehensive solution existed.[9]

[8] Surg, ECA Medical Group Annual Rpt, 1944, sec. 3, p. 11.

[9] Rpt to CO, 1st ECA Regiment, 30 Nov 44, sub: Assistance at Channel Base Section, Corresp fldr, file 816541, box 59, RG 338/332, NARA.

During the breakout and pursuit the number of people for whom civil affairs was responsible expanded with the size of the liberated area. Yet its medics seemingly kept abreast of civilian needs, if only because the bitter fighting of the Battle of Normandy was over. The major diseases were enteric infections—dysentery, diarrhea, and typhoid fever. Other widespread ills—venereal disease, diphtheria, tuberculosis, and scabies—reflected the conditions of the German occupation and the presence of both enemy and Allied armies. Lack of penicillin for combating venereal disease among civilians was a persistent difficulty. The wartime spread of diphtheria, caused by the lapse of vaccinations, was more easily met. Civil affairs personnel labored to stimulate programs of immunization, especially among children, using military supplies of toxoid until civilian laboratories could reopen and reestablish production.

Paris fell with little fighting. Alarming forecasts of mass hunger proved to be greatly exaggerated, though deficiencies were real enough and civil affairs officers dispatched 11,000 tons of food in truck convoys as an emergency measure. Shortages of fuel were serious notwithstanding the summer weather, for without fuel the city could not cook its food, pump its water, light its streets, or flush out its sewage. Yet Paris' own resources were great, and were quickly applied to its medical needs. The Pasteur Institute supplied serums, medical and surgical equipment was abundant, and trained personnel were numerous and sophisticated. Meanwhile, in southern France an ECA regiment accompanying the Seventh Army labored at Nice and Cannes, fighting a typhoid epidemic traceable to broken sewer lines. Despite the impact of war, however, the public health situation had begun to stabilize by autumn in both the cities and the rural towns of liberated France.[10]

While ECA detachments operated in localities affected by war, other civil affairs organizations offered advice to the governments of liberated nations as they sought to restore normal conditions. SHAEF established special missions to provide liaison between national governments and the Allied military authorities. Headed by an American or British officer, each mission had two medical officers plus a variety of specialists (venereologists, sanitary engineers, nutritionists), who were added as needed. The missions served under two headquarters: ETOUSA, for France and Luxembourg; and the 21 Army Group, for the conquered nations of northern Europe. However, the European Civil Affairs Division loaned the British twenty-four American experts—fourteen doctors and ten Sanitary Corps officers—to serve with Montgomery's headquarters.

Problems varied from nation to nation. Belgium requested consultants in nutrition, while France wanted experts in veterinary medicine and

[10] John W. Bailey, "An Outline Administrative History of Civil Affairs in the ETO" (hereafter cited as "Civil Affairs Hist"), p. 198, file 314.7-2; Rpt, Lt Col H. R. Hennessy, G-5, COMZ, 30 Dec 44, sub: Summary of Public Health, COMZ, ETO, box 1, H. R. Hennessy Papers, MHI; Harry L. Coles and Albert K. Weinberg, *Civil Affairs: Soldiers Become Governors*, United States Army in World War II (Washington, D.C.: Office of the Chief of Military History, Department of the Army, 1964), pp. 722 and 759-82; Surg, ECA Medical Group, Annual Rpt, 1944, sec. 3, p. 13.

narcotic drug control, among others. In all nations the missions determined from civilian authorities what medical supplies were needed and sought to obtain adequate quantities from military depots and other sources. They also recruited medical workers for refugee camps, investigated sanitary conditions, and monitored disease outbreaks. The commonest problems among civilians were those classic accompaniments of war, malnutrition and venereal disease, and both entailed policy recommendations to Allied governments as well as efforts to obtain supplies of food and medication. At the top as at the bottom, civil affairs medics proved an essential lubricant in the process of starting once more the paralyzed wheels of civil government health care. By September French public health departments had resumed operation in many areas, and officials had once again begun to collect communicable disease reports.[11]

To this point success keynoted the civil affairs story, for much good was accomplished with modest means. Yet organizational problems lingered. Contradictory directives emanated from ETOUSA and SHAEF. In late September ETOUSA attempted to clarify the chief surgeon's civil affairs responsibilities. Hawley was thenceforth to be responsible for the requisitioning, storage, and bulk issue of medical supplies for civilian use; for supervising public health and sanitation, as necessary, to safeguard the health of the military command; and for furnishing tactical advice and support to civil affairs personnel. Apparently, the distinction between military and civil affairs medicine was breaking down at the ETOUSA level. At the level of the field forces, however, unit surgeons continued to resent the civil affairs medics who operated in their commands, demanding their assistance but on occasion rejecting their advice.

For their part, civil affairs medical officers sometimes expressed foreboding over the inadequacy of their organization in view of the monumental tasks that lay ahead. "I feel," emphasized one high-ranking officer of the Public Health Branch, G-5, SHAEF, "that the Tables of Organization have been totally inadequate from the top to the bottom in our public health program. They have been inadequate in SHAEF and at every staff level below us." As the reconquest of Europe proceeded, men and supplies not only were spread thinner but encountered worse problems. In the late autumn severe fighting began again, and in December the Ardennes attack fell with full fury upon disordered regions, where recovery had only begun.[12]

The German eruption during one of Europe's coldest winters pushed hordes of suffering refugees and DPs into the region just behind the lines, already crowded with Allied troops. In front-line cities like Liege, bombing forced the homeless into underground air raid shelters that were potential incubators of epidemic louse-borne typhus. Food stores were lost; freezing weather impeded transport; military needs monopolized

[11] Hoff, ed., *Civil Affairs/Military Government*, pp. 427–29 and 452–67.

[12] Interv, OSG with Lt Col Leonard A. Scheele, USPHS, 8 Dec 44, file HD 000.71, CMH.

whatever vehicles still moved on rail or road; and the waterways were frozen. Some local officials, fearing German reprisals if recaptured, hastily decamped, and at least one military government detachment was overrun and captured.[13]

Public health efforts continued through the attack, though under great difficulties. In the hard-hit First Army area an ECA detachment surveyed the hospitals and moved injured civilians into facilities at Verviers and Liege or, when none were available, into private homes. Its public health officer drew up a sanitation plan, and military and civilian police strove to enforce it. When diphtheria broke out, the First Army provided antitoxin. Civilians gave critical assistance to the slender civil affairs cadres by helping to care for themselves; the local Red Cross provided evacuation, and some local doctors braved the battle to aid survivors. As the enemy withdrew, soldiers aided in reopening local hospitals, and the SHAEF mission turned over supplies of drugs, dressings, and ambulances to Belgian public health workers. But even as the battle ended, a new and unprecedented challenge loomed as the invasion of Germany impended.[14]

Military Government

American troops seized small areas of western Germany as early as September 1944. The first military government teams were at work in Aachen, "a fantastic, stinking heap" of snow-clad ruins, as the Ardennes offensive swept close by.[15] Widespread occupation of enemy territory, however, followed the collapse of the Bulge in January 1945. During February almost the entire Rhineland fell, and invasion of the German heartland followed in March. Hitherto the chief duty of civil affairs personnel had been that of advising and assisting friendly governments. Now it became that of helping to rule a conquered people.

Policy guidance for the effort was less than satisfactory. A handbook prepared by SHAEF was rejected by President Roosevelt as too lenient. Guided by the ideas of Secretary of the Treasury Henry J. Morganthau, Jr., the Joint Chiefs of Staff determined to treat Germany as a conquered, not a liberated, territory; not to rehabilitate its economy, except as required by military necessity; and not to provide any relief to its people, except to prevent disease or disorder. Immediately following the conquest of German soil, the Supreme Commander was to become responsible for establishing military government. He was to delegate his power to army group commanders, and so on down the line; in short, military units were to administer the areas they occupied. At some time following the surrender, power was to pass to a control commission representing the United States, Great Britain, and the U.S.S.R. Meanwhile, order had to be reestab-

[13] Hoff, ed., *Civil Affairs/Military Government*, p. 451; Study No. 35, G–5, USFET, Report of General Board on Displaced Persons, Refugees, and Recovered Allied Military Personnel, p. 9, file HD 319.4.

[14] Hoff, ed., *Civil Affairs/Military Government*, pp. 451–52.

[15] Robert Wolfe, ed., *Americans as Proconsuls: United States Military Government in Germany and Japan, 1944–1952* (Carbondale, Ill.: Southern Illinois University Press, 1977), p. 56.

lished, the will of the Allies imposed, Naziism eliminated, war criminals apprehended, and a civil administration free of Nazi taint set up to work under military direction. Contacts, other than necessary official ones, between Americans and Germans were forbidden, to the end that aloof and formally correct behavior might make the conquered sensible of the detestation in which they were held by all decent peoples.[16]

Under these general provisions, Nazi party members and ardent sympathizers were to be removed from public health organizations. Medical care would be extended to civilians to the extent necessary to control communicable disease and to prevent its spread across German boundaries. As far as possible, German supplies were to be used, and German needs to be met only after the wants of the occupiers and DPs had been satisfied. While austere, this prescription was by no means barbarous, and in some respects worked fairly well; in others, it proved highly unrealistic, as medcial personnel soon discovered. According to Deputy Military Governor General Lucius D. Clay, the planners of American policy had led a "cloistered and academic life" and none had gotten out into the "mud." But now theory had to be tested against German realities.[17]

But who was to direct medical policy during this first phase of the Occupation, when field armies still fought on German soil? Already inadequate for their task, the ECA regiments were divided—two to Germany, one to Belgium, and one to France. The tasks in Germany proved to be familiar ones, for the distinction between conquered and liberated territory, which seemed so clear to planners in London and Paris, amounted to much less on the ground. As before, public health personnel provided emergency care to sick and wounded civilians, restored sanitation, tried to rebuild civilian medical services, arranged for the transport and distribution of medical supplies, cared for DPs and refugees, and fought against real and threatened epidemics.

German problems differed, however, in their magnitude, their political dimension, and their entanglement with the policies of multiple occupying powers. Local governments were full of Nazis, and purges deprived them of their most experienced workers at the time when the collapse of the central government made their functions more than ever important. Similarly, the German health professions had never had more urgent tasks, but all, especially the medical profession, were tainted with Naziism. Western Germany was large and contained heavily industrialized areas, where the infrastructure of power, water, and sewage disposal lines was forbiddingly complex, hard to com-

[16] Directive, G5, HQ, 12th Army Group, sub: Military Government of Germany Prior To Defeat or Surrender, in Rpt No. 33, General Board, USFET, sub: Procedures Followed by Civil Affairs and Military Government in the Restoration, Reorganization and Supervision of Indigenous Civil Administration, p. 21.

[17] Quotation from John Gimbel, *The American Occupation of Germany: Politics and the Military, 1945–1949* (Stanford, Calif.: Stanford University, 1968), p. 7. See also HQ, SHAEF, Handbook for Military Government in Germany, 15 Sep 44, paras. 396–430; Ziemke, *Occupation of Germany*, pp. 31–33 and 89–90; Hoff, ed., *Civil Affairs/Military Government*, pp. 468–69.

prehend and to repair. As a whole, the region conquered by the Western Allies was a food-deficit area, accustomed to draw sustenance from the East, now devastated by war and occupied by the Russians.

To meet such unprecedented difficulties, SHAEF was obliged to turn to the field forces because they alone had the necessary medical troops, trucks, and supplies. The change came quickly in the early spring of 1945. Apparently the immediate cause was pressure form the field force surgeons, notably Colonel Gorby of the 12th Army Group and his preventive medicine officer, Col. Tom F. Whayne, MC. These two persuaded General Kenner, already convinced by his own observation that civil affairs could not meet its new responsibilities, to seek new directives from the Supreme Commander. In orders issued on 12 and 14 April SHAEF determined that "partial ECLIPSE conditions" existed and concluded that civilian health must henceforth be a command responsibility.[18]

Field army surgeons now took direct supervision and control of ECAD medical personnel. The responsibility for achieving results also passed to the field forces, for each commander became responsible for plans, policies, and supervision of public health work in his area within the existing framework of policy. This departure was and remained controversial. Some G–5 officers were bitter, for they were well aware of the many essential tasks still performed by trained military government personnel. They still provided guidance and advice, worked with the field forces in a variety of jobs, investigated reports of disease outbreaks, and aided in medical supply. Through G–5, SHAEF, they retained a direct wire to the Supreme Commander and through European Headquarters, United States of America Typhus Commission, a direct connection to the organization that provided most of the vaccine and other antityphus supplies used in the theater. Unworthy gloating by some of those who had now taken charge did nothing to salve their feelings. Hawley himself averred that "the medical service of Civil Affairs broke down completely at the first small problems," perhaps the only time that the difficulties of conquered Germany were described as small.[19]

Implementation of the new arrangement varied in detail from one headquarters to another. In the 12th Army Group, discussion between Colonel Gorby and the G–5, Brig. Gen. Cornelius E. Ryan, led to an amicable agreement. On 26 April 12th Army Group G–5 medical officers

[18] Directive, HQ, SHAEF, to CGs, 6th and 12th Army Groups, and HQ, 21 Army Group and COMZ, ETO, 14 Apr 45, sub: Public Health Functions in Occupied German Territory, file G–5/OMGUS Records, PHB/PWB, box 471, RG 260, NARA.

[19] Quoted words from Ltr, Hawley to TSG, 20 Apr 45, file HD 024 ETO O/CS (Hawley-SGO Corresp). See also Ltr, Draper to "Steve" [Brig Gen James S. Simmons, Chief, Preventive Medicine Service, OSG, WD], 9 Apr 45; Rpt, Col Philip R. Beckford, Surg, 99th Infantry Division, to Chief, Public Health and Welfare Branch, OMGUS, 3 May 46, sub: Experiences in and Impressions of Military Government Public Health Operations in Germany, May 1945 to May 1946; 12th Army Group Report of Operations, vol. XIII (Medical Section), pp. 238 and 240; Hoff, ed., *Civil Affairs/Military Government*, pp. 472–81.

shifted over to Gorby's medical section, and on 1 May a Public Health Branch was established under Colonel Whayne. In the Ninth Army active management of public health passed to the corps surgeons, and the corps boundaries became the basic geographical limits of control. The Ninth Army surgeon's Operations Branch supervised public health, and his preventive medicine staff submitted communicable disease reports. In the Third Army Patton's surgeon assumed direct control over all public health personnel attached to the army; he established a public health subsection in his own office and organized three public health teams, attaching one to each corps. Each team consisted of one medical officer, one Sanitary Corps officer, three Army nurses, and two drivers with vehicles. Under operational control of the corps surgeons, the teams organized and supervised health work at DP camps, found German health workers to assist, advised the corps on civil public health problems, and aided lower echelons down to regimental level in meeting day-to-day crises.

The division of responsibility had ended, and the medical resources of the field forces, relieved from many customary duties by rapidly falling casualty rates, became available to aid in the care of noncombatants. For all the ill feeling it had caused, the change was right and timely. Even as the reorganization took place, field forces and military government personnel alike were meeting major challenges posed by epidemic disease among liberated captives within the Reich.

The Typhus Epidemic

For centuries, epidemic louse-borne typhus had been a classic disease of disorderly times. Caused by rickettsiae—pathogenic organisms intermediate in size between bacteria and viruses—typhus was typically a disease of winter, when people seldom bathed or removed their clothing. Anything that made cleanliness more difficult, caused crowding, or increased privation might contribute to an outbreak. Hence its ancient association with war. Often victims infected themselves by scratching louse bites, rubbing the feces of the insects into the abrasions in their skin. Rickettsiae in dry louse feces carried on the skin or hair of others might also be inhaled. The course of the disease featured high fever; a rash on the body; and, in severe cases, delirium, stupor, and death. Prevention was difficult, requiring elaborate machinery to bathe large numbers of people and to steam their clothing. During and after World War I the disease had caused millions of deaths in eastern Europe and Russia.

The American government launched the fight against typhus early in the war, establishing the United States of America Typhus Commission in 1942 and staffing it with medical officers drawn from the Army, Navy, and Public Health Services. Prevention must be the key, for the disease could not be effectively treated with any existing drug. Experimental work by the commission, and especially by the Rockefeller Foundation in North Africa, established a new method of controlling the disease by dusting fully clothed people with an insecticide, DDT, whose lethality and staying power had recently been proven in Department of Agriculture laboratories. A crucial test of the method came during a major outbreak in Naples during the winter of 1943–44. Originating among refugees huddled in caves and crowded tenements, the epidemic threatened wholesale loss of life. The commission organized a campaign, with the assistance of the Rockefeller Foundation and the military occupation authorities, that applied control measures to the whole population of Naples. The outbreak was halted in midwinter and in the midst of war—an extraordinary episode in the history of preventive medicine. Now, however, a new and more severe test loomed in Germany, for conditions there, as much as any that history records, favored the spread of typhus.[20]

Attacking prisoners and laborers from the endemic regions of eastern Europe, the disease had increased steadily in Germany from 1939 on. Some 2,700 cases were reported to the Nazi government in 1942 and 3,300 the following year. Though typhus struck German soldiers on the Eastern Front, and spread widely among concentration camp inmates, as long as the Reich held together normal control measures sufficed to keep incidence to a relatively low level. In 1944, however, failure of the system for reporting typhus foreshadowed a coming debacle, as the once excellent public health system buckled under the pressures of war. Failing transport meant malnourishment among military and civilians alike—and typhus had always been a disease especially dangerous to the ill-fed. As the final collapse began, louse-infested slave laborers, many of whom were already infected, escaped from their pens and took to the roads. In cities devastated by bombing, hungry people huddled for warmth in cellars and tunnels or abandoned their homes to become refugees. "Here were the Four Horsemen, riding abreast, on the move," wrote Lt. Col. Sanford V. Larkey, chief of Hawley's Historical Division, "and the third [pestilence] was in the lead." [21]

The Allies first met typhus in the Rhineland, the part of Germany, shaped like a mutton bone, that lies west of the river. "The Rhineland in these days of March 1945," wrote Colonel Larkey, "could scarcely be believed by those who saw it—it cannot be appreciated by those who did not. It was [the] Wild West, [the] hordes of Genghis Khan, the Klondike Gold Rush and Napoleon's retreat from Moscow all rolled up into one." The region seethed with people wandering this way and that, heading for home or simply seeking food and shelter. Roving bands moved mostly on foot, pulling carts loaded with their belongings. DPs gathered in

[20] Ebbe Curtis Hoff, ed., *Communicable Diseases: Arthropodborne Diseases Other Than Malaria*, Medical Department, United States Army in World War II (Washington, D.C.: Office of the Surgeon General, Department of the Army, 1964), pp. 176–94; Sir Arthur Hurst, *Medical Diseases of War* (Baltimore: Williams & Wilkins, 1944), pp. 235–60; Wiltse, *Mediterranean*, pp. 362–65; Charles M. Wheeler, "Control of Typhus in Italy, 1943–1944, by Use of DDT," *American Journal of Public Health* 36 (February 1946): 119–29.

[21] Quoted words from Larkey "Hist," ch. 14, p. 56. See also Hoff, ed., *Arthropodborne Diseases Other Than Malaria*, p. 233.

great camps, sometimes 15,000 or more together, building little fires to warm themselves and cook their food.[22]

In early March a party of Italian laborers trekking home from a camp in Holland fell into the hands of the Ninth Army. Four who were sick were turned over to the 91st Evacuation Hospital and later transferred to a civilian maternity hospital in Aachen. Here, a First Army medical officer spotted them, made a quick diagnosis of typhoid or typhus, sent the men to a local contagious disease hospital, and forwarded sera to the 10th Medical Laboratory. The laboratory confirmed that all four—now in convalescence and out of personal danger—had typhus.[23]

A few more cases turned up in Aachen, all among DPs who had entered the city when already ill. But on 5 March Ninth Army troops encountered more in Moenchen-Gladbach, 30 miles to the northeast. A Dutch laborer, misdiagnosed as a diphtheria victim, died after passing on his real illness to the staff and patients at the local hospital. In turn, he may have brought the disease from Neuss, a city on the Rhine across from industrial Duesseldorf, where it had been introduced the preceding November by Russians working for the Nazi labor office, Organization Todt. In Moenchen-Gladbach the Americans counted 183 cases among the heavy concentrations of foreign labor brought by the Germans to work on the defenses of the West Wall. Suspicions that the disease might still be active in Neuss were confirmed when an officer looking for hospital space found 21 more cases at the city hospital, where their illness had been misdiagnosed as paratyphoid. Typhus then spread rapidly to the hospital staff.

General Hawley, learning of the outbreak, sent two officers to the Ninth Army to guide typhus control, while a representative of the United States of America Typhus Commission was attached to the First Army. The system of military government public health teams proved useful in meeting the typhus threat; doctors did on-the-spot examinations of suspect cases, and team members dusted and isolated contacts of the victims. Ninth Army medical officers, aided by German doctors and police, sought to isolate the centers of infection by mass dusting and selective vaccination. Meanwhile, the First Army discovered serious conditions in Cologne. Here public health officers carried out a typhus survey and found 65 cases scattered throughout the bomb-wrecked city in air raid shelters, prisons, and hospitals. Most were DPs or former inmates of a Gestapo prison; the remainder were German civilians. Members of the local police, in conveying prisoners to the Buchenwald Concentration Camp, had become infected; 20 fell ill. By early March a total of 120 cases had developed, 35 of whom died.[24]

---

[22] Quoted words from Larkey "Hist," ch. 14, p. 56. See also ibid., p. 55; Rpt, Military Government Detachment E1-H2, Co H, 2d ECA Regiment, to CSurg, HQ, ETOUSA, 28 May 45, sub: Typhus Epidemic, Koln, Germany, 1945.

[23] Preventive Medicine Division, OofCSurg, HQ, ETOUSA, Semiannual Rpt, January-June 1945, pp. 5-7.

[24] Hoff, ed., *Arthropodborne Diseases Other Than Malaria*, pp. 242-43.

DIAGRAM 6—DDT DUSTING PROCEDURE

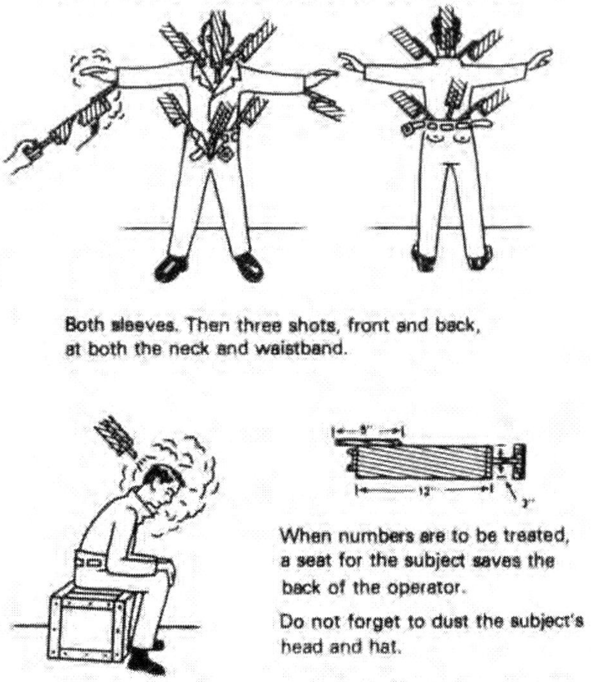

Source: Adapted by authors from Hoff, ed., *Arthropodborne Diseases Other Than Malaria*, p. 218.

The Americans cleaned out the Gestapo prison, moving the sick to hospitals and dusting and immunizing the healthy former inmates *(Diagram 6)*. German civilians were organized into teams to assist. Spot checks on the streets of Cologne showed that typhus was commoner among laborers and prisoners simply because they were far more likely than German civilians to be infested with lice. Again and again, the spread of the disease proved to be directly caused by the large drifting population. A party of Ukrainian laborers left Cologne early in March and stopped for two days in the town of Hermuelheim, sleeping in a small air raid shelter. On 24 March thirty residents who shared the shelter came down with the disease. Hurriedly, the military government teams dusted the entire town and immunized those who had used the shelter.

Other outbreaks flared in the Moselle region and the Palatinate, only to be stamped out by similar quick action. Reports of new cases declined rapidly during April and May and vanished during June. About 700 cases had been spotted in all. By the first week of summer the Rhineland was substantially free of the disease. Two-thirds of the cases occurred among DPs, a group only one-tenth the size of the German population. But because previous infections had served to create some degree of immunity, the DPs who became sick were more than ten times as likely to survive as infected Germans (3 percent mortality as against 35 percent).[25]

For the result, credit went to DDT, the accidents of battle, and the reorganized medical service. The Ardennes battle had delayed the eruption of the Allied armies until the end of winter, allowing the Reich to maintain some measure of control through the season when typhus might have been most devastating. When the Rhineland fell, Americans were ready to take charge. Adequate personnel, guided by experts and employing the technique of isolating contacts, mass dusting, and selective immunization, had knocked out the epidemic. Only two Americans caught typhus. Both were medical officers engaged in control work, and their cases were mild.

As the military government took hold, orders were issued to keep DPs in their camps pending repatriation to their own countries. The roads emptied, except for necessary military and civilian traffic, and the turmoil of the late winter and early spring came to an end. The Allies now turned the Rhine itself into a barrier against the reintroduction of typhus. The danger that the disease might spread westward, created by the first crossing at Remagen on 7 March, caused the chief surgeon's office to seek a verbal agreement with the First and Ninth Armies to prohibit movement of civilians across the river. On the twentieth the armies established a cordon sanitaire from the Swiss border to the North Sea along the east bank of the Rhine and its distributary, the Waal. All who crossed from east to west, except Allied military personnel, were dusted with DDT. Anyone showing symptoms was sent at once to U.S. Army medical installations. Shortly afterward, Brig. Gen. Leon A. Fox, field director of the Typhus Commission, met with representatives of ETOUSA and the 12th Army Group at Hawley's office in Paris to formalize the policy, and a SHAEF directive followed on 31 March. Hundreds of thousands of refugee Rhinelanders returning from the inner Reich were deloused at ports of entry established in Oberkassel, Wiesbaden, Mannheim, and Wesel. POWs were deloused in prison enclosures, and sometimes issued dust guns and taught to delouse their comrades. But even as these measures took shape, medical personnel knew that a new test would come to the east of the river.[26]

Uncovering the Reich

"It was France all over again," wrote an American medic in April 1945, "save that this time the end was in sight. Across the Rhine were the famous autobahns . . . , speed came back to travel, and distances were not so important anymore." American forces liberated Allied soldiers who had endured anything from days to years as POWs. Not surprisingly, most were in poor condition. The Germans had moved prisoners about on forced marches, trying to prevent them from falling into Allied hands; those who were sick or injured they

[25] Essential Technical Medical Data, HQ, ETOUSA, April 1945, pp. 3–4.

[26] Preventive Medicine Division, OofCSurg, HQ, ETOUSA, Semiannual Rpt, January–June 1945, pp. 28–29; Ltr, HQ, ETOUSA, to CGs, Section Cdrs, and COs, 12 Apr 45, sub: Establishment of a "Cordon Sanitaire," file 383.7 (DPs: General Policies and Procedures).

left behind, to be overtaken by the invaders and to become a burden upon them. In either case, a new medical task fell to American field units and to ADSEC and COMZ hospitals: Wounded, ill, or hungry, the RAMPs required quick attention.[27]

What nearly all had in common was malnutrition. But differences were marked between Westerners and east Europeans. Both the Germans and their own nations had treated the two groups quite differently. Western countries had attempted to support their soldiers in enemy hands, manifesting interest in their welfare and sending them great quantities of supplies through the Red Cross. The Soviet Union, on the other hand, had not signed the Geneva accords; disowned its prisoners; and, until the end of the war, showed no concern for their fate. Poles, Serbs, and many other captives had no spokesman at all, for their nations had disappeared before the Nazi invaders.

The experiences of American POWs were complex and contradictory. Within the camps poor and inadequate food was a perennial problem, perhaps the worst that prisoners faced. Moreover, the ration declined steadily from the fall of 1944, as air strikes disrupted German transport. Red Cross packages provided an essential supplement (supposedly 1,000–2,000 calories a day), but delivery was irregular and became less reliable as the ration declined, for the same cause. Sanitary conditions varied greatly from camp to camp, but they were generally deficient and, in combination with overcrowding and an erratic diet, produced much sickness. Medical treatment usually conformed to Geneva Convention norms; the less serious cases were treated in camp by Allied medics, the more serious in well-equipped German hospitals. But generalization is difficult in the face of variations so great that a prisoner's life, as well as his comfort, might depend on whether he was sent to the "remarkably well equipped" Stalag II–B or to the "notorious Stalag IX–B," where "one needle holder, one pair of forceps, one pair of scissors, and a spool of black cotton thread" were said to represent all the surgical equipment available. Overall, however, American prisoners did well in German camps; only about one-half of 1 percent died.[28]

A report by three army doctors, repatriated in September 1944, provided a glimpse of life in an *Oflag* (officers camp) in the Polish Corridor. Red Cross and YMCA packages arrived regularly. In consequence, Americans could buy delicacies on the black market with cigarettes, trading with Polish laborers in the camps or through friendly guards. "The prisoner of war," reported Capt. H. J. Weintraub, MC, "is the richest man in Germany." Though buildings were ill-heated, clothing was old and poor, and medicine was in short supply, Americans were constantly reminded of their relatively prosperous lot by

[27] Quoted words from 110th Evacuation Hospital Semiannual Rpt, January–June 1945, pp. 5–6. See also Surg, Third U.S. Army, Semiannual Rpt, January–June 1945, p. 35.

[28] David A. Foy, *For the War Is Over: American Prisoners of War in Nazi Germany* (New York: Stein and Day, 1984), pp. 114–15. See also pp. 17–81. By comparison, about 38 percent died in Japanese prison camps.

observing their fellow prisoners. The British were worse off in their camps; the French and Poles fared miserably; and "horrible conditions" existed among the Russians, caused by starvation, tuberculosis, and typhus. When Russians were sent to the American camp as hospital workers, the doctors put the worst cases to bed, ignoring German orders to make them work.[29]

Beginning with the Ardennes, however, treatment of American prisoners declined and soon approximated that endured by the Russians for many years. The reason lay not in any change of policy, but in the advanced state of disintegration of the German Army and nation. Americans captured in the Bulge were in poor condition when retaken. "Many," noted a hospital report, "were nothing more than wraiths of skin and bone, too weary to rise from their cots, and too emaciated to be able to eat a solid meal." Ceaseless marching without sufficient food or rest was the basic cause. "We marched, starved, froze, scratched lice, suffered from sickness and . . . marched some more," recalled one American. "We lived in fields, slept in barns or fields, and dodged aerial strafings. We covered 600 miles in 87 days, and I had joined the Air Force so I wouldn't have to walk." [30]

As prisoners of a retreating army, they had also been subjected to random brutality by individual guards or officers. At Heppenheim the Seventh Army overran a German camp for Allied prisoners, where 283 American patients were found in "terrible condition due to brutal treatment rendered by a German Major, Medical Corps, who admitted his hate for Americans." After a Good Friday visit by General Devers, the 6th Army Group commander, the men were quickly transferred to general hospitals. In custody, the German medical officer committed suicide.[31]

Initially, policy emphasized holding all RAMPs in place, as long as military operations continued. Responsibility fell upon the American and British medical services, but other Allied nations were encouraged to provide medical assistance, to the extent possible, and to evacuate their compatriots "expeditiously" in order to relieve the two principal western Allies to the burden. Because no Russian or Yugoslav hospitals existed, their RAMPs were cared for in German facilities. Russians were retained in the western zones of Germany, pending the junction of American and British forces with the Soviet armies. By international agreement the Russians were separated from others, granted special privileges, and placed in camps where soldiers and civilians were mixed together.[32]

[29] Quoted words from Interv, ETO with Capt H. J. Weintraub, 30 Sep 44, file 383.6 (Intervs, Repatriated POWs) ETO. See also W. Paul Havens, Jr., ed., *Infectious Diseases*, Medical Department, United States Army in World War II (Washington, D.C.: Office of the Surgeon General, Department of the Army, 1963), pp. 390–92; Larkey "Hist," ch. 14, p. 15; Havens, ed., *Medical Consultants*, pp. 452–55.

[30] First quotation from 110th Evacuation Hospital Semiannual Rpt, January–June 1945, p. 5. Second and third quotations from Foy, *For You the War Is Over*, p. 144.

[31] Surg, Seventh U.S. Army, Semiannual Rpt, January–June 1945, p. 7.

[32] Admin Memo No. 48, HQ, SHAEF, 26 Feb 45, sub: Hospitalization and Evacuation of RAMPs, in Book II, Planning Branch, Operations Division, OofCSurg, HQ, ETOUSA, 1945, file 383.6 (ETO); ADSEC Hist, p. 158; Historical Division, European

Continued

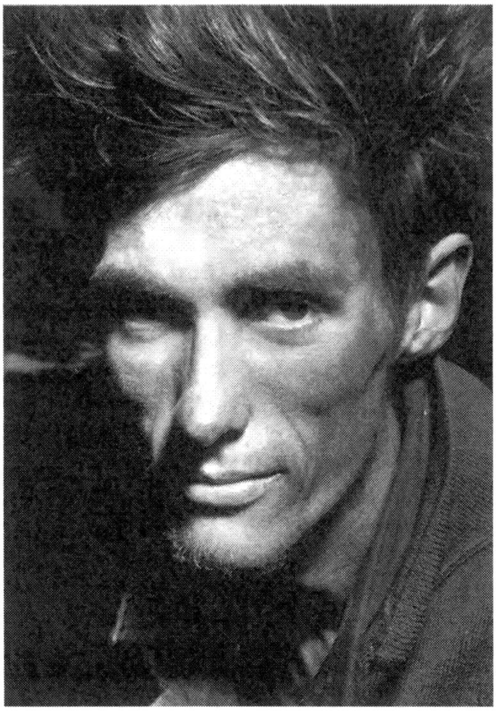

MALNOURISHED AMERICAN RAMP

In March 1945, however, a staff conference in the Office of the Assistant Chief of Staff, G–4, ETOUSA, modified the policy by providing for quick evacuation of British and American RAMPs. A system of "buffer camps" was set up in Belgium and France—at Liege, Epinal, Stenay, Le Havre, and Rouen—and at Bournemouth, England, to receive 60,000 to 70,000 men. For Americans, Camp Lucky Strike in the Normandy Base Section near Rouen became the largest reception center. Here the 77th Field Hospital opened on 8 April, with an initial capacity of 350 beds. Patients arrived in such numbers, however, that the 306th General Hospital moved in to care for convalescents—an additional 1,000 beds. Of the first 12,000 RAMPs to arrive at Camp Lucky Strike, 18 percent required hospitalization. As usual, malnutrition, with its many complications, was the root cause.

Some problems developed in handling these cases. A newspaper report alleging intolerable conditions at the camp brought General Eisenhower and five visiting U.S. senators on an inspection trip. Complaints among the physically fit centered on their urgent desire to go home. Some men were dissatisfied with the food, particularly the bland diet served to new arrivals without salt or seasoning. The problem with diet reflected the lack of knowledge among well-fed Americans of how to handle starvation victims. Earlier, the Red Cross and the post exchanges, with misguided kindness, had plied RAMPs with candies and other food their depleted systems were unable to handle. Reacting to the bad results, doctors at Camp Lucky Strike enforced small though frequent feedings of food that seemed tasteless to men whose dreams, for many months, had featured rich and heavy meals. Medical personnel also may have exaggerated the condition of their charges. Despite the long lapse, their digestive processes revived with use. Men ate in four successive messes, each presenting a more elaborate menu; they took between-meal feedings of cocoa and eggnog and swallowed multivitamins with their food. A daily intake of some 5,000 calories brought a rapid gain in weight, while enteric symp-

Command, "RAMPs: The Recovery and Repatriation of Liberated Prisoners of War," 1947, pp. 38–74, Ms. no. 8-3.1 CA 8, CMH.

toms disappeared under the regimen. The high-powered inspection team, finding no basis for the charges, departed satisfied.[33]

By May the treatment of RAMPs had become less pressing. The malnourished had been fed; the sick had either recovered or died. Even in the last phase of the story the Russians faced the hardest fate, for upon repatriation to their own country the prison camps of the *Gulag* apparently received not only collaborators who had served the enemy but also soldiers and laborers merely suspected of collaboration. For the ETO medical service, however, the emphasis was shifting noticeably. In the summer of 1945 the Third Army operated 237 hospitals: 3 for RAMPS; 13 for DPs; and the rest for German POWs, who by then constituted the main burden of care.[34]

The POWs

German soldiers had been taken prisoner in increasing numbers since the first days of the invasion, but the collapse of the Ruhr pocket in April 1945 signaled a new avalanche: 325,000, in place of an anticipated 150,000. This was, however, only a downpayment on the vast tactical triumph to come. In the same month the First Army took 389,000 prisoners; the Third Army, 237,000; and the Ninth Army, 324,000. By 2 June 1945 more than 3 million prisoners were in American hands; nine days later a SHAEF report placed the total at more than 4 million. What was to be done with a whole captured army? [35]

Despite good intentions, years of planning for the assault on Europe had not provided an answer. The obligations of the United States toward enemy prisoners were defined in the Geneva accords of 1929 and embodied in the 1940 field manual *Rules of Land Warfare.* Both enjoined humane treatment of POWs, and provided for their medical care. ETOUSA consigned its POWs to the Services of Supply, with actual responsibility resting upon the theater provost marshal. He, in turn, adopted high-minded rules for the medical care of prisoners. They were to receive a physical examination upon their arrival in camp; to be immunized; and, when ill, to be cared for on the same basis as American troops. Rigorous sanitary measures also were prescribed to prevent the spread of disease in POW camps.[36]

---

[33] MFR, Planning Branch, Operations Division, OofCSurg, HQ, ETOUSA, 16 Mar 45, sub: Handling of RAMPs, in Book I, Planning Branch, Operations Division, OofCSurg, HQ, ETOUSA, 1944–45, file 383.6 (ETO); MFR, Operations Division, OofCSurg, HQ, ETOUSA, 9 Apr 45, sub: Policy Pertaining to Evacuation of Allied Prisoners of War, file 383.6; Eisenhower, *Crusade in Europe*, pp. 420–21; Bayne-Jones Interv, 1966, vol. 4 p. 773, NLM; Essential Technical Medical Data, HQ, ETOUSA, April 1945, apps. 22–29.

[34] 298th General Hospital Annual Rpt, 1945, pp. 118 and 255; Surg, Third U.S. Army, Semiannual Rpt, July–December 1945. See also Coles and Weinberg, *Civil Affairs*, pp. 854–55.

[35] Eisenhower, *Crusade in Europe*, p. 406; OofTPM, HQ, ETOUSA, Weekly PW Status Rpt, 2 Jan 45, file 383.6, box 316, RG 112, NARA; Rpt, G–1, SHAEF, 11 Jun 45, sub: Totals on Prisoners of War Taken and Disarmed Enemy Forces Rounded Up, file 383.6/1–3, box 26, RG 331, NARA.

[36] Field Manual 27–10, *Rules of Land Warfare*, 1940; Technical Manual 19–500, *Prisoners of War*, 5 Oct 44, pp. 1–3; Ltr, HQ, SOS, ETOUSA, to Provost Marshal, SOS, and Cdr, SOS, 26 Nov 42, file 383.6 (POW Hospitalization, 1942–44); in same file, Regulations Governing Prisoners of War, OofTPM, HQ, ETOUSA, 10 Jul 43.

Before D-Day Axis prisoners were transported to remote rear areas, including Great Britain and the United States, where their treatment was in general excellent. Similarly, the first prisoners taken after the invasion were shipped back across the Channel. But when large numbers began to fall under the Army's control during the breakout and pursuit, POW camps were set up on the Continent, some in the very buildings earlier used by the Germans to house Allied prisoners. Military police units ran the camps, and provisional POW overhead detachments saw to the prisoners' medical needs, which were usually great. POWs arrived in masses, many ill or injured in battle. Camp construction went slowly, and overcrowding, insufficient shelter, and cold rations were the rule. For these camps in liberated France, the coming of the year 1945 at first meant vastly improved conditions of life, while establishment of the POW hospital center near Cherbourg offered expert treatment for those needing medical or surgical care.[37]

Yet some basic problems were not addressed. Field forces often stripped POWs of their personal equipment, including tents and even mess gear, apparently in order to cram the maximum number into the available transport. Because the camps often had no equipment to issue, many prisoners lived without shelter and ate canned rations with sticks for spoons. Enteric and respiratory illnesses followed. Major lacks existed in the medical support system through the early stages of capture, detention, and transport to the rear. Neither the military police battalion, the escort guard company, nor the POW processing company had organic medical elements. Added to the confusion and disorder of war, and the battered state of many railways, the lack of professional advice to commanders helped to make for some rough journeys. Prison trains rolled for days without adequate provisions for water, sanitation, rest, or even ventilation, and their arrival in the rear threw new waves of sick and exhausted men upon the prison camps.[38]

The masses who surrendered in the spring of 1945 presented a new and stunning challenge. ETOUSA planners had failed either to foresee the dimensions of an unconditional surrender or to allow for the disintegration of the German Army that accompanied it. Treatment of German prisoners by Americans mirrored the experience of Americans in enemy hands: Those captured last suffered most. Improvisation became the rule in Germany and resulted in the creation of POW transient enclosures—institutions that did no credit

[37] On POW camp conditions, see 2029th PWOD Annual Rpt, 1944, pp. 2–3, and Semiannual Rpt, January–June 1945, pp. 7–8. See also 2021st PWOD Annual Rpt, 1944, p. 5; 2018th PWOD Periodic Rpt, April–December 1944, p. 3; 6832d PWOD Periodic Rpt, 25 Aug 44–30 Jun 45, pp. 2–3; and 2024th PWOD Semiannual Rpt, January–June 1945, p. 2. All in box 383, RG 112, NARA. Information on POW general hospitals will be found in file 319.1–2, box 440, RG 112, NARA.

[38] For the makeup of military police formations, see T/O&E 19–35 (August 1943), T/O&Es 19–47, 19–55, 19–57, 19–237 (November 1943); T/O&E 19–500 (April 1944); and T/O&E 19–7 (September 1944). In March 1945 124 POWs suffocated in transit, provoking an IG investigation and an American apology to the German High Command. See report of investigation in file 383.6/3–16, box 26, RG 331, NARA.

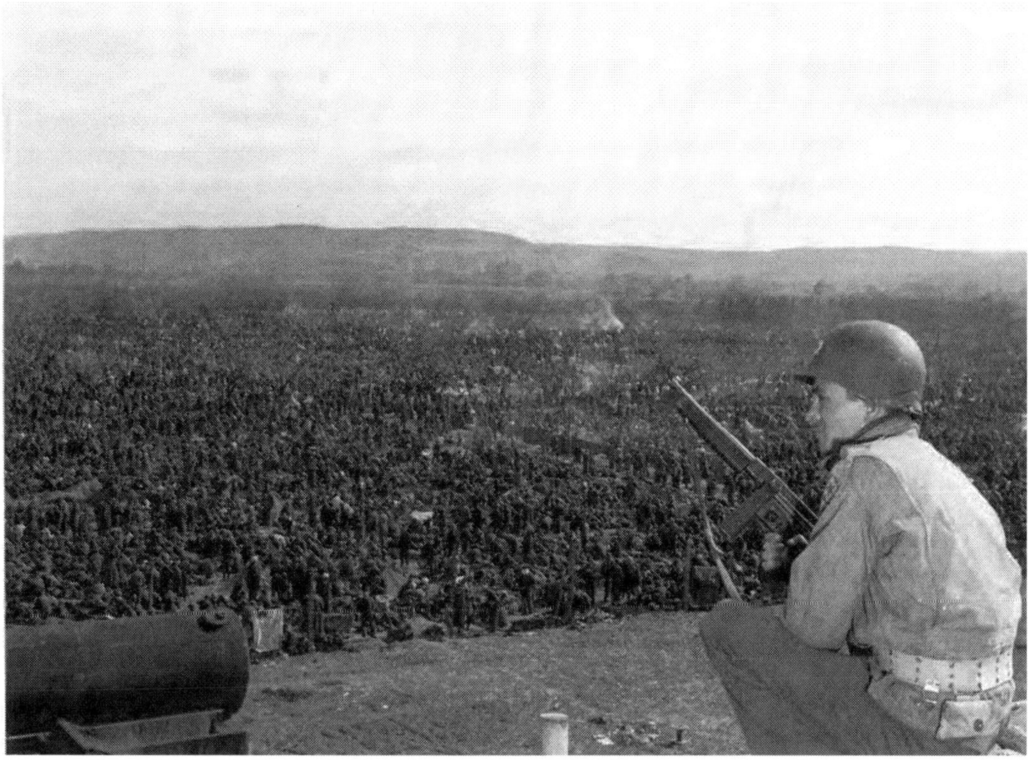

PRISONER-OF-WAR TRANSIENT ENCLOSURE AT REMAGEN

to the humanity or competence of the victor.

Early in April the theater provost marshal decided that the approaching inundation (which he underestimated by almost 2 million) would have to be absorbed in great part by four enclosures to be established along the Rhine. The surrenders of that month and May, however, soon raised the number of transient enclosures to seventeen (*see Map 24*). In most if not all, sanitary conditions were wretched; "the dysenteric feces of the penned-in thousands were trampled and emulsified in the muddy surface of the ground." In one barbed-wire pen near Remagen a mass of louse-infested men, ranging in number up to 169,000, endured the cold European spring with no shelter whatever. Their guards, untrained for the task, were temporary-duty men pulled from infantry units. Colonel Mason, the ADSEC deputy surgeon, viewed the result with amazement:

April 20th was a blustery day with alternate rain, sleet and snow and with bone chilling winds sweeping down the Rhine Valley . . . over the flats where the enclosure was located. Huddled close together for warmth, behind the barbed wire was a most awesome sight—nearly 100,000 haggard, apathetic, dirty, gaunt, blank-staring men clad in dirty field gray uniforms and standing ankle deep in mud. Here and there were dirty white blurs which, upon

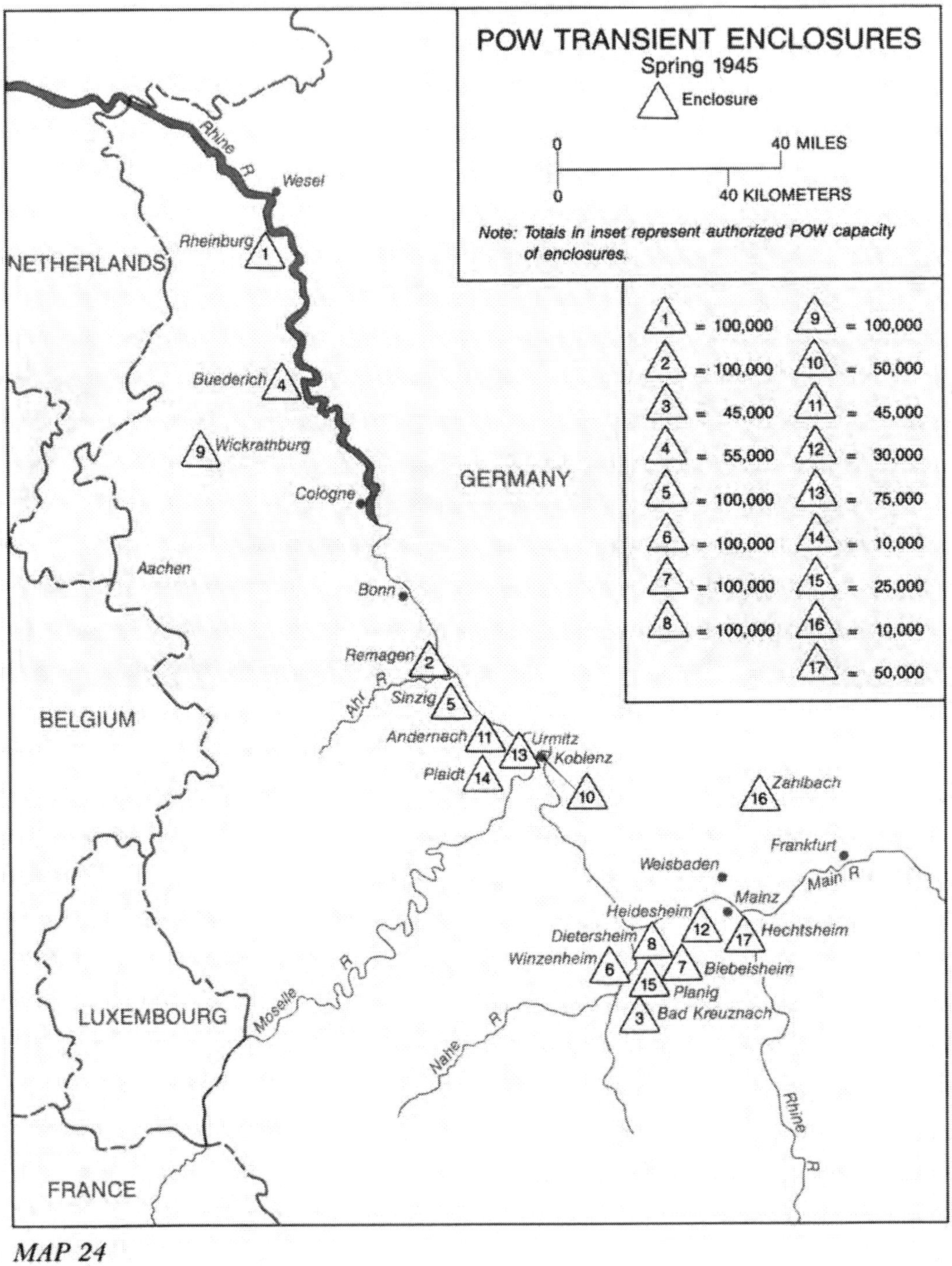
POW TRANSIENT ENCLOSURES
Spring 1945
Enclosure
0
40 MILES
0
40 KILOMETERS
Note: Totals in inset represent authorized POW capacity of enclosures.
1 = 100,000
2 = 100,000
3 = 45,000
4 = 55,000
5 = 100,000
6 = 100,000
7 = 100,000
8 = 100,000
9 = 100,000
10 = 50,000
11 = 45,000
12 = 30,000
13 = 75,000
14 = 10,000
15 = 25,000
16 = 10,000
17 = 50,000
NETHERLANDS
GERMANY
BELGIUM
LUXEMBOURG
FRANCE
Rhine R
Wesel
Rheinburg
Buederich
Wickrathburg
Cologne
Aachen
Bonn
Remagen
Ahr R
Sinzig
Andernach
Urmitz
Koblenz
Plaidt
Zahlbach
Frankfurt
Weisbaden
Main R
Mainz
Heidesheim
Hechtsheim
Dietersheim
Winzenheim
Biebelsheim
Planig
Bad Kreuznach
Moselle R
Nahe R
Rhine R

MAP 24

a closer look, were seen to be men with bandaged arms or standing in shirt sleeves! The . . . that the men had not eaten for at least two days, and the provision of water was a major problem—yet only 200 yards away was the Rhine River running bank full.[39]

Conditions in the transient enclosures bore heavily upon men already malnourished and ill-clad, and caused extraordinary sick rates. From 1 May to 15 June POW admissions to hospitals were about eight times those of American troops; the POW death rate from disease was about 20.5 times as great. Almost a quarter of all prisoners in the Advance Section showed up on sick call every week. The fact that the sick could be hospitalized was a tribute to Colonel Beasley, the ADSEC surgeon. Strengthened by a command decision giving him control of the medical units within the command, Beasley established dispensaries within the enclosures—in buildings, if available, or in tents—and staffed them with German medics. Field hospital sections moved up to the wire and made a practice of holding patients until doctors were convinced that they could endure life in the open. When a case of typhus appeared at the Remagen camp, Beasley assigned three officers from ADSEC's Preventive Medicine Division and sixteen five-man teams, drawn from the 423d and 480th Fumigation and Bath Companies, to dust all the prisoners and the Americans who had been in contact with them. While the pen was quarantined for twenty-one days, the dispensaries segregated and sent to the hospitals for observation any sick who appeared likely to have typhus.[40]

In view of the harsh conditions in the transient facilities, medical intervention may have prevented mass deaths. Elements of the 9th, 50th, 61st, 62d, 78th, and 83d Field Hospitals supported the enclosures, and new POW hospital centers were established with German medics working under the general superintendence of American medical battalions. During the period from 1 May to 15 June American medics reported a death rate among POWs in the enclosures of 35.6 per thousand, or 3.6 percent per year, with diseases—diarrhea and dysentery heading the list—as primary causes of mortality.[41]

With the end of the fighting, running the transient enclosures became the mission of several divisions of the field armies, but ultimately of the 106th Infantry Division alone. The primary duty of providing medical care fell to the division surgeon. The burden was great. Food was "not plentiful"; sanitation remained poor. According to the surgeon, "PWTEs containing up to 160,000 louse infested people, a high percentage of whom were either sick or wounded,

[39] First quotation from Ebbe Curtis Hoff, ed., *Special Fields*, Medical Department, United States Army in World War II (Washington, D.C.: Office of the Surgeon General, Department of the Army, 1969), p. 375. Second quotation from James B. Mason and Charles H. Beasley, "Medical Arrangements for Prisoners of War En Masse," *The Military Surgeon* 107 (December 1950): 345.

[40] Hoff, ed., *Special Fields*, p. 394; ADSEC Hist, p. 162; Surg, ADSEC, COMZ, Semiannual Rpt, January-June 1945, pp. 6–7; Gordon Hist, vol. 1, pt. 3, p. 19, CMH.

[41] Memo, Seventh U.S. Army, 13 May 45, sub: Consolidated List of PW, PWX & DP Installations, box 316; Surg, ADSEC, 13 May 45, sub: Report on PWTEs, box 313. Both in RG 112, NARA. See also Eesential Technical Medical Data, HQ, ETOUSA, July 1945, pp. 4–5 and encl. 11.

crammed into spaces initially meant for 20 to 50 thousand was not a pleasant picture." Shelter was nonexistent, even for the old and young. Rain soaked the prisoners, and the nighttime cold indirectly caused the deaths of a few by carbon monoxide from the small fires they had built inside the foxholes where they lived.[42]

Medical progress was halting—rich in personnel, poor in supplies. German medics were rapidly screened and organized, and delousing teams were set to work. But neither the 106th Division nor the camp commanders could obtain medical supplies from higher headquarters during April and May, though all the vehicles controlled by the division surgeon and the medical battalion "were on a constant 24-hour medical supply hunt." The division obtained some civilian nurses through the German Red Cross and local officials. Hospitals were set up in buildings or tents. All were in close proximity to the enclosures, and all had an adequate supply of water. The primary causes of admission were dysentery and upper respiratory infections, as might be expected. "Thank God for this mercy!" exclaimed a POW who found himself in a hospital on 28 May. "I rest again—for the first time since the beginning of April—in a bed! I can cover myself with a good big brown American blanket!"[43]

By June the 106th Division was running all seventeen POW transient enclosures, two of which contained not POWs but Russian and Czech DPs. The surgeon counted 10,000 beds in the fifteen attached hospitals, staffed largely by German medics. On the twelfth the British took over the enclosures, with some 200,000 inmates, in their zone. Rapid discharges in the camps that remained combined with warm weather to bring about a sharp decline in sick rates. On 10 July the French 10th Infantry Division took over the remaining POW enclosures along the Rhine in what was now the French Zone. Adding up the totals of its prisoner patients, the 106th Division recorded 1,817,393 cases on sick call and 1,697 deaths, of which 1,404 had occurred in May, 214 in June, and 79 in July.[44]

Complicating prisoner health problems in the European Theater were changes in the food ration. During the early fighting on the Continent prisoners had been more than adequately fed, receiving under Geneva rules rations equivalent to those of American soldiers. As a result, even nonworking prisoners ate better than Allied civilians. In response to an outcry against coddling POWs, the ration was reduced in December 1944. Yet prisoners were still reported to be gaining weight in captivity. They were also increasing in number,

[42] Surg, 106th Infantry Division, Annual Rpt, 1945, pp. 5–6, file 319.1–2, box 392, RG 112, NARA.

[43] First quotation from ibid., p. 8, file 319.1–2, box 392, RG 112, NARA. Second quotation from Kurt W. Boehme, *Die deutschen Kriegsgefangenen in amerikanischer Hand: Europa* (Munich: Verlag Ernst and Werner Gieseking, 1973), p. 316.

[44] Surg, 106th Infantry Division, Annual Rpt, 1945, p. 17, file 319.1–2, box 392, RG 112, NARA. On the internal economy of the camps, see policy memoranda in ibid., plus Daily PWTE situation reports in Medical Branch, COMZ, ETO, POW Enclosure Rpts, box 17, RG 332, NARA. See also Fred Clinger, Arthur Johnston, and Vincent Masel, *The History of the 71st Infantry Division* (Augsburg: E. Kieser KG, Druckerei und Verlag, 1946), p. 101.

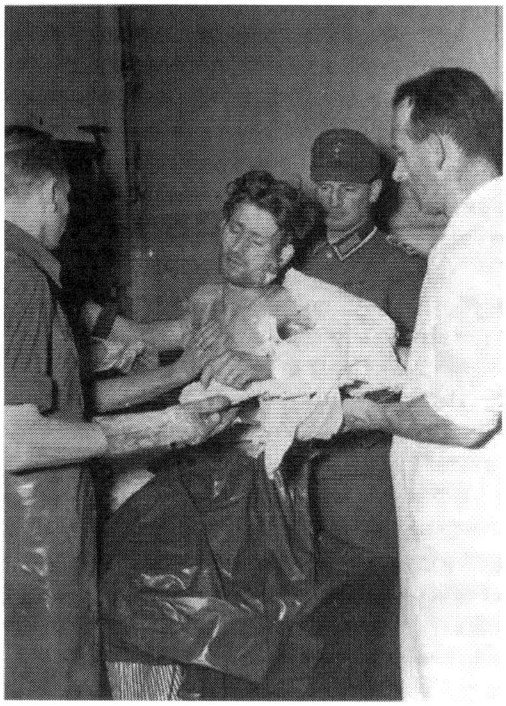

GERMAN MEDICS TREATING A GERMAN POW *in a military hospital*

for optimism among the Allies over a quick end to the war caused outshipments of POWs to the United States and England to be suspended from October 1944 to February 1945.

Then in the spring of 1945 a worldwide food shortage, caused in great measure by transport problems, brought warnings from the War Department. In March ETOUSA ordered strict food conservation in U.S. Army messes. The question of how to feed the German Army when it surrendered also became acute, especially in view of the Geneva rules to which all Allied nations had committed themselves. Realizing the problems that impended, SHAEF's Prisoner-of-War Division proposed to hold Germans who surrendered after the capitulation as disarmed enemy forces, rather than as POWs, feeding them a reduced ration drawn as far as possible from the German economy. General Eisenhower recommended paroling farm and industrial workers promptly, not only to relieve the Army but also to get the German economy moving again. Yet this sensible proposal, which was reminiscent of Lt. Gen. Ulysses S. Grant's method of handling the Confederate Army in the spring of 1865, ran afoul of denazification requirements, under which each POW had to be interviewed several times by G–2 officers, and of the continental Allies' demands for POW labor to speed up postwar reconstruction.[45]

In mid-May SHAEF met the problem by defining the prisoners as workers or nonworkers, placing the former on a 1,500–2,000-calorie ration and the latter on a 2,900-calorie ration. While the nonworker ration was about the same as the official civilian issue, civilians were able to supplement their dole by bargaining or keeping gardens, options not usually open to prisoners.

The consequences were quick to appear. Carrying out the orders of SHAEF's chief medical officer, General Kenner, a nutrition survey team in May inspected the POW transient enclosures and reported that the condition of the prisoners was good. Some POW detachment surgeons in the same month even boasted of weight gains among their prisoners. By the

[45] Staff Mins, Col P. C. Bullard, SHAEF-PWX, 19 Mar 45; Msg, Eisenhower to G–1, SHAEF-PWX. Both in file 383.6/3–17, box 26, RG 331, NARA.

end of the month, however, a report from the Koblenz camp surgeon revealed that nonworkers were receiving inadequate rations. Extensive malnutrition was recorded in the stockades of the Third and Seventh Armies and the Communications Zone in August. Avitaminosis appeared in florid deficiency syndromes, caused by not only the reduced ration but also the fact that fine-ground unenriched American flour formed a large part of it. Prisoners showed early symptoms of pellagra and beriberi, and weight loss was common. Conditions also varied widely from one camp to another, making a mockery of official policy. A new survey, ordered in August by Kenner with the concurrence of the provost marshal, found that nonworkers received anywhere from 1,250 to 2,040 calories a day, workers from 1,450 to 2,882. Furthermore, worker and nonworker were variously defined. In some camps young prisoners received dietary supplements in recognition of their greater metabolic needs; in others they did not.[46]

This survey resulted in immediate action. Kenner issued a letter ordering the surgeons of all major commands to provide multivitamin capsules to all prisoners with signs of malnutrition. At his instance Eisenhower's headquarters sent a letter to all commanding generals, revising the categories of prisoners into workers, light workers, and nonworkers, and prescribing menus for feeding each group. Working rations were ordered for all prisoners under 21 years of age, and dietary supplements were specified for all prisoners found by medical officers to be malnourished. A survey team was ordered to make periodic checks to ensure compliance.[47]

With many hospitals under their control, and a variety of liberated peoples to provide care for, the armies continued to use both captured supplies and captive labor. German medical supplies were inventoried and consolidated, and ETOUSA notified its units that captured stocks were available for POW enclosures, DP camps, RAMP facilities, and German civilian hospitals, and set forth a standard procedure for ordering needed items.

Under Geneva rules enlisted POWs could be required to work at specified jobs, and many found employment in the hospitals. Hospital centers housed German laborers in their own compounds, or drew them daily from local POW enclosures. DPs served also, sometimes as guards for the Germans. By and large the captive workers made good records, and on occasion were rewarded with letters

[46] Kenner became theater chief surgeon in July. See Rpt, Nutrition Survey Team, SHAEF, to CSurg, ETOUSA, 15 May 45, sub: Nutritional Survey of German Prisoners of War Under Control of United States Army on the European Continent, p. 2, in Essential Technical Medical Data, HQ, USFET, July 1945; Hoff, ed., *Special Fields*, pp. 389–94; Memo, Nutrition Survey Team, SHAEF, to Chief, Preventive Medicine Division, OofCSurg, ETO, 31 Aug 45, sub: Report of Nutritional Survey of German Prisoners of War and Disarmed Enemy Elements Under Control of the United States Army on the European Continent, box 327, RG 112, NARA; CampSurg, PWTE A-10 [Koblenz], Weekly Sanitary Rpt, 21 May 45, box 392, RG 112, NARA.

[47] Ltr, CSurg, TSFET, to Surgs, All Major Commands and Sectors, 15 Sep 45, sub: Multivitamin Capsules for Prisoners of War and Disarmed Enemy Elements, and Ltr, HQ, USFET, to CGs, 25 Sep 45, sub: POW Menu #2, Fifth Revision. Both in box 36, RG 112, NARA.

of appreciation from grateful commanders. Some kept hospital medical records, but apparently none provided hands-on care to Allied soldiers. When in May Kenner complained to Hawley of the great number of POW and DP workers, Hawley pointed out that the command had no alternative to employing them. "Demands upon the enlisted personnel of fixed hospitals," he wrote, "have made it impossible to operate . . . on an acceptable standard without additional help." Because many prisoners were only too happy to work under the better living conditions of the hospitals, and to eat the more abundant food, and because the hospitals needed the prisoners, there was in fact no alternative to the system, even if one had been desirable.[48]

DPs and Slave Laborers

Wherever they went in Germany during the spring of 1945, Americans wondered at the numbers of displaced persons. The historian of the 108th Evacuation Hospital remarked upon "the great migration of these liberated people" as they "made haste to leave this hateful country which had been their prison for many years." Some trudged afoot; others rode bicycles; some crowded into German Army vehicles. Some dragged rickety homemade carts, heaped with personal belongings—or with loot, for the DPs were not scrupulous in dealing either with German property or with German lives. Neither tractable nor gentle, the wanderers exhibited what Americans came to call the "Liberation Complex," a mingling of hunger, exultation, and vengefulness that made them a danger to their onetime rulers and a burden to their liberators.[49]

DPs had been drawn into Germany from almost every nation of Europe to labor for Hitler's war effort. Some had been volunteers, some conscripts, some little better than slaves. Their treatment varied widely. Farm laborers fared best, sharing the food they helped to raise or, at worst, finding opportunities to glean or steal sustenance. In Prussia a Western correspondent covering the Russian advance heard a Frenchman boast, "It was we . . . who ran the agriculture of East Prussia in the last two years." At Hadamar, in the state of Hesse, a former insane asylum turned Gestapo prison held both well-fed Poles and starving Germans. The Poles were farm workers; the Germans were political prisoners restricted to the prison ration. Civilian and military prisoners were often found mixed together, for some RAMPs had been compelled to labor and some had sought it as an alternative to starvation. Though the overall state of millions of individuals defies summary, DPs and RAMPs in good physical

[48]Quoted words from Ltr, Hawley to Kenner, 1 May 45, box 2, Hawley Papers, MHI. See also GO No. 29, Oise Section, COMZ, 4 Mar 45, sub: Estimate of Labor Service Companies, file 383.6; 803d and 819th Hospital Centers Semiannual Rpts, January–June 1945; Cady, "Notes on the 21st General Hospital (AUS)," p. 585, Cady Papers, MHI; Gorby Interv, 1962, CMH. On SHAEF opposition to allowing POWs to provide medical care for Allied soldiers, see Ltr, HQ, ETOUSA, to Section Cdrs, COMZ, 9 Feb 45, sub: Utilization of German Protected Medical Personnel. For information on earlier POW service in hospitals, see Chapter XIV of this volume.

[49]The 108th Evacuation Hospital Travelogue, June 1945.

condition were rare, with the Russians among them having suffered the worst.[50]

Dealing with severely malnourished and often tubercular patients in the midst of war proved a difficult task. With their own wounded to care for, the field forces often turned for assistance to doctors and nurses among the DPs. They also moved patients into German hospitals and, in some cases, when Allied nurses and doctors were available, set up special hospitals. More rarely, mobile hospital units took on the task of caring for sick and starving DPs.[51]

Typhus was common east of the Rhine, just as it had been to the west. Every effort was made to delouse DPs in their camps and at shipping points, where they gathered to go home. Teams equipped with power dusters set to work at Neubau, where many western Europeans were evacuated by air, or at Wuerzburg and Bamberg, where rail transport to countries east of the Rhine was centered. As the number of hospitals for POWs and American military fell, those for DPs increased, reaching a total of twenty-two in the Third Army area in September 1945. But depleted American manpower made consolidation of the patients and the discharge of as many as possible to their own countries desirable. An international organization, the United Nations Relief and Rehabilitation Administration (UNRRA), began making plans to assume control of the remaining DP hospitals, except those holding Soviet citizens who were to be returned to their own nation.[52]

With the end of the fighting, the field armies became occupying forces responsible for defined regions in the American Zone of Occupation. Their division surgeons were now responsible for the DP, RAMP, and POW hospitals in their division areas and for medical care of the camps. Even with the advent of UNRRA, the Army found itself still in charge of many facilities—even of the DP camps, because the international organization could not at first find the manpower to assume full responsibility. Thus the surgeon of the 2d Armored Division was still charged with two RAMP hospitals, ten DP hospitals, and fifty-three German military hospitals. Because Army personnel were clearly inadequate to handle the load—645 RAMP patients, 937 DPs, and 11,409 POWs—dependence upon the various groups to help care for their own members also continued. DP dispensaries were maintained by camp inmates under the eye of the division surgeon, and the Americans viewed with gratification and surprise the "high standards of sanitation . . . maintained by the same people who had been taken out of the indescribable filth of the concentration camps

---

[50] Quoted words from Alexander Werth, *Russia at War* (New York: E. P. Dutton, 1964), p. 958. See also Coles and Weinberg, *Civil Affairs*, p. 858, and surveys at end of Larkey "Hist," ch. 14, pp. 104 et seq. General policy is set forth in Ltr 383.7-1, AG, SHAEF, to HQ, 21 Army Group (Rear), CG, 6th Army Group (Rear), and CG, COMZ, 27 Mar 45, sub: Medical Care for DPs and Refugees in Germany, in ETOUSA.

[51] Havens, ed., *Infectious Diseases*, pp. 347–48; Rpt, SrConsultant in TB to CSurg, ETOUSA, 3 Apr 45, sub: Tuberculosis in Russian RAMPs at 46th General Hospital, p. 1.

[52] Surg, Third U.S. Army, Semiannual Rpts, January–June 1945, pp. 90 and 140, and July–December 1945, pp. 1–2 and 33–34.

and [prison] hospitals under German control." [53]

Yet DP camps, because discipline was less severe and because they contained many women, formed a tougher problem for the occupation authorities than either the hospitals or the POW camps, especially as the postwar VD rate began to rise. DPs were not responsible for all, or even most, of the venereal disease that afflicted defeated Germany: American troops and German civilians were the most numerous victims and carriers. Yet, of the ten DP hospitals in the 2d Armored Division area, one was for venereal disease alone. The atmosphere of the camps was not conducive to high personal standards in any respect. DPs differed greatly from one another in culture and education; intellectuals and plain folk mingled with peasants from the most primitive regions of eastern Europe. Inevitably, though unfairly, the image too many Americans carried away was of an indistinguishable mass of "sleeping, eating and scratching people," infested with lice and defecating at random. Though systematic attention to cleanliness changed the picture in some camps, others, especially those marked for transients, showed little lasting improvement. The soldiers were happy to see UNRRA take over care of the DPs in the fall of 1945 and still happier to see the majority of the displaced depart to their homes.[54]

[53]Surg, 2d Armored Division, Semiannual Rpt, January-June 1945, p. 7.

[54]Quoted words from Surg, 29th Infantry Division, Semiannual Rpt, January-June 1945, p. 8. See also Surg, 5th Armored Division, Semiannual Rpt, January-June 1945, and Surg, 4th Armored Division, Semiannual Rpt, July-December 1945.

Mingled with the DPs, Americans also began to find concentration camp inmates. Some were on the roads, in flight with their guards from advancing Russian spearheads: In the small south German town of Cham, Third Army units found 6,000 survivors of a march from the Flossenbuerg Concentration Camp and assigned the 120th Evacuation Hospital to their care. Others had reached a temporary haven. At a *Luftwaffe* airfield in Austria, designated by military government units to receive the liberated, the 121st Evacuation Hospital found about 14,000 people whose condition was that of "starved, half-crazed animals." Thousands had already been hospitalized in hangars and barracks by the 646th Clearing Company, the first medical unit on the scene. The evacuation hospital admitted 3,000 patients during the first week. Medics drew supplies from a large consolidated depot at St. Florian and also scoured the countryside for milk and food. Over 300 cases of typhus were identified, as well as tuberculosis and dysentery. Despite all efforts, the mortality rate was high during the first days, and a tenth of the patients died overall. But many survivors owed their lives to the American units and to a German Army field hospital that had arrived to give assistance. "Order replaced chaos," reported the commander of the evacuation hospital, "and it was gratifying to see the improvements in the patients, both physically and mentally." [55]

[55]Quoted words from the 121st Evacuation Hospital Semiannual Rpt, January-June 1945. See also 120th Evacuation Hospital Semiannual Rpt, Janu-

Continued

Most inmates, however, were still behind wire when the Americans arrived. April brought the opening of two major concentration camps, or rather camp systems, around Buchenwald and Dachau. In early May Army units "uncovered" (as the records usually say) Mauthausen, near the Austrian town of Linz, where Adolf Hitler had spent much of his boyhood. Meanwhile, British troops captured two large camps at Bergen-Belsen in Hannover (*Map 25*). Medical conditions among many inmates were outside the experience of the medical personnel compelled to deal with them; the tasks they faced proved to be loathsome and laborious in the extreme.

The general history of the concentration camps is well known. The first, the main camp at Dachau, was established in 1933, a few months after the Nazis took power. During the 1930s concentration camps served no purpose but to confine, torment, and destroy enemies of the regime and members of groups defined as antisocial. Inmates produced little, in order not to compete with free labor. When war came, German conquests brought an international influx of prisoners. By 1942 increasing shortages of manpower in the Reich began to transform camp inmates into true slave labor. Satellite camps sprang up. At the war's end Dachau and many other camps ran industries that were profitable to the SS and important to the war effort. Among the prisoners, conditions of life remained bad because endless new labor was available to replace the dead. While none of the western camps was an extermination facility, like Auschwitz and other camps in the east, killing undesirables remained an important function. Russian POWs were shot on occasion and, like Poles and Jews, used by Nazi doctors as human guinea pigs in bizarre experiments.

In the spring of 1945 the primitive discipline of the camps enforced by the SS broke down. The food ration, always inadequate, apparently fell from about 1,000 calories a day to 600 or less. Mains, broken in some cases by Allied bombs, ceased to deliver water. The invasion of the Reich caused the SS to shuffle prisoners from one camp to another in unheated boxcars or in forced marches afoot, to prevent their capture. Overcrowding increased in the barracks, where the well, the sick, and the dead sprawled together indiscriminately. Fuel shortages slowed the incineration of bodies. Filled with people who were starving and ill, the remaining camps became charnel houses, whose images confronted an unbelieving world in the photographs and newsreels made by journalists who followed the Allied armies.[56]

Administratively, the concentration camps fell first under the field armies. The early days following liberation were chaotic. Quarantine was imposed, and available medical units

ary-June 1945. Both in file 319.1-2, box 408, RG 112, NARA.

[56] Heinz Hoehne, *The Order of the Death's Head: The Story of Hitler's SS* (New York: Coward-McCann, 1970), pp. 88 and 199–203. On Buchenwald, see Rpt, 3 May 45, sub: Visit to Buchenwald Concentration Camp, Weimar, Germany, file 383.6 ETO (Buchenwald Camp). On Bergen-Belsen, see William A. Davis, "Typhus at Belsen," *The American Journal of Hygiene* 46 (July 1947): 66–83. Information on the medical experiments in the camps may be found in Chapter XVII of this volume.

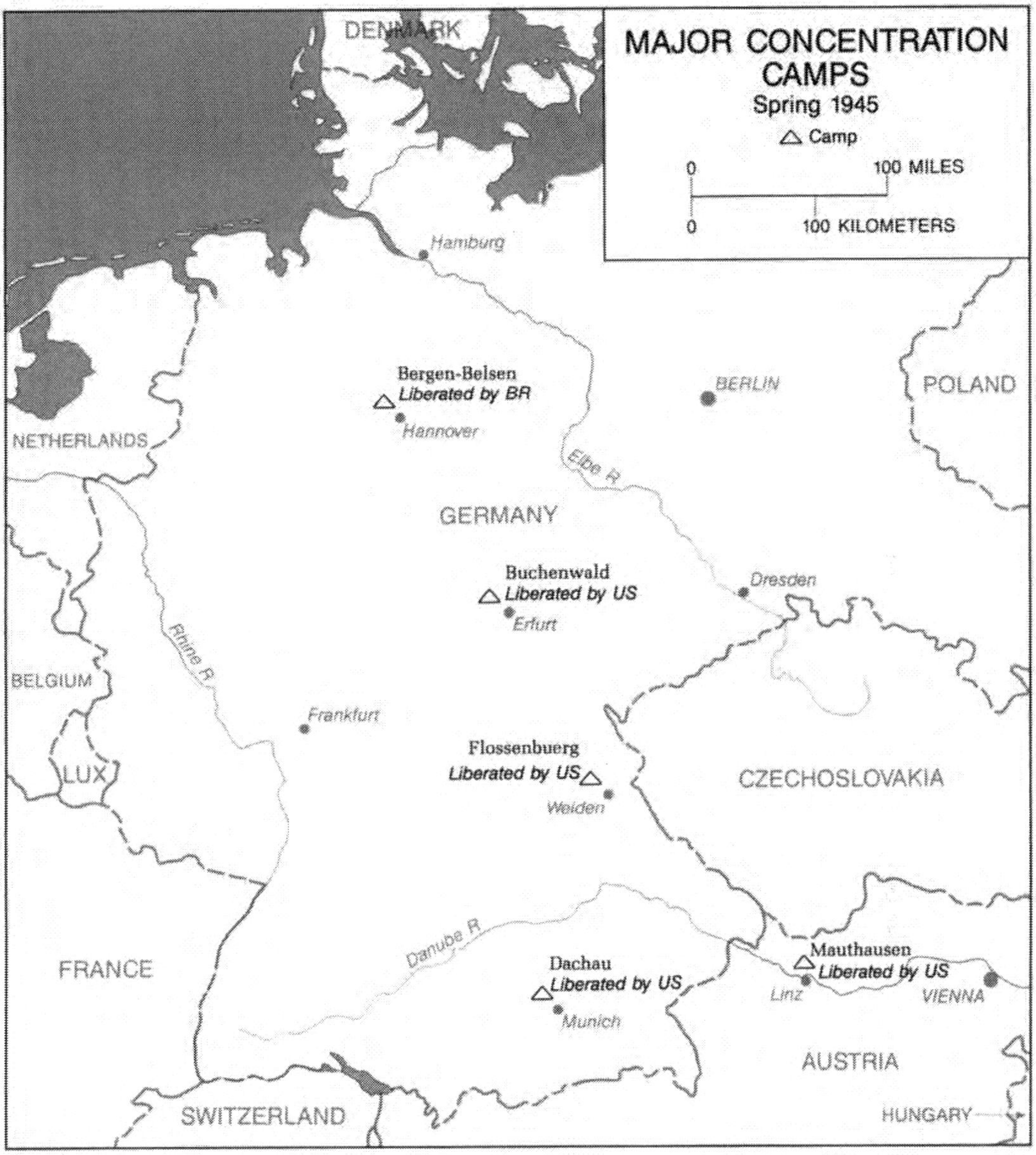
MAJOR CONCENTRATION CAMPS
Spring 1945
Camp
0
100 MILES
0
100 KILOMETERS
DENMARK
Hamburg
Bergen-Belsen
Liberated by BR
Hannover
BERLIN
POLAND
NETHERLANDS
Elbe R
GERMANY
Buchenwald
Liberated by US
Erfurt
Dresden
Rhine R
BELGIUM
Frankfurt
Flossenbuerg
Liberated by US
Weiden
LUX
CZECHOSLOVAKIA
Danube R
Dachau
Liberated by US
Munich
Mauthausen
Liberated by US
Linz
VIENNA
FRANCE
AUSTRIA
SWITZERLAND
HUNGARY

MAP 25

were thrown in, using their own supplies and calling on the armies for rations to feed the starving. At some camps German medics were brought in; at others inmates were sent to civilian or German Army hospitals. Throughout, former prisoners with medical training were called upon to help their fellows. Inmate doctors, who had been working for years with virtually no supplies, provided knowledgeable assistance.[57]

Liberated prisoners suffered from complex interacting pathologies, advanced starvation, and frequently traumatic injury as well. Those at Buchenwald were the first in a haunting army tens of thousands strong. "There was no adipose tissue on these people," reported the Third Army surgeon, "and nutritional edema . . . was present in all individuals." At Dachau the workers had received enough food for survival, but other prisoners were in poor shape. Many exhibited ulcerated gums, pallor, and swollen feet; their skin, thin and fragile, had been worn by the hard wooden slabs they slept upon. Abrasions became infected, resulting in boils, abscesses, and ulcers. Small local infections, under camp conditions, resulted in "massive nonpurulent edema . . . with sloughing and gangrene." Tuberculosis was widespread, diarrhea ubiquitous. Some inmates, shot or beaten, bore injured limbs in makeshift slings. Morbidity ran about 25 percent of the 32,000-odd men and 300 women in the main camp. The prison hospital, wrote one of the first doctors into Dachau, was surprisingly clean and orderly under inmate control.[58]

Autopsies on the bodies of typhus victims revealed widespread and varied ills: local hemorrhages, liver and kidney damage, the mucosa of the colon and rectum eroded or deeply ulcerated, tuberculosis of the lungs, and pneumonia. "The heart," reported the 116th Evacuation Hospital commander, "was generally pale and very soft so that a finger could easily be thrust through it." Doctors concluded that the patients' typhus was fairly mild, but superimposed upon tuberculosis, severe malnutrition, and chronic diarrhea. Under such conditions the ubiquity of death was hardly surprising. Troops of the 42d Infantry Division entering Dachau found the last shipment of prisoners still at the railhead—apparently Polish Jews from Birkenau who were sent west to evade the Red Army. Flatcars and open boxcars held about 2,500 emaciated bodies, piled on one another. "Their cadaverous arms and legs seem[ed] disproportionately long compared to their sunken abdomens, narrowed bony chests, visible ribs, protruding shoulder blades, and withered necks. . . ."

---

[57] 120th Evacuation Hospital Semiannual Rpt, January-June 1945, file 319.1-2, box 408, RG 112, NARA; Havens, ed., *Medical Consultants*, p. 452; Press Release, "Underground Medical Unit Operated in Nazi Prison Camp," file 383.6 ETO (Buchenwald Camp). The head inmate surgeon at Buchenwald had unique status: The SS guards, respecting his skill, had required him to treat their own men.

[58] First quotation from Surg, Third U.S. Army, Semiannual Rpt, January-June 1945, p. 139. Second quotation from Rpt, 1st Lt Marcus J. Smith, MC, to PostSurg, Dachau Concentration Camp, 5 May 45, sub: Health and Sanitation Rpt, file 383.6 ETO (Dachau Camp), in Source Materials Collected by Col M. P. Rudolph, MC, box 312, RG 112, NARA. See also Marcus J. Smith, *The Harrowing of Hell: Dachau* (Albuquerque: University of New Mexico Press, 1972), p. 91.

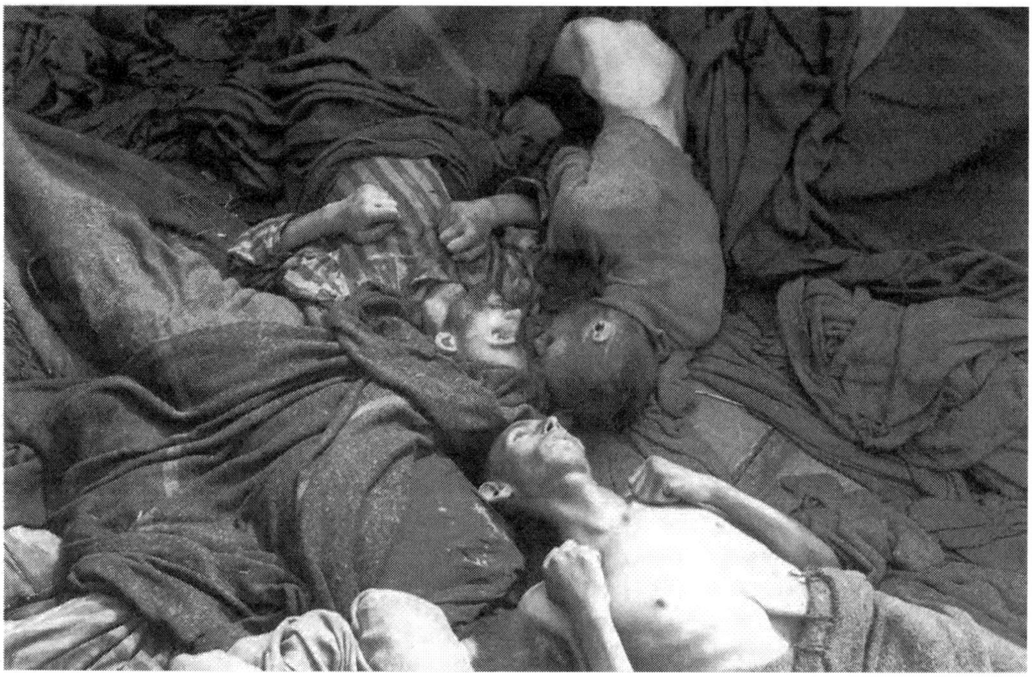

LAST SHIPMENT TO DACHAU. *The bodies of starved prisoners, who died en route from another camp, lie grotesquely in a boxcar.*

Some wore striped pajama-like garments; many were naked. Bodies and freight cars were lightly coated with white morning frost.[59]

Survivors gave their liberators guided tours of the camps. Living quarters were squalid: "The well, the sick, the dying, and the dead lie next to each other in . . . poorly ventilated, unheated, dark, stinking buildings." The dead were everywhere. A nurse at Dachau saw bodies in "huge stacks like so much kindling wood." Each camp had a crematory, for, as the universal joke went, the only way out was through the chimney. At Flossenbuerg a little hand-operated railway ran from the camp to the crematory. Each morning, those who had died the night before were collected, dumped into the cars, and pushed to the furnace. When the Americans arrived, fifteen or twenty naked skeletal bodies lay stacked and waiting to be burned. "It was a weird place," recalled a battalion surgeon, "the crackling furnace and the naked corpses with their lolling heads and stiff arms and legs. . . . I opened the door of the blazing furnace and inside I saw three corpses sizzling and burning."[60]

[59] First quotation from 116th Evacuation Hospital Semiannual Rpt, January-June 1945, an., p. 12. Second quotation from Smith, *Dachau*, p. 79.

[60] First quotation from 116th Evacuation Hospital Semiannual Rpt, January-June 1945, an., p. 2. Second quotation from Smith, *Dachau*, p. 80 (see also pp. 90-91). Third quotation from William M. McConahey, *Battalion Surgeon* (Rochester, Minn.: Privately published, 1966), p. 145. See Surg, Seventh U.S. Army, Semiannual Rpt, January-June 1945.

Burial parties—mainly German civilians, working under duress—disposed of the bodies. A journalist at Dachau shortly after liberation saw peasants climb the mounts of corpses, bring down bodies and "heave-ho" them into wagons. Such unwilling sextons had to work from the tops of the heaps—"they could not pull the bodies out from lower down because pieces would come off." Wagonload by wagonload, they were moved to mass graves. Among the dead were former guards. In the first hours of freedom able-bodied prisoners had taken revenge on their onetime tormentors, holding hunts for SS men and beating to death those they found. Some accounts of the Dachau liberation assert that American troops machine-gunned several hundred guards.[61]

Care of the sick followed essentially the same pattern in all camps. At Buchenwald the 120th Evacuation Hospital took over the SS barracks as a hospital: sturdy buildings, with latrines and heated showers. Inmates had already occupied the barracks, however, and in consequence the furniture, rugs and bedding were infested with lice. Hospital personnel stripped the rooms and scrubbed walls and tile floors with soap and water. Canvas cots were moved in and covered with German or American army blankets. German civilians were drafted and instructed in the use of DDT hand dusters. When everything was ready, patients were brought by ambulance, unloaded, and dusted under their clothing. They were carried into the hallway of the barracks, stripped, and bedded down. Their clothes either were burned or put through a steam delousing machine. By the third day someone—possibly Army engineers—had repaired the water system, and the admission procedure changed to include a thorough bath after the first delousing. Americans handling the sick doused themselves and their bedding with powder, and no cases of infestation or sickness occurred.[62]

At Dachau the 116th and 127th Evacuation Hospitals worked in the SS barracks, after tearing out partitions to make large wards. The kitchens of the excellent SS mess hall provided food for patients and staff. From this center, order began to spread to the shambles outside. Thirty-two thousand prisoners were crowded into an area intended for about 10,000; water, sewers, and lights had all failed; starving inmates had broken into SS warehouses and gorged themselves on food they could not digest. A sanitary company, a quartermaster laundry, an engineer unit, and a fumigation and bath unit arrived to help out. Healthy inmates set up an International Prisoners Committee to present their grievances to the Americans, to defuse national antagonisms, and to assist the cleanup. Inmates removed rubbish, and the committee ensured that all

[61] 116th Evacuation Hospital Semiannual Rpt, January–June 1945, an., p. 5. See also Howard A. Buechner, *Dachau: The Hour of the Avenger* (New Orleans: Thunderbird Press, 1986), and Nerin E. Gun, *The Day of the Americans* (New York: Fleet Publishing Co., 1966). Buechner was a 45th Division medical officer, and Gun was an inmate of Dachau at the time.

[62] 120th Evacuation Hospital Semiannual Rpt, January–June 1945, p. 20, file 319.1–2, box 408, RG 112, NARA.

water was boiled, until chlorination of a restored water supply could begin. By the end of May it was possible to assume, for the first time in Dachau's twelve-year history as a concentration camp, that the well would not needlessly become sick.

Yet scenes within the hospitals were grim. When the Seventh Army liberated the camp, about 140 inmates were dying every day. The 127th Evacuation Hospital admitted about 1,900 patients during May, of whom 900 had multiple diseases, and another 260 in June. From early May until mid-June the unit lost 246 patients. The 116th Evacuation Hospital admitted over 2,000 patients, of whom nearly 1,800 either had typhus or were suspect. Bacillary dysentery was common. During May 140 patients died of typhus, 28 of tuberculosis, 15 of starvation, and 7 of enteritis (inflammation of the bowels). Malnutrition was a contributory factor in all deaths, and the hospital staff struggled not only to feed their patients—at first GI rations supplemented by milk chocolate, and eggnog, and later German Army rations—but also to keep them from eating too much. Multivitamins were given to counteract the effects of starvation, plasma to increase body proteins, and intravenous fluids to reestablish fluid balance. All who survived gained weight rapidly, and within two weeks the living skeletons that had filled the camp at the end of April had recovered their human appearance.[63]

The typhus threat caused the Seventh Army, upon taking over the camp, to quarantine it and appoint a camp surgeon. Soon representatives of the Typhus Commission arrived to observe, investigate, and assist. A commission officer reached Dachau in May and took over a section of one ward for study and treatment of selected cases. The commission arranged for supplies of vaccine and para-aminobenzoic acid, then the most effective medicine known for treating the disease. Another of its officers assisted the British at Bergen-Belsen. Abandoning an early attempt to do research under the conditions of Dachau, the commission instead emphasized measures of treatment and especially of prevention. General Fox, its field director, declared that the concentration camp represented a "menace to the whole of northwestern Europe" because of conditions outside the barbed wire as well as within.[64]

As stories of the camp spread, Allied journalists arrived to explore the homes of the SS officers and the scoured but still oppressive and ill-smelling barracks. A woman reporter, Elizabeth May Craig, penned a description of the place on V–E Day. At the 116th Evacuation Hospital the nurses wore olive drab trousers and shirts, aprons and gauze masks. As a penicillin squad was giving injections, its blonde leader complained: "I can't

[63] 116th Evacuation Hospital Semiannual Rpt, January-June 1945, an., p. 8.

[64] Ibid., an., p. 7; Hoff, ed., *Arthropodborne Diseases Other Than Malaria*, pp. 206–07; Davis, "Typhus at Belsen." In Records of the USA Typhus Commission, RG 112, NARA, see Ltr, Brig Gen Bayne-Jones to Col K. R. Lundeberg, 7 Sep 44, box 69, and Ltr (source of quotation), Fox to Bayne-Jones, 18 May 45, box 70.

find enough muscle to get a hypodermic in." A surgeon remarked that he could not perform operations; the shock would kill the patients. The chief nurse, in a soft South Carolina drawl, told Craig that as yet no hospitalized patients had recovered. "There is no disposition except death," she said.[65]

Gradually Dachau was cleared, the epidemic controlled, the living placed under treatment, and the dead buried. Cheering groups of prisoners began to depart for home. Allied soldiers who had liberated the camp and Army medics who had worked there were left to record in official reports, private letters, and diaries their recollections of a situation that is fortunately without an exact parallel in recent, or perhaps any, history.

A system of organized inhumanity fell apart in a chaos almost worse than what had gone before. Uncovering the camps and political prisons of the Third Reich revealed conditions to which even a war-jaded world responded with disbelief. Medical work was grim and summary, but its significance went beyond even the saving of lives. The compassionate treatment of the camp survivors marked the restoration of moral order amid the worst scenes that Nazi tyranny had been able to devise.

[65] 116th Evacuation Hospital Semiannual Rpt, January–June 1945, an.

CHAPTER XVII

From War to Occupation

On 8 May 1945 the war that had devastated Europe and claimed millions of human lives came to an end with the unconditional surrender of the German forces. For many medical personnel in the American Army, the tasks of reconstruction had already begun. During the spring and summer military government detachments were hard at work throughout the American Zone—"the harbingers of a new order and the only stable influence in a world turned upside down."[1]

Composed of three or four officers and five enlisted men apiece and equipped with two jeeps with trailers, the detachments represented the Occupation to Germans everywhere except in the big cities. They arranged burial for corpses lying in the streets, restored a system of rationing that guaranteed civilians a small basic allowance of food, returned local police to their duties, and sought to restore electricity and water supplies. American public health officers surveyed the disease situation, spotted potential sources of infection, and recommended remedial action. Since the American Zone comprehended all of Bavaria, part of Berlin, and parts of prewar Wuerttemberg, Baden, Hesse, Kurhessen, Nassau, and the cities of Frankfurt, Bremen, and Bremerhaven (*see Map 26*), some 19 million Germans, millions of POWs, and a large but decreasing number of DPs had become dependent upon the American Army.[2]

Despite earlier fears of guerrilla warfare, German armed resistance was over by the end of May. But problems were immense, and were not made easier by upheaval within the Army itself. On 1 July ETOUSA was redesignated United States Forces, European Theater (USFET); on 16 July SHAEF was inactivated; and on 1 August COMZ became Theater Service Forces, European Theater (TSFET). The change of names was accompanied by a change in personnel that began at the top but permeated all ranks. On 1 August General Hawley departed for the United States, and a distinguished postwar career in civilian medicine. For the month of July General Kenner bore

[1] Ziemke, *Occupation of Germany*, p. 186.

[2] See Hoff, ed., *Civil Affairs/Military Government*, p. 494; Wolfe, ed., *Americans as Proconsuls*, pp. 52–57; Medical Plan for Preliminary [*sic*] Occupation of Germany, in Miscellaneous file, Shambora Papers, MHI. Military government detachments were organized in July and August 1944, and the first entered Germany on 15 September of that year.

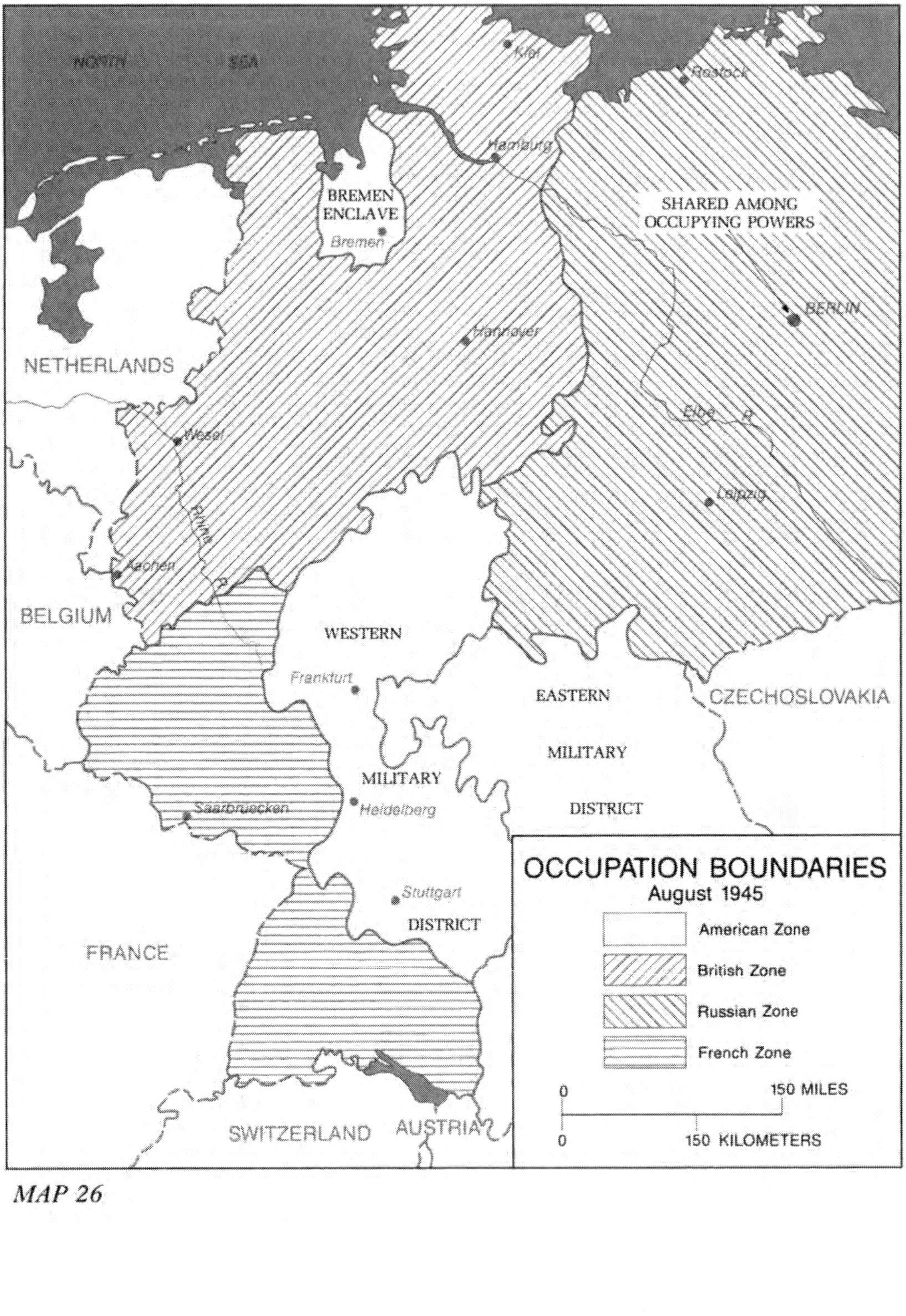
NORTH SEA
Kiel
Rostock
Hamburg
BREMEN
ENCLAVE
Bremen
SHARED AMONG
OCCUPYING POWERS
BERLIN
Hannover
NETHERLANDS
Wesel
Elbe R.
Rhine
Leipzig
Aachen
BELGIUM
WESTERN
Frankfurt
EASTERN
CZECHOSLOVAKIA
MILITARY
MILITARY
Saarbruecken
Heidelberg
DISTRICT
Stuttgart
DISTRICT
FRANCE
SWITZERLAND
AUSTRIA
OCCUPATION BOUNDARIES
August 1945
American Zone
British Zone
Russian Zone
French Zone
0
150 MILES
0
150 KILOMETERS

MAP 26

the title of Surgeon, Occupation Forces, Germany. On the day Hawley left, Kenner became both TSFET and USFET surgeon, and chief medical adviser to his old commander, General Eisenhower, who now commanded USFET. To Kenner fell the duties of guiding the medical service through a time when it must give direction to a conquered nation while undergoing constant change itself.[3]

Public Health

The danger of disease was acute. Food and fuel were in short supply for civilians, and homelessness was common in a land of shattered buildings. Great movements of population continued as DPs left the country and Germans expelled from the east trekked in. Cold and hungry, the mass of wanderers faced the danger of epidemics, even in rural areas. Refugees from the cities thronged many country towns, drinking water from shallow wells fouled by the runoff from latrines and manure piles. In May an outbreak of typhoid occurred at Moringen, a town of 2,000, which was accommodating twice that number of people. But the greatest problems afflicted the bombed cities.

Nowhere were they greater than in Berlin. When the Western Allies entered the former capital to share occupation duties with the Soviets who had conquered it, they had to cope with the ruin wrought by 75,000 tons of British and American bombs, plus Russian artillery shells. Over the rubble hung the stink of unburied dead. Four of every five dwellings were in ruins, transport was at a standstill, bridges over the many canals had been destroyed, and broken sewers poured their contents into the water below. The canals and the water-filled bomb craters were nurseries for clouds of mosquitoes, and a plague of flies beset the city as the weather warmed. In the first months of the Occupation, epidemics of dysentery, typhoid, and diphtheria swept the population. Most adults and older children survived, but dysentery, which the people called hunger typhoid, killed 65 percent of the newborn babies. Berliners subsisted on about 800 calories a day.

Remarkably, the city's Central Health Office still existed, with subsidiary organizations in each administrative district. All services, however, were at a standstill when the Americans arrived in July. Of 240 peacetime hospitals, only 150 were in operation, and these lacked ether, narcotics, alcohol, and sulfa drugs. There was little transport and no telephone service. Communicable disease reports had to be delivered by messenger, and patients were borne to hospitals through rubble-mounded streets on stretchers or primitive carts. The city's water supply was still potable at the source, but contamination from some 1,600 breaks in the mains caused the Central Health Office to order all drinking water to be boiled. The four-power government of Berlin agreed on some basic actions to prevent disease, especially typhus. The Russians began to isolate and treat

[3]On the change in command, see GO No. 3130, HQ, ETOUSA, 20 Jun 45, and GO No. 167, HQ, USFET, 21 Jul 45. Hawley became, in turn, chief medical director of the Veterans Administration, chief executive officer for Blue Cross and Blue Shield, and president of the American College of Surgeons.

typhus cases, and Maj. David Greely of the United States of America Typhus Commission drew up a comprehensive program that, once accepted by the Americans, Russians, British, and French, became part of the city's law. Under direction of the Central Health Office, dusting teams and medical workers in every district were immunized; refugees and bathhouses were deloused; all cases were isolated; and their contacts were dusted and observed.[4]

By such vigorous action the occupying powers suppressed the immediate threat of epidemic outbreaks. Aiding them was the tradition of discipline among the Germans, who, to the surprise of the Americans, remained law-abiding except in the areas of prostitution and the black market. Encouraged by the Potsdam agreement, the military government sought the maintenance of good health and medical services by the Germans. With combat over and conditions less threatening, the influence of military government specialists grew steadily, and in August Kenner decided to relieve the field commands of direct responsibility for public health.

The result was the emergence in late summer of a reorganized medical service and the reemergence of a civil public health establishment. Kenner made public health a function of the ECA detachments attached to the two military districts into which the American Zone had been divided—the Western, under the Third Army, with headquarters at Munich; and the Eastern, under the Seventh Army at Heidelberg. G–5, USFET, set policy; the chief surgeon provided overall technical supervision. Each district commander, through his own G–5 section, set policy for public health work in his own area, while the military district surgeon, who was also the field army surgeon, provided technical oversight. To ensure adequate personnel, General Eisenhower ordered that field command medical personnel were to be made available to the military government as necessary. With the approval of military public health experts, the German system of organizing public health began to revive at the local level, and by September 1945 efforts were under way to reestablish the German Red Cross.[5]

But the revival of the German medical profession—an absolutely essential element in restoring and safeguarding public health—was a more complex problem. Many factors conspired to weaken the profession's

[4] Ziemke, *Occupation of Germany*, p. 304; Rpt, USA/MG, 3 Aug 45, app. A, file U.S. Group Control Council, and Ltr, Greely to Bayne-Jones, 24 Aug 45, file Paris #III, box 70, Records of the USA Typhus Commission, RG 112, NARA; Memo, HQ, USFET, 7 Sep 45, sub: Program for the Prevention and Control of Typhus Throughout Berlin, file Preventive Medicine, box 471, and HQ, USFET, Weekly MG Rpt, 20 Jul 45, file Weekly CA/MG Rpts, box 541, OMGUS, PHB/PWB, RG 260, NARA. For a general study of bombing and German health, see Special Rpt, HQ, USFET, January 1947, sub: The Effect of Bombing on Health and Medical Care in Germany, file Preventive Medicine (General), box 541, OMGUS, PHB/PWB, RG 260, NARA.

[5] Directive, HQ, USFET (to CGs, Eastern and Western Military Districts and Berlin District), 6 Aug 45, sub: Public Health Functions in the U.S. Zone of Germany, in Kenner Diary, bk. 3, following p. 408. See also Memo, Wilson, DepC, PHB, G–5, USFET, to DepACofS, G–5, USFET, 21 Aug 45, sub: Military Government Conference, 9 August 1945, file Public Health, box 471; HQ, USFET (OMGUS), Weekly Rpts, 9 Aug and 21 Sep 45, file Weekly CA/MG Rpts, box 541. Both in OMGUS, PHB/PWB, RG 260, NARA.

ability to serve its people at a time of great need. Before Hitler's rise to power German medicine had written a distinguished record, especially in research, winning, up to 1930, thirty-five Nobel prizes, more than any other nation to that time. Freedom of inquiry had prevailed in the universities. After 1933 the profession was forcibly organzied by the Nazis, provided with subsidies, and given a national leader and a party-line publication. Doctors in administrative posts were usually compelled to join the Party, and after September 1938 Jews were purged from the profession's ranks. During the war military demands increased; at a conference with General Kenner, the assistant chief surgeon of the German Supreme Headquarters averred that 45 percent of the German doctors were in the Wehrmacht, 55 percent in civil practice. Hence, at the war's end many doctors were in POW pens, and many others were deeply compromised for political reasons. The 6th Army Group captured the personnel files of the medical association of the State of Baden, whose membership comprised all the doctors and dentists and many of the public health officials. Less than a quarter lacked significant Party connections. Of all professions, the medical had one of the highest percentages of Nazis, leading law, teaching, and even public administration.[6]

In consequence, denazification hit the medical profession particularly hard, especially when a major purge of former Nazis began at the end of September 1945. In the town of Wasserburg a military government detachment, acting on new regulations, disqualified twenty medical doctors, fifteen dentists, fifty-one teachers, ten mail carriers, and twenty policemen. In the rural township of Alzenau the detachment operating there found only three of seventeen local doctors politically clean. In Baden the efficiency of medical and public health services was "greatly reduced"; in Pforzheim a tuberculosis center had to be closed; and in Karlsruhe the directors of both hospitals were dismissed. The large industrial city of Stuttgart faced a "serious public health problem" because twenty-two of the twenty-five top members of the public health staff, as well as most of its hospital chiefs, had been ousted. "The situation [in Stuttgart]," reported the military government, "threatened to become chaotic," for no replacements were found despite a prolonged search.[7]

Supposedly, Germans who had been active party members or ardent supporters were forbidden to practice any profession, to hold any post of honor, or to perform any work above the level of manual labor. But reality intruded. The sick could hardly be allowed to die because their doctors had joined the Nazi party. In practice, therefore, the situation rapidly became more destructive to the denazification law than to the medical profession. The military government detachments issued so-called temporary work permits to people whose services were needed, and because the permits were never revoked, doctors

[6] Bailey, "Civil Affairs Hist," pp. 201–30, file 314.7-2; Kenner Diary, bk. 3, pp. 333–34.

[7] Quoted words from HQ, USFET (OMGUS), Weekly CA/MG Field Rpt, 1 Nov 45. See also ibid., 11 Oct 45. Both in file Weekly CA/MG Rpts, box 541, OMGUS, PHB/PWB, RG 260, NARA.

and dentists continued to care for their patients as before.[8]

The efforts of all health workers were needed. Long-term problems demanded attention. Public health laboratories had to be rebuilt and pharmacies reopened. Veterinary services also were needed, for, in a nation short of food, control of animal diseases was more than ever essential. Drugs and sera for inoculating farm animals were hard to obtain, and a wartime lapse in efforts to combat tuberculosis left much milk infected. Moreover, one of the postwar epidemics continued, and indeed intensified. Venereal disease emerged as a complex and durable problem, one closely intertwined with American occupation policy.

Experts had long predicted a sharp rise in venereal diseases when hostilities ended. Events soon proved them right. Among the remaining DPs, poor and demoralized females yielded readily to their liberators, whose mood, after months of battle, was to enjoy as much sex as possible as soon as possible. Rape by American soldiers was common, often requiring neither violence nor threats. ("A man who enters a strange house, carrying a rifle in one hand," ruled the judge advocate general of the Seventh Army, "is not justified in believing he has accomplished a seduction."[9]) Military courts punished soldiers convicted of rape, but found the crime hard to prove. The German women were needy, and susceptible to the food and other gifts soldiers could provide. The VD rate among former combat troops, only a fourth that of COMZ forces while the fighting continued, rose rapidly after V–E Day, equaling and then surpassing the rate among support troops.[10]

The end of the war, however, tended to change the character of many liaisons. Peaceful rather than armed conquest became the rule, and relationships developed that were based on personal preference, mutual pleasure, and the hope of marriage. This biological and human process soon caused the Army's nonfraternization policy to collide head-on with its policy on venereal disease. The notion that American soldiers could be transformed into aloof poster figures had never borne much relation to reality. Nonfraternization continued after the war in response to the vengeful feelings of American public opinion, and not to that of the soldiers, some of whom were soon grousing that "the policy is just to give the brass the first crack at all the good looking women." Immured behind barbed wire, American military compounds caused the Germans to remark that their conquerors were the only people in the world who put themselves into concentration camps.[11]

Meanwhile, the rising VD rate mocked the ability of officialdom to enforce nonfraternization. Efforts by the chief surgeon's office to get a ruling from the high command on whether venereal disease could be

[8] Ziemke, *Occupation of Germany*, pp. 182 and 387–88.

[9] As quoted in ibid., p. 220.

[10] 12th Army Group Report of Operations, vol. XIII (Medical Section), pp. 244–45 and 256–58; Padget Interv, 1 August 45, box 223, RG 112, NARA.

[11] As quoted in Ziemke, *Occupation of Germany*, p. 324.

considered evidence of fraternization at first produced no clear policy. Some commanders refused to set up prophylactic stations lest soldiers be encouraged to fraternize, and some men were court-martialed and fined $65 merely for going on sick call with venereal disease. Contradictions abounded, as SHAEF's judge advocate pointed out in May:

> The very establishment of prophylactic stations and the directives requiring reports of the contraction of venereal disease are indicative of the realistic view which the Army has heretofore taken of the problem. Soldiers will fraternize in the manner indicated, in spite of any rules to the contrary, and should they, fearful of being tried by court martial for such fraternization, avoid the use of prophylaxis or checkup, venereal disease may become rampant and completely out of control.[12]

In fact, the VD rate among troops in the theater rose from 56 in April to 177 per 1,000 per year in August 1945, and to 233 in January 1946.

On 4 June, bowing to the inevitable, SHAEF issued orders that contracting venereal disease could not be used either directly or indirectly as evidence of fraternization. In July General Eisenhower modified theater rules to allow fraternization in public places, and on 1 October the policy ended. Nonfraternization split and sank upon the reef of sex, but not until it had allowed the Germans, during the particularly trying year, to enjoy the spectacle of their conquerors "engaged in the most widespread violation of their own laws since Prohibition." [13]

The end of nonfraternization did not, however, halt the VD epidemic. Despite the rapid repatriation of hundreds of thousands of DPs during the summer, some 500,000 remained in Germany, at least half nonrepatriable for political reasons. The fundamental source of the epidemic, however, was the poverty of the Germans that made sex easy to obtain, as well as the confusion and upheaval that attended the organizational changes in the theater and the dispatch of troops to the Pacific or to home. Commands disappeared, boundaries shifted, new organizations were erected in the place of old, and green troops replaced veterans. Control of venereal disease had always depended upon command responsibility. For the moment, lines of authority were hopelessly confused, and low-score men were undisciplined and disorderly.[14] To add to the problem, the War Department suddenly withdrew the familiar V-Packette prophylactic kit and substituted a new, supposedly more effective, item without providing adequate supplies. Only penicillin therapy prevented venereal disease from becoming a serious drain on job performance, for personnel turbulence, supply failures, and the conditions of postwar Germany defeated the traditional methods of prevention.

---

[12] Ibid., p. 325.

[13] Ibid., p. 324. See also Preventive Medicine Division, OofCSurg, HQ, ETOUSA, Semiannual Rpt, January–July 1945, VD Control Branch sec., p. 1; Ltr, HQ, ETOUSA, to CGs of Major Commands, 4 Jun 45, sub: Policy on Relations Between Allied Occupying Forces and Inhabitants of Germany, in 12th Army Group Report of Operations, vol. XIII (Medical Section), pp. 225–29. VD rates are given in Essential Technical Medical Data Rpts, HQ, TSFET, October 1945 and April 1946, boxes 36 and 37, file 350.05, RG 112, NARA.

[14] The subject of redeployment is covered later in this chapter.

With good reason, the military government sought to attack the VD problem among civilians. In August USFET directed compliance with a 1927 public health law, enacted by the Weimar Republic. As a result, facilities for isolation and treatment of victims were established in hospitals, physicians were ordered to report cases, and German health officials were tasked with promoting a VD education program. Because penicillin was not yet available for German use, treatment for syphilis followed the old course, with patients taking arsenicals or mercury preparations. Gonorrhea patients received sulfa drugs; unfortunately, many cases resisted treatment, and hospital space set aside for venereal disease cases filled rapidly, all the more so because shelter and food were available there. On 28 October the Army made penicillin available to the detention hospitals on the grounds that curing gonorrhea was essential to the protection of American troops.[15] The detention wards and buildings now cleared rapidly, and soon cases were being treated on an outpatient basis, enabling workingmen who caught the disease to seek treatment without leaving their families to starve. One ironic side effect of penicillin treatment was noted: Prostitutes were able to ply their trade with briefer interruptions because their "turn-around time" in hospitals had been shortened.[16]

The most serious long-run danger to German health was the shortage of food. The medics could do little but monitor the situation. Apparently, occupation authorities did not at first grasp the dimensions of the problem. During the war German civilians had fared better than those of conquered nations. Especially in towns and small cities that had escaped bombing, survey teams in the spring and summer had found shops well stocked with basic foods and streets thronged with people who appeared adequately clothed and nourished.

However, wrecked transport systems had, in fact, created a spotty pattern of local excess and local need. Early reports from the cities were bleak. In April a nutrition survey team, sent by ETOUSA, had found only a ten-day supply of food on hand in major cities; in industrial Duesseldorf and Essen children were in poor condition and civilians were receiving a basic ration of only 1,000 calories a day. But Allied policy-makers at the time were convinced that the problem of the German economy was to prevent its resurgence, rather than to restore it to meet the calamitous changes that defeat entailed.

The Occupation intensified supply problems by drawing arbitrary military boundaries that divided farm from market areas. Remaining food stocks in the cities were looted by Allied troops, DPs, and the Germans themselves. And throughout western

---

[15] Because penicillin also cured other and more serious illnesses, the military government instituted strict controls to prevent German physicians from diverting it for unauthorized purposes.

[16] Quoted words from Ziemke, *Occupation of Germany*, p. 422. See also Directive, HQ, USFET (to CGs, Western and Eastern Military Districts and Berlin District), 28 Oct 45, sub: Penicillin for Treatment of Gonorrhea Among Civilians, file Penicillin Directives, box 539, OMGUS, PHB/PWB, RG 260, NARA; Morrison C. Stayer and William A. Brumfield, Jr., "Venereal Disease Control in the United States Occupied Zone of Germany," *The Military Surgeon* 100 (May 1947): 375–81.

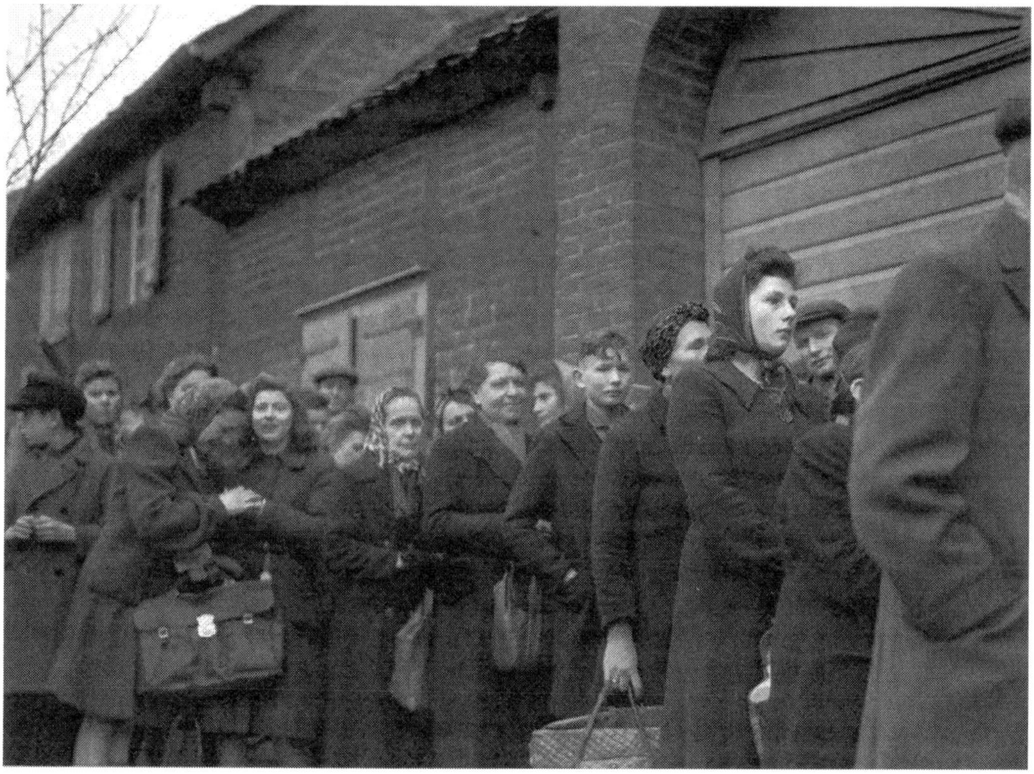

GERMAN CIVILIANS AWAITING THEIR FOOD RATIONS

Germany, an area too heavily populated to feed itself even in normal times, fields lay abandoned while the DPs who had worked them took to the roads and the German men who had plowed and harvested them before the war sat in prison pens.[17]

At the end of August Maj. Gen. Morrison C. Stayer, director of Public Health and Welfare for the military government, reported that nutritional survey teams had found "60 percent of the Germans living on a diet that would inevitably lead to diseases caused by malnutrition." Though workers doing heavy labor got up to 2,800 calories a day, normal consumers received rations whose caloric value apparently varied from about 800 to about 1,150. As a result of quantitative and qualitative deficiencies, avitaminosis and marked weight loss had already appeared in both adults and children. The inevitable consequence of hunger was a vast black market, to which farmers sent their surplus crops and city dwellers sacrificed their prized possessions. GIs, too, were quick to make money by selling food and cigarettes, and as a consequence Quartermaster depots suffered major losses. In this way Americans supported Germans with Army food supplies, but in such a way

[17] 12th Army Group Report of Operations, vol. XIII (Medical Section), pp. 267–74 and 280–82.

as to allow both German and American criminals to profit in the process.[18]

In October G–5, USFET, summarized bleakly the nutritional state of the civil population in the American Zone: The worst conditions were among children, pregnant and nursing women, and city dwellers. Street weighing indicated losses among males of up to 13 percent of body weight, depending on age, and up to 15 percent among women. Vitamin and protein deficiencies were also observed. The worst conditions were in Berlin; the best, as might be expected, in the rural regions of Bavaria.

> In general, no reserves of body weight exist and caloric intakes remain inadequate. Protein is often relatively, if not absolutely, inadequate. Such improvement as has occurred is mainly in vitamins and minerals, the cumulative effect of the summer's supply of non-rationed fruit and vegetables, a source which cannot be depended on in the coming months. The effects of deficiencies are cumulative and often not at once apparent.[19]

Vigorous efforts by Clay and the Germans produced supplies to raise the ration to an official 1,550 calories. Yet, as matters developed, the American Zone squeaked past the time of worst privation as much by luck as by policy. In contrast to the previous year, the winter was mild. The harvest was unexpectedly good. Washington provided imports to maintain the new ration. An expected influx of German refugees from the East did not materialize until late in the winter. Many individual Americans proved to be more generous to their former enemies than the formal policies of their government might have suggested. Private contributors in the United States organized under the Council of Relief Agencies Licensed To Operate in Germany and, with official sanction, consigned substantial tonnages of food and medical supplies to German church and labor groups. By the spring of 1946 a German Central Committee for the Distribution of Foreign Charitable Gifts was in operation, and the military government had begun to accept contributions from non-American voluntary agencies, notably in Switzerland. Most gifts came from people of German background and language, and from labor and religious groups, many of which—like the Mennonites and Lutherans—had ties to a Germany that long antedated Hitler.[20]

Nevertheless, hand-to-mouth living was the rule. By March 1946 food stocks were available for only sixty days, and on 1 April Clay was obliged to reduce the ration again, under pressure from a worldwide food shortage caused by the disruptions of the war. In May and June the normal consumer received only about 1,180 calories a day, and even this low level

[18] As quoted in Ziemke, *Occupation of Germany*, p. 352. See also p. 353. Stayer's position is misidentified in this source. On Stayer, see Name-Rank file, CMH.

[19] Special Rpt, HQ, USFET, 3 Oct 45, sub: Summary of Nutritional State of the Civilian Population in the American Zone of Germany, file CA/MG Rpts, box 541, OMGUS, PHB/PWB, RG 260, NARA.

[20] Ltr, Edward M. O'Connor to Lt Col Alden E. Bevier, PH&W Branch, OMGUS, 25 Mar 46, sub: CRALOG, in file Public Health, box 472. See also Memo, PH&W Branch, OMGUS, 4 Mar 46, sub: Importation of Relief Supplies, in file Centre d'Entr'Aide, box 477. Both in OMGUS, PHB/PWB, RG 260, NARA.

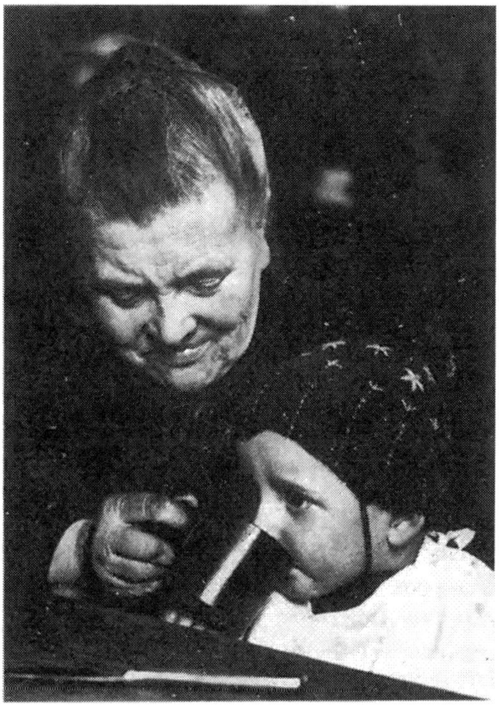

FOOD ASSISTANCE FOR GERMAN REFUGEES *from the East*

could be sustained only by distributing Army surplus stocks. In May a health survey in Mannheim showed that 60 percent of infants had rickets, and random weighing of adults provided evidence of malnutrition in the general population as well. A famine had been avoided, but only a general revival of the German economy could prevent recurrence of the danger. Though a new crisis would strike in the spring of 1947, the best sign for the future of the American Zone was that the United States government had tacitly come to accept the need for such a revival.[21]

Medical Intelligence

While most Army medical personnel concerned themselves with the health of the troops, or with that of the civil population, a select group helped to carry out an elaborate program of technical intelligence. During the war medical intelligence units had developed both in the surgeon general's office and in the medical sections of theater and field commands. In Washington the wartime mission of collecting health information on foreign countries grew into a complex effort, highly integrated with the Army Staff's other technical intelligence-gathering programs. Ultimately, the once modest files of the surgeon general's unit constituted a worldwide geography of disease. On the war fronts medical materiel was collected and forwarded to the Medical Equipment Laboratory at Carlisle Barracks, Pennsylvania, where captured drugs, biologicals, and equipment were assembled, tested, and analyzed. In ETOUSA Hawley's Medical Intelligence Branch sought out information on German diseases and methods of control, on enemy casualty statistics, and on the Nazi biological warfare program. In the 12th Army Group an elaborate field program developed, as army surgeons attached technical intelligence teams to their S–2 sections and the gathering of information and materiel extended down to the medical groups and battalions.[22]

[21] Lucius D. Clay, *Decision in Germany* (Garden City, N.Y.: Doubleday, 1950), pp. 266–69.

[22] See Preventive Medicine Division (or Service), OSG, WD, Annual Rpts, 1943–45, boxes 17 and 18, RG 112, NARA; James M. Simmons et al., *Global Epidemiology: Geography of Disease and Sanitation* (Philadel-

Continued

A second effort developed in quite a different way and for different purposes. Interest in Germany's industrial and technical secrets was not wholly a concern of the military. The potential economic value of enemy discoveries aroused the interest of the American research establishment, and of drug and medical supply manufacturers, among many others. By the end of the war the Allies had determined to treat ideas, processes, and to some extent the personnel of the German industrial and scientific machine as prizes of war.

During preinvasion planning SHAEF set up the T (for Technical) Subdivision in its G–2 section to plan the exploitation of scientific and industrial targets, a term which included both technical processes and individuals who might possess useful knowledge. A detention center for special prisoners was set up, first in Paris and then in Kransberg Castle outside Frankfurt, and code-named DUSTBIN. The prime catch were the rocket builders from Peenemuende, but medical experts, like Dr. Karl Brandt, the Reich's commissioner for sanitation and health, were likewise sought out. Ultimately a broad progam emerged, guided by the inter-Allied Combined Intelligence Operations Subcommittee, headquartered in London, which included both theater personnel and experts sent by the Technical Industrial Intelligence Committee, an agency of the Joint Chiefs of Staff.[23]

Biological warfare remained a topic of great interest. Wartime had seen much Allied concern over reports of German efforts in the field. The British and American governments, overestimating Nazi interest in such weapons, justified elaborate programs for the research, development, manufacture, and stockpiling of biological weapons on the need to defend and retaliate against an enemy attack. In preparing for the invasion of Europe the Medical Department collected blood samples from German prisoners, with the aim of learning whether group immunizations had been given against botulism, plague, cholera, epidemic typhus, psittacosis, and lymphocytic choriomeningitis, as a prelude to infecting Allied soldiers. No evidence was discovered. For a time considerable excitement reigned west of the Atlantic over stories spread by a refugee doctor in Switzerland that the Germans planned to use the toxin of botulism in shells. Supplies of toxoid had been developed at the main American biological warfare installation in Camp Detrick, Maryland, and Surgeon General Kirk urged the inoculation of all Allied soldiers destined to participate in the D-Day landings. But American and British authorities in England both discounted the stories, and Hawley recommended only that the toxoid be stockpiled in case of need.[24]

The fall of Germany produced a flurry of activity by the Americans and British, aimed at uncovering the whole story of the German biological

phia: J. B. Lippincott Co., 1944); Hoff, ed., *Special Fields*, pp. 288–89; Surg, 12th Army Group, Hist, January–June 1945, pp. 18–19.

[23] Ziemke, *Occupation of Germany*, p. 314.

[24] Ltrs, Col John E. Gordon to Col Karl E. Lundeberg, Chief, Preventive Medicine Service, OSG, WD, 24 Jun 44, and Lundeberg to Gordon, 7 Jun 44, file 17, box 4, RG 112, NARA.

warfare effort. The results were disappointing. A research office existed within the *Heerensanitaets Inspektion*, the German equivalent of the surgeon general's office, under Prof. H. Kliewe. About 45 years old, Kliewe was an agreeable and informative prisoner, "unassuming and talkative," who impressed his captors as "a good hard [scientific] worker without much imagination." The program he headed had received little encouragement from either Hitler or the Wehrmacht high command, who viewed biological weapons as impractical and hard to control. Kliewe's files, seized intact in the vault of a monastery at Niederviehbach, Bavaria, yielded a detailed picture of a confused and ineffectual effort, carried out largely under the patronage of Hermann Goering. Until 1940 Germany had been wholly inactive in the field. But in 1943 intelligence reports of Allied work led Hitler to order the study of defensive measures. A committee was set up under the German Army's Ordnance Department; but, in view of Goering's interest, the State Research Council also took a hand, and Heinrich Himmler, ever ready to expand the functions of his own empire, offered to provide experimental facilities at a concentration camp.[25]

Though Hitler forbade research in offensive weapons, work began under a committee code-named *BLITZABLEITER* (Lightning Rod). "In order to give suitable protective regulations," its members explained, "the enemy's technique of introduction must be tested. Therefore the experiments planned are not at variance with the Fuehrer's order." Himmler's influence may have appeared as one member of the committee urged "experiments on human beings." Trials were actually scheduled with agents that might damage agricultural production, including hoof and mouth disease, potato beetles, and Japanese beetles.[26]

But meetings of the committee were irregular, and various research groups went their own way without central direction. Kliewe carried out studies with aerosols, the method most favored by American researchers at Camp Detrick, Maryland. Goering's man in the field, a Dr. Blome,[27] was chief of cancer research for the State Research Council. When the organization took over the Nesselstedt Monastery for cancer studies, Blome planned to construct laboratories nearby for biological warfare experiments, as well. Work began in 1944, but little had been accomplished by the following year, when the Red Army arrived. Another experimental station at Gersberg had barely been started; when the Americans captured the site, they found only a few excavations among a stand of pine trees. All in all, the German program amounted to very little compared with American, British, and (presumably) Russian endeavors, and to almost nothing compared with the contemporary Jap-

[25] See Rpt, ALSOS, 12 Sep 45, sub: A Review of German Activities in the Field of Biological Warfare, in file 22, RG 112, NARA. Quotation on p. 20. This comprehensive report was prepared by American and British medical intelligence officers.

[26] Ibid., p. 26, file 22, RG 112, NARA.

[27] It is unclear whether the "Doctor Blome" mentioned here is identical with Kurt Blome, a longtime Nazi.

anese development and use of biological warfare agents against China.[28]

More portentous was a surprise development: the German invention of nerve gases. In May 1945 Colonel Beasley, the ADSEC surgeon, received from a liaison officer with the Ninth Army a report of a large, well-camouflaged chemical warfare plant at Lossa. A new war gas, believed to be an organic phosphorus compound, had been found in cylinders and bombs. "The chemical is very persistent with a very distinctive 'bon-bon' odor," the officer wrote, and atropine sulphate was the only known antidote. Neither German nor American gas masks offered adequate protection, and rubber clothing was needed to prevent it from penetrating the skin. Japanese chemical warfare officers were said to have visited the plant and "undoubtedly have the gas." [29]

Later, after grilling I. G. Farbenindustrie employees at the cartel's Frankfurt headquarters, a team representing the Combined Intelligence Operations Subcommittee was able to develop a basic picture of the new weapon, its chemical structure, production methods, and medical effects. Of the lethality of the gases the Germans had invented—Tabun, Sarin, and Soman—there could be no doubt: In the Farben plant at Dyhernfurth, later seized by the Russians, four pipefitters had died in convulsions despite protective clothing. According to the Farben workers, the first gas, Tabun, had been discovered in the 1930s during routine studies of organophosphate insecticides. A chemist had complained of difficulty with seeing and feared that he was losing his sight. A chemical he was working with proved to be affecting his nervous system, causing contraction of his pupils, and the military implications of the discovery were realized soon after.

Officers of the Chemical Warfare Service and their British counterparts led the investigation, but the nerve gases posed an evident medical problem. Their physiological effects were little short of spectacular. The gases prevented the body from breaking down acetylcholine, a chemical produced by the motor nerves to contract the muscles. Because a victim's muscles could contract but could not relax, violent cramps, nausea, and involuntary defecation and urination occurred, followed by convulsions and death when paralysis reached the muscles that control breathing. Tabun's lethality was twenty times that of phosgene, a common agent of World War I; Sarin was twice as toxic as Tabun; and Soman was two to three times as toxic as Sarin. The Russians also discovered the nerve gases in Germany and quickly dismantled and shipped east a plant devoted to their manufacture. Thus a new and deadly weapon entered the arsenals

---

[28] On Allied and Japanese endeavors, see Robert Harris and Jeremy Paxman, *A Higher Form of Killing: The Secret Story of Chemical and Biological Warfare* (New York: Hill and Wang, 1982), pp. 83–135, 141–43, and 152–54. See also Intel Rpt C-H/30A, sub: Resume of Russian BW Intelligence Gathered by German Intelligence Organization, pp. 53–56, file 14 (BW), box 3, ETO-Surgical Section, RG 332, NARA.

[29] Memo, George R. Gallagher to Surg, ADSEC, [May 1945], in Ninth U.S. Army Liaison Rpts file, Burwell Papers, MHI. The story that the Japanese had the gas was false.

of all the major powers that survived the war.[30]

Medical intelligence officers were also interested in the once splendid German medical profession, its fate in wartime and its recent discoveries. Investigators reported that medical institutions were in sad shape. Many hospital buildings, schools, and laboratories had been heavily damaged and medical faculties militarized or dispersed. The Luitpold Hospital of the University of Wuerzburg had been battered by an air raid in March 1945; at Marburg the surgical and ophthalmological building had been destroyed and some laboratories looted. The famed medical faculty of the University of Vienna had been dispersed, most into the lake region of Upper Austria, and other skilled workers and teachers had likewise been scattered by the war.[31]

Nevertheless, research continued, though isolated from international medicine. The most striking evidence of the provincialism of the Germans was their relative ignorance of penicillin, which they knew only from reprints of British and American journal articles. Progress occurred in laboratories, but the secrets of large-scale production had never been learned. Yet able men, despite all difficulties, had continued to make interesting discoveries. American doctors interviewed Prof. Dr. Gerhardt Kuentscher, who had made his name as an orthopedic surgeon by developing the use of nails in treating fractures of the long bones. Kuentscher, 45 years old, spoke English fairly well and was very cooperative. Basically, his method was to drive V-shaped nails down the marrow channels of the broken bones, where they served as internal splints, eliminating the need for postoperative traction, casts, and exterior support. Kuentscher emphasized the need for caution and for special training before surgeons used the technique, which in inexpert hands had produced many failures. Though attracted, the Americans continued to view his method with reserve, remarking with a touch of chauvinism that "the method needs extensive trial in American hands."[32]

Examination of the well-equipped Physiology Institute at the University of Goettingen, where aeromedical research had been carried on, brought out the extent to which the war, by dividing the scientific world, had induced duplication of effort. The American and British investigating team—medical officers of the Army, Navy, and Air Force of both countries—concluded that German aviation medicine was largely inferior to that of the Allies. Nevertheless,

[30] Intel Rpts, CIOS, subs: The Medical Aspects of German Chemical Warfare, app. III of Chemical Warfare Installations in the Munsterlager Area, file XXXI-86, box 687; Chemical Warfare, I. G. Farbenindustrie A. G., Frankfurt/Main, file XXX-19, box 681; Technical Information on Tabun and Sarin, file XXIII-24, box 672. All in Army Staff G-2-P Records, 1946-51 (CIOS), RG 319, NARA. See also John Cookson and Judith Nottingham, *A Survey of Chemical and Biological Warfare* (New York: Monthly Review Press, 1969), pp. 213-20. On the discovery of Tabun, see also Harris and Paxman, *A Higher Form of Killing*, p. 53.

[31] A Series of Interviews With Members of German Medical Schools, Research Institutes and Hospitals, file XXVI-32, box 676. See also Intel Rpt, CIOS, sub: German Medical Schools, file XXX-50, box 681. All in Army Staff G-2-P Records, 1946-51 (CIOS), RG 319, NARA.

[32] Miscellaneous Interviews on Medical Practice and Research in Germany, file XXIX-13, box 679, Army Staff G-2-P Records, 1946-51 (CIOS), RG 319, NARA.

USSTAF found ongoing experiments on high-speed jet and rocket flying of sufficient interest to take over a wing of the Kaiser Wilhelm Institute in Heidelberg, permitting German scientists to continue their work under American direction. In this case German aircraft technology had outstripped the Allies, and medical research had followed suit.[33]

The many misuses of medicine fostered under the Third Reich emerged in a series of war crimes trials, notably the "doctors' trial" at Nuernberg in 1946–47 and, almost twenty years later, the Auschwitz trial prosecuted by the Federal Republic of Germany. Doctors had taken part in human experimentation and in attempts to devise quick methods of mass sterilization—as one defendant put it, "not only to defeat the enemy but to exterminate him." Though the full story of these atrocities lies outside the scope of this study, Army doctors played a role in the preliminary investigations, in gathering evidence, and in attempting to assess the medical value of experimental results that had been gained at terrible cost.[34]

Experimentation on the living had been a feature of several concentration camps. At Buchenwald First and Third Army medical officers heard stories, later confirmed, of experiments on prisoners aimed at standardizing a typhus vaccine. At Dachau experimental work had been carried out in Bunker No. 5, from which few prisoners emerged alive. Favored guinea pigs had been Russian prisoners of war, German and Polish Jews, and Polish Roman Catholic priests. After sufficient training in the camp, the victims proved to be excellent experimental subjects, obeying orders "*wie auf Draht gezogen, widerspruchslos*"—like puppets, making no objection. Brought close to suffocation by one experiment, a prisoner continued to beg permission to breathe: "One moment, please . . . may I breathe? Is it all right if I breathe?" He took a deep breath and said, "Thank you very much. . . ."[35]

The doctors who carried out the experiments were a varied lot. Seventy-four-year-old Dr. Klaus Schilling, director of the SS Malaria Experimental Station at Dachau, had in happier years been chief of the Department of Tropical Diseases at the Robert Koch Institute in Berlin. In the concentration camp he accepted the prisoners chosen for him by the commandant—

[33] Intel Rpt, CIOS, sub: Aviation Medicine, General Medicine, Veterinary Medicine, Chemical Warfare, p. 19, file XXVIII–59, box 679, Army Staff G–2–P Records, 1946–51 (CIOS), RG 319, NARA. See also Ltr, Col J. B. Gordon, AG, USAFE, to CG, USFET, 1 Aug 45, sub: Exploitation of German Aviation Medicine Research, file Aviation, box 471, OMGUS, PHB/PWB, RG 260, NARA.

[34] On Nazi medical atrocities, see Andrew C. Ivy, *Doctors of Infamy* (New York: Henry Schuman, 1949); Jack S. Boozer, "Children of Hippocrates: Doctors in Nazi Germany," *The Annals of the American Academy of Political and Social Science* 450 (July 1980): 83–97 (quotation on p. 85); *Trials of War Criminals Before the Nuernberg Military Tribunals Under Control Council Law No. 10, October 1946–April 1949*, Washington, D.C., vols. I–II; Bernd Naumann, *Auschwitz: A Report on the Proceedings Against Robert Karl Ludwig Mulka and Others Before the Court at Frankfurt*, intro. Hannah Arendt (New York: Frederick A. Praeger, 1966); and Robert Jay Lifton, *The Nazi Doctors: Medical Killing and the Psychology of Genocide* (New York: Basic Books, 1986).

[35] First quotation from Intel Rpt, CIOS, sub: The Treatment of Shock From Prolonged Exposure to Cold, Especially in Water, p. 40, file XXVI–37, box 675. Second quotation from Intel Rpt, CIOS, sub: Aviation Medicine, General Medicine, Veterinary Medicine, Chemical Warfare, p. 12, file XXVIII–59, box 679. Both in Army Staff G–2–P Records, 1946–51 (CIOS), RG 319, NARA.

"definitely not volunteers," his interrogators noted. Schilling sought to produce immunity to malaria by repeated infections; as soon as the patient's temperature rose, he instituted therapy with Atabrine or quinine. Though admitting that "these afebrile attacks of malaria were pretty hard on the patients," he protested that "only a few" had died. Emphasizing that the experimental subjects had better treatment than the average prisoner, he claimed to have known nothing of the horrors of the camp in which he worked. "It was difficult," said one interrogator, "to get a straight story from him." [36]

Some of the most horrifying experiments had been carried out during 1942 with a low-pressure chamber. The aim, as the two doctors involved explained in a secret report to Himmler, was to clarify the question of how the human body would respond to a blowout in a pressurized aircraft cabin. To answer this "purely scientific" question, victims were subjected to rapid decompression, inducing agonizing cases of the bends. Among other results, the experimenters noted "severe symptoms of anoxic cerebral dysfunction . . . clonic convulsions, respiratory disturbances similar to the convulsive respiration of agony, temporary blindness and paralysis of limbs, and severe post-hypoxemic confusional 'twilight' states." Recommending that all involved in the experiments be tried as war criminals, medical officer Maj. Leo Alexander remarked that the suffering involved had "failed to add one iota" to what other investigators had already learned from more conventional methods of scientific inquiry.[37]

A series of experiments directed by an SS doctor, Sigmund Rascher, represented another venture into aviation medicine—in this case, with the aim of discovering the best means to revive crash victims downed at sea. Some features of the protocol approached a kind of satanic farce. After long immersion in ice water, naked victims were placed between the bodies of women from the brothel at Ravensbrueck Concentration Camp. In the background hovered Doctor Rascher, rectal thermometer in hand, ready to take the temperature of any who revived enough to attempt intercourse. Yet, under the direction of another and more competent physiologist, experiments with hot baths turned up useful experimental data. "The method of rapid and intensive rewarming in a hot water bath of 45°C of people in shock from exposure to cold, especially in water," wrote Major Alexander, "should be immediately adopted as the treatment of choice by the Air-Sea Rescue Services of the United States Armed Forces." [38]

---

[36] Quoted words from Intel Rpt, CIOS, sub: Tropical Medicines and Other Medical Subjects in Germany, p. 11, file XXXV. See also Miscellaneous Interviews on Medical Practice and Research in Germany, file XXIX-13. All in box 679, Army Staff G-2-P Records, 1946-51 (CIOS), RG 319, NARA.

[37] First quotation from Intel Rpt, CIOS, sub: Miscellaneous Aviation Medical Matters, app. 20, p. 139. Second quotation from ibid., p. 14. See also pp. 12-13. In file XXIX-21, box 680, Army Staff G-2-P Records, 1946-51 (CIOS), RG 319, NARA. Those involved became defendants in the "doctors' trial"; some were executed.

[38] Quoted words from Intel Rpt, CIOS, sub: The Treatment of Shock From Prolonged Exposure to Cold, Especially in Water, p. 68, file XXVI-37, box 675, Army Staff G-2-P Records, 1946-51 (CIOS), RG 319, NARA. Rascher was shot two weeks before

Continued

Who Goes Where, When, and How?

The work done by Army doctors ranged from protecting the health of the German people to uncovering the details of war crimes. But for most medical personnel, officers and enlisted alike, the months that followed V–E Day had little to do with the conquered people. For the majority the central concerns were the war that still went on in the Pacific, and the seemingly endless processes of redeployment and readjustment that accompanied the transfer of troops to battlegrounds on the other side of the world.

Invasion of the Japanese home islands impended, and the desperate struggle waged by the defenders of Okinawa in the spring of 1945 promised resistance of suicidal fury. But for some fortunate veterans of the European and African fighting, demobilization rather than a new war seemed to be in the cards. In particular, the surgeon general was feeling "urgent pressure by Congress and civilian communities to relieve from active duty all medical officers not actually professionally engaged." Faced with demands both from the Pacific and from the home front, General Kirk drew the obvious conclusions: "ETO repeat ETO—MTO repeat MTO—alone is [*sic*] surplus."[39]

Medical Department personnel formed, of course, only a small part of the vast redeployment that impended. The logistical problem was immense, but official policy made it more complex still. For years the Army had been developing a scheme based on the general principle that those who had fought longest and hardest should be returned home for discharge. Termed readjustment, this attempt at fairness led quickly to monumental practical difficulties and endless paperwork. When combined with the transfer of units, it created a logistical nightmare.[40]

The Army divided units of the European Theater into four categories. In the first were those (like the Third and Seventh Armies) designated as occupation forces. In the second were those overseas less than one year that were to be transferred to the Pacific, either directly or by way of the United States. In the third were units to be organized in the theater, either as occupation forces or as transferees to the Pacific. In the fourth were units with long overseas service that were to remain in the theater only while needed and then to be returned to the zone of interior for demobilization. Green troops from American training camps would arrive to replace departing veterans. Millions of tons of equipment awaited crating

the liberation of Dachau, apparently on Himmler's orders, either because he had attempted to fake experimental results or because he knew too much. See also ibid., pp. 41 and 47; A. Mitscherlich and F. Mielke, *The Death Doctors,* trans. James Cleugh (London: Elek Books, 1962), pp. 23–91.

[39] TWX Conference, 7 Aug 45.

[40] On the planning process for redeployment, see Readjustment Regulation 1–1, WD, 15 Feb 45, sub: Personnel Plan for Readjustment of Military Personnel After the Defeat of Germany; Readjustment Regulation 1–2, WD, 15 Sep 44 and 5 Mar 45 (rev.), sub: Personnel Procedures for Readjustment Movements, file HD 300, HQ, ETOUSA; and Basic Plan for Redeployment for Readjustment, 31 May 45. All in file Redeployment Directives ETO '45. See also Rpt, Richards and Fenton to CSurg, HQ, ETOUSA, 15 Apr 45, sub: Visit to Headquarters, Army Service Forces, on Redeployment Problems, file 334 (Redeployment Problems).

and shipment to the Asian battlegrounds.[41]

Some inevitable blunders occurred in the movement of units. Through a War Department error, affiliated hospital units like Harvard's 5th General Hospital, some of which had served in the theater for years, were placed in Category II (transfer to the Pacific) rather than IV (marked for demobilization). Often medical personnel were pulled out of the redeployment process to lend a hand in forwarding other units. On 9 April 1945 COMZ established the Assembly Area Command to operate the camps and staging areas designated to receive units marked for redeployment and to house them during processing. Each camp in each assembly area needed a dispensary, and fixed hospital beds equal to 4 percent of the troop capacity had to be provided and staffed. The new command had its own medical personnel, but too few for the job to be done. Hence, Medical Department transients joined the work as they passed through the camps on their way either to home or to the Pacific.

Some of the assembly areas were huge, and their medical support needs considerable. One of the largest operated near Marseilles under the Delta Base Section. Here in late May Kenner found, overlooking the port city, three engineer regiments more than halfway finished with the construction of a cantonment that sprawled over 10.5 square miles of high arid terrain. Buildings were a mixture of prefabricated and cement block structures and tents; in a nearby quarry, German POWs labored to produce the blocks. About 12,000 people were already staging for departure—not only American military but liberated Russians bound for Odessa. A camp population of 60,000 was expected when construction was complete. A 250-bed central infirmary handled short-term cases, while the seriously ill were evacuated to the 43d General Hospital at St.-Pons. The engineers had erected concrete-block showers, and were laying out athletic fields, tennis courts, a horseshoe pitch, PXs, a beer garden, Red Cross clubs, and an open-air theater seating 10,000. In the base section as a whole 60,000 Americans waited for their orders; 150,000 German POWs worked, if not at jobs, then at suntans. The Germans had their own 2,000-member medical establishment—doctors, nurses, and enlisted men. Eventually the Delta Base Section had five general and three station hospitals operating between Biarritz and Nice, most to serve the transients—more than 13,000 beds, of which almost 9,000 were occupied.[42]

Yet with all its difficulties, the movement of units was simply a large version of a familiar task. What raised it to a new level of complexity was the Army's determination to deal fairly

[41] On redeployment plans and methods, see SOP, OofCSurg, HQ, ETOUSA, 15 May 45, sub: Readjustment of Medical Department Officers for Redeployment, and also AGO, WD, 4 Nov 44, sub: War Department Policies and Procedures Governing the Redeployment of the Army Upon the Cessation of Hostilities in Europe. Both in file HD 370.5 (Redeployment Directives), box 307, RG 112, NARA.

[42] Memo, Kenner to ACofS, G–4, SHAEF, 10 Jun 45, sub: Report of Inspection of Medical Service, Delta Base Section, during Inclusive Period 14–22 May 1945, in Medical Division, COSSAC/SHAEF, War Diary, July 1945; Surg, Delta Base Section, Annual Rpt, 1945, p. 7.

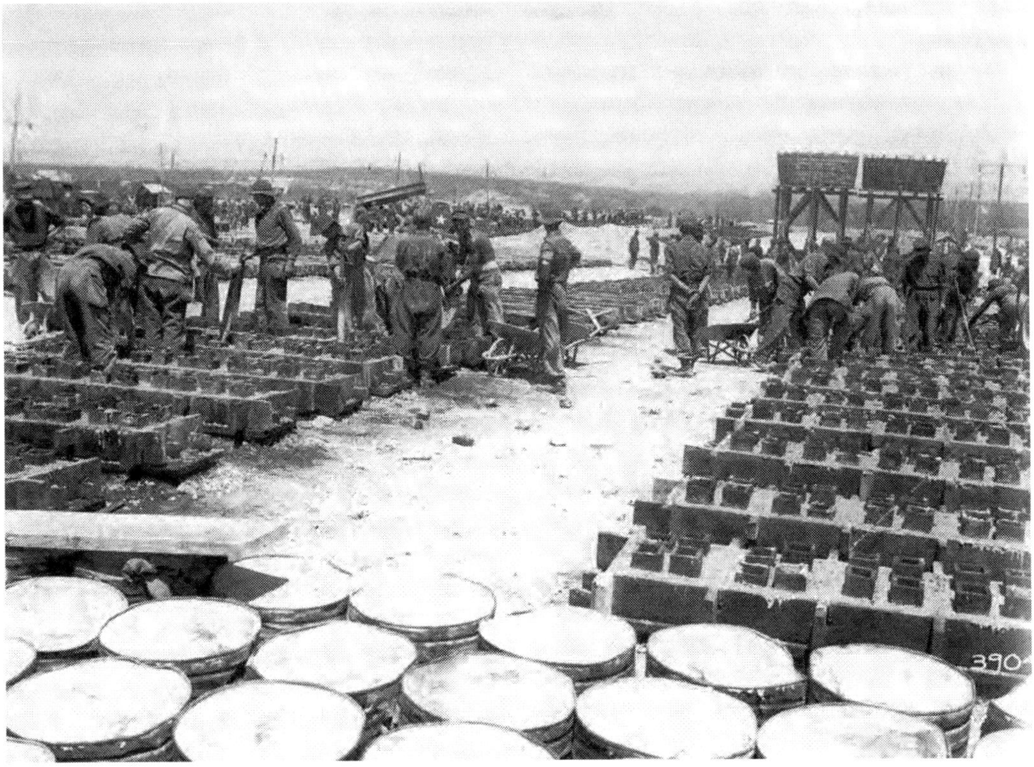

POW LABORERS AT DELTA BASE SECTION STAGING AREA *near Marseilles*

with the individual soldier, by demobilizing those with the longest and most difficult service. The Army planned a partial demobilization of about 1 million men to follow the defeat of Germany. Not only units but men and women had to be categorized, on the basis of individual adjusted service ratings (ASR). Elements of this point score included total time of service since 1941, number of months served overseas, combat service, decorations, and number of dependent children. With 85 points an enlisted man or woman would be discharged; with fewer, further service would be required. While no similar critical score was established for officers before the surrender of Japan, their point score had to be taken into account in determining whether they would serve again in combat. Provided that no pressing need existed, the high-score officer might reasonably hope for early discharge.[43]

But how, in practice, was readjustment to be combined with redeployment? Personnel officers from major commands—the Army Air Forces, the field armies and army groups, and the

[43] John C. Sparrow, *History of Personnel Demobilization in the U.S. Army*, DA Phamphlet 20-210 (Washington, D.C., 1954), pp. 64-84. The critical score was reduced to 80 points after V-J Day and, in response to political pressures, repeated downward revisions followed.

Ground Force Reinforcement Command—got a look at the theater's plan at a conference held in Paris on 15 May 1945. Individuals with lower than the critical score first had to be shifted from Category IV units to Categories I or II, that is, either to the occupation forces or to those marked for the Pacific. Similarly, high-score men and women had to be moved from Category I and II units to Category IV. In preparing a unit for the Pacific, personnel experts first withdrew all who were physically unqualified for combat; then transferred the high-score people; then filled their places with low-score soldiers or, in the case of officers, with other high-score men who were to be retained on the grounds of their essential qualifications.[44]

Much confusion resulted. By 1945 most units were composites of regulars and draftees, veterans and replacements. The long-service men were far more likely to be in positions of authority, and disproportionate losses in experience and skill, leadership and expertise loomed on every side. "You suddenly lost the chief of surgery," complained a senior medical officer who had observed the effect on the hospitals. "You suddenly lost the chief of medicine. . . . And they were ordered to Camp Lucky Strike or they were ordered to Camp Chesterfield, where they sat, in many cases." [45] One hard-hit example was the 127th General Hospital at Nancy, France, which lost the assistant chief of the surgical service, the chief of the orthopedic section, the chief of the general surgical section, an orthopedic ward officer, and an anesthetist.

Some exceptions to the redeployment rules had to be taken into account. A special case was represented by the so-called Green Project, under which 38,000 men and women with skills needed at home were selected and dispatched to the zone of interior by air. For evident reasons, many were medical personnel required by the Army hospitals inundated by the huge lift of battlefield casualties. An early task of the chief surgeon's office was to select 1,000 medical officers of especially long service or urgently needed skills.[46]

For nurses, a critical score of 55 separated those who could be transferred to the Pacific from those who could not. Nurses who had been overseas for two years, or in two theaters of operations, were not required to serve further in combat (though they might, of course, volunteer, and many did—at the 127th, 14 nurses volunteered for duty in the China-Burma-India Theater). Volunteers, however, could not meet the demands of the War Department; 5,300 nurses in all asked for service in the Pacific theaters, but 8,900 were required. Theater policy required that married

[44] OofCSurg, HQ, TSFET, Quarterly Report of Operations, 8 May–30 Sep 45, pp. 26–28; HQ, ETOUSA, 2 Jun 45, sub: Report of G–3 Training Conference, p. 2, file HD 370.5 (Redeployment Training).

[45] Shambora Interv, 8 Oct 62, p. 32, CMH.

[46] See Draft Directive, COMZ, ETOUSA (to CGs, Seine, Delta, and United Kingdom Base Sections), 11 May 45, sub: Green Project for Return of Military Personnel From Europe to ZI, in box 311, RG 112, NARA; Memo, TSG to ACofS, Operations Division, WD, thru CG, ASF, 19 May 45, sub: Period I Requirements of Medical Department Personnel Within War Department Readjustment and Redeployment Regulations, file Green Project.

nurses be placed in occupation or reserve units, setting off a flurry of weddings.[47]

Between War Department policy, theater rules, and the needs of the Pacific War, personnel officers struggled with a system that was as complex as a Bach fugue but far less harmonious. As of V–E Day the mere calculation of ASR scores, on which everything else depended, was slow and imperfect. The chief surgeon's office found itself drawing upon a pool of less than half its medical officers—those for whom scores were available—to meet demands for immediate full staffing of units scheduled for departure. Lack of information worked injustice at both ends of the scoring range; because their scores had not been computed, some low-point men escaped reassignment to the Pacific and some high-point soldiers missed going home.

On 12 July 1945 the situation reached gridlock. Reassignment of Medical Department officers came to a halt, while the chief surgeon's harassed staff tried to discover which officers were available, where they might be found, and what their scores might be. A central card file was set up by military occupational specialty (MOS). Thereafter, a requisition for a Category II unit—direct transfer to the Pacific—could be met simply by selecting the lowest-score men from the required MOS. The fact that the system was again functional did not, however, make it just. No individual officer could predict his fate on the basis of his score, and those deprived of an anticipated visit home by direct reassignment were apt to be unhappy soldiers.

Moreover, MOS numbers did not really reflect exact gradations of professional skill and experience. Some medical units continued to be readjusted by nonmedical personnel officers at the major commands and, as a result, showed up at assembly areas with professionally unbalanced staffs, requiring new rounds of reorganization that lasted in some cases up until the very moment of sailing. Nurses received separate but not equal treatment; their problems were shunted to the Nursing Division to handle, and "special readjustments of nurses occurred only when deficiencies were noted and reported." Despite such problems, Kenner's staff contrived to impose a measure of rough justice upon readjustment. Nothing, however, could alter the fact that the reassignment process tore veteran units to pieces and destroyed, all too often, the morale it was meant to sustain.[48]

Throughout the upheaval medical personnel, even as they attempted to straighten out their own problems, also examined and provided physical profiles for all troops. Because the profile was essential in determining fitness for future combat service, the theater called for all soldiers to be rated by 1 July. The method in use contained six elements, abbreviated PULHES—physical condition, upper extremities, lower extremities, hearing, eyes, and psychiatric diagnosis. Ratings from one to four were given

[47] 127th General Hospital Annual Rpt, 1945, p. 5; Army Nurse Corps Division, HQ, USFET, Report of Activities, 8 May–30 Sep 45, pp. 15–16.

[48] Army Nurse Corps Division, HQ, USFET, Report of Activities, 8 May–30 Sep 45, pp. 34–40. Quotation on p. 39.

for each element on a scale that ran from "normal" to "serious defect." The resulting score, in turn, was translated into the profile: A or B indicated General Assignment troops; C, Limited Assignment troops; and D, disqualified for future assignment. Doctors involved in the work needed sharp eyes, not only to spot malingerers but to prevent collusion between commanding officers and unit surgeons who sought to rid their units of men who were physically fit but maladjusted. While profiling implied much tedious routine work, and while errors did occur (the chief surgeon cited a frostbite victim whose L-3 rating did not prevent a reinforcement depot from rating his general condition P-1), the system was fundamentally simple and workable, a fortunate circumstance under the conditions that existed in the theater during the summer of 1945.[49]

A New Upheaval

Army planners anticipated that a year would elapse between the surrender of Germany and the fall of Japan. The explosion of two atomic bombs during August 1945 left the whole structure of planning—for partial demobilization, systematic readjustment, the Pacific buildup, and the invasion of the enemy's home islands—one ruin among many.

The vast medical establishment built for the war must now, in large part, be collapsed like a tent and disposed of. The first task was to reverse the schedule of deployment. Instead of hastening low-score units to the Pacific, the theater must retain them. High-score units took their place in the pipeline, bypassing the Assembly Area Command and moving directly to ports for shipment home. While most Category II units returned to their former commands, a few, already in transit to the Pacific, were diverted home to the indignation of high-score men still awaiting transportation in Europe. By the end of September the categories had been abandoned, and the War Department redesignated its units in Europe as occupation forces; as redeployment forces, whose next stop was home; or as liquidation forces, technical service units whose special task consisted in closing out facilities that were no longer needed.[50]

Under the new dispensation, the ASR continued to be of some importance. Those with the highest scores supposedly returned home; those with the middling scores (60–79 points) served as liquidation forces; and those with the lowest scores, along with professional soldiers who volunteered to stay in Europe, entered the Occupation. However, theory often failed to square with practice. Because the theater had precipitately shipped out its lowest-score men, many were now permanently lost to the occupation forces that needed them. Their loss, the departure of high-score personnel, and normal attrition caused by sickness, compassionate leaves, and

[49] Charles M. Wiltse, ed., *Physical Standards in World War II*, Medical Department, United States Army in World War II (Washington, D.C.: Office of the Surgeon General, Department of the Army, 1967), pp. 68–71; Surg, Channel Base Section, Hist, January–June 1945, p. 6.

[50] Resume of Activities of Divisions of Medical Section, HQ, TSFET, p. 1; Directive, HQ, USFET, 6 Oct 45, Redeployment and Readjustment Following Cessation of Hostilities.

so forth, seriously compromised some essential services. Among medical specialists, orthopedic surgeons in particular were depleted by the process, a misfortune for many young soldiers whose method of driving jeeps resulted in large numbers of broken bones. By the end of 1945 shortages also developed or threatened in otolaryngology, ophthalmology, and radiology.

Overall, however, the worst effect was the continuing loss of experienced line officers and NCOs. Green men, ill-led, accumulated in occupation units, and the results showed up through the medical and legal statistics in high rates of disorder, crime, and venereal disease. Quantitatively, however, medical personnel were able to keep up with those they served. Of 15,770 medical officers in the theater on V–E Day, 14,012 returned home by the end of December 1945. In all, some 224,000 officers and men departed by the year's end, and the 258,000 medical troops present when Germany surrendered shrank to 34,000. Yet similar changes transformed the forces they served. At year's end theater strength still topped 600,000 and authorized beds numbered 24,400, but the chief surgeon reckoned the supply of doctors, nurses, and dentists adequate to the reduced demand. Though further reductions were on the way for the theater's medical personnel, the troop basis too was destined to shrink by one-half during the first six months of 1946.[51]

Helping to offset losses of medical officers was the arrival in early 1946 of about 200 replacements, most of them products of the Army Specialized Training Program (ASTP). Established during the war to ensure a continuing supply of new doctors and other professionals, the ASTP since 1942 had provided a free education and living expenses to selected draftees. In return, the 13,000-odd young physicians graduated under the program owed the nation three years of active military service. A godsend during the throes of readjustment, the new arrivals were "enthusiastically received at the various hospitals" of the European Theater.[52]

More serious was the drain on MAC officers. As separation criteria were lowered, personnel officers calculated that by the end of March the theater would have less than half the MACs required to fill its T/O vacancies. Though 150 replacements were dispatched from the zone of interior, the gap that remained obliged the chief surgeon's office to utilize officers without special medical training. An adequate supply of administrative officers could have relieved some of the pressure on the physicians, but in 1945–46 the number of MACs was small. Continuing losses to civilian

[51] Professional Services Division, OofCSurg, HQ, USFET, Periodic Rpt, 8 May–30 Sep 45, p. 5, file 319.1-2, Shambora Papers, MHI. On VD in the occupation units, see below. See also Resume of Activities of Divisions of Medical Section, HQ, TSFET, pp. 3–5.

[52] Quoted words from Essential Technical Medical Data Rpt, HQ, TSFET, March 1946, p. 5, file 350.05, box 37, RG 112, NARA. On the ASTP program, see Marvin A. Kreidberg and Merton G. Henry, *History of Military Mobilization in the U.S. Army, 1775–1945*, DA Pamphlet 20-212 (Washington, D.C., 1955), p. 635; Col Francis M. Fitts, MC, "Training in Medicare, Dentistry, and Veterinary Medicine . . . Under the Army Specialized Training Program, 1 May 1943 to 31 December 1945, Ms no. 3-4BA, RG 319, NARA.

life were especially painful because the war had demonstrated the value of these officers as never before.[53]

Hospitalization and Evacuation

Hospitals throughout the theater were also caught in the successive upheavals of 1945. At a conference on 30 April medics and engineers had agreed to hold planned construction to a minimum in view of the impending end of the war. Bed requirements, equal to 6 percent of troop strength on V-E Day, were projected as being equal to 5.5 percent on D+30, the same on D+60, and to 4 percent on D+90. In May the theater established an evacuation policy of 60 days to speed the movement of the war-wounded home. Immediately after V-E Day a second conference resulted in an agreement to end all construction in Great Britain and the liberated countries, except for two facilities near Le Havre that were intended to receive patients awaiting shipment to the zone of interior.

Meanwhile, the theater sought to utilize its best plants as long as possible, restaffing when the units originally in possession were redeployed. In Germany fixed hospitals were established only as needed to support the Army of Occupation. Pending their departure, the large forces marked for redeployment sent their sick and injured to mobile hospitals or to facilities along the line of communications that had not yet been closed. As troop strength fell, many mobile units also left, until only the minimum needed by the occupation forces remained. In practice, the so-called mobile hospitals that remained in Germany worked out of fixed installations and provided service to area commands; their mobility consisted in the capability to move to the field on short notice, if the units they served were suddenly called out. Whenever possible, the Army used German civilian or military plants to house its patients, though the chief surgeon had first call on other buildings if needed for medical use.

As matters worked out, twenty sites for fixed hospitals were quickly acquired, thirteen in existing civilian or military buildings (*see Map 27*). The work of making the structures suitable for use involved a great deal of scrounging; plumbing, for example, often had to be salvaged from bombed-out structures to enable repairs to get under way at once. Food was cooked on field stoves, until regular fuel shipments could be restored, and Quartermaster laundry platoons continued for the time being to clean pajamas, bedding, and other supplies.[54]

In the Allied nations hospital closures were the order of the day. As previously noted, both POW and civilian labor had become essential to the operation of many large hospitals, both on the Continent and in the United Kingdom Base. An example was the 819th Hospital Center at Verdun. In January 1945 the headquarters, housed in a "spacious, well

[53] Personnel Division, OofCSurg, HQ, TSFET, Hist, 10 Oct–31 Dec 45, p. 2. On the postwar personnel problems of the Army Medical Department, see Albert E. Cowdrey, *The Medics' War* (Washington, D.C.: U.S. Army Center of Military History, 1987), ch. I.

[54] OofCSurg, HQ, TSFET, Quarterly Report of Operations, 8 May–30 Sep 45, pp. 13–16.

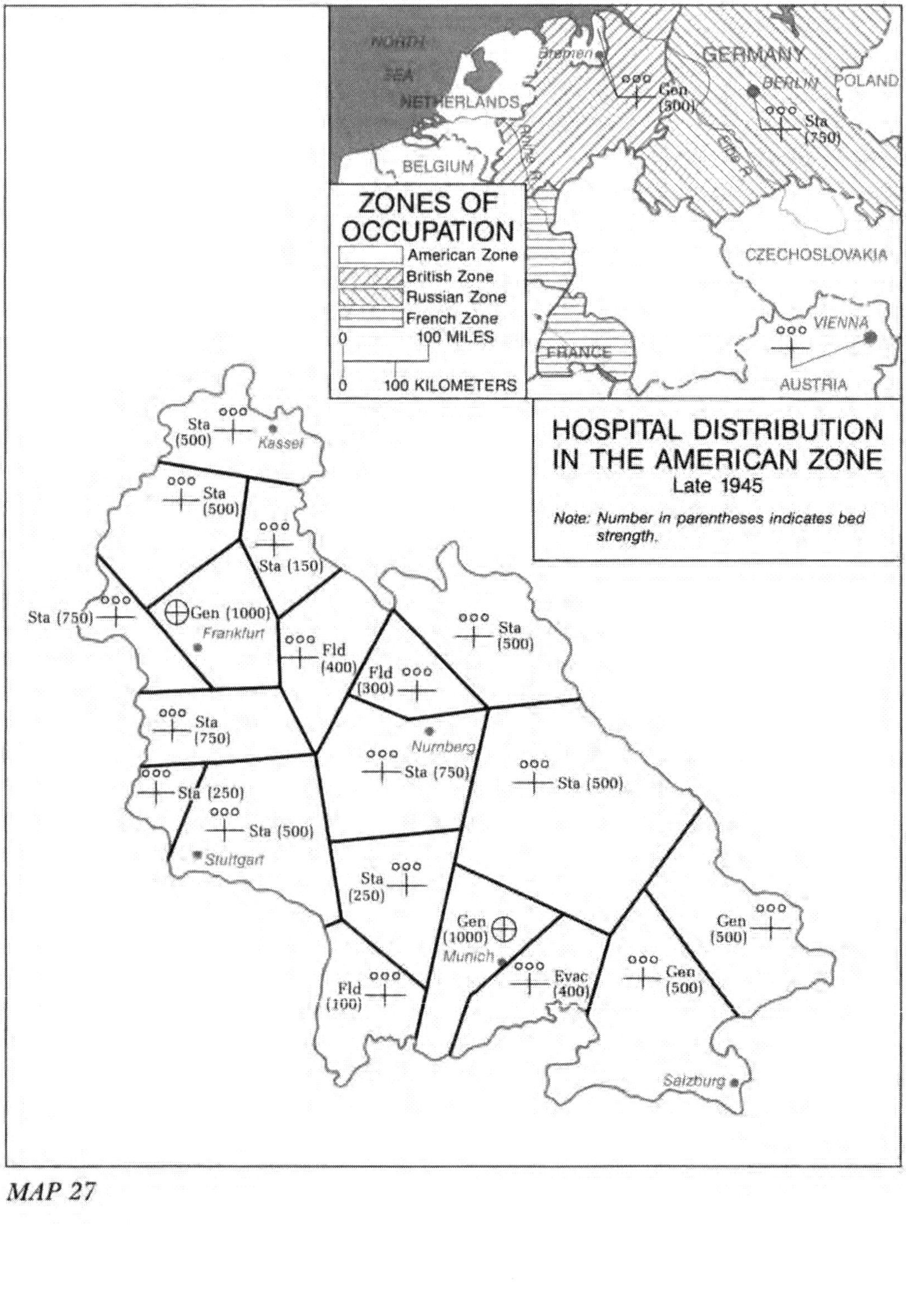
NORTH SEA
NETHERLANDS
BELGIUM
Bremen
GERMANY
BERLIN
POLAND
Gen (500)
Sta (750)
CZECHOSLOVAKIA
VIENNA
AUSTRIA
FRANCE
ZONES OF OCCUPATION
American Zone
British Zone
Russian Zone
French Zone
0 100 MILES
0 100 KILOMETERS
HOSPITAL DISTRIBUTION IN THE AMERICAN ZONE
Late 1945
Note: Number in parentheses indicates bed strength.
Sta (500)
Kassel
Sta (500)
Sta (150)
Sta (750)
Gen (1000)
Frankfurt
Fld (400)
Fld (300)
Sta (500)
Sta (750)
Numberg
Sta (750)
Sta (500)
Sta (250)
Sta (500)
Stuttgart
Sta (250)
Gen (1000)
Munich
Gen (500)
Evac (400)
Gen (500)
Fld (100)
Salzburg

MAP 27

appointed" chateau at Bar-le-Duc, supervised the operation of eight general hospitals with a combined bed capacity that grew to exceed 13,000. Each hospital had its own 500-man POW enclosure, the Germans supplying "many services including those of a technical nature." DPs guarded the captives, and some 300 French civilians worked in each hospital. Every hospital had farms—in all, over 300 acres were in cultivation, and DPs and POWs worked together, planting, tending, and harvesting fresh vegetables for the hospital patients and staff, with the surplus going to the local Quartermaster depot for general issue to the troops. After V–E Day the center became a staging area for medical units destined for the Pacific and also for the Army of Occupation. Here general and station hospitals were processed by center personnel, whose regular duties had disappeared as occupied beds plummeted below 2,000. But the center was a part of the process its staff guided. Hence the month of June was taken up, not with preparing others to move, but with internal redeployment and readjustment. The center's hospitals had varied fates. One, the 95th General Hospital, went to strategic reserve; two went directly, and one indirectly, to the Pacific; one replaced another unit leaving the Continent; and two remained in operation where they were. The prisoners were sent to camps and the DPs to their homes, and the French civilians were dismissed gradually "in order not to disturb the economic stability of the [neighboring] communities." [55]

As closures took place, plants were often returned to the host nation on a lend-lease basis, some with their American equipment intact. In the United Kingdom a few closings preceded V–E Day in response to British requests for the return of specific buildings, but many more resulted from the end of the fighting. Evacuation from the Continent to Great Britain ceased in May, and during that month eight facilities were returned, followed by twenty-six in June. By autumn sixty-eight hospital plants had been closed in Great Britain and forty-four on the Continent; in the Allied countries only fifty-six remained operational in American hands and fourteen others, already empty, awaited formal disposition. Provisional POW hospitals in France were either closed down or concentrated in the Oise Base Section. In June redeployment of units emptied building after building, as ten 1,000-bed general hospitals and twenty-six smaller units departed. During July, August, and September the outflow was continuous and very large. [56]

The closure of large units with intricate equipment charged to their accounts was anything but easy. In England personnel equipped with checklists, issued by the United Kingdom Base, went through a complex ritual. A vexing problem, especially noticeable after V–E Day, when numbers of units were on the move simultaneously, was the lack of timely information from higher headquarters. "On one occasion," noted General

[55] 819th Hospital Center Semiannual Rpt, January–June 1945, p. 3.

[56] Memo, Col S. B. Hays to Beers, Pappas, and Parker, 10 May 45, sub: June Redeployment, file Redeployment, box 304, RG 112, NARA.

Kenner, "ten hospital units were ordered to be ready for movement within ten days." Indecision, followed by sudden demands for mass movement, posed special problems to medical units that had to assist the processing of others.[57]

Disposition of patients depended primarily on whether or not they were battle casualties. The latter departed quickly for home, 42,000 in May alone. RAMPs likewise headed for the zone of interior. On the other hand, the theater had obvious reasons to retain patients from among its occupation troops and, despite the hospital closings, ample resources to do so. Normally, few who were injured during peacetime found any quick road home. For this reason, evacuation totals fell rapidly after the departure of the battle wounded. By autumn the theater was virtually empty of the men whose injuries had helped to bring the victory. However, a considerable patient load remained. Theater hospitals were filled with not only the sick and those with commonplace injuries but also collectors who shot themselves with souvenir weapons and new replacements who were ill-trained and unhandy in the use of firearms. The disorderly state of Germany was also a source of injuries, for some casualties resulted from "skirmishes with the civil population or Displaced Persons."[58]

After the defeat of Japan the pace of hospital closures slowed. In Germany the system stabilized at a level much reduced since the war; in Austria it expanded. In August 1945 the American Zone of Occupation was created in Hitler's homeland, bringing the 124th General Hospital to Salzburg, the 110th Station Hospital to Vienna, and a medical depot to Wels. Revised post-V–J Day plans for hospitalization in Germany provided 38 hospital units to serve the occupation forces, including 8 general hospitals, 10 field hospitals, and 1 convalescent facility. This was a far cry from V–E Day, when the theater had contained 200 fixed hospitals, with 195,000 beds; 118 evacuation, field, and convalescent hospitals, with 63,000 mobile T/O beds; and over 700 other medical units of all types. And in time the new estimates were revised downward as well. By January 1946 the theater held 35 evacuation, field, and convalescent hospitals, with 19,955 beds; of these, 16 were nonoperational, awaiting redeployment or inactivation. By mid-1946 only 4 such units remained, with 1,600 beds, and 17 fixed hospitals, with 10,400. With declining numbers went consolidation, as USFET took over the remaining medical services of the Mediterranean Theater.[59]

Medical training was obliged to keep pace with the rapidly changing course of redeployment and readjustment. With the coming of V–E Day, special courses began to prepare doctors, nurses, administrators, and enlisted men for service in the Pacific. Tropical medicine, the effects of Japanese weapons, and the problems of sanitation and preventive medicine in the Pacific were taught until 15

[57] OofCSurg, HQ, TSFET, Quarterly Report of Operations, 8 May–30 Sep 45, p. 31.

[58] Chief Consultant in Surgery Rpt, January–June 1945, file Professional Services 1945/1, Shambora Papers, MHI.

[59] Resume of Activities of Divisions of Medical Section, HQ, TSFET, Operations Division sec., p. 3.

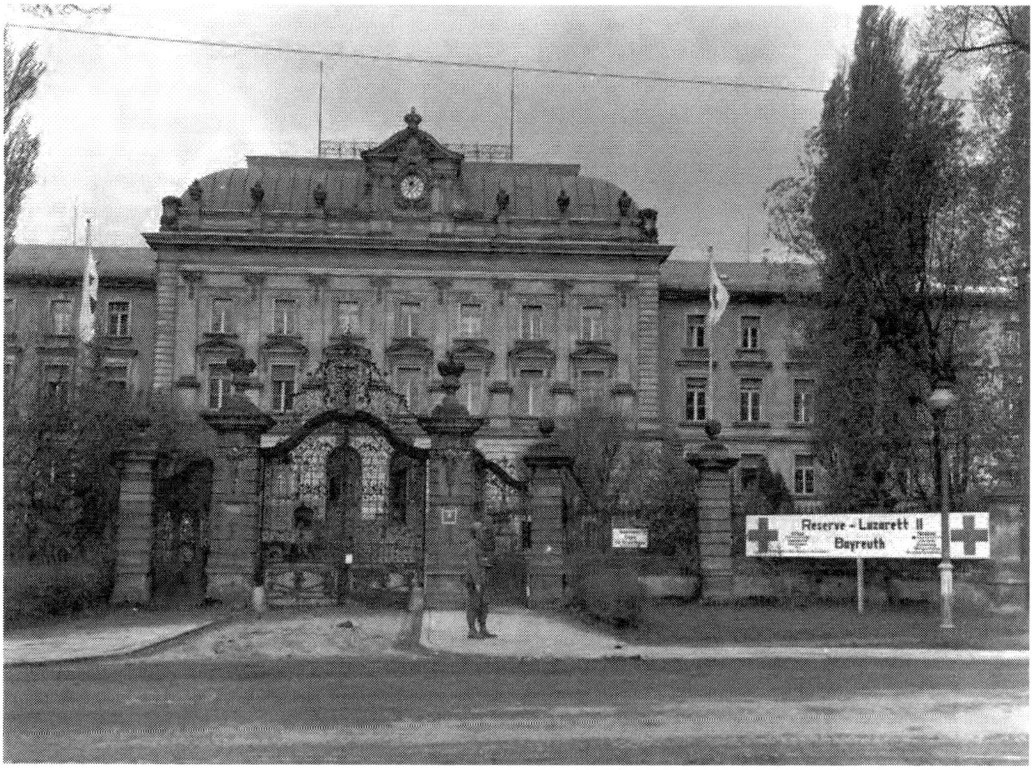

GERMAN HOSPITAL TAKEN OVER BY OCCUPATION FORCES

August 1945, then dropped. But the main theme and most significant problems of the time were those connected with the training of new arrivals in the theater. Of these there seemed to be no end. Heavy emphasis upon on-the-job training reflected the haste and confusion of the process, which left no time (and very often, no qualified instructors) to give formal courses in the many duties the newcomers had to learn. The rapid loss of experts in all fields and in all ranks made training more and more burdensome and difficult as the year advanced. Not only were veteran Americans leaving the hospitals, but the German POW workers who had proven so useful were being rapidly sent to their homes. Some discharged Americans also stayed in the theater to work as civilians in Army installations. But this, too, was a stopgap.

To fill the gaps, hospitals turned increasingly to German civilians, especially for record-keeping and secretarial work. Thus the 101st General Hospital at Berlin on 10 July opened a civilian labor office, which quickly hired 125 Germans as kitchen helpers, laborers, typists, electricians, plumbers, cabinetmakers, tailors, and carpenters, among other jobs. As personnel losses continued, more were hired, and by early December 651 civilians were being "used in almost every department of the hospital." General Kenner recognized the need that existed, and throughout the occupation zone German civilians took clinical as well as support positions, serving as laboratory, X-ray, and dental technicians and as male nurses.[60]

Meanwhile, however, the War Department had announced two policy changes: The total bed allotment for the theater was reduced to 4 percent of the total troop strength, formerly the allotment for fixed beds alone; and the troop basis for the Army of Occupation was shortly afterward reduced to 300,000. The theater's efforts to speed construction and Washington's troop reductions appeared to be headed in opposite directions. Kenner began to reduce the number of field and evacuation hospitals in order to retain his fixed beds, and sought to hold on to hospital sites by limiting the size of the units (station and general hospitals) that were to occupy them. He knew that War Department authorizations took no account of 90,000 civilian dependents expected to arrive during the spring and summer of 1946. Hence, he sought to keep actual beds, to satisfy War Department demands by paper reductions, and to equip his permanent hospitals (if necessary from local sources) for the ten-year period that Army planners then viewed as the minimum length of the Occupation. Amid daily and almost hourly changes in personnel, plans, readjustment standards, and the like, the physical basis for a long-term American presence began to take form.[61]

Medical Supply

Medical supply was a tangle of difficulties. At V–E Day the job of supplying the armies became secondary to the transshipment of supplies to the Pacific. Depot workers, instead of handing out items as needed, turned to a thousand complex details of documentation, marking, and packing. In the process seemingly insignificant matters—obtaining wood for crating was an example—became baffling obstacles for men working amid war-battered civilian economies. Then in September the goal changed again. Allocation to occupation troops remained a duty, but most supplies were either to be returned to the United States or handed over to the liberated nations. Despite the shift in course, the mastery over medical supplies established long ago under ETOUSA was still in evidence, aided by a variety of technical improvements. The field armies consolidated their depots under four major centers—Bremen, Berlin, Weinheim, and Furth. A centralized stock system was set up in August. When TSFET took over, medical supply was centralized in the Office of the Chief Surgeon (*Chart 12*), and electric accounting machines kept tabs, through bimonthly reports from the depots, of stocks on hand and issues throughout the theater.

During redeployment, units on their way to the four main ports of

[60] 101st General Hospital Annual Rpt, 1945, pp. 21–22.

[61] OofCSurg, HQ, TSFET, Quarterly Report of Operations, 1 Oct–31 Dec 45, pp. 9–10.

CHART 12—ORGANIZATION OF THE OFFICE OF THE CHIEF SURGEON, TSFET, OCTOBER 1945

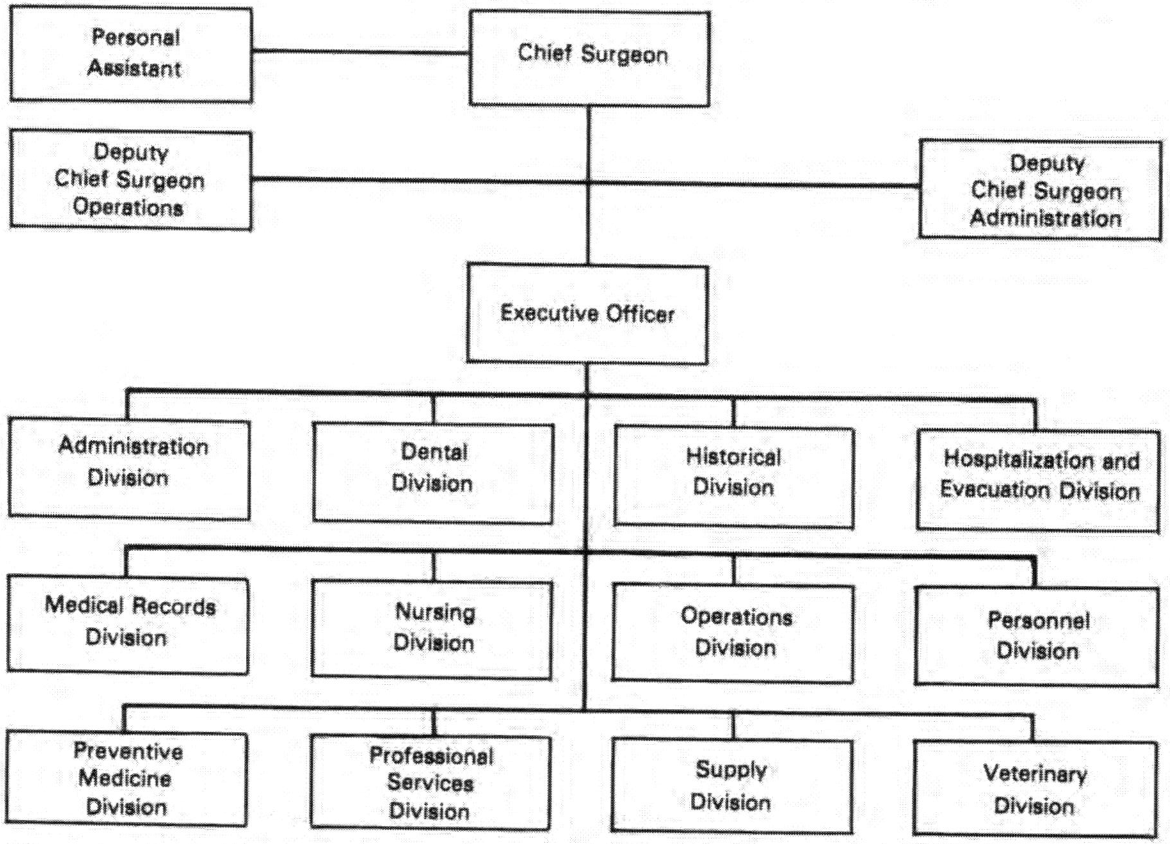

Source: OofCSurg, HQ, TSFET, Quarterly Report of Operations, 11 Oct–31 Dec 45, App. 4.

Marseilles, Rouen, Le Havre, and Antwerp carried their authorized equipment with them, replacing lost or unserviceable items from base section depots in the staging areas. Hospitals turned in their equipment and, in exchange, received complete prepacked assemblies that were prepared at the main depots and shipped to the ports. Some of these procedures changed after the Assembly Area Command began to function, but the general shape of redeployment remained unchanged until V–J Day. After that units no longer needed any but basic equipment, for they no longer faced the possibility of combat. The outmovement of supplies dwindled, and tonnages on hand in medical depots rose dramatically.[62]

Until V–J Day the War Department, after receiving reports of goods on hand, forwarded shipping orders to guide their redistribution. But after V–J Day most of the orders were canceled. The theater now forwarded to the Government Procurement Agency declarations of surplus items. Goods obtained under reverse lend-lease were especially likely to be in this category, because the implements and supplies were unsuitable for use in the United States. The wartime Allies were the main beneficiaries of surpluses, though arranging for payments with their financially strapped governments interposed many delays. Nevertheless, even in 1945 USFET turned over fifty 1,000-bed general hospital assemblies to the French government, eight to the Belgian, and three to the Dutch.

Additionally, mountains of captured German war materiel required control. Between July and October the Supply Division prepared a master catalogue of some 6,400 medical items, with standard nomenclature and stock numbers. Instead of handling out supplies as needed, medical supply officers brought to former Wehrmacht stocks the same sort of centralized management that now characterized the handling of American goods, and with it more effective means of preventing losses and supplying the needs of German civilians through the military government. Captured stocks were consolidated, first to nine and then to six installations; by the end of September the total tonnage of medical supplies on hand had sunk from a high of 31,000 tons to about 18,000.

In the onetime arsenal of Great Britain the seventeen depots of early 1945 were rapidly consolidated to six after V–E Day. As the almost 100 hospitals and dispensaries that had drawn upon them began to close, and as troops were shipped away, the familiar outflow of materiel reversed. Closing hospitals turned in their equipment, and the depots used turn-ins, plus stocks on hand, to fabricate new assemblies for shipment to the Pacific and returned British items to the Government Procurement Agency. While the three major duties of receiving equipment, constructing assemblies, and issuing supplies went on, the workers were themselves being pulled away for redeployment. German POWs were essential during this period, readying equipment for use against their former allies. Their numbers rose steadily at Depot M–24, the last to survive, until 1,200 prisoners and their American supervisors

[62] Wiltse, ed., *Medical Supply*, pp. 383–87.

were working around the clock. At V-J Day all except routine activity ceased for a month, then resumed—now with the object of closing the whole wartime medical establishment down for good.[63]

Health of the Troops

Personnel turbulence and loss of manpower also dominated the field of preventive medicine among the occupation forces. Stability was the great need, for whenever it could be attained, the health of the troops improved. Settled cantonments were a plus because area control was possible, and the attention of commanders, engineers, and medics could be concentrated upon enforcing the rules of sanitation, obtaining a potable water supply, and so forth. A rapid decline in the case rate of infectious hepatitis, from 22.8 per 1,000 per annum in March to 6.4 in June, reflected the fact that troops again were drinking chlorinated water. Theater forces were reimmunized against typhus and—a novelty—against influenza as well, in a move dictated by memories of the pandemic that had followed World War I and the development of a vaccine during wartime by the Army Epidemiological Board. Close cooperation with the Typhus Commission and the military government helped to ensure both civilians and military against the development of any new foci of the disease. During all of 1945 only five cases of typhus were reported among Americans, and some doubt existed as to the diagnosis in two of these. The prime Army concern was to guard against complacency. A pool of personnel trained in control had to be maintained, power dusters stockpiled, and DDT supplies kept on hand. Such vigilance was warranted, not by conditions within Army cantonments, but by the presence of a cold, hungry, and crowded civilian population outside.[64]

The chief negative factor was the continuing personnel upheaval. The redeployment camps, the staging and assembly areas, the troop trains, and the arrival and departure points all presented problems in disease control. A mitigating circumstance was the fact that more space was available to house the troops who remained. By the time cold weather arrived in 1945 most American soldiers were living in permanent buildings, and those still under canvas—primarily men in the assembly and staging areas—kept warm in winterized quarters.

American troops, healthy during the fighting, in general remained so in peacetime, except for continuing problems with diphtheria and venereal disease. Common diarrhea among the troops increased during the summer of 1945, but not enough to cause alarm. In the Mediterranean area an old enemy, malaria, posed a threat because one of the major ports through which troops were funneled

[63] Above paragraphs based upon OofCSurg, HQ, TSFET, Quarterly Report of Operations, 8 May–30 Sep 45, pp. 59–69; Wiltse, ed., *Medical Supply*, p. 374.

[64] OofCSurg, HQ, TSFET, Quarterly Report of Operations, 8 May–30 Sep 45, p. 73; Resume of Activities of Divisions of Medical Section, HQ, TSFET, Preventive Medicine Division sec., p. 6; Rpt, OofCSurg, HQ, TSFET (to Theater CSurg), 19 Jan 46, sub: Brief Resume of Major Items of Interest and Activities in Preventive Medicine Division Since VE Day, pp. 1–2.

was Marseilles. Lying amid an endemic malarious region, the old port city of southern France and its environs were filled with natural breeding places for Anopheles mosquitoes. The theater launched an all-out malaria prevention program, employing airplanes to spray the local area with DDT and forming a provisional malaria control unit with Italian POWs to augment the effort on the ground. The program, supplemented by an information campaign among the troops and by French authorities among the population, forestalled an outbreak.

Diphtheria, a nagging problem since the previous year, remained a medical burden during the Occupation. No epidemic broke out, but incidence remained high and the illness was highly virulent and life-threatening, especially because of complications such as myocarditis (inflammation of the heart muscle). Indeed, thirty-eight deaths were recorded among the 1,195 cases that occurred among American troops in the first ten months of 1945—a case fatality rate of 3 percent. Immunization programs among German children seemed the best bet for long-term control of a disease that had grown steadily on the Continent during the war years. For soldiers, early diagnosis and quick treatment were essential, and medical efforts were largely directed toward this end.[65]

Exacerbating the medical problems was the heavy influx of green troops during early 1946. Struggling to find quick replacements for the departing veterans, the Army reduced the length of the basic training cycle for new recruits and pushed them quickly through the training centers. Crowding, rapid turnover, and cold weather resulted in epidemic outbreaks of respiratory complaints and childhood diseases—chiefly measles, German measles, scarlet fever, mumps, and meningitis. Many men who were incubating such complaints filed aboard the troopships bound for Europe. Here crowding was at its maximum during voyages prolonged by bad weather. Either on shipboard or soon after arrival many fell ill, spreading their contagions to others. To this situation there was no fundamental answer, except to isolate and treat the sick. By April the declining incidence in zone-of-interior training centers promised a healthier crop of young soldiers to fill depleted formations overseas.[66]

In general good health, Americans settled down to enjoy the amenities of the Continent. Despite the ruin of war, much remained undestroyed in the European treasure house. Medical officers, hoping to improve their professional skills, studied at dozens of institutions, including the universities of Oxford, Edinburgh, and Paris. Nurses found educational opportunities in France and Great Britain. In a less weighty vein, the Third and Seventh Armies opened ski schools. Winter sports in Switzerland and the summertime beaches of the Riviera beckoned. Men and women who had come to make war stayed to learn and

[65] Cir Ltr No. 69, OofCSurg, HQ, TSFET, 28 Sep 45; Resume of Activities of Divisions of Medical Section, HQ, TSFET, Professional Services Division sec., p. 3.

[66] Ltr, TSG to CG, USFET, 26 Apr 46, box 1497, RG 112, NARA.

to enjoy. The troops began a long, peaceful residence in Germany, first as occupiers and later as allies, that continues at this writing, when those who were young men and women in 1945–46 have reached the threshold of old age.[67]

---

[67] See, for example, Army Nurse Corps Division, HQ, USFET, Report of Activities, 8 May–30 Sep 45, pp. 7–8.

EPILOGUE

The Theater in Retrospect

The American medical service that supported the invasion of Europe and the conquest of Hitler's Germany was a successful but paradoxical organization. Given the unresolved problems of command that afflicted not only the medics but the whole theater, it probably worked better than it should have. Hawley's position under the service forces required strengthening before he could exercise fully the prerogatives of a theater chief surgeon. The creation of SHAEF, establishing Kenner in a supranational headquarters, might have made for serious trouble. Practical accommodations and the sheer force of Hawley's personality resolved issues that, under a less able or less personable chief surgeon could have led to bitter jurisdictional conflicts but—except in the case of the fledgling air forces, struggling toward independence—did not. Similarly, the position of the chief surgeon vis-a-vis base section and ground force commanders and their surgeons might have led to sterile or destructive squabbles. There can be little doubt that the history of Army medicine in the European Theater was given an ineradicable stamp by Paul Hawley's strength and by Albert Kenner's forbearance.

The ETO medical service differed from that of other combat theaters in the long period of preparation that preceded the fighting.[1] Even granting the hiatus caused by the North African invasion, the buildup in Great Britain was elaborate and lengthy. Here inter-Allied cooperation received its first test, as a vast American army took up residence in the British Isles. Hawley's early contacts with British military leaders and physicians helped to establish a successful pattern of professional interaction that continued throughout the war. Yet some serious problems surfaced. The logistics of the medical buildup were staggeringly complex, and the resolution of the supply problems that developed proved to be beyond the capacity of the chief surgeon and his staff, requiring expert help from the United States. But the adoption and implementation of reforms put the medics ahead of the game: In later days, when the theater supply problems on the Continent were most tangled, the medical system worked well.

[1]The contrasting situation in the Pacific theaters will be explored in Mary Ellen Condon-Rall and Albert E. Cowdrey, *The Medical Department: Medical Service in the War Against Japan*, United States Army in World War II (Washington, D.C.: U.S. Army Center of Military History, forthcoming).

Other aspects of the buildup caused sharp, though transient, difficulties. The program of American hospital construction in England burdened the resources of the host nation, and the ensuing delays strained Hawley's patience. Demands by the theater for medical personnel were large, perhaps excessive, and the priorities accorded to service troops in general and to medics in particular were low. The result was a buildup that moved by fits and starts. In succession, the theater had too few medical facilities for the rapidly expanding army; then too few professionals to staff its hospitals; and, finally, too many and too much of everything to support forces largely engaged in training, not fighting.

In its prime mission—the accumulation of overwhelming forces to strike a knockout blow—the buildup was a great success, in which the medical service shared fully. Yet some of Hawley's decisions cast long shadows. Presented with some two and a half years to prepare his forces, the chief surgeon was able to devise and implement a correspondingly elaborate plan of medical support. One of the most questionable parts of the plan provided for the transportation of large numbers of fixed hospitals to the Continent after D-Day and for their utilization as far forward as the Advance Section of the Communications Zone. Early movement forward was essential for such units, because general hospitals required time to make their bed strength operational. But the effort to advance their complex equipment and marry it to the units encountered great difficulties. Hawley consistently overestimated the ability of the bomb-shattered European transport system to handle the demands of war. Many general hospitals became separated from their gear, and when they arrived near the front, they were difficult to house and subject to enemy attack. In the event, the advanced general hospitals were used in ways that had not been foreseen, some as "little more than holding units." [2] Hawley's somewhat cumbersome and grandiose conceptions, based perhaps on the experience of World War I, might have fared better under a commander like Britain's Montgomery than under Bradley and Patton, masters of improvisation and the armored thrust.

Indeed, as the chief surgeon's Operations Division admitted after the war, the struggle waged in Europe was so unlike World War I that "comparison is hardly of value." The Medical Department learned that availability of fixed beds meant little in the absence of transport. Hence, reported the medical section of the General Board established after the war to analyze the theater's accomplishments and failings, "the experience of the European Theater of Operations indicates that field hospitals and semimobile, 750-bed evacuation hospitals can be used much more effectively by the Advance Section . . . and that general hospitals should be established only in the base, and possibly the intermediate, section of the Communications Zone." [3]

---

[2] Study No. 95, General Board, USFET, sub: Medical Service in the Communications Zone in the European Theater of Operations, Medical Section, p. 4, file HD 334.

[3] Ibid., p. 3, file HD 334. The General Board was established in ETOUSA in June 1945 and continued by USFET. See GO No. 128, HQ, ETOUSA, 17 Jun 45; GO No. 128, HQ, USFET, 7 Aug 45; and GO No. 312, HQ, USFET, 20 Nov 45.

Aircraft provided essential support to the medical system, speeding evacuation both within Europe and from the Continent to Great Britain. Though Hawley launched planning in November 1943, skepticism extended up to the Supreme Commander, and air evacuation began as an emergency measure and no more. Yet it proved to be a logical complement to the armored thrusts that carried line units beyond the reach of the railroads. Despite fickle weather and the lack of dedicated medical aircraft, the speed and the advantage of a smooth ride to the patient ultimately caused the whole theater to become "completely 'air conscious.'" On the ground as well, increased mobility demanded innovations that ETOUSA planners foresaw only in part. While they grasped the need for holding units at airfields, the extent of the need there and at every transfer point along the lines of evacuation was not fully appreciated. Many units had to be improvised during the breakout and pursuit, field and evacuation hospitals frequently being pressed into service. The fact that the theater had prepared for gas warfare and that none occurred freed the medical gas treatment battalions to become holding units—a happy accident. Meanwhile, those mobile hospitals that followed the armies often proved in fact to be less than their designation implied. The whole question of mobility deserved reconsideration. Perhaps significantly, when the surgeon general in August 1945 issued a T/O&E for a forward hospital to treat nontransportables, the new sixty-bed unit bore the name of mobile army surgical hospital (MASH). The experience of the European Theater in hospitalization and evacuation alike pointed to the need for a medical service as supple as the shifting battlefields of mechanized war.[4]

Other problems arose because the theater's obsessive demands for more and more medical units seemingly took little account of the war going on in the Pacific or the needs of the home front. A mixture of high clinical standards, bureaucratic empire building, and reluctance to see the wounded pass beyond theater control evidently contributed to Hawley's resistance to the evacuation of casualties on troopships. Of a piece with his other aims was Hawley's endeavor to hold the theater evacuation policy as high as possible. All these policies tended to maximize the need for American medical personnel in the European Theater; in the end, direct orders from the War Department were needed in late 1944 to speed evacuation, to turn over prisoners to the care of their own medical service, and to limit the commitment of new medical manpower from a declining national pool. Yet, in the Ardennes crisis, the sheer redundancy of medical units proved the key factor in enabling the straining system to handle the influx of wounded.

Some problems similar to those of the American medical service also afflicted the wartime Allies. The establishment inherited by the British from World War I was not mobile enough, a lesson driven home in the opening days of the war in Europe when medical units and supplies were overrun

---

[4] Quoted words from Operations Division, OofCSurg, HQ, ETOUSA, Semiannual Rpt, January-June 1945, pp. 4–5. See also Table of Organization and Equipment No. 8–571, August 1945.

and all too many wounded were abandoned to the enemy. Persistent shortages in vehicles and fuel stymied attempts to improve mobility. A special case was the air transport of the wounded. The Royal Air Force blocked efforts by the British Army to gain dedicated aircraft for medical use. Ad hoc air evacuation developed anyway during the African campaigns, with Britain's wounded riding transport planes—many of them American—on return trips. The usual problems had to be faced in moving the wounded to airfields, in holding them, and in responding to the often unpredictable arrivals and departures of nondedicated aircraft. In the event, reforms in the British medical service were not fully implemented in any theater prior to the D-Day invasion, and throughout the war dedicated medical aircraft never played the role they might have. The British Army as a whole adapted less to the era of the blitzkrieg than that of any other major combatant, and the Americans, during their years of residence in Great Britain, may well have learned bad lessons from their hosts as well as good ones.[5]

Uniquely American, however, was the way that replacement policy interacted with the stresses of the European fighting to produce a large and, in substantial part, probably preventable burden of neuropsychiatric casualties. While some units had been hard used in all American wars, the experience of continuous combat by large forces against a determined, well-equipped enemy was rare in the nation's annals. The lessons that other armies, including the British, had learned on the Western Front in World War I seemingly had little effect on the Americans in the European Theater. Here the same units were committed to battle, month after month, by a theater that possessed a huge support system but few reserve combat forces. The result was extremely wearing on the men who bore the brunt of the fighting.

In February 1945 the 12th Army Group surgeon, Colonel Gorby, invited the attention of his superiors to the "continued high loss of manpower from combat exhaustion." Key personnel were beginning to be affected, including small unit leaders with excellent records in combat. Studies carried out in the harassing conditions of the Italian campaign had already shown that healthy men could endure combat stress only for 200–240 days, after which their efficiency declined sharply. Studies in the European Theater confirmed these findings, and Gorby compared the needs of men to those of trucks: "Relief after 130 to 150 combat days," he wrote, "is comparable to the 10,000 mile overhaul." He argued that rotation was necessary to retain men in service. The British rotated personnel out of the line after 12 days, for a rest period of 4 days, and the U.S. Air Force rotated fliers home after a certain number of combat missions. The medical service in various units made provision for its own personnel, so far as it was able, returning doctors in front-line units to COMZ hospitals and replacing them with men who had not seen combat, and in some cases rotating hard-pressed unit medics at least out of the range of enemy shells. But no comprehensive

[5] Crew, *AMS, Administration,* 1:462–505

system of rotation for the troops was installed during World War II in the theater.[6]

Despite its errors, the theater could point to a superlative achievement in lifesaving under what were often most difficult circumstances. The job it did was of staggering size. Direct hospital admissions for all causes between 6 June 1944 and 11 May 1945 totaled 1,052,659, by far the highest for any theater of operations. A total of 381,433 patients were evacuated to the United Kingdom during that time: 148,229 by sea and 233,204 by air. Of 183,121 patients carried to the zone of interior, 154,383 went by sea and 28,738 by air. The First Army, with 249,090 casualties from all causes, suffered far more than the other field forces. The Third Army had 139,240; the Seventh Army, 80,099; and the Ninth Army, 54,877. Despite the evacuation crisis of the winter, the theater could properly boast at the end of 1944 that "at no time have any of the armies we supported been embarrassed, hindered, or their combat efficiency adversely affected by an inability to clear themselves of casualties." The European Theater enjoyed the lowest nonbattle and disease death rates of all overseas theaters. Of 393,987 battle wounded admitted to its hospitals, 12,523 died—a mortality rate of 3.2 percent, the lowest for any theater of operations.[7]

Not all of this distinguished record can be credited to the medical system that Hawley built. The European Theater profited by the experience of other theaters in many respects, including the care of neuropsychiatric casualties. Above all, it was fortunate in its environment, despite the cold injuries that marked its one great failure to heed and apply preventive measures. Northwestern Europe was comparatively compact, contained many friendly people who aided their liberators, lacked jungles, and possessed (even if in damaged form) all the physical substructure of industrial civilization.

Nevertheless, medical organization and clinical skill exploited the advantages and compensated for many of the failings of the wartime environment. In the early critical phases of evacuation, when the wounded man had to be dragged, carried, or assisted to safety under fire, the basic contribution of the medics was physical strength and raw courage. Hailing the aidman at the end of the struggle, Hawley's headquarters declared that he "must face the same danger as armed troops without recourse or dependence upon weapons of any sort. He 'takes,' he never 'gives'—except that he gives himself in order that his mission may be accomplished." [8]

[6] Quoted words from Surg, 12th Army Group, Hist, January–June 1945, an. 18, p. 1. See also ibid., an. 19. A limited policy of granting leaves to the United States and to rear areas was in force in the European Theater at the time. On neuropsychiatric rates, see Albert J. Glass and Robert J. Bernucci, eds., *Zone of Interior*, Medical Department, United States Army in World War II (Washington, D.C.: Office of the Surgeon General, Department of the Army, 1966), p. 406.

[7] Quoted words from Extract, Operations Rpt, 1944, attached to Study No. 95, General Board, USFET, sub: Medical Service in the Communications Zone in the European Theater of Operations, Medical Section, file HD 334. See also Reister, ed., *Medical Statistics*, pp. 32 and 322–23.

[8] Operations Division, OofCSurg, HQ, ETOUSA, Semiannual Rpt, January–June 1945, p. 6. The fact

Continued

Above all, the technical competence of the Medical Department could hardly be faulted. "In the ETO," Hawley was to admit later, "I never hurt for clinical talent but I was constantly hurting for leadership of this talent half as good as the talent itself." Throughout the theater Regular Army medical officers assumed command positions, turning over hands-on care to the highly qualified civilians who, as reserve officers or as wartime volunteers, brought to the Army a multitude of sophisticated skills. Their efforts on behalf of the wounded and sick were eased immensely by new discoveries that either accompanied the war or immediately preceded it. The development of sulfa drugs in the late 1930s by French researchers exploiting a German discovery "opened the treasure house of bacterial chemotherapy," in the words of a recent historian of medicine. During the early 1940s mass production methods turned penicillin, discovered in 1928, into a revolutionary new weapon against bacterial infections and made it available to the theater from D-Day on. The discovery in 1938 of the insecticidal properties of DDT made control of typhus incomparably easier than in the past, and aided the control of mosquito-borne and fly-borne diseases as well. The number of lives saved by these innovations alone was beyond computation. The introduction of synthetic antimalarials and advances in vascular surgery likewise impacted upon the battlefield. The development of the blood program was a landmark, and the increased use of whole blood as well as plasma was fundamental to medical success in saving the lives of wounded men.[9]

A distinctive feature of the theater was the fact that virtually all its fighting was done in heavily populated areas. Among the Allied nations of Europe, close ties developed between the civil and military medical establishments. Venereal disease control was a sensitive sociomedical issue that demanded tactful handling on the Continent, as it had in Great Britain, in the face of social norms that varied drastically from one nation to the next. Devastation by Allied bombs, as well as by German shells, left formidable problems in public health and disease prevention. Army medics trained in civil affairs took the lead in confronting these problems, but command responsibility and the intervention of the field forces was essential to their solution.

In Germany the Medical Department met a situation new to American armies: the surrender and imprisonment of a whole enemy army, numbering in the millions; the liberation of other millions of prisoners and displaced persons; and the care of a conquered people who were both industrialized and highly urbanized. Official American policy in the form of nonfraternization and the initial deci-

that the European Theater was the last theater to see major combat apparently was the reason why the basic studies on combat stress and preventive psychiatry, which helped to prepare the way for later rotation policies, were all based on data from the Mediterranean and Pacific theaters.

[9] First quotation from Press Release, "Better Federal Medical Service," 13 Dec 49, box 5, General Green's Office Reference Files, AGO, RG 112, NARA. Second quotation from Harry F. Dowling, *Fighting Infection: Conquests of the Twentieth Century* (Cambridge, Mass.: Harvard University Press, 1977), p. 107.

sion to impose a harsh peace obstructed medical efforts to suppress disease. The practice of giving POW doctors and nurses charge of their sick and injured countrymen proved to be more important than ever in the last days of the war—and would have been even more so if the desperate last-ditch resistance foreseen by American policy-makers had materialized. American medical personnel were freed to work among DPs, RAMPs, and concentration camp inmates; to aid civilians; and to guide the German hospital system during the transition to peace. By the summer of 1945 all efforts were being hampered by the demands of the ongoing Pacific war and partial demobilization. Forces had to be dispatched halfway around the world, experienced men and women readied for discharge, and mountains of supplies disposed of in accord with rapidly changing demands from Washington. In meeting these complications, Kenner's quiet hand was no less important than Hawley's brusque one had been earlier.

Throughout, the doctors, nurses, corpsmen, administrators, and specialists of the Medical Department were privileged to repair much of the human havoc wrought by the war. On the Normandy beaches, among the hedgerows, in hospital wards that filled the grand hotels of Paris, in the cellars of battered Liege, and among the living skeletons of Dachau and Buchenwald, they brought a measure of practical compassion into the most ruinous of wars. For that, all who were concerned in the prodigious effort could, in the glow of victory, look back upon their work and find it good.

Bibliographical Note

The Medical Department: Medical Service in the European Theater of Operations is a volume that had a long gestation in the Historical Unit of the Office of the Surgeon General (OSG). Though an earlier draft by George Garand, Hubert D. Potter, and Pauline Vivette was frequently consulted by us, this volume was written under the aegis of the U.S. Army Center of Military History largely from primary sources collected by the Historical Unit, and now in the custody of the Center in Washington, D.C., and from Army records in the custody of the National Archives and Records Administration (NARA) in Suitland, Maryland. Most of the NARA records, unless otherwise noted, are located in Record Group (RG) 112, Records of the Office of the Surgeon General (Army). Identification of sources, by depository codes, is explained in Chapter I, footnote 1.

The variety and sheer bulk of available primary sources at NARA are somewhat daunting. The footnotes to this volume detail the various types of periodic reports consulted for a wide range of medical offices, activities, and units, ranging from the ETO chief surgeon's staff downward to the smaller field units. We also made extensive use of the comprehensive medical history of the European Theater, prepared by Lt. Col. Sanford V. Larkey of the chief surgeon's office, and of the many official documents it reproduces. Col. John E. Gordon's manuscript history of preventive medicine in the theater provided a reliable guide to this area of military medicine. A collection of letters representing backchannel communications between the theater chief surgeon and the surgeon general (Hawley-Kirk Correspondence) was most helpful in gaining perspective on the ETO medical service, its accomplishments and its failings. The Medical Division, COSSAC/SHAEF, War Diary, covering the years 1943–45, was also exceptionally useful. The chapters that deal with the opening of the Reich were enhanced by the reports of the units that aided the concentration camp survivors; by the records of various intelligence organizations, notably those of the Combined Intelligence Operations Subcommittee; and by the records of the Office of the Military Government (OMGUS), which may be found in RG 260, Records of United States Occupation Headquarters, World War II. The records of the United States of America Typhus Commission are voluminous and well organized. RG 112 also contains transcripts of interviews with medical personnel, completed in the European Theater at the end of the war; these supply many personal touches and much operational detail. Division combat narrative files, in RG

407, Records of the Adjutant General's Office, 1917–, provided extensive human interest detail on division-level medical service. The reader should note that, upon publication of this volume, all materials deposited in the Center of Military History will be returned to the Army collection at NARA for refiling into the appropriate record groups in accordance with NARA's record-keeping system.

The sources in other repositories are less voluminous but no less valuable. The collections of the U.S. Army Military History Institute at Carlisle Barracks, Pennsylvania, were essential in many ways. This repository contains numerous medical unit histories and also the papers of Paul R. Hawley, Charles H. Beasley, John C. Burwell, William E. Shambora, and Lee Cady, which are both of a personal and an official nature. No one writing on medical history can fail to take advantage of the remarkable collections of the National Library of Medicine in Bethesda, Maryland. Here we found many important insights in the William S. Middleton Papers, diary, and interview transcript. Further materials on the fight against typhus are abundant in the Stanhope Bayne-Jones Collection.

The Center of Military History has in its custody, in addition to the Historical Unit's collection of documents, other pertinent records. These include several groups of oral history materials. The oldest are memoranda of interviews with key medical personnel, completed by the Historical Unit, OSG, as well as transcripts of the discussions of the Editorial Advisory Board during the early planning stages of this volume. This material offered revealing insights into personalities and policy at a time when the theater's problems were still fresh in the minds of those who had been its leaders. In addition, we conducted other very helpful interviews with Honorable Elliot Richardson, Col. Virginia Brown, Col. Tom F. Whayne, Brig. Gen. Crawford F. Sams, Maj. Gen. Thomas J. Hartford, Brig. Gen. Sam F. Seeley, Maj. Gen. Collin F. Vorder Bruegge, Jane Lee, Joseph A. Gosman, M.D., Lester Wallman, M.D., and Herbert F. Wing. General Sams also supplied a valuable manuscript autobiography. Again, with the publication of this volume, these documents (except Sams' manuscript) will be transferred to Carlisle or retired to NARA.

The emphasis upon primary sources should not obscure the importance of secondary materials as well. The vast literature that covers the military history of the European Theater offered us a framework within which the medical events could be made meaningful. While a variety of sources will be found in the footnotes, we must emphasize the special importance of the earlier volumes in the Center's United States Army in World War II series. Especially useful in gaining an understanding of strategy, theater structure, and logistics were Roland G. Ruppenthal's two-volume work *Logistical Support of the Armies*; Maurice Matloff and Edwin M. Snell's *Strategic Planning for Coalition Warfare, 1941–1942*; and Maurice Matloff's *Strategic Planning for Coalition Warfare, 1943–1944*. The combat histories were used as guides to the course of events, once the invasion had begun. Essential to this study were Gordon A. Harrison's *Cross-*

Channel Attack, Martin Blumenson's *Breakout and Pursuit*, Charles B. MacDonald's *The Siegfried Line Campaign* and *The Last Offensive*, and Hugh M. Cole's *The Lorraine Campaign* and *The Ardennes: Battle of the Bulge*. Of great importance in shaping this volume were the earlier medical works in the series by Charles M. Wiltse, *The Medical Department: Medical Service in the Mediterranean and Minor Theaters*, and by Clarence McKittrick Smith, *The Medical Department: Hospitalization and Evacuation, Zone of Interior*. We also drew extensively upon the forty-odd volumes of the Medical Department, United States Army in World War II, series. These exhaustive accounts, written in great measure by physicians who were participants in the events they describe, provided the clinical and technical background for this volume. Finally, the volumes of Wesley Frank Craven and James Lea Cate, *The Army Air Forces in World War II*, were used as appropriate, as were Mae Mills Link and Hubert A. Coleman's *Medical Support of the Army Air Forces in World War II* and the official histories of the Royal Army Medical Services and the Emergency Medical Services published by Her Majesty's Stationery Office.

List of Abbreviations

AAF	Army Air Forces
ACofS	Assistant chief of staff
ADSEC	Advance Section
AFHQ	Allied Force Headquarters
AG	Adjutant general
AFG	Army Ground Forces
An	Annex
Anon	Anonymous
App	Appendix
ASR	Adjusted service rating
ASTP	Army Specialized Training Program
ATC	Air Transport Command
Bde	Brigade
Bn	Battalion
BTNI	British Troops in Northern Ireland
CAdminOff	Chief administrative officer
CATOR	Combined Air Transport Operations Room
CCWOff	Chief chemical warfare officer
Cdr	Commander
CEngr	Chief engineer
CG	Commanding general
Chron	Chronological
CIOS	Combined Intelligence Operations Subcommittee
Cir	Circular
CMedOff	Chief medical officer
CMH	Center of Military History
CO	Commanding officer
COMZ	Communications Zone
CONAD	Continental Advance Section
CofOpns	Chief of operations
COrdOff	Chief ordnance officer
Corresp	Correspondence
COSSAC	Chief of Staff to the Supreme Allied Commander (Designate)
CofPMS	Chief of Preventive Medicine Service, OSG
CQM	Chief quartermaster
CSigOff	Chief signal officer

CsofSupSvcs	Chiefs of Supply Services
CSurg	Chief surgeon
CTransOff	Chief transportation officer
Dep	Deputy
DPs	Displaced persons
DUKW	Amphibian truck
ECAD	European Civil Affairs Division
EMS	Emergency Medical Service
EMT	Emergency medical tag
Engr	Engineer
ETO	European Theater of Operations
ETOUSA	European Theater of Operations, United States Army
FECOMZ	Forward Echelon, Communications Zone
G–1	Personnel officer or section of divisional or higher staff
G–2	Intelligence officer or section of divisional or higher staff
G–3	Operations officer or section of divisional or higher staff
G–4	Supply officer or section of divisional or higher staff
G–5	Civil affairs officer or section of divisional or higher staff
GFRC	Ground Force Reinforcement Command
GO	General Order
Hist	History
HC	Hospital center
Hosp	Hospital
HU	Holding unit
JAGD	Judge Advocate General's Department
LC–1	Landing craft
LCI	Landing craft, infantry
LCT	Landing craft, tank
LCVP	Landing craft, vehicle/personnel
LOI	Letter of instruction
LST	Landing ship, tank
LVT–1	Landing vehicle, tracked ("Alligator")
MAC	Medical Administrative Corps
MC	Medical Corps
MedGasTr	Medical Gas Treatment Battalion
Memo	Memorandum
MFR	Memorandum for the Record

MHI	U.S. Army Military History Institute
MISP	Medical in-transit storage point
MOS	Military occupational specialty
NARA	National Archives and Records Administration
NATOUSA	North African Theater of Operations, United States Army
OofCSurg	Office of the Chief Surgeon
OofTPM	Office of the Theater Provost Marshal
Opns	Operations
OSG	Office of the Surgeon General
POW(s)	Prisoner(s) of war
PROCO	Special project for continental operations
ProvESBGp	Provisional Engineer Special Brigade Group
PWOD	Prisoner-of-War Overhead Detachment
RAF	Royal Air Force
RAMP	Recovered Allied military personnel
Regt	Regiment
Rpt	Report
S–2	Intelligence officer or section of regimental or lower staff
S–3	Operations officer or section of regimental or lower staff
SC	Sanitary Corps
Sec	Section
Sess	Session
SHAEF	Supreme Headquarters, Allied Expeditionary Force
SO	Special Order
SOLOC	Southern Line of Communications
SOS	Services of Supply
Spec	Special
SPOBS	Special Observers Group
SS	*Schutzstaffel* (Elite Guard)
TAG	The Adjutant General
T/E(s)	Table(s) of equipment
T/O(s)	Table(s) of organization
T/O&E(s)	Table(s) of organization and equipment
TSFET	Theater Service Forces, European Theater
TSG	The Surgeon General
UNRRA	United Nations Relief and Rehabilitation Administration
USAFBI	United States Army Forces in the British Isles
USANIF	United States Army Northern Ireland Force

USFET	United States Forces, European Theater
USPHS	United States Public Health Service
USSTAF	United States Strategic Air Forces
VD	Venereal disease
WAAC	Women's Army Auxiliary Corps

Basic Military Map Symbols[1]

Basic Medical Symbols

Medical treatment facility, operating [2]	+
Medical treatment facility, not operating [2]	⊞
Medical supply unit	⊕
Veterinary treatment facility, operating [2]	V
Veterinary treatment facility, not operating [2]	⊠
Hospital train	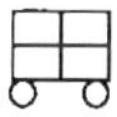
Hospital ship	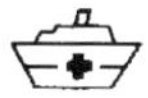
Other medical units [3]	⊞

Basic Military Symbols

Section	••
Platoon or detachment	•••
Company	I
Battalion	II
Regiment or group; combat team (CT following identifying numeral)	III
Brigade	X
Division; command of an air force	XX
Corps; Air Force	XXX

[1] For complete listing of symbols in use during World War II period, see FM 21-20, dated October 1943, from which these are taken.

[2] Includes collecting and clearing elements.

[3] Includes nontreatment facilities, other than supply, such as laboratories and headquarters of various medical facilities.

Army XXXX

Army group XXXXX

Service command, department, or section of a communications zone . . . . OOO

Communications zone . . . . OOOO

Airfield . . . .

EXAMPLES

9th Evacuation Hospital, assigned to a corps . . . .

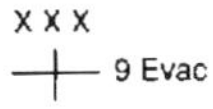

16th Field Hospital, assigned to a service command . . . .

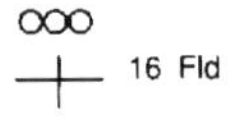

3d Convalescent Hospital, assigned to an army . . . .

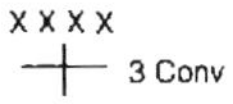

6th Station Hospital, assigned to a base section (not operating)

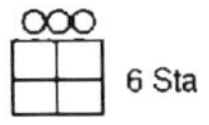

38th General Hospital, assigned to a communications zone . . . .

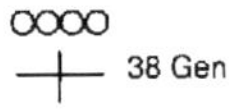

Fifth Army Medical Depot . . . .

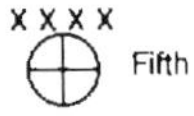

17th Veterinary Evacuation Hospital, assigned to an army . . . . . .

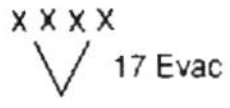

213th Veterinary General Hospital (Italian), assigned to a base section . . . .

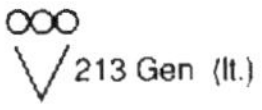

41st Hospital Train . . . .

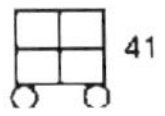

Hospital ship *Acadia* . . . .

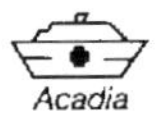

54th Medical Battalion . . . .

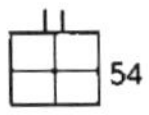

Company B, 47th Armored Medical Battalion . . . .

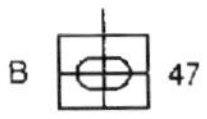

309th Airborne Medical Company . . . .

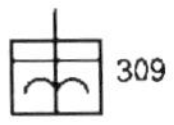

Company A, 3d Medical Battalion . . . .

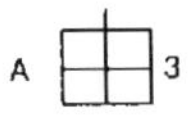

Clearing Station, 34th Division (2d platoon, clearing company, organic medical battalion) . . . .

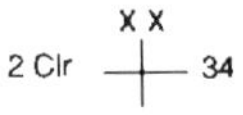

15th Medical General Laboratory, assigned to a base section .

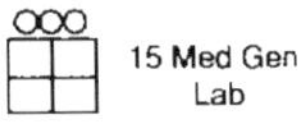

Index

☆ U.S. GOVERNMENT PRINTING OFFICE: 1992 275-131

PIN : 068164-000